Rights and Resources

The International Library of Medicine, Ethics and Law
Series Editor: Michael D. Freeman

Titles in the Series

Death, Dying and the Ending of Life
Margaret P. Battin, Leslie Francis and Bruce Landesman

Abortion
Belinda Bennett

Ethics and Medical Decision-Making
Michael D. Freeman

Children, Medicine and the Law
Michael D. Freeman

Health and Human Rights
Lawrence O. Gostin and James G. Hodge Jr.

Mental Illness, Medicine and Law
Martin Lyon Levine

The Elderly
Martin Lyon Levine

The Genome Project and Gene Therapy
Sheila A.M. McLean

Rights and Resources
Frances H. Miller

AIDS: Society, Ethics and Law
Udo Schüklenk

Women, Medicine, Ethics and the Law
Susan Sherwin and Barbara Parish

Legal and Ethical Issues in Human Reproduction
Bonnie Steinbock

Medical Practice and Malpractice
Harvey Teff

Human Experimentation and Research
George F. Tomossy and David N. Weisstub

Medicine and Industry
George F. Tomossy

Rights and Resources

Edited by

Frances H. Miller

Boston University School of Law, USA

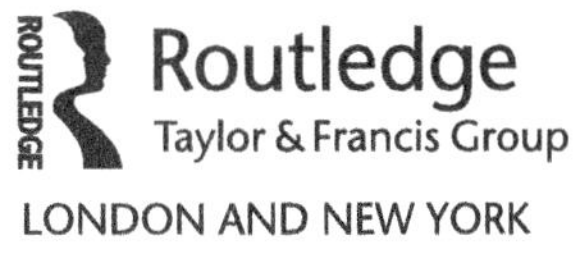

LONDON AND NEW YORK

First published 2003 by Dartmouth Publishing Company and Ashgate Publishing

Reissued 2018 by Routledge
2 Park Square, Milton Park, Abingdon, Oxon OX14 4RN
711 Third Avenue, New York, NY 10017, USA

Routledge is an imprint of the Taylor & Francis Group, an informa business

A Library of Congress record exists under LC control number: 2002074721

ISBN 13: 978-1-138-71899-9 (hbk)
ISBN 13: 978-1-315-19435-6 (ebk)

Contents

Acknowledgements

The editor and publishers wish to thank the following for permission to use copyright material.

American Association for the Advancement of Science for the essay: Michael A. Heller and Rebecca S. Eisenberg (1998), 'Can Patents Deter Innovation? The Anticommons in Biomedical Research', *Science*, **280**, pp. 698–701.

American Society of Law, Medicine & Ethics for the essays: Susan M. Wolf (1994), 'Shifting Paradigms in Bioethics and Health Law: The Rise of a New Pragmatism', *American Journal of Law and Medicine*, **20**, pp. 395–415. Copyright © 1994. Reprinted with the permission of the American Society of Law, Medicine & Ethics and Boston University. All rights reserved; Daniel Callahan (1992), 'Symbols, Rationality, and Justice: Rationing Health Care', *American Journal of Law and Medicine*, **18**, pp. 1–13. Copyright © 1992. Reprinted with the permission of the American Society of Law, Medicine & Ethics and Boston University. All rights reserved; Christopher Newdick (1997), 'Resource Allocation in the National Health Service', *American Journal of Law and Medicine*, **23**, pp. 291–318. Copyright © 1997. Reprinted with the permission of the American Society of Law, Medicine & Ethics and Boston University. All rights reserved.

George J. Annas and Frances H. Miller (1994), 'The Empire of Death: How Culture and Economics Affect Informed Consent in the U.S., the U.K., and Japan', *American Journal of Law and Medicine*, **20**, pp. 357–94. Copyright © 1994 George J. Annas and Frances H. Miller.

Arizona State Law Journal for the essay: Ellen A. Waldman (2000), 'Disputing Over Embryos: Of Contracts and Consents', *Arizona State Law Journal*, **32**, pp. 897–940. Copyright © 2000 Ellen Waldman.

Case Western Reserve University for the essay: Robert L. Schwartz (1993), 'Life Style, Health Status, and Distributive Justice', *Health Matrix*, **3**, pp. 195–217.

Hastings Center for the essays: Robert A. Burt (1996), 'The Suppressed Legacy of Nuremberg', *Hastings Center Report, September–October*, **26**, pp. 30–33; Leonard H. Glantz, George J. Annas, Michael A. Grodin and Wendy K. Mariner (1998), 'Research in Developing Countries: Taking "Benefit" Seriously', *Hastings Center Report, November–December*, **28**, pp. 38–42; Nancy M.P. King (1995), 'Experimental Treatment: Oxymoron or Aspiration?', *Hastings Center Report, July–August*, **25**, pp. 6–15.

Houston Law Review for the essay: Henry T. Greely (1997), 'The Control of Genetic Research: Involving the "Groups Between"', *Houston Law Review*, **33**, pp. 1397–430.

McGill Law Journal and Copibec for the essay: Ronald Dworkin (1993), 'Justice in the Distribution of Health Care', *McGill Law Journal*, **38**, pp. 883–98. Copyright © 1993 Ronald Dworkin.

Melbourne University Law Review for the essay: Belinda Bennett (1999), 'Posthumous Reproduction and the Meanings of Autonomy', *Melbourne University Law Review*, **23**, pp. 286–307.

O'Brien Center for Scholary Publications for the essay: Timothy Stoltzfus Jost (1998), 'Health Care Rationing in the Courts: A Comparative Study', *Hastings International and Comparative Law Review*, **21**, pp. 639–714. Copyright © 1998 University of California, Hastings College of the Law. Reprinted by permission.

Oxford University Press for the essays: Margaret Brazier and José Miola (2000), 'Bye-Bye Bolam: A Medical Litigation Revolution', *Medical Law Review*, **8**, pp. 85–114. Copyright © 2000 Oxford University Press; Don Chalmers and Robert Schwartz (1993), '*Rogers* v. *Whitaker* and Informed Consent in Australia: A Fair Dinkum Duty of Disclosure', *Medical Law Review*, **1**, pp. 139–59. Copyright © 1993 Oxford University Press; Margaret Brazier and John Harris (1996), 'Public Health and Private Lives', *Medical Law Review*, **4**, pp. 171–92. Copyright © 1996 Oxford University Press; Gerald Dworkin and Ian Kennedy (1993), 'Human Tissue: Rights in the Body and its Parts', *Medical Law Review*, **1**, pp. 291–319. Copyright © 1993 Oxford University Press. By permission of Oxford University Press.

Princeton University Press for the essay: Norman Daniels and James Sabin (1997), 'Limits to Health Care: Fair Procedures, Democratic Deliberation, and the Legitimacy Problem for Insurers', *Philosophy and Public Affairs*, **26**, pp. 303–50. Copyright © 1997 Princeton University Press. Reprinted by permission of Princeton University Press.

Wake Forest Law Review Association, Inc. for the essay: Maxwell J. Mehlman (1999), 'How will we Regulate Genetic Enhancement?', *Wake Forest Law Review*, **34**, pp. 671–714. Copyright © 1999 Wake Forest Law Review Association, Inc.

Every effort has been made to trace all the copyright holders, but if any have been inadvertently overlooked the publishers will be pleased to make the necessary arrangement at the first opportunity.

Series Preface

Few academic disciplines have developed with such pace in recent years as bioethics. And because the subject crosses so many disciplines important writing is to be found in a range of books and journals, access to the whole of which is likely to elude all but the most committed of scholars. The International Library of Medicine, Ethics and Law is designed to assist the scholarly endeavour by providing in accessible volumes a compendium of basic materials drawn from the most significant periodical literature. Each volume contains essays of central theoretical importance in its subject area, and each throws light on important bioethical questions in the world today. The series as a whole – there will be fifteen volumes – makes available an extensive range of valuable material (the standard 'classics' and the not-so-standard) and should prove of inestimable value to those involved in the research, teaching and study of medicine, ethics and law. The fifteen volumes together – each with introductions and bibliographies – are a library in themselves – an indispensable resource in a world in which even the best-stocked library is unlikely to cover the range of materials contained within these volumes.

It remains for me to thank the editors who have pursued their task with commitment, insight and enthusiasm, to thank also the hard-working staff at Ashgate – theirs is a mammoth enterprise – and to thank my secretary, Anita Garfoot for the enormous assistance she has given me in bringing the series from idea to reality.

MICHAEL FREEMAN
Series Editor
Faculty of Laws
University College London

Introduction
Patient Rights and Health Care Resources: Two Sides of An Irregular Coin

In an ideal world, health care rights would be perfectly matched to health care resources, and their joint implementation would be seamless. But in the disorder of the real world, things are far more complicated. Moral significance attaches to society's articulation of health care rights, and imparts momentum towards realizing them. Yet, society rarely articulates rights with one clear voice. Moreover, realizing rights in a world of scarce resources is a complex and uncertain process at best, and success in achieving that goal usually tends to vary depending on the eye of the beholder. Even if resources could be found to fulfil some abstract ideal, the inevitable static emanating from politics and economics would interfere with its accomplishment (cf. Winslow, 2001). Moreover, scientific uncertainties permeating medicine, which patients, judges and politicians alike often fail to comprehend, guarantee a less-than-perfect fit between enunciating health care as a right and any benefits that universal access to resources might contribute towards realizing that objective.

Patients' legal and ethical rights associated with health care are little more than rhetoric when the resources needed to implement them are elusive, so, in that sense, insufficient or inaccessible resources can make up the dark underside of the ephemeral rights coin. Rights to health care ring equally hollow when the medical, and increasingly the pharmaceutical, communities give lip service to their legitimacy but fail to acknowledge responsibility for the economic and social ramifications of trying to fulfil them. But most importantly, an institutional or a societal failure to understand both the obvious and the more subtle ramifications of articulating rights, or a simple lack of will to accept the financial and social costs of enforcing them, effectively undermines the likelihood that they will be realized.

The rights of individual patients to obtain or decline health care resources are inextricably intertwined with these and other complex legal, ethical and economic issues, and this volume of the International Library of Medicine, Ethics and Law explores various aspects of these paradoxes. A short collection of essays like this one can only hope to scratch the surface of the rich literature on patients' rights as interwoven, however tangentially, with health care resources. The selections which follow attempt to achieve a balance between evolutionary changes in old jurisprudential chestnuts like informed consent and newer thinking about the rights–resources tension as related to such emerging issues as patenting biotechnology, property ownership of human tissue, and genetic testing, therapy and enhancement. Although many of these essays explore common-law responses to patients' assertion of rights and claims to resources, legislatures have become increasingly active participants in these continually fascinating legal, bioethical and societal dilemmas. As technology spawns ever more sophisticated and expensive therapies, a shift towards more implicit and explicit schemes for allocating resources seems inevitable. Patients' right theory will have to adapt to new realities or risk the possibility of irrelevance.

Background to the Essays

Patient rights did not become a high-profile issue for health care until well after the mid-1900s, but the topic has achieved impressive prominence since that time. Although courts articulated a right for patients to insist upon giving an informed consent before submitting to medical treatment at least as far back as 1911,[1] it took almost half a century before medicine had much to offer patients beyond care and comfort of the sick and dying. In the aftermath of the Second World War, however, technological advances began to spur changes in the way we think about disease, and the prospect of finding cures for human ailments became more widely accepted. A diagnosis of serious disease now tends to function, at least in the USA, as more of a catalyst for patient action than as a trigger for depressed resignation.

At the beginning of the twenty-first century, patient rights associated with such clinical issues as abortion, treatment for mental illness, death and dying, genetic testing, treatment and enhancement, and participation in experimental trials of new drugs and devices constitute only a few of the many areas where reasonable minds can still differ on the appropriate scope of legal protection. Further out towards the periphery of clinical care, patients' rights to medical privacy are just now being fleshed out by statute and the common law to comport with electronic medical records and data transmission.[2] On the resources side of the equation, controversies concerning xenotransplants (Bach *et al.*, 2001), appropriate allocation of human organs for transplantation (Mahoney, 2000), and reimbursement for experimental therapies (Hoffman, 1999; Holder, 1994) continue unabated. Overt and more covert rationing schemes also seem inevitable in the light of the staggeringly high costs of technological advance.

Some of the most divisive political issues bedeviling US President George W. Bush's first year in office, for example, involved health care rights and resources. On the domestic front, these included controversies with international repercussions involving embryonic stem cell research[3] and human cloning,[4] as well as the failed enactment of a Managed Care Patients Bill of Rights.[5] Although politicians of all shades purport to support making insurers more accountable to patients, partisan disagreement over enforcement provisions – whether health insurance subscribers should be able to sue managed care organizations (MCOs) directly for alleged violations – proved a stumbling block from the outset. Guaranteeing MCO patients rights to require accountability from their health insurers plays well to the action-oriented US electorate, and enabling legislation will undoubtedly be passed sooner or later. Any rights purportedly guaranteed by statute nonetheless ring hollow when subscribers' ability to enforce them remains weak and government hesitates to impose meaningful sanctions for violations. Such politically 'charged' US controversies pale into insignificance, however, when enforcement of human rights on a global scale is at issue (Annas, 1998a; Annas and Grodin, 1999).

The Rights–Resources Relationship

In the opening essay in Part I, 'Shifting Paradigms in Bioethics and Health Law: The Rise of a New Pragmatism' (Chapter 1), Susan Wolf reminds us that, when we speak of 'rights' associated with health care, we must be ever mindful of context. Every Western-trained bioethicist and health lawyer can recite, at the drop of a hat, the dominant principle governing patient rights – autonomy, leavened to a greater or lesser extent with beneficence. But a closer look at the way in which the autonomy principle plays out in actual practice reveals an altogether more complex and layered picture. Wolf points to empirical studies on such subjects as advance directives and to feminist and race-attentive scholarship to demonstrate that the reasoning actually employed in clinical settings often bears little or no resemblance to rationalist legal and ethical 'rules'. She contends in this thought-provoking essay that such factors as race, ethnicity, gender and source of payment matter greatly to anyone seeking to understand patient rights, and that a more pragmatic approach will contribute more towards their realization than ever-more-elegant articulation of abstract ethical–legal principles such as 'autonomy' and 'beneficence'.

Chapter 2, George Annas and Frances Miller's 'The Empire of Death: How Culture and Economics Affect Informed Consent in the U.S., the U.K., and Japan', examines the influence of cultural attitudes towards truth-telling and death on legal rules. The authors analyse the impact of those attitudes on three countries' willingness to expend financial resources on health care, finding that attitudes and economics influence the legal rules about the kind and depth of information doctors are required to impart to patients in the course of the consent process. The USA, with its historically robust protection for the rights of individuals, views illness as a problem to be solved and is prepared to spend vast sums of money to ward off death. Its informed consent doctrine is accordingly patient-centred and expansive.

Japan's citizens, on the other hand, seem to fear death less. Public discourse about striving to avoid death whenever possible is accordingly muted and fewer resources are allocated to warding it off. Since individual choice with respect to therapy has traditionally been downplayed, Japanese informed consent doctrine has tended in practice to be not only highly paternalistic, but verging on the duplicitous. The historically hierarchical British have also been more accepting of illness and debility than are US patients, as evidenced by the fact that the British consistently devote only half the percentage of GDP to health care than their former colony does. They literally cannot afford the broadly expansive patient-centred doctrine of informed consent that prevails in the USA under this state of economic affairs, and the British standard of disclosure has thus also tended towards the paternalistic. Miller and Annas believe that cultural attitudes towards death affect the resources that a society is willing to allocate to the health sector and that patients' rights to information under informed consent doctrine in these three countries reflect those underlying value choices.

Patient Rights

Informed Consent

Margaret Brazier and José Miola (Chapter 3) view the evolution of patients' rights through a wide analytical lens in their essay 'Bye-Bye Bolam: A Medical Litigation Revolution?'. The authors believe that the House of Lords' landmark *Bolam*[6] decision of almost half a century ago established a professional standard of care for physicians that erroneously came to dominate medical ethics as well as clinical practice. In Brazier and Miola's opinion the House of Lords' recent pronouncement reasserting the judiciary's primacy over the medical standard of care,[7] along with parallel regulatory and professional developments curbing physician hegemony, herald a 'velvet revolution' for patients' rights in litigation involving informed consent. The decision also portends change for the treatment of mature minors and the mentally incapacitated.

Brazier and Miola contend that in the aftermath of *Bolam*, in which McNair J, famously stated, 'A doctor is not guilty of negligence if he has acted in accordance with a practice accepted as proper by a responsible body of medical men skilled in that particular act . . .',[8] courts in essence disregarded the qualifying word 'responsible' and handed over patients' rights to the medical profession, lock, stock and barrel. As a result, paternalistic professional judgments, including those suffused with moral and social agendas, came to dominate not only informed consent litigation, but death and dying and reproductive rights cases, *inter alia*, as well.

The authors point out that evidence-based medicine and the rapid adoption of practice guidelines have considerably demystified medical therapy, making it easier for judges themselves to evaluate what 'responsible' medical practice (including the standard of disclosure for informed consent cases) might be – or at least to identify what might constitute *irresponsible* practice. Moreover, the General Medical Council (1999), the Law Commission (1995) and the Human Rights Act 1998 have all recently reinforced the importance of human rights concerns in the medical care context. In Brazier's and Miola's view, it is not a minute too soon for courts to abandon 'inappropriate deference to medical opinion' and to compel physicians to justify their practices with evidence rather than escaping censure merely because a small body of their peers might also happen to rely on outmoded notions of care.

In '*Rogers* v. *Whitaker* and Informed Consent in Australia: A Fair Dinkum Duty of Disclosure' (Chapter 4), Don Chalmers and Robert Schwartz analyse the Australian High Court's 1992 rejection of the UK's physician-oriented *Bolam* standard of disclosure in informed consent litigation.[9] The High Court opted instead for its own version of the patient-centred 'American' rule,[10] whereby a physician must disclose all information that a reasonable patient would find material to a decision about whether to proceed with recommended therapy. The *Rogers* decision was silent on whether an objective or a subjective patient standard should apply on the issue of causation, but both lower courts had used the subjective criterion.

Chalmers and Schwartz point out a little appreciated fact: plaintiffs rarely win when causation in an informed consent claim is evaluated according to an objective standard. Whatever legal doctrine might require, when *necessary* medical procedures are at stake the 'reasonable patient' is unlikely to reject her doctor's advice no matter what she might have been told about risks and alternatives. For example, whenever a patient is in serious pain or seems to require immediate medical intervention, fact-finders are unlikely to discern a causal relationship between her physician's failure to disclose all material risks and that patient's agreement to undergo exploratory or ameliorative surgery. Few juries would believe that, under urgent circumstances, a reasonable patient would refuse apparently necessary surgery had she been fully informed of all risks associated with most surgical procedures.

In the authors' view, 'only truly elective procedures can give rise to successful informed consent actions' (p. 113) in a jurisdiction having the reasonable patient standard of disclosure. But in Australia, where the High Court subsequently confirmed explicitly that the subjective standard applies,[11] fact-finders are permitted to determine whether a *particular* patient would have refused a procedure which in fact resulted in injury had she been better informed about risk. That is a far easier question for a jury to conclude in the plaintiff's favour in any given case. Although the decision means that Australian physicians have a broader duty to disclose than do doctors in other common-law jurisdictions (Miller, 2000, pp. 36–38), the authors did not expect a sharp increase in litigation alleging a failure to secure informed consent. They predicted that the continuing lack of a widespread contingent fee system for litigation (Ponte, 2000, pp. 341–42), a fairly strong social safety net and the tight fiscal realities of the Australian health care system would avert a flood of lawsuits. That prediction seems accurate thus far; nine years later only seven reported opinions in all Australian federal courts and state territorial supreme courts have discussed informed consent even tangentially.

Reproductive Rights

Frozen Embryos 'Disputing Over Embryos: Of Contracts and Consents' (Chapter 5) is Ellen Waldman's effort to sort out the troublesome contract disputes that increasingly seem to afflict those separating couples for whom the prospect of joint parenthood now resides only in their frozen embryos. Sidestepping the public policy and constitutional issues that have persuaded at least two US courts to hold that parenthood should not be forced on unwilling parties on the basis of any agreement they might have achieved at the time when the embryo was created,[12] she concentrates her analysis on the contractual rights which the majority of courts considering the issue have thus far found persuasive. Waldman believes that parties' contractual claims relating to jointly-created embryos – the essential resource for their joint reproduction, as it were – depend for their validity on the agreement's complete separation and independence from medical consent documentation and procedure.

Since the creation of frozen embryos requires non-trivial invasive procedures for women, medical informed consent is an inevitable aspect of any infertility clinic's *modus operandi*. But consent to medical intervention is a distinct volitional act firmly grounded in principles of personal autonomy. The author believes that medical consent should be entirely separated from any agreement the parties might come to concerning the future disposition of frozen embryos – their joint resource, in a crude sense – created from their gametes. She considers any contract relating to embryo disposition arrived at in conjunction with the medical consent process fatally suspect and would not urge the judiciary to endorse it. Instead, she would require a completely independent process for making dispositional decisions. This process should focus sharply on the ramifications of creating human embryos in the light of possible changes in the parties' circumstances and should be designed to ensure that both gamete donors participate fully and voluntarily in any decision. Then, and only then, would she ask a court to hold the parties to their bargain concerning future use of their biological resource.

Posthumous Reproduction Belinda Bennett tackles the thorny ethical dilemmas associated with taking gametes from corpses for artificial conception in her essay, 'Posthumous Reproduction and the Meanings of Autonomy' (Chapter 6).[13] Using as a springboard three recent and highly-publicized cases from Australia, Britain and France wherein widows had sperm removed from their husbands' corpses posthumously for the purpose of conception, she explores the philosophical underpinnings of dead people's interests in their own reproductive material. She concludes that those cases were probably wrongly decided, because the courts failed to consider the husbands' special relational interests inherent in the concept of reproductive autonomy.

Bennett maintains that gametes are fundamentally different from any other type of human tissue because they contain reproductive potential, and that difference affects the way the law should regard what may be done with them after death. Posthumous reproduction creates whole new relationships, and changes the way people think about prior ones. The author approves of courts who have found the property model inadequate for analysing human interests in bodily tissue,[14] and pinpoints the special death-transcending value of gametes to the individuals whose bodies produced them. She advocates a special analytical category for gametes post death, articulated not in rights-based terminology but in autonomy-enhancing relational ones instead. Asserting that '[p]osthumous reproduction using assisted conception techniques is not simply about whether a widow has a right to have her dead husband's child', she concludes that the widow's desires are not the legal issue. Instead, the critical legal focus should be on the deceased spouse's 'relational autonomy', and by that criterion 'there are very few cases in which posthumous reproduction using assisted conception techniques can be justified'.[15]

Research Subjects' Rights

Robert A. Burt's 'The Suppressed Legacy of Nuremberg' (Chapter 7) asks why on earth the first principle emanating from the Nuremberg trials should have been that 'the voluntary consent of the human [research] subject is absolutely essential' (Annas and Grodin, 1992, p. 102). The Nazi physicians on trial there had conducted incomprehensibly barbaric 'medical research' on concentration camp inmates, including such atrocities as deliberately confining inmates to pressure chambers and raising the simulated altitude to the point where their lungs exploded. Why did the Nuremberg judges think it so important to address the rights of research subjects to withhold consent when the Nazi doctors' experiments were stunningly unethical under *any* conceivable criteria?

Burt's answer is a troubling one. The Nuremberg judges were forced to recognize that they could not rely on 'the self-restraining decency of traditional embodiments of social authority' (p. 194), most pointedly including professional ethics, to prevent such horrific brutality from being visited on research subjects. Observance of the first Nuremberg principle requiring the human subject to consent would at least make clear to the world that the human resources essential to such diabolical experiments – of no possible benefit to the subjects themselves and exposing them to unimaginable agony – must never again materialize. In theory, no sane person would ever agree to submit to torture in order to satisfy unethical researchers' warped notions of scientific inquiry, and no civilized society should permit such immoral 'research' to take place within its borders.

In Chapter 8 Leonard Glantz, George Annas, Michael Grodin and Wendy Mariner then take on the exploitation of clinical research subjects in developing countries in their thoughtful essay, 'Research in Developing Countries: Taking "Benefit" Seriously'. Picking up on recent controversies over the exploitation of vulnerable populations to obtain clinical research subjects for new drugs and vaccines (Belkin, 1998; Varmus and Sacher, 1997), the authors believe that, for experimental studies on the citizens of undeveloped countries to be ethically justifiable, any benefits identified by those investigations must be made economically available to people within those countries. This means that research protocols must address not only the relevant scientific and medical issues raised by the proposed studies, but must also set forth realistic financial plans for distributing any therapeutic fruits stemming from those investigations within the subject country. The authors assert that, when underdeveloped societies contribute human resources towards resolving the health problems of the world's sick people, fundamental ethical principles mandate that their contribution entitle those countries to full participation in any resulting scientific benefits. In essence, those societies have 'paid in advance' for the therapy made possible through their citizens' sacrifices as resources for the research enterprise.

Nancy King's 'Experimental Treatment: Oxymoron or Aspiration?' (Chapter 9) deftly pinpoints the manner in which patient and clinician perceptions become distorted when participation in medical research goes forward under the indeterminate banner of 'experimental therapy'. Experimental *research* is generally defined as a systematic inquiry intended to produce scientific knowledge which can be generalized (National Commission, 1978, pp. 2–3) and the term applies to investigations designed to discover evidence about what works and what doesn't work in health care. Medical *therapy*, on the other hand, is usually defined as those health care interventions scientifically demonstrated to benefit patients. The compound term, *experimental therapy*, confuses the objectives underlying those two quite different concepts and undercuts clear thinking about the true human stakes involved in clinical research.

When clinical investigators go forward with research professing a dual intent – both to acquire scientifically generalizable information through an experimental protocol and, at least hypothetically, to deliver therapy which may benefit the health of individual research subjects – both subject and researcher are likely to formulate differing perceptions of the exercise. To the investigative scientist, the primary objective is to collect evidence about the validity of the scientific hypothesis. Any benefit to the subject – however deeply desired by the researcher – is simply a bonus. To any research subject with a disease, however, the dominant motivation is usually the hope of benefiting personally from a medical intervention. Any advance in scientific knowledge that her participation as a resource for the experiment might permit is distinctly secondary. King highlights the conflicts inherent in their perspectives and suggests abandoning labels and moving towards a joint and more candid decision-making process, individualized by context. She would require physicians to offer patients 'meaningful justification' for recommending their participation in clinical research.

Genetics

In Chapter 10 Henry Greely considers the rights of people sharing similar genetic characteristics in his essay, 'The Control of Genetic Research: Involving the "Groups Between"'. He points out that, for more than two decades, government has regulated US biomedical research indirectly at two levels: through its massive research funding programmes and by way of its power to approve new drugs and devices before they can be marketed across state lines.[16] Clinical investigators receiving federal funding have to submit their proposals for experimentation on human subjects to expert panels who must approve both study design and protections for the human resources necessary for the study before funding will be approved. Thus the government has an initial and powerful say in whether specific research proposals go forward at all. The subjects of that research (or of experimental protocols whose results will be submitted to the Food and Drug Administration) also have a say: they must be fully informed of all study ramifications that might affect them and give voluntary consent to their participation before the study be implemented. This double-pronged federal oversight creates a ripple effect observed throughout the rest of the world's research communities, because all drugs and devices seeking to be marketed in the USA must meet the same standards for the protection of human subjects.

Greely notes that genetic research is almost always focused on groups of people rather than on individuals, because genetic knowledge is gained only by comparing the genomes of people who share some condition thought to have a genetic origin with those who do not. The knowledge thus gained can have both positive and negative implications for members of the larger group regarding autonomy, reputation and commercialization potential. Although researchers often encounter structural and strategic difficulties in affording a group itself a say in research design and participation, Greely believes that, for such a study to pass ethical muster, the group must always be given the opportunity for input (Weijer and Emanuel, 2000; Davis, 2000).

Next, Maxwell Mehlman addresses the not-so-distant future of genetics in his essay, 'How will we Regulate Genetic Enhancement?' (Chapter 11). He defines genetic enhancement as the use of genetic techniques to introduce or improve characteristics in people generally deemed to be within the category of 'normal' for that characteristic. Mehlman takes as a given that, as soon as these techniques permit, some healthy people will employ genetics for elective rather than simply for therapeutic purposes. Those individuals will seek to increase their presumed attractiveness, physical abilities and intelligence in much the same way that some people today choose to undergo cosmetic surgery to improve appearance, or take drugs to enhance athletic performance. Moreover, some parents will elect to subject their offspring to genetic manipulation in order to enhance such socially rewarded characteristics as appearance, intelligence and sports prowess, in much the same way that some parents have sought injections of human growth hormone for their non-hormone-deficient children who just happen to be shorter than the parents would like them to be. Mehlman sees no feasible way of proscribing the use of genetics for enhancement purposes once the scientific genie has escaped from that bottle, but he is very much concerned about giving the genie appropriate rules to play by.

Apart from having safety and efficacy concerns for the patients themselves relating to the non-therapeutic use of genetics, he sees three serious negatives – visited primarily on third parties – resulting from the widespread application of genetic enhancement techniques. The most important is the threat to social equality, because enhancement is unlikely to be subsidized by public or private insurance. The enhancement resource will thus be employed primarily by the wealthy to improve their already privileged economic and social status. This will inevitably widen the gulf between society's haves and have-nots, further jeopardizing democratic political and social structures held together – however tenuously – by the promise of equality of opportunity. Related to the threat to social equality is the unfairness problem encountered by those forced to compete with enhanced individuals for such societal benefits as jobs, education, marriage partners and sports championships. Mehlman also sees threats to personal autonomy when genetic enhancement is forced on non-consenting individuals, such as children and the unborn, who are affected by germ-cell manipulation.

Mehlman reviews the existing regulatory mechanisms which might be brought to bear on the harmful societal problems widespread genetic enhancement would spawn – personal and professional self-regulation, third-party payers, pharmaceutical regulation and direct legislative control of professionals – and finds them less than ideal for the purpose. He briefly examines tort and fiduciary law for analogies to ways in which we might seek to level the societal playing field when power imbalances stemming from genetic enhancement are deemed to affect relationships between parties unfairly. Finally, he concludes that no single method will constitute a panacea for the social problems created by genetic enhancement, but urges attention to the issue now, as well as a search for creative regulatory response before the enhancement genie wriggles too far from the confining strictures of his bottle.

Balancing Rights: Individuals versus Society

In the final essay of Part II, Margaret Brazier and John Harris walk the philosophical tightrope between an individual's right to personal autonomy and society's need to restrain it in the interests of public health, in their exploration, 'Public Health and Private Lives' (Chapter 12). This essay was intended to prompt reform of the UK's still relatively standardless Public Health (Control of Diseases) Act of 1984,[17] enacted in light of the HIV/AIDS pandemic. Under that statute, public health officers have discretionary power to curtail individual liberties drastically to stop the spread of disease. Although current better and more widespread understanding of the way in which HIV infection is transmitted reduces the possibility that public health officers would exercise their powers to the limit in an effort to halt the proliferation of AIDS cases, the authors' discussion nonetheless raises issues equally relevant to *any* analysis of constraints on personal liberty designed to protect society from the acts of individuals that could spread communicable disease. The initial reaction to the post-11 September anthrax scare in the USA, which prompted the issuance of an ill-conceived Model Emergency Health Powers Act,[18] comes to mind. Brazier and Harris basically ask how far society can – or should – go to 'recognize and enforce an obligation not to expose others to infection' (p. 297).

Health Care Resources

Legal scholarship focusing on health care resources tends to cluster primarily around hot-button rationing[19] issues associated with micro-level decision-making, particularly when it comes to naturally scarce medical resources – the sharp end of the resource allocation stick, as it were. Scores of legal essays deal with organ allocation to individuals, for example.[20] Many other essays examine denials of medical care when economic concerns limit access to all the care that could conceivably offer some benefit for the human condition (see, for example, Havighurst, 1992). Yet, relatively few legal scholars examine macro-resource allocation decisions – the blunt end of the stick – in any detail, although occasionally some will explore what the law has to say about allocating health care resources for specific purposes or to general population groups (cf. Elhauge, 1994). Their usual answer? Not all that much, except for the state of Oregon's path-breaking experiment in explicit rationing for Medicaid patients (Kalb, 1992; Leichter, 1999; Rai, 1997), and an occasional essay exploring the implications of QALYs[21] and their analogues (Harris, 1987; Williams, 1985).

Aggregate choices about health care resources are customarily thought to belong more properly to the realms of politics and economics than to the law, because such policy choices tend to reflect societal values more than to emanate from abstract legal principles *per se* (Rai, 1997, p. 1097, n. 75). The law usually becomes involved in resource allocation issues only when implementation problems surface after those broader policy choices have been made, whether by government or through markets. Part III starts off with a series of essays by philosophers and a doctor, which establish the ethical and economic and ground rules for health care resource allocation against which the more purely legal issues are later played out.

Resource Allocation Theory

The first essay in the Resources section is 'Justice in the Distribution of Health Care' by Ronald Dworkin (Chapter 13) which constitutes a philosopher's take on both the macro- and the micro-aspects of health resource allocation as seen through the lens of the justice principle. Dworkin attempts to devise a model that fits the contemporary world, wherein technological progress offers seemingly limitless – and limitlessly expensive – opportunities to pursue the Holy Grail of perfect health. He rejects the ancient ideal of insulation, which postulates that health care is *the* most important way for society to spend its resources. That ideal also proposes that for any member of society to die merely because life-saving resources are unavailable is intolerable, and that medical care should be distributed in an egalitarian manner regardless of ability to pay. Dworkin finds such an ideal clearly unworkable because modern technology – particularly at the dawn of the pharmacogenomics era – demonstrates a continuing genius for devising new ways whereby a country could end up allocating its entire GDP to health care if it chose to do so (cf. Lave and Lave, 1970). Moreover, the insulation ideal offers no guidance on what principles should guide distribution at the micro-level.

Dworkin offers instead an alternative approach for achieving justice in resource allocation, which 'integrates health care into competition with other goods'. His model posits that, if all members of society had equal financial worth and that each had to choose how to spend those resources on personal health care, very few people would choose to spend their resources on life-saving treatment in the late stages of Alzheimer's disease, for example, or on life-sustaining treatment once a persistent vegetative state had set in. Instead, they would devise institutional arrangements to reflect their preferences. Those for whom 'life at all costs' was a more important value than enhancing current enjoyment of life would spend their (equal) resources on insurance to accomplish that goal. Whatever the deficiencies in such a model, Dworkin argues that at least it cannot be faulted for failing to achieve justice.

Professor Dworkin goes on to argue that, if one could be reasonably sure what arrangements people would make if they had to make their own allocation decisions, then we could institute a single-payer system to replicate those basic medical services for all of society. But to the extent we were unsure, we would opt for a managed competition scheme with enough flexibility to accommodate individual preferences through additional insurance coverage beyond a set of basic benefits. He acknowledges the many defects in achieving his model, but posits that '[h]ealth might not be more important than anything else – but the fight for justice in health might well be' (p. 336).

In Chapter 14 another philosopher cautions us that we have no choice but to recognize that economic reality must temper medical judgement and political choices about health resource allocation at both the macro- and the micro-levels.[22] Daniel Callahan's 'Symbols, Rationality, and Justice' reminds us that health care is a far cry from the only good that society needs and values, and that systematic limits on health care spending are unavoidable. Callahan's essay advocates (surely belated) universal health insurance coverage for the USA, with a sufficiently high baseline of 'decent care' to eliminate glaring economic disparities among beneficiaries. He argues that, although rationing in such a system would be inevitable, '[r]ationing should be understood as a symbol of reasoning and restraint' (p. 338). He connects individual rights with such health care rationing and argues that, if the allocation system chosen meets the tests of fairness and rationality, it will be morally defensible.

Two other non-lawyers, philosopher Norman Daniels and physician James Sabin, pick up on these themes in 'Limits to Health Care: Fair Procedures, Democratic Deliberation, and the Legitimacy Problem for Insurers' (Chapter 15). Focusing on the USA's shift in private decision-making authority over health care resources from patients and physicians to private insurers and employers, they explore the fairness and legitimacy of the relatively remote institutional decision-making processes through which managed care seeks to limit medical services. They recognize the economic necessity for limits, but maintain that, even where moral disagreement about the utility of therapies exists, justice and accountability can be accommodated when decisional procedures are acknowledged by all stakeholders as fair. Once the broad policy decisions concerning health resource allocation have been made, the law comes more directly into play with regulation and litigation to protect rights stemming from those policy decisions.

Property Rights in Health Care Resources

The two essays by lawyers that follow explore the issue of property rights in the resource allocation context. First, in Chapter 16, 'Can Patents Deter Innovation?', Michael Heller and Rebecca Eisenberg examine the impact of patent protection on biotechnology research, utilizing the Tragedy of the Anticommons metaphor. They also make an analogy with free markets in post-socialist economies to illustrate the way in which patent monopolies make biotechnology resources artificially scarce. These authors worry that biotech resources will end up being underproduced because the financial and transaction costs of amalgamating the fragmented property rights necessary for future scientific progress (or to produce competing products that could add capacity) are often insurmountable (see Stolberg, 2001; cf. 'Scramble', 2001). In the wake of President Bush's pronouncement that federal funding for embryonic stem cell research will be allowed only on those cell lines already patented by mid-2001 (Wade, 2001), their concerns could prove well justified in the USA sooner than they may have imagined. Presumably Heller and Eisenberg would oppose that policy decision because it intensifies the patent monopoly problem. In any event, they advocate more selective federal regulation to ensure that upstream patent monopolies do not unduly stifle downstream medical product advances.

The second essay in this sub-section, Gerald Dworkin and Ian Kennedy's 'Human Tissue: Rights in the Body and its Parts' (Chapter 17), explores, among other things, whether humans should have equitable or intellectual property protection for their own tissue. Focusing on English law, the authors review the rights of individuals with regard to their own bodies during their lifetime, and of third parties to dispose of their corpses after death. They then consider the sale of human tissue. Acknowledging that sales of 'renewable tissue' such as blood and semen have long been quietly tolerated, they note that 'commercial dealings with human tissue' nonetheless raise society's ethical antennae. Thus sales of human organs have been banned for years in the UK[23] and the USA[24] (and in many other countries), although illegal markets in body parts nonetheless flourish surreptitiously all over the world (Finkel, 2001, p. 6). The current ethical debates over embryonic stem cell research[25] and human cloning (Annas, 1998; Robertson, 1998) further underscore the validity of the authors' point.

Dworkin and Kennedy believe that English law would not follow the landmark California Supreme Court decision in *Moore* v. *University of California*[26] which gave the the plaintiff – whose tissue had been immortalized by researchers without his knowledge or permission in a commercialized cell line – no proprietary claim. They predict that English courts would instead accord such a plaintiff some form of direct compensation from researchers for the unauthorized use of property unique to him. The essay concludes with a plea for a deliberate societal consensus about permissible uses of human tissue, so that scientific advances will remain available for the full benefit of society.

Legislative and Judicial Approaches to Health Resource Allocation

In Chapter 18 Christopher Newdick zeroes in on the judicial review of health resource allocation in the UK, with its government-controlled single-payer scheme, in his essay, 'Resource Allocation in the National Health Service'. Tracing the centralized process by which the British government adopts macro-economic policies which limit (in comparison with other countries) the economic resources available to health authorities, Newdick observes that 'for practical purposes the level of resources invested in health by the central government is beyond the supervision of the courts' (p. 443). When it comes to identified patients harmed when NHS consultants cannot be found to deal with emergency cases, however, English courts are showing greater willingness to intervene on behalf of those sustaining injury.[27] Newdick closes his essay with a plea for a standing commission to foster ongoing dialogue about how to achieve the difficult 'balance between clinical and allocative efficacy in the allocation of health resources' (p. 464).

Timothy Jost carries the same analytical theme into comparative context with his essay on 'Health Care Rationing in the Courts: A Comparative Study' (Chapter 19). Focusing on the very different health care and judicial review systems in Germany, the UK and the USA, Jost demonstrates that judge-made law casts a long shadow over resource allocation decisions at both the macro- and the micro-levels in all those countries, notwithstanding the relatively small number of cases that ever make it to trial. Jost advocates retaining judicial oversight of contested denials of care, notwithstanding the judiciary's lack of expertise in medical and economic matters, but using intermediate review bodies to evaluate these disputes in an administrative setting first. Courts would ordinarily defer to the findings of these expert bodies, but would nonetheless have the final say on the justness of particular resource allocation decisions. In Jost's view such a system would build on the strengths of both administrative and judicial processes, yet temper the recognized deficiencies of relying on either system alone to make critical decisions about health resource allocation.

Resource Allocation and Vulnerable Groups

The final two essays in the volume consider controversial issues that some contend ought to count substantially where health care rationing at the level of individuals is concerned: lifestyle and age. 'Life Style, Health Status, and Distributive Justice' by Robert Schwartz delves into the notoriously contentious question of whether people's self-destructive behaviour should count against them when it comes to claiming 'their share' of medical resources. Schwartz ticks off a surprisingly broad range of lifestyle decisions which could conceivably have a negative impact on health, ranging from obvious candidates like substance abuse, unprotected sex, obesity and failure to obtain vaccinations or medical treatment, to less obviously deleterious activities like extreme sports, refusal to wear seat belts or bicycle helmets, engaging in *protected* sex, and the choices of what occupations to engage in and where to live. His point is to demonstrate that few of us live lives devoid of behaviour that might be considered in some way destructive to perfect health.

Schwartz examines the traditional justifications for making people 'pay' for their lifestyle choices that threaten health: deterrence, punishment and equity. He finds them based on faulty presumptions about voluntariness, causation and whether a given lifestyle choice is warranted by other societal considerations. Schwartz asserts that volition is a myth with regard to many lifestyles. Genetics, family and social environments, gender, ethnicity, education and wealth, to name some of the relevant factors, all play a role beyond the immediate control of the individual, notwithstanding whatever element of volition may also be involved. As far as causation is concerned, the link between a particular health event and its causative agent is usually tenuous at best. Finally, countervailing liberty interests and societal considerations having to do with dangerous occupations like firefighting and military service weigh against blanket penalization of lifestyle choices that could be considered inimical to health.

Finally, Marshall Kapp's essay, '*De Facto* Health-Care Rationing by Age: The Law has no Remedy' (Chapter 21), tackles the perennial question of whether age can – or should – be a criterion for limiting health services against the wishes of elderly patients who 'rage against the dying of the light' (Thomas, 1952). Kapp forthrightly acknowledges that explicit rationing on the basis of age cannot be defended politically – senior citizens constitute a formidable voting bloc in all countries – and examines some of the small number of overt proposals to limit medical care for the elderly. These include Daniel Callahan's 'setting limits' concept (1987), Robert Veatch's 'fair innings' idea (1988), and Norman Daniels' 'Prudential Lifespan Account' theory (1985, pp. 86–113). Kapp attempts to show that the usual justifications for rationing health care on the basis of age do not stand up to close ethical scrutiny because 'old age by itself has no predictive value in individual situations' (p. 580).

Although Kapp takes the pragmatic view that overt health care rationing for the elderly is a political impossibility, and labels it an ethical transgression, he maintains that it nonetheless flourishes out of sight in all societies under cover of 'soft' bedside neglect. He then proceeds to demonstrate why the law has precious little to offer the elderly by way of either prospective intervention when covert rationing is imminent, or reparation once medical care has been denied on the basis of age alone. He concludes that, with the law of little help, at the end of the day caregivers are still left pretty much alone with the ongoing ethical struggle to define the concept of 'appropriate' medical care for the elderly.

Conclusion

Working through rights/resources issues in health care and formulating ethical responses to the dilemmas they raise is critically important to the future of a just society. The foregoing essays were chosen to provide different views about a range of thorny health care rights questions, at least peripherally related to health care resource problems, in the twenty-first century. Not all these dilemmas may appear pressing in many societies now, but eventually they all will be. We can sweep them untidily under the carpet and muddle through or we can face them head-on and think deeply and creatively about devising broadly-supported solutions before more avoidable societal damage takes place. The better choice should be clear.

Acknowledgement

My grateful thanks to Ruth Miller, Boston University School of Law Class of 2002 and Jennifer Norton, Boston University School of Law Class of 2003, for invaluable research assistance.

Notes

1 *Schloendorff* v. *Society of the N.Y. Hospital*, 105 NE 92 (NY 1914).
2 Health Insurance Portability and Accountability Act of 1996 (HIPAA), Pub. L. No. 104–191, 110 Stat. 1936) (1996); Council Decision 88/557/EEC of 4 November 1988 on a Community action in the field of information technology and telecommunications applied to health care, art. 2, 1988 OJ (L 314). *Burger* v. *Lutheran General Hospital*, 759 NE 2d 533 (Ill. 2001) (upholding state statute allowing disclosure of medical records intrahospital and to hospital's counsel); *Koudsi* v. *Hennepin County Medical Centre*, 317 NW 2d 705, 708 (Minn. 1982) (noting that although information regarding plaintiff's status as a patient in the hospital is not confidential, improving technology creates potential harm to privacy); *Weld* v. *Glaxo Wellcome*, 746 NE 2d 522 (Mass. 2001) (class certification is proper in cases regarding pharmacy's use of prescription data for marketing purposes).
3 See, further, Vastag (2001), describing international attempts to foster stem cell research despite US limitations; Wade (2001a), noting that the USA and many Western European countries lagged behind in stem cell research because of ethical debates; McNeil (2001).
4 See, further, Leggett and Regalado (2002), describing China's progress towards cloning humans.
5 See, further, Pear (2001), describing the negotiations between the White House and the House regarding the bill's language.
6 *Bolam* v. *Friern Hospital Management Committee*, [1957] 2 All ER 118, [1957] 1 WLR 582.
7 *Bolitho* v. *City and Hackney Health Authority*, [1997] All ER 771; [1998] AC 232, (HL).
8 *Bolam*, 1 WLR at 587.
9 *Rogers* v. *Whitaker* (1992) 175 CLR 479.
10 *Canterbury* v. *Spence*, 464 F. 2d 772 (DC Cir. 1972).
11 *Rosenberg* v. *Percival* (2001) 178 ALR 577; *Chappel* v. *Hart* (1998) 156 ALR 517.
12 *A.Z.* v. *B.Z.*, 725 NE 2d 1051 (Mass. 2000); *J.B.* v. *M.B.*, 751 A.2d 613 (NJ 2000).
13 23 *Melbourne University Law Review*, 286 (1999).
14 *Moore* v. *Regents of California*, 793 P. 2d 479 (1990).
15 *Id.*, at 306.
16 45 *Code of Federal Regulations* § 46 (1999); see also 'Federal Policy for Protection of Human Subjects', *Federal Register*, **56**, 28003-28032 (1991).
17 Public Health (Control of Diseases) Act (1984) ch. 22, s. 1 et seq.
18 Centers for Disease Control and Prevention, Model State Emergency Health Powers Act (draft 23 October 2001) (drafted by the Center for Law and the Public's Health at Georgetown and Johns Hopkins University).
19 Rationing is defined here as deliberately denying medical services to particular patients in order to use those resources elsewhere to better effect.
20 See, for example, Mahoney (2000), a fairly comprehensive market-friendly essay advocating regulation rather than abolition of competitive markets in human tissue.

21 QALYs = Quality Adjusted Life Years.
22 For a symposium exploring what British health economists have to say about these issues, see *Journal of Medical Ethics*, **27** (4) (2001).
23 Human Organ Transplants Act 1989, c. 31 § 7 (UK).
24 42 USCA § 274e (2001) (enacted in 1984). See also Finkel (2001).
25 'President Bush Backs Federal Funding for Limited Embryonic Cell Study' (2001) *BNA Health Law Reporter*, **10**, 16 August, p. 289.
26 793 P.2d 479 (Cal. 1990).
27 *Bull* v. *Devon Area Health Authority*, 22 BMLR 79 (Eng. CA 1989).

References

Annas, George J. (1998a), 'Human Rights and Health: The Universal Declaration of Human Rights at 50', *New England Journal of Medicine*, **339**, p. 1778.

Annas, George J. (1998b), 'Why We Should Ban Human Cloning', *New England Journal of Medicine*, **339**, p. 122.

Annas, George J. and Grodin, Michael A. (1992), *The Nazi Doctors and the Nuremberg Code*, Oxford and New York: Oxford University Press, pp. 94–107.

Annas, George J. and Grodin, Michael A. (1999), 'Medical Ethics and Human Rights: Legacies of Nuremberg', *Hofstra Law and Policy Symposium*, **3**, p. 111.

Bach, Fritz H., Ivenson, Adrian J. and Weeramantry, Judge Christopher (2001), 'Ethical and Legal Issues in Technology: Xenotransplantation', *American Journal of Law and Medicine*, **27**, p. 283.

Belkin, Lisa (1998), 'The Clues are in the Blood', *New York Times*, 26 April, § 6 (Magazine), p. 46.

Callahan, Daniel (1987), *Setting Limits: Medical Goals in an Aging Society*, New York: Simon & Schuster.

Daniels, Norman (1985), *Just Health Care*, Cambridge: Cambridge University Press.

Davis, Dena S. (2000), 'Groups, Communities, and Contested Identities in Genetic Research', *Hastings Center Report*, **30** (6), p. 38.

Elhauge, Einer (1994), 'Allocating Health Care Morally', *California Law Review*, **82**, p. 1449.

Finkel, Michael (2001), 'Complications', *New York Times*, 27 May, § 6 (Magazine), p. 6.

General Medical Council (1999), *Seeking Patients' Consent: The Ethical Considerations*, London: GMC.

Harris, John (1987), 'QALYfying the Value of Life', *Journal of Medical Ethics*, **13**, p. 117.

Havighurst, Clark C. (1992), 'Prospective Self-Denial: Can Consumers Contract Today to Accept Health Care Rationing Tomorrow?', *University of Pennsylvania Law Review*, **140**, p. 1755.

Hoffman, Sharona (1999), 'A Proposal for Federal Legislation to Address Health Insurance Coverage of Experimental and Investigational Treatments', *Oregon Law Review*, **78**, p. 203.

Holder, Angela R. (1994), 'Funding Innovative Medical Treatment', *Albany Law Review*, p. 795.

Kalb, Paul E. (1992), 'Defining an "Adequate" Package of Health Care Benefits', *University of Pennsylvania Law Review*, **140**, p. 1987.

Lave, Judith R. and Lave, Lester B. (1970), 'Medical Care and its Delivery: An Economic Appraisal', *Law and Contemporary Problems*, **35**, p. 252.

Law Commission (1995), *Mental Incapacity*, Report 231, London: Law Commission.

Leggett, Karby and Regelado, Antonio (2002), 'Fertile Ground: As West Mulls Ethics, China Forges Ahead in Stem Cell Research', *Wall Street Journal*, p. A1.

Leichter, Howard M. (1999), 'Oregon's Bold Experiment: Whatever Happened to Rationing?', *Journal of Health Politics, Policy and Law*, **24**, p. 147.

McNeil, Donald G. jr (2001), 'In a Tiny Room in Sweden, a Large Trove of Stem Cells', *New York Times*, 29 August, p. A1.

Mahoney, Julia D. (2000), 'The Market for Human Tissue', *Virginia Law Review*, **86**, p. 163.

Miller, Frances H. (2000), 'Health Care Information Technology and Provider Accountability: A Symbiotic Relationship', in M. Freeman and A.D.E. Lewis (eds), *Law and Medicine: Current Legal Issues*, Oxford: Oxford University Press, p. 27.

National Commission of Human Subjects of Biomedical and Behavioral Research (1978), *The Belmont Report: Ethical Principles and Guidelines for the Protection of Human Subjects of Research*, DHEW Publication No. (OS) 78-0012, Washington, DC: DHEW Publications.

Pear, Robert (2001), 'Measure Defining Patients' Rights Passes in House', *New York Times*, 3 August, p. A1.

Ponte, Lucille M. (2000), 'Reassessing the Australian Adversarial System: An Overview of Issues in Court Reform and Federal ADR Practice in the Land Down Under', *Syracuse Journal of International Law and Commerce*, **27**, p. 335.

Rai, Arti Kaur (1997), 'Rationing Through Choice: A New Approach to Cost-Effectiveness Analysis in Health Care', *Indiana Law Journal*, **72**, p. 1015.

Robertson, John A. (1998), 'Human Cloning and the Challenge of Regulation', *New England Journal of Medicine*, **339**, p. 119.

'Scramble Over Stem Cells', *Wall Street Journal*, 13 August, p. B1.

Stolberg, Sheryl G. (2001), 'Patent on Human Stem Cell Puts U.S. Officials in Bind', *New York Times*, 17 August, p. A1.

Thomas, Dylan (1952), 'Do Not Go Gentle into That Good Night', *Collected Poems*, London: J.M. Dent & Sons.

Varmus, Harold and Sacher, David (1997), 'Ethical Complexities of Conducting Research in Developing Countries', *New England Journal of Medicine*, **337**, p. 1003.

Vastag, Brian (2001), 'Seeding the World with Stem Cells', *Journal of the American Medical Association*, **286**, 4 July, p. 33.

Veatch, Robert (1988), 'Justice and the Economics of Terminal Illness', *Hastings Center Report*, **18** (4), p. 34.

Wade, Nicholas (2001a), 'List of Stem Cell Researchers Shows Hands Had Been Tied', *New York Times*, 28 August, p. A10.

Wade, Nicholas (2001b), 'Scientists Divided on Limit of Federal Stem Cell Money', *New York Times*, 16 August, p. A16.

Weijer, Charles and Emanuel, Ezekial J. (2000), 'Protecting Communities in Biomedical Research, *Science*, **289**, p. 1142.

Williams, Alan (1985), 'The Value of QALYs', *Health and Social Sciences Journal*, **94**, p. 4967.

Winslow, Ron (2001), 'Intensive Care: One Patient, 34 Days in Hospital, a Bill for $5.2 Million', *Wall Street Journal*, 2 August, p.1.

Part I
The Rights–Resources Relationship

[1]

Shifting Paradigms in Bioethics and Health Law: The Rise of a New Pragmatism

Susan M. Wolf†

Neither bioethics nor health law is old as an established discipline. Modern bioethics dates from the late 1960s or early 1970s.[1] Health law as a domain characterized by its own casebooks, courses, and specialists arguably began somewhat earlier.[2] While

---

† Associate Professor of Law & Medicine, University of Minnesota Law School, and Faculty Associate, Center for Biomedical Ethics, University of Minnesota; A.B. Princeton University; J.D., Yale Law School. This Article originated as a presentation at the American Society of Law, Medicine & Ethics 1994 Health Law Workshop. I am grateful to workshop participants plus George Annas, Allan Brandt, Daniel Farber, Philip Frickey, Michael Grodin, and Suzanna Sherry for their suggestions. Terrence J. Dwyer of the University of Minnesota Law School provided helpful research assistance. I am also deeply indebted to Professor Melvin Tumin, who introduced me to Dewey's work over twenty years ago. I write in fond memory of both Jay Healey and Mel.

[1] *See* DAVID J. ROTHMAN, STRANGERS AT THE BEDSIDE: A HISTORY OF HOW LAW AND BIOETHICS TRANSFORMED MEDICAL DECISION MAKING (1991); Albert R. Jonsen, *The Birth of Bioethics*, HASTINGS CTR. REP., Nov.-Dec. 1993, at S1. One could argue that the birth of modern bioethics was the promulgation on the Nuremberg Code in 1949, the first major pronouncement of the ethics of human subjects research. However, modern bioethics as a field did not really get under way in the U.S. until later. On the Nuremberg Code's impact and its limits in the U.S., see THE NAZI DOCTORS AND THE NUREMBERG CODE: HUMAN RIGHTS IN HUMAN EXPERIMENTATION (George J. Annas & Michael Grodin eds., 1992).

Bioethics is the study of ethical problems in health care and the biological sciences. I eschew the use of "biomedical ethics" or "medical ethics" as the overarching term because of their excessive emphasis on medicine, to the exclusion of nursing and other health care ethics.

[2] The rise of health law as a discipline apart from forensic medicine, a rise that seems to have started around 1960 and certainly gathered steam in the 1970s and 1980s, can be roughly gauged from the publication dates of its casebooks. *See* WILLIAM J. CURRAN ET AL., HEALTH CARE LAW, FORENSIC SCIENCE, AND PUBLIC POLICY (4th ed. 1990) (first published in 1960 as LAW AND MEDICINE); DAVID J. SHARPE ET AL., CASES AND MATERIALS ON LAW AND MEDICINE (1978); WALTER WADLINGTON ET AL., CASES AND MATERIALS ON LAW AND MEDICINE (1980); MICHAEL H. SHAPIRO & ROY G. SPECE, JR., CASES, MATERIALS, AND PROBLEMS ON BIOETHICS AND LAW (1981 & Supp. 1991); JUDITH AREEN ET AL., LAW, SCIENCE AND MEDICINE (1984 & Supp. 1989); BARRY R. FURROW ET AL., HEALTH LAW (2d ed. 1991 & Supp. 1994) (first published in 1987); CLARK C. HAVIGHURST, HEALTH CARE LAW AND POLICY (1988 & Supp. 1992); GEORGE J. ANNAS ET AL., AMERICAN HEALTH LAW (1990). *See also* Joseph M. Healey, *William J. Curran and American Health Law*, 55 CONN. MED. 313 (1991). George Annas writes that "[i]n the 1950s and 1960s, 'Law and Medicine' courses in law schools were almost exclusively concerned with . . . forensic psychiatry and forensic pathology. . . . In the late 1960s, some . . . courses began concentrating on broader medicolegal issues. . . . In the 1970s, . . . at least some . . . courses expanded to include public policy . . . ." George J. Annas, *Health Law at the Turn of the Century: From White Dwarf to Red Giant*, 21 CONN. L. REV. 551, 551 (1989). As the contents of the casebooks reflect, health law covers a wide array of legal and policy problems in health care, ranging from informed consent and medical malpractice, to issues of access to health care, health care finance, and employment relations in health care. On the rise of health law and the field's relationship to bioethics, see generally Alexander Morgan Capron & Vicki Michel, *Law and Bioeth-*

each has far older precursors,[3] the two fields have seen a modern resurgence in the last thirty years or so. Yet each in these three decades has been dominated by a certain method or paradigm.[4] In bioethics that has come to be known as "principlism," deductive reasoning from a limited set of middle-level ethical principles, albeit with some reciprocal attention to the implications of the case at hand for those principles.[5] No comparable term has emerged in health law, and the field has arguably been less enamored of philosophical abstraction.[6] But the pattern

---

ics, 27 LOY. L.A. L. REV. 25 (1993).

Commentators have mapped the relationship of bioethics to health law variously. George Annas has argued that health law drives bioethics. GEORGE J. ANNAS, JUDGING MEDICINE 3 (1988). *See also* Carl E. Schneider, *Bioethics in the Language of the Law*, HASTINGS CTR. REP., July-Aug. 1994, at 16 [hereinafter *Language of the Law*]. However, Capron and Michel argue that "[r]eciprocally, bioethics has shaped the law." Capron & Michel, *supra*, at 32. They maintain that the two fields are distinct, even if closely interrelated. This is supported by the fact that there are now journals primarily devoted to one or the other (for example, on bioethics: the *Hastings Center Report, Kennedy Institute of Ethics Journal, Cambridge Quarterly of Healthcare Ethics*, and *Bioethics* versus on health law: the *American Journal of Law & Medicine, Annals of Health Law*, and *Health Matrix: The Journal of Law-Medicine*—though *Law, Medicine & Health Care* recently muddied the waters by switching its name to the *Journal of Law, Medicine & Ethics*). But there is certainly tremendous overlap; nonlawyer bioethicists regularly discuss law, and lawyers have long joined in the multidisciplinary collaboration to create modern bioethics.

[3] Medical ethics is millennia old, of course, including the Hippocratic oath and corpus. William Curran finds the earliest western medicolegal texts to be 16th- and 17th-century Italian works. He recounts that Harvard established a professorship in legal medicine in 1877, but the field was dominated by forensic medicine at least into the 1950s. William J. Curran, *Titles in the Medicolegal Field: A Proposal for Reform*, 1 AM. J. L. & MED. 1, 10 (1975). In the first issue of the *American Journal of Law & Medicine* in 1975, Curran proposed the term "'health law,' to cover the wide range of legal aspects of medicine, nursing, dentistry, and other health service fields including public health and the environment." *Id.*

[4] "Paradigm" is, of course, borrowed from THOMAS S. KUHN, THE STRUCTURE OF SCIENTIFIC REVOLUTIONS 10-11 (2d ed. 1970). I am not the first to apply the term to current bioethics debates. It is used, for example, in *Symposium: Emerging Paradigms in Bioethics*, 69 IND. L.J. 945 (1994). See especially Carl E. Schneider, *Bioethics With a Human Face*, 69 IND. L.J. 1075, 1085 & n.46 (1994) ("the centerpiece of bioethics—its autonomy paradigm" [hereinafter *With a Human Face*]). *See also* Arthur L. Caplan, *Autonomy and Long-Term Care*, 343 LANCET 1024, 1024 (1994) ("the dominant paradigm of autonomy in bioethics"); Juan Carlos Tealdi, *Teaching Bioethics as a New Paradigm for Health Professionals*, 7 BIOETHICS 188 (1993); Leslie P. Francis, *The Roles of the Family in Making Health Care Decisions for Incompetent Patients*, 1992 UTAH L. REV. 861, 880 ("the predominant liberal paradigm of bioethics"); Bruce Jennings et al., *Ethical Challenges of Chronic Illness*, HASTINGS CTR. REP., Feb.-Mar. 1988, at S1, S4 (the "autonomy paradigm" in bioethics).

Daniel Farber and Philip Frickey note that Kuhn's "term is almost always misused to mean something like 'world-view.' ... For [Kuhn], a paradigm was not a set of assumptions or a perspective, but rather an actual example of scientific work which served as a model ...." Daniel A. Farber & Philip P. Frickey, *Practical Reason and the First Amendment*, 34 UCLA L. REV. 1615, 1629 (1987) (footnote omitted). I use the term to refer to the model of bioethics analysis supplied by TOM L. BEAUCHAMP & JAMES F. CHILDRESS, PRINCIPLES OF BIOMEDICAL ETHICS (4th ed. 1994). Roger B. Dworkin agrees in *Emerging Paradigms in Bioethics: Introduction*, 69 IND. L.J. 945, 946 (1994).

[5] *See* BEAUCHAMP & CHILDRESS, *supra* note 4, at 37; PRINCIPLES OF HEALTH CARE ETHICS (Raanan Gillon & Ann Lloyd eds., 1993); K. Danner Clouser & Bernard Gert, *A Critique of Principlism*, 15 J. MED. & PHIL. 219 (1990). The reciprocal inductivism in Beauchamp & Childress is more recent, as comparison of the current fourth edition to earlier editions shows.

[6] There is an empiricist history in modern health law on certain topics, such as malpractice, investigating law's clinical effects. *See, e.g.*, SYLVIA A. LAW & STEVEN POLAN, PAIN AND PROFIT: THE POLITICS OF MALPRACTICE (1978); SYLVIA A. LAW, BLUE CROSS: WHAT WENT WRONG? (2d ed. 1976). More recently, see PAUL C. WEILER ET AL., A MEASURE OF MALPRACTICE: MEDICAL INJURY, MALPRACTICE LITIGATION, AND PATIENT COMPENSATION (1993).

has often been similar: the creation of middle-level rules (on informed consent, surrogate decision-making, advance directives and so on) and then their downward application with insufficient attention to the clinical context, the specific characteristics of the disputants (such as insurance status, race or ethnicity, and gender), and whether the rules will actually work in medical settings.[7] In truth, both have been "applied" disciplines concerned not so much with ethical and legal theory per se, but with ethics and law in health care and the biological sciences. Yet the dominant approach in each has been to develop middle-level rules.[8]

These related paradigms are now under attack from a number of quarters. In bioethics, a plethora of alternative methods has recently been put forth, a new empiricism has challenged the content of previously accepted principles, and burgeoning feminist and race-attentive work has rendered suspect any bioethical approach geared to the generic "patient." A new crop of publications trumpets these challenges to the old order and attests to fundamental shifts under way.[9]

Less widely recognized is the comparable challenge brewing in health law. Courts and legislatures have long enunciated the rules of informed consent, ad-

---

[7] The pattern has not been invariable. For example, informed consent doctrine has occasioned considerable empirical investigation. *See, e.g.*, Alan Meisel & Loren H. Roth, *Toward an Informed Discussion of Informed Consent: A Review and Critique of the Empirical Studies*, 25 ARIZ. L. REV. 265, 340 (1983) (but cautioning that "the studies . . . are, as a whole and with some notable exceptions, worse than anecdote and speculation"). Despite these studies, Jay Katz could reaffirm in 1984 his earlier assessment that "'[T]he law of informed consent is substantially mythic and fairy tale-like as far as advancing patients' rights to self-decisionmaking is concerned.'" JAY KATZ, THE SILENT WORLD OF DOCTOR AND PATIENT 83 (1984) (footnote omitted).

There is also some attention to patient characteristics such as insurance status to be found in health law writings before the recent shift. *See, e.g.*, Rand E. Rosenblatt, *Dual Track Health Care—The Decline of the Medicaid Cure*, 44 CIN. L. REV. 643 (1975) (book comment); SYLVIA A. LAW, THE RIGHTS OF THE POOR 80-110 (1974).

[8] Beauchamp and Childress actually place both rules and more general principles at the middle level, between more abstract theory and particular judgments about cases. BEAUCHAMP & CHILDRESS, *supra* note 4, at 15, 38. I use "middle-level rules" here to apply to both rules and principles, distinguishing them from higher-order theory.

[9] Methodologic challenges include John D. Arras, *Getting Down to Cases: The Revival of Casuistry in Bioethics*, 16 J. MED. & PHIL. 29 (1991); Albert R. Jonsen, *Of Balloons and Bicycles or the Relationship between Ethical Theory and Practical Judgment*, HASTINGS CTR. REP., Sept.-Oct. 1991, at 14; Clouser & Gert, *supra* note 5; Ronald M. Green, *Method in Bioethics: A Troubled Assessment*, 15 J. MED. & PHIL. 179 (1990); Henry S. Richardson, *Specifying Norms as a Way to Resolve Concrete Ethical Problems*, 19 PHIL. & PUB. AFF. 279 (1990); ALBERT R. JONSEN & STEPHEN TOULMIN, THE ABUSE OF CASUISTRY: A HISTORY OF MORAL REASONING (1988); Stephen Toulmin, *The Tyranny of Principles*, HASTINGS CTR. REP., Dec. 1981, at 31. Collections of essays on the methodology ferment include META MEDICAL ETHICS: THE PHILOSOPHICAL FOUNDATIONS OF BIOETHICS (Michael A. Grodin ed., 1995); A MATTER OF PRINCIPLES? FERMENT IN U.S. BIOETHICS (Edwin R. DuBose et al. eds., 1994); PRINCIPLES OF HEALTH CARE ETHICS, *supra* note 5. *See generally* David DeGrazia, *Moving Forward in Bioethical Theory: Theories, Cases, and Specified Principlism*, 17 J. MED. & PHIL. 511 (1992).

Race-attentive challenges include essays in "IT JUST AIN'T FAIR": THE ETHICS OF HEALTH CARE FOR AFRICAN AMERICANS (Annette Dula & Sara Goering eds., 1994) [hereinafter "IT JUST AIN'T FAIR"], and in AFRICAN-AMERICAN PERSPECTIVES ON BIOMEDICAL ETHICS (Harley E. Flack & Edmund D. Pellegrino eds., 1992).

Gender-attentive and feminist challenges include FEMINISM & BIOETHICS: BEYOND REPRODUCTION (Susan M. Wolf ed., forthcoming) [hereinafter "FEMINISM & BIOETHICS"]; FEMINIST PERSPECTIVES IN MEDICAL ETHICS (Helen Bequaert Holmes & Laura M. Purdy eds., 1992); SUSAN SHERWIN, NO LONGER PATIENT: FEMINIST ETHICS AND HEALTH CARE (1992); CHRISTINE OVERALL, ETHICS AND HUMAN REPRODUCTION: A FEMINIST ANALYSIS (1987).

vance directives, and surrogate decision-making, for example. We now are investigating with greater intensity how those rules and attendant legal practices (such as the use of forms) play out in the clinic, what empirical data provide in support or critique of the law, and whether all of this affects some groups differently.[10]

This growing attention to context, to empirical realities, and to difference has been diagnosed as "inductivism" or sometimes Rawlsian "coherentism" in bioethics.[11] However, placed side-by-side with the comparable shift in health law, it seems part of larger trends. This is not just parochial ferment in the limited ranks of bioethicists. Instead, it seems linked to the rise of a new pragmatism.[12] John Dewey, William James, and Charles Sanders Peirce have come to visit the clinic and find much to criticize.[13]

The problem with this diagnosis is that pragmatism is a slippery beast—hard to define and seemingly all things to all people, as others have long noted.[14] Yet the rejection of deduction from grand and universal principles in favor of detailed attention to context, empirical realities, and differences among individuals and groups supports the diagnosis.[15] The advantage of considering this diagnosis is

---

[10] *See, e.g.*, *With a Human Face*, *supra* note 4; FURROW ET AL., *supra* note 2, at 375-77.

[11] *See* BEAUCHAMP & CHILDRESS, *supra* note 4, at 17-28.

[12] Susan H. Williams seems to agree in *Bioethics and Epistemology: A Response to Professor Arras*, 69 IND. L.J. 1021, 1021 (1994) ("[I]n bioethics . . . [t]he move from theory-based systems of ethics to narrative-based systems of ethics is paralleled by shifts in several related fields. In legal theory, one can see this development in the rise of legal pragmatism . . . .").

On the revival of interest in pragmatism generally, outside of bioethics and health law, see, for example, *Symposium on the Renaissance of Pragmatism in American Legal Thought*, 63 S. CAL. L. REV. 1569 (1990) (subsequently published as ARTICLES AND COMMENTS PRESENTED AT THE SYMPOSIUM ON THE RENAISSANCE OF PRAGMATISM IN AMERICAN LEGAL THOUGHT (1990)); RICHARD POSNER, PROBLEMS OF JURISPRUDENCE (1990); CORNEL WEST, THE AMERICAN EVASION OF PHILOSOPHY: A GENEALOGY OF PRAGMATISM (1989) (especially chs. 5, 6); RICHARD RORTY, CONTINGENCY, IRONY, AND SOLIDARITY (1989); Daniel A. Farber, *Legal Pragmatism and the Constitution*, 72 MINN. L. REV. 1331 (1988); RICHARD RORTY, CONSEQUENCES OF PRAGMATISM (1982); RICHARD RORTY, PHILOSOPHY AND THE MIRROR OF NATURE (1979).

[13] This is not their first visit. Karen Hanson notes that "one of Dewey's favorite examples [of the connection between facts and values] is drawn from . . . medical practice." Karen Hanson, *Are Principles Ever Properly Ignored? A Reply to Beauchamp on Bioethical Paradigms*, 69 IND. L.J. 975, 976 (1994) (citing John Dewey, *Theory of Valuation*, *in* 13 THE LATER WORKS 191, 210-11 (Jo Ann Boydston ed., 1988)).

[14] *See, e.g.*, Daniel A. Farber & Suzanna Sherry, *The 200,000 Cards of Dimitri Yurasov: Further Reflections on Scholarship and Truth*, 46 STAN. L. REV. 647, 647 n.3, 649-50 (1994) [hereinafter "*The 200,000 Cards*"; Daniel A. Farber & Suzanna Sherry, *Telling Stories Out of School: An Essay on Legal Narratives*, 45 STAN. L. REV. 807, 820-22 (1993) [hereinafter "*Telling Stories Out of School*"].

[15] Joseph Singer writes,

> Pragmatists argue that philosophers and legal theorists miss the point if we spend our time worrying about the internal coherence of systems of abstract principles . . . . Rather, pragmatists counsel attention to the actual workings of law in particular settings in social life . . . .
>
> . . . .
>
> . . . . Rather than worrying primarily about how a new practice fits with established conceptual structures or rule systems, pragmatists concentrate on satisfying human needs. This focus . . . measures the justice of established legal institutions and reform proposals by what they do, rather than whether they cohere with an already existing ideal vision.

Joseph William Singer, *Property and Coercion in Federal Indian Law: The Conflict Between Critical and Complacent Pragmatism*, 63 S. CAL. L. REV. 1821, 1822 (1990). Though I diagnose the bioethics and health law shifts as "pragmatist," Daniel Farber and Philip Frickey suggest additional pos-the link it establishes to a vibrant intellectual tradition now enjoying resurgence, and to a multidisciplinary literature considering the implications.[16] As I conceded above, bioethics and health law have always been "applied" or practical. But in shifting their respective approaches increasingly away from something principle- or rule-driven to something more inductivist and empirical, their approach to the practical becomes pragmatist.[17]

My goal here is first to analyze the paradigm shift under way in bioethics. I then analyze the less discussed shift I discern in health law. Finally, I consider what is gained by seeing both shifts as part of the pragmatist revival, and where bioethics and health law should go from here.

With the other authors in this symposium, I write in memory of Joseph Healey. Jay, I think, would approve the diagnosis. He was a student of the realities of health care,[18] attentive to the background importance of the power differential between doctors and patients[19] and to the larger context,[20] critical of the adequacy of any general principle (including patient self-determination),[21] and laboring to discern the proper future of health law.[22] I argue that the future of both health law and bioethics lies in the clinic, more than in the philosopher's study or law professor's library.[23] Jay spent his too short life working in clinical settings. If he could, he would welcome us back.

I. THE SHIFT IN BIOETHICS

For the bulk of its short history, modern bioethics has been dominated by what has come to be known as "principlism." This approach owes much to the pervasive influence of Tom Beauchamp and James Childress's *Principles of Biomedical*

---

sible rubrics in noting that "[a]n impressive array of recent legal commentary has suggested a movement away from grand theory toward something new, variously called 'intuitionism,' 'prudence,' and 'practical reason.' . . . [A]ll share some fundamental characteristics . . . ." Farber & Frickey, *supra* note 4, at 1645-46 (footnotes omitted). Of course, some of the new more inductivist approaches in bioethics might try to lend their own names to the diagnosis instead, especially casuistry. My goal is not to adjudicate among these competitors, but to diagnose the larger trend of which they are a part.

16 *See supra* note 12.

17 *Cf.* Daniel C. K. Chow, *A Pragmatic Model of Law*, 67 WASH. L. REV. 755, 757-58 (1992) (contrasting a pragmatic view with a deeper pragmatism).

18 *See* Joseph M. Healey, *Bridging the Gap II*, 56 CONN. MED. 703 (1992) ("physicians are expressing their frustration with ethical and legal analysis that seems remote from the practice of medicine. . . . There needs to be . . . an attempt to inform public policy with the experience of the participants.").

19 *See* Joseph M. Healey, *Health Law in Connecticut: Historical Perspectives, Contemporary Concerns, and Future Directions*, 21 CONN. L. REV. 723, 726-30 (1989) (on "the rise of medical power" [hereinafter *Health Law in Connecticut*]).

20 *See* Joseph M. Healey, *Moving Beyond Futility*, 56 CONN. MED. 270 (1992) ("While the futility issue will remain an important focus, . . . the context for discussion is likely to shift to the larger societal level.").

21 *See Health Law in Connecticut*, *supra* note 19, at 739-40.

22 *See id.*

23 One could argue, of course, that there are many different ways to do both bioethics and health law, and that we need remote theoreticians as well as those involved in the clinic. While it is certainly true that there are different ways of value, I am arguing in this Article that bioethics and health law grounded in clinical realities and concerned about the fate of vulnerable patients and research subjects is better.

Ethics, now in its fourth edition.[24] Principlism is an approach to reasoning about ethical problems that proceeds in the main not deductively from higher-order theory, or inductively from fine-grained attention toward the situation presented, but from middle-level principles down to the case presented. The four principles offered in the book have become the most familiar litany recited in bioethics: autonomy, beneficence, nonmaleficence, and justice. The *Principles* book did not originate them; they were first offered by the National Commission for the Protection of Human Subjects in *The Belmont Report*.[25] The book, however, gave them great currency. To some extent, Beauchamp and Childress stand wrongly accused of promulgating principlism. Their ethical approach is more complex, some critics have been guilty of caricaturing it, and the latest edition of their book includes new material to address the critics.[26] Yet it is fair to say that in a great many quarters the book has been taken to advance a principlist approach.

The four principles and indeed principlism—reasoning and justification from such principles—had until recently so permeated the bioethics literature, bioethics clinical practice, and bioethics education, that there seemed to be little fundamental intellectual movement. We were dotting i's and crossing t's, doing what Thomas Kuhn might call "normal science."[27] We were in a period of quiescence.

That has now changed. We are in the midst of a paradigm shift, as Edmund Pellegrino noted not long ago.[28] We see fundamental challenges to the method of reasoning downward from middle-level principles, to the content of those principles, and to the failure of bioethics to attend to differences associated with gender, race, ethnicity, and insurance status. There is a proliferation of alternatives to principlism: a demand for even more abstract moral theory deductively applied,[29] advocacy of specified principlism,[30] a revival of casuistry,[31] the call for an inductivism based on empirical information or ethnography,[32] interest in narrative bioethics,[33] and the articulation of care-based ethics.[34] There are also challenges

[24] *See* BEAUCHAMP & CHILDRESS, *supra* note 4. *Cf.* Dworkin, *supra* note 4, at 946 ("If any work in bioethics may be said to be truly paradigmatic, it is Tom L. Beauchamp's and James Childress' seminal *Principles of Biomedical Ethics*." (citation omitted)).

[25] *See generally* THE BELMONT REPORT: ETHICAL GUIDELINES FOR THE PROTECTION OF HUMAN SUBJECTS OF RESEARCH (National Commission for the Protection of Human Subjects of Biomedical and Behavioral Research ed., 1978).

[26] *See* BEAUCHAMP & CHILDRESS, *supra* note 4, chs. 1 & 2,

[27] KUHN, *supra* note 4, at 5.

[28] Edmund D. Pellegrino, *The Metamorphosis of Medical Ethics: A 30-Year Retrospective*, 269 JAMA 1158 (1993).

[29] *See* Clouser & Gert, *supra* note 5.

[30] *See* Richardson, *supra* note 9. Beauchamp and Childress argue that specified principlism is not an alternative but a salutary amendment to their approach. *See* BEAUCHAMP & CHILDRESS, *supra* note 4, at 28-32, 104-11.

[31] *See* JONSEN & TOULMIN, *supra* note 9.

[32] *See, e.g.*, Barry Hoffmaster, *Can Ethnography Save the Life of Medical Ethics?*, 35 SOC. SCI. & MED. 1421 (1992).

[33] *See, e.g.*, HOWARD BRODY, STORIES OF SICKNESS (1987). *See also* KATHRYN HUNTER, DOCTORS' STORIES: THE NARRATIVE STRUCTURE OF MEDICAL KNOWLEDGE (1991).

[34] The literature on care-based approaches to ethics without specific focus on bioethics is voluminous. *See, e.g.*, AN ETHIC OF CARE: FEMINIST AND INTERDISCIPLINARY PERSPECTIVES (Mary Jeanne Larrabee ed., 1993); JEFFREY BLUSTEIN, CARE AND COMMITMENT: TAKING THE PERSONAL POINT OF VIEW (1991); FEMINIST ETHICS (Claudia Card ed., 1991); Lawrence Blum, *Gilligan and Kohlberg: Implications for Moral Theory*, 98 ETHICS 472 (1988); Annette Baier, *What Do Women Want in a Moral Theory?*, 19 NOÛS 53 (1985); NEL NODDINGS, CARING: A FEMININE APPROACH TO ETHICS AND MORAL

from a variety of perspectives to the content of the usual four principles.[35]

We simultaneously see the rise of empiricism in bioethics,[36] with attention to differences of race, ethnicity, and gender. Two prominent collections, for example, now explore African American perspectives on bioethical problems.[37] Empirical studies increasingly look for differences by race or ethnicity in attitudes toward advance directives and other aspects of medical decision-making.[38] We also see increasing empirical exploration by gender,[39] as well as the emergence of a feminist literature on bioethics.[40] And authors now explore the intersection of race, gender, and economic status.[41]

Thus, the period of quiescence in bioethics has yielded to one of great ferment. Yet what is most remarkable about this shift is how long it took to come about. The new debates on method and attention to gender arrived late compared to the fields whose interdisciplinary collaboration gave birth to modern bioethics. In law, for example, it would be difficult to have a serious debate now about whether there is any merit to feminist and other gender-attentive work,[42] or to Critical Race scholarship and other race- and ethnicity-attentive writing.[43] And, people who write on jurisprudence and philosophy of law would laugh at the idea that our method of traveling between cases and normative propositions is settled; witness the ongoing

---

EDUCATION (1984) [hereinafter "CARING"]; CAROL GILLIGAN, IN A DIFFERENT VOICE: PSYCHOLOGICAL THEORY AND WOMEN'S DEVELOPMENT (1982). On care-based approaches in bioethics, see, for example, SHERWIN, *supra* note 9, at 42-57; Hilde Lindemann Nelson, *Against Caring*, and Nel Noddings, *In Defense of Caring*, in 3 J. CLIN. ETHICS 8 (1992).

My list of challenges to "principlism" is not exhaustive. For example, there is a revival of interest in virtue theory. *See, e.g.*, Pellegrino, *supra* note 28.

[35] See, e.g., Rebecca J. Cook, *Feminism and the Four Principles*, in PRINCIPLES OF HEALTH CARE ETHICS, *supra* note 5, at 193, as well as other essays in that volume. *But see* Ruth Macklin, *Women's Health: An Ethical Perspective*, 21 J. L. MED. & ETHICS 23 (1993) (defending the adequacy of the four principles for gender analysis).

[36] See, e.g., *Empirical Research in Medical Ethics* (Robert M. Arnold & Lachlan Forrow eds.), 14 THEORETICAL MED. 195 (1993), and studies cited therein.

[37] *See* "IT JUST AIN'T FAIR", *supra* note 9; AFRICAN-AMERICAN PERSPECTIVES ON BIOMEDICAL ETHICS, *supra* note 9.

[38] One important such study is under way at the Pacific Center for Health Care Ethics at the University of Southern California, resulting thus far in Leslie J. Blackhall et al., Ethnicity and Attitudes Toward Patient Autonomy (1994) (unpublished manuscript, on file with the Pacific Center for Health, Policy and Ethics, University of Southern California Law Center). Another is reported in Celia J. Orona et al., *Cultural Aspects of Nondisclosure*, 3 CAMBRIDGE Q. HEALTHCARE ETHICS 338 (1994). *See also* Jeremy Sugarman et al., *Factors Associated with Veterans' Decisions about Living Wills*, 152 ARCHIVES INTERNAL MED. 343 (1992); articles in Special Issue, *Cross Cultural Medicine: A Decade Later*, 157 W. J. MED. 213 (1992).

[39] *See, e.g.*, Susan M. Rubin et al., *Increasing the Completion of the Durable Power of Attorney for Health Care: A Randomized, Controlled Trial*, 271 JAMA 209 (1994); Jaya Virmani et al., *Relationship of Advance Directives to Physician-Patient Communication*, 154 ARCHIVES INTERNAL MED. 909 (1984).

[40] *See, e.g.*, FEMINISM & BIOETHICS, *supra* note 9; FEMINIST PERSPECTIVES IN MEDICAL ETHICS, *supra* note 9; SHERWIN, *supra* note 9.

[41] *See, e.g.*, Dorothy E. Roberts, *Reconceiving the Patient: Starting With Women of Color*, *in* FEMINISM & BIOETHICS, *supra* note 9.

[42] The feminist and gender-attentive literature is now copious. Collections include FEMINIST LEGAL THEORY: FOUNDATIONS (D. Kelly Weisberg ed., 1993); FEMINIST LEGAL THEORY: READINGS IN LAW AND GENDER (Katharine T. Bartlett & Rosanne Kennedy eds., 1991).

[43] This literature too has become abundant. *See generally* Richard Delgado & Jean Stefancic, *Critical Race Theory: An Annotated Bibliography*, 79 VA. L. REV. 461 (1993); Symposium, *Minority Critiques of the Critical Legal Studies Movement*, 22 HARV. C.R.-C.L. L. REV. 297 (1987).

debates about storytelling and the uses of narrative.[44] So, there is something to explain in the slowness and reluctance of bioethics to face these issues.

I argue elsewhere that this reluctance is a function of the deep structure of bioethics.[45] First, it is a product of the field's early embrace of a liberal individualism largely inattentive to social context. This not only has made individual autonomy the pivotal value in bioethics, but has generally led to an overly simplistic vision of what autonomy and liberty entail. Only in recent times have communitarians, empiricists, and others rebelled, claiming that the picture of a monadic individual armed with her rights erases too much of her context and invites moral bankruptcy.[46]

Second to blame is the field's early embrace of Kantianism. This yielded requirements of universal norms, and an impartial perspective inattentive to relationships and community. It also privileged abstract reasoning over virtue, character, and the moral emotions. Thus we saw the rise of deductivism and moral systems building.

Third, bioethics has demonstrated a tendency to think of the patient or research subject generically, without attention to race, gender, or insurance status. The literature on the termination of life-sustaining treatment, for example, was until recently largely devoid of considerations of who the patient was, special barriers to communication that the doctor and patient might encounter, and different ways of thinking about ethical problems that some patients might embrace. Indeed, for lack of focusing on real characteristics of real patients, this abstract patient has often been thought of as someone without problems of race, gender, or resources. The result, I have suggested, has been a bioethics for the privileged patient.[47] This is a bioethics that has been strong on proclaiming individual autonomy to choose, but weak on insisting on access to health care and the creation of choices for those who have few.

Finally, the reluctance to face problems of method and difference even as related fields have assumed that challenge can be traced to the failure of bioethics to be self-critical.[48] This may well be rooted in the need for bioethicists to be accepted in the world of medicine and medical schools. Now that empirical research is demonstrating medicine's differential treatment of patients by race, gender, and insurance status, we have to wonder what critical edge and independence bioethics

---

[44] *See, e.g.*, Marc A. Fajer, *Authority, Credibility, and Pre-Understanding: A Defense of Outsider Narratives in Legal Scholarship*, 82 GEO. L.J. 1845 (1994); *The 200,000 Cards*, *supra* note 14; William N. Eskridge, Jr., *Gaylegal Narratives*, 46 STAN. L. REV. 607 (1994); Richard Delgado, *On Telling Stories in School: A Reply to Farber and Sherry*, 46 VAND. L. REV. 665 (1993); *Telling Stories Out of School*, *supra* note 14; Kathryn Abrams, *Hearing the Call of Stories*, 79 CAL. L. REV. 971 (1991); Symposium, *Legal Storytelling*, 87 MICH. L. REV. 2073 (1989).

[45] I offer an extended discussion in Susan M. Wolf, *Introduction: Gender and Feminism in Bioethics*, *in* FEMINISM & BIOETHICS, *supra* note 9.

[46] *See, e.g.*, Roger B. Dworkin, *Medical Law and Ethics in the Post-Autonomy Age*, 68 IND. L.J. 727 (1993); articles in *Individualism & Community: The Contested Terrain of Autonomy*, HASTINGS CTR. REP., May-June 1994; Marion Danis & Larry R. Churchill, *Autonomy and the Common Weal*, HASTINGS CTR. REP., Jan.-Feb. 1991, at 25; Charles W. Lidz & Robert M. Arnold, *Institutional Constraints on Autonomy*, 14 GENERATIONS 65 (1990); Daniel Callahan, *Autonomy: A Moral Good, Not a Moral Obsession*, HASTINGS CTR. REP., Oct. 1984, at 40.

[47] *See* Susan M. Wolf, *Health Care Reform and the Future of Physician Ethics*, HASTINGS CTR. REP., Mar.-Apr. 1994, at 28, 32 & n.36.

[48] For an exploration of this, see Rebecca Dresser, *What Bioethics Can Learn from the Women's Health Movement*, *in* FEMINISM & BIOETHICS, *supra* note 9.

may have surrendered in striving so hard to be accepted in medical settings. Nor has the field of bioethics come to grips with the fact that bioethicists have been predominantly white, able-bodied, and insured, with few bioethicists explicitly writing from nondominant perspectives.[49]

Given this sociological and analytic history, the reluctance to face the challenges of method and difference should be no surprise. Nor should the ensuing anguish. What may be most surprising is that the challenges are finally being heard.

They are being heard in large part due to three developments: the rise of a robust empirical literature on what actually goes on in the clinic in ethically sensitive domains, the emergence of feminist work, and the development of race-attentive analysis. Each of these merits closer scrutiny.

A. The Rise of Empiricism

Part of the challenge to bioethics method comes from an empirical literature provoking fundamental questions about the agreed wisdom. Though there were relevant empirical studies earlier,[50] beginning in the 1980s there was a growing volume of empirical studies on a range of bioethics topics.[51] These included informed consent, the use of do not resuscitate (DNR) orders, other decisions about forgoing life-sustaining treatment, the use of advance directives, and surrogate decision making for incompetent patients.

Such empirical studies have suggested that the dominant modes of bioethics analysis may bear little relationship to the ethical reasoning actually used in clinical situations. For example, a study of genetic counseling and the ensuing reproductive decisions showed counselees ignoring probabilities and instead taking a binary view ("it either will or will not happen"), imagining scenarios to ask "'Can I cope . . . ?'" and "'trying out the worst.'"[52] Moreover, Nancy Rhoden described obstetricians neither honoring women's refusals of cesareans nor acting on the probability of fetal harm, but instead pursuing a "maximin" strategy of minimizing the chance of a worst-outcome scenario regardless of its actual probability.[53] These sorts of studies suggest that the analytic method bioethics has embraced, most importantly principlism, is at best a means of post hoc rationalization. It is often not an accurate reflection of actual decisional processes in bioethics. Nor is it necessarily a good prescription for how bioethics decisions should be made; it

[49] Exceptions to this include Roberts, *supra* note 41; Adrienne Asch, *Reproductive Technology and Disability*, *in* REPRODUCTIVE LAWS FOR THE 1990s at 69 (Sherrill Cohen & Nadine Taub eds., 1989); and Fred Rosner, *The Traditionalist Jewish Physician and Modern Biomedical Ethical Problems*, 8 J. MED. & PHIL. 225 (1983).

[50] *See, e.g.*, Meisel & Roth, *supra* note 7.

[51] For a discussion of the emergence and content of these studies, see Susan M. Wolf, *Quality Assessment of Ethics in Health Care: The Accountability Revolution*, 20 AM. J. L. & MED. 105, 119-23 (1994); *Empirical Research in Medical Ethics*, *supra* note 36. These studies use a variety of methodologies; by "empirical" I do not mean to exclude observational studies by medical anthropologists and sociologists. An especially large empirical study now under way is described in *Support: Study to Understand Prognoses and Preferences for Outcomes and Risks of Treatments*, 43 J. CLINICAL EPIDEMIOLOGY v (Supp. 1990).

[52] Abby Lippman-Hand & F. Clarke Fraser, *Genetic Counseling: Parents' Responses to Uncertainty*, *in* RISK, COMMUNICATION, AND DECISION MAKING IN GENETIC COUNSELING, PART C OF ANNUAL REVIEW OF BIRTH DEFECTS, 1978, at 325, 332-34 (Charles J. Epstein et al. eds., 1979).

[53] *See* Nancy K. Rhoden, *The Judge in the Delivery Room: The Emergence of Court-Ordered Cesareans*, 74 CAL. L. REV. 1951 (1986).

may be exceedingly rationalist and theory-driven, ignoring the role of emotions and the realities of how bioethical decisions are made.[54]

Moreover, empirical work has begun to show problems with the content of the key values and principles used in bioethics analysis. For example, respect for autonomy has surely been the central value or principle championed. But empirical studies show that a sizeable number of people do not want to make treatment decisions for themselves.[55] Moreover, empirical studies now emerging on different ethnic and racial groups show a diversity of values and approaches to treatment decisions.[56]

Finally, empirical research has challenged the standards developed through the conventional bioethics analysis. Surrogate decision-making for incompetents is an apt example. The conventional wisdom has been that a patient's loss of competence should not extinguish her decisional rights. Rather, a surrogate decision maker should take over, deciding as the patient would.[57] But empirical studies now indicate that surrogate decision makers do little better than chance at replicating the patient's own choice. So the conventional rationale for surrogate decision-making—that the surrogate could stand in the patient's stead and speak for that now incompetent person—seems problematic in the face of this data.

Bioethics' belated engagement with empiricism thus has offered challenges to key dimensions of the old bioethics paradigm. That empiricism has made problematic the dominant analytic method, the values and principles usually applied in the analysis, and the resultant standards.

B. Feminist Work

A burgeoning feminist literature has challenged the reigning bioethics paradigm as well. Early on, feminist literature relevant to bioethics concerned mainly reproductive issues—abortion, reproductive technologies, surrogate motherhood, and the like.[58] More recently, feminist work has taken on the full range of bioeth-

[54] My genetics and obstetrics examples suggest the role of emotions and cognitive strategies in patient and physician decision-making. William James similarly suggests the role of "temperament" in philosophers' theorizing. *See* Thomas C. Grey, *Hear The Other Side: Wallace Stevens and Pragmatist Legal Theory*, 63 S. Cal. L. Rev. 1569, 1588 (1990) ("Almost uniquely among philosophers, James believed that philosophical disputes were the intellectual formulations of temperamental differences . . . ." (footnote omitted)).

[55] *See, e.g.*, Lesley F. Degner & Jeffrey A. Sloan, *Decision Making During Serious Illness: What Role Do Patients Really Want to Play?*, 45 J. Clinical Epidemiology 941 (1992); Jack Ende et al., *Measuring Patients' Desire for Autonomy: Decision Making and Information-Seeking Preferences Among Medical Patients*, 4 J. Gen. Internal Med. 23 (1989); William M. Strull et al., *Do Patients Want to Participate in Medical Decision Making?*, 252 JAMA 2990 (1984). These and other studies are discussed in *With a Human Face*, *supra* note 4, at 1091-104.

[56] *See supra* note 38.

[57] Specifically, the surrogate is supposed to apply a three-tier decisional standard. She should enforce the patient's express wishes, if known; should otherwise extrapolate from what is known of the patient's wishes and values, in an exercise of substituted judgment; and when not enough is known to ground an exercise of substituted judgment, should decide in the patient's best interests. *See, e.g.*, Allen E. Buchanan & Dan W. Brock, Deciding for Others: The Ethics of Surrogate Decision Making 93-134 (1989).

[58] The feminist literature on each of these reproductive topics is large. Indeed, when Hypatia published two special issues in 1989 devoted to feminism and health care ethics, one entire issue was devoted to reproduction. *See Ethics and Reproduction*, Hypatia, Fall 1989; *Feminist Ethics and Medicine*, Hypatia, Summer 1989.

ics issues, not just those that have to do with women's reproductive capacities. Thus we see feminist writing on AIDS, the allocation of health care resources, death and dying, genetics, the patient-physician relationship, and so on.[59]

Two overlapping types of gender-attentive work have offered challenges to mainstream bioethics: work on the treatment of women, and feminist theory. The former is older. There is a long-standing critique of the treatment of women as patients and research subjects in medicine and the biological sciences.[60] That critique is now augmented by data on the exclusion of women from research, inadequate research on women's health problems, and women's lesser access to cardiac and other treatments.[61] These studies of gender have prompted the American Medical Association (AMA) to issue a report and ethical guidelines,[62] the National Institutes of Health (NIH) to create an Office of Research on Women's Health,[63] and other government and quasi-governmental bodies to begin considering questions of gender equity in biomedicine.[64]

All of this offers important challenges to the usual bioethics focus on the genderless generic patient. By showing that gender should not be ignored and indeed may be a pivotal category of analysis, this gender-attentive work suggests that a highly abstract bioethics that ignores context and individuals' characteristics is inadequate. But this gender-attentive challenge ought to be distinguished from the challenges offered by feminist theory in bioethics. The latter challenges may ultimately prove more fundamental and controversial.

Turning then to the application of feminist theory to bioethics, the first question is, of course, which theory. There are a plurality of feminist approaches, as Rosemarie Tong and Alison Jaggar have illuminated.[65] Though some bioethicists now looking at feminist work seem to focus on the ethics of care,[66] a number of feminists working in bioethics have rejected the notion that a feminist bioethics would necessarily embrace an ethics of care. Tong herself contrasts feminine ethics, which she takes to valorize caring, and feminist ethics, which may criticize

---

[59] *See, e.g.*, FEMINISM & BIOETHICS, *supra* note 9; Leslie Bender, *A Feminist Analysis of Physician-Assisted Dying and Voluntary Active Euthanasia*, 59 TENN. L. REV. 519 (1992); Steven Miles & Allison August, *Courts, Gender and "The Right to Die"*, 18 L. MED. & HEALTH CARE 85 (1990).

[60] *See, e.g.*, BARBARA EHRENREICH & DIEDRE ENGLISH, FOR HER OWN GOOD: 150 YEARS OF EXPERTS' ADVICE TO WOMEN (1978).

[61] *See, e.g.*, Leslee J. Shaw et al., *Gender Differences in the Noninvasive Evaluation and Management of Patients with Suspected Coronary Artery Disease*, 120 ANNALS INTERNAL MED. 559 (1994); Anthony Orencia et al., *Effect of Gender on Long-Term Outcome of Angina Pectoris and Myocardial Infarction/Sudden Unexpected Death*, 269 JAMA 2392 (1993). *See generally* Council on Ethical and Judicial Affairs, *Gender Disparities in Clinical Decision Making*, 266 JAMA 559 (1991), and studies cited therein. *But see* Anita M. Arnold et al., *Gender Differences for Coronary Angioplasty*, 74 AM. J. CARDIOLOGY 18 (1994) (showing some gender differences that favor women); Daniel B. Mark et al., *Absence of Sex Bias in the Referral of Patients for Cardiac Catheterization*, 330 NEW ENG. J. MED. 1101 (1994).

[62] *See* Council on Ethical and Judicial Affairs, *supra* note 61.

[63] *See* Vivian W. Pinn, *Women's Health Research: Prescribing Change and Addressing the Issues*, 268 JAMA 1921 (1992).

[64] *See, e.g.*, FUNDING HEALTH SCIENCES RESEARCH: A STRATEGY TO RESTORE BALANCE (Floyd E. Bloom & Mark A. Randolph eds., 1990) (Institute of Medicine report).

[65] *See* ROSEMARIE TONG, FEMINIST THOUGHT: A COMPREHENSIVE INTRODUCTION 1 (1989) (distinguishing liberal, Marxist, radical, psychoanalytic, socialist, existentialist, and postmodern approaches to feminist work); ALISON M. JAGGAR, FEMINIST POLITICS AND HUMAN NATURE 8-13 (1983) (discussing liberal feminism, traditional Marxism, radical feminism, and socialist feminism).

[66] *See, e.g.*, BEAUCHAMP & CHILDRESS, *supra* note 4, at 85-92.

the association of caring traits with female gender as being a function of the historical subordination of women and our concomitant need to demonstrate caring toward those in greater power.[67] Susan Sherwin explicitly rejects the notion that a feminist bioethics would necessarily be an ethics of care at all.[68]

Indeed, there is a much richer variety of feminist approaches relevant to bioethics than simply an ethics of care. For example, Lawrence Blum explicates eight different ways in which an ethics of justice and an ethics of care might interrelate in forming an overall ethical approach.[69] Sandra Harding, Nancy Hartsock, and others elaborate feminist standpoint theory, borne of the notion that those who have experienced oppression have an especially important perspective on societal arrangements and wrongs;[70] Mary Mahowald investigates the application of this to bioethics.[71] Seyla Benhabib's turn on Jürgen Habermas's communicative ethics, with Benhabib's urging to analyze ethical problems with reference to concrete rather than generalized others, has implications for bioethics that Janet Farrell Smith explores.[72]

Out of the rich array of feminist approaches now being developed, we see three basic claims emerge. The first is that sexism in medicine and science *is* an ethical problem. This means that the workings of gender are not only appropriate but also inescapable problems for bioethicists to engage. The second claim is that bioethical analysis requires attention to power in biomedical settings: who has it, how it works, and how to fix the current inequities. The third claim is that analysis of power and morality cannot proceed without careful attention to context and difference. Thus we must ask how does the problem at hand manifest differently for a woman, for a Latina, for a Latina who is without health insurance, and for this particular Latina by her own account. As Susan Sherwin argues, feminist analysis must pay attention to more than gender—to race, ethnicity, and resources.[73] There is no such thing as a woman without race or ethnicity and without resource limitations (or strengths). As Elizabeth Spelman warns, we must avoid the trap of essentialism, the trap of thinking that all women experience the same thing, as if race, resources, and other factors have no impact.[74]

C. Race-Attentive Work

As new as gender analysis is in bioethics, attention to race and ethnicity is even newer. Two important collections of essays were published in 1992 and 1994,

---

[67] *See* Rosemarie Tong, Feminine and Feminist Ethics (1993).

[68] *See* Sherwin, *supra* note 9, at 42-57. *See also* Nelson, *supra* note 34. *But see* Caring, *supra* note 34.

[69] *See* Lawrence A. Blum, *supra* note 34.

[70] *See* Sandra Harding, Whose Science? Whose Knowledge? Thinking from Women's Lives 119-33 (1991); Nancy C. M. Hartsock, *The Feminist Standpoint: Developing the Ground for a Specifically Feminist Historical Materialism*, *in* Feminism and Methodology: Social Science Issues 157 (Sandra Harding ed., 1987). *See also* Martha Minow & Elizabeth V. Spelman, *In Context*, 63 S. Cal. L. Rev. 1597 (1990).

[71] *See* Mary B. Mahowald, *On Treatment of Myopia: Feminism, Standpoint Theory, and Bioethics*, *in* Feminism & Bioethics, *supra* note 9.

[72] *See* Janet Farrell Smith, *Communicative Ethics in the Physician-Patient Relationship*, *in* Feminism & Bioethics, *supra* note 9.

[73] Sherwin, *supra* note 9, at 10, 222-40.

[74] Elizabeth V. Spelman, Inessential Woman: Problems of Exclusion in Feminist Thought (1988).

both focusing on African American health problems and perspectives.[75] These are catalyzing dialogue, as witnessed by Anita Allen's critique of the first collection.[76] She mixes praise for the volume with the complaint that it includes little data on African American views and on differences among African Americans. She also remarks that the book seems to be a colloquy among black and white academics for consumption by other academics.

In the essay that Allen finds the intellectual linchpin of the book, Jorge Garcia grapples with the question of what it might mean to develop an African American bioethics.[77] To analyze that, he distinguishes three clusters of questions. First, what does it mean for an ethical position to involve an ethnic perspective? Is this just relativism? And does it make sense to associate someone's ethical perspective with race, when identity is affected by multiple factors?[78]

Second, Garcia asks what the content of an African American perspective might be. In deriving an answer, he explores how racial stereotypes can be avoided, and what the relevance of African American history and experiences should be.

Finally, he asks how an African American perspective should be used. Should it be used to create a uniquely African American ethics, or be adopted by society at large? Should it valorize all done by African Americans, or establish community limits on acceptable actions? And should it be used primarily to emphasize past suffering by African Americans in the name of medicine and science,[79] or to cast African Americans as effective agents in the world wielding real power?

While Garcia explores what it would mean to develop an African American bioethics, others pursuing race-attentive work have advanced different projects. One project is to document and analyze differences in health care by race and ethnicity. There is now an outpouring of this empirical literature,[80] prompting the AMA to issue a report urging the abolition of racial bias in medicine.[81] Another project is to investigate whether there are different perspectives associated with race and ethnicity when people consider bioethical problems. Thus a group of

---

[75] *See* AFRICAN-AMERICAN PERSPECTIVES, *supra* note 9; "IT JUST AIN'T FAIR," *supra* note 9.

[76] Anita L. Allen, *Book Review of African-American Perspectives on Biomedical Ethics*, 104 ETHICS 404 (1994).

[77] *See* Jorge L. A. Garcia, *African-American Perspectives, Cultural Relativism, and Normative Issues: Some Conceptual Questions*, *in* AFRICAN-AMERICAN PERSPECTIVES, *supra* note 9, at 11.

[78] On the effect of multiple factors and what she calls "intersectionality," see Kimberlé Crenshaw, *Demarginalizing the Intersection of Race and Sex: A Black Feminist Critique of Antidiscrimination Doctrine, Feminist Theory and Antiracist Politics*, 1989 U. CHI. LEGAL F. 139 (1989).

[79] Dorothy Roberts justifiably argues that only some of that suffering—primarily the Tuskegee Syphilis study—has been acknowledged thus far by bioethicists. Roberts, *supra* note 41. On the horrors of medical treatment and experimentation on African Americans in the time of slavery, see, for example, Todd L. Savitt, *The Use of Blacks for Medical Experimentation and Demonstration in the Old South*, 48 J. S. HIST. 331 (1982); TODD L. SAVITT, MEDICINE AND SLAVERY: THE DISEASES AND HEALTH CARE OF BLACKS IN ANTEBELLUM VIRGINIA (1978). For further historical analysis, see also Vanessa Northington Gamble, *A Legacy of Distrust: African Americans and Medical Research*, 9 AM. J. PREVENTIVE MED. 35 (1993); Vernellia R. Randall, *Racist Health Care: Reforming an Unjust Health Care System to Meet the Needs of African-Americans*, 3 HEALTH MATRIX 127, 146-48 (1993). On Tuskegee, see, for example, JAMES H. JONES, BAD BLOOD: THE TUSKEGEE SYPHILIS EXPERIMENT (1981).

[80] *See, e.g.*, John Z. Ayanian et al., *Racial Differences in the Use of Revascularization Procedures After Coronary Angiography*, 269 JAMA 2642 (1993); Jeff Whittle et al., *Racial Differences in the Use of Invasive Cardiovascular Procedures in the Department of Veterans Affairs Medical System*, 329 NEW ENG. J. MED. 621 (1993). *See generally* Council on Ethical and Judicial Affairs, *Black-White Disparities in Health Care*, 263 JAMA 2344 (1990), and studies cited therein.

[81] *See* Council on Ethical and Judicial Affairs, *supra* note 80.

researchers at Johns Hopkins and Georgetown Universities, for example, is investigating the reproductive decisions of women infected with the HIV virus many of whom are from racial and ethnic minority groups.[82] Another group at the University of Southern California is studying end-of-life decisions, looking for different perspectives associated with race and ethnicity.[83] Both of these projects are distinct from Garcia's project of conceiving an African American bioethics. After all, one could analyze empirical disparities by race using the Beauchamp and Childress model of bioethics, condemning racism in medicine as a violation of their principle of justice. One could also stick with such a model while acknowledging that different people and even different groups may exercise their autonomy by adhering to different values.

But there is yet another race-attentive project of fundamental importance: critiquing the currently dominant models of bioethics from the standpoint of those people arguably most harmed by the health care system—people of color. This is Dorothy Roberts's project in an essay that focuses on the experiences of women of color.[84] Roberts looks at the dominant model of bioethics and finds it wanting, a set of principles (such as respect for patients' autonomous decisions and for patient confidentiality) that may apply when the patient is white and privately insured, but not when the patient is a poor woman of color receiving health care in a public setting. Roberts's project is not to make marginal revisions in the current model of bioethics, or to supplement it with an African American perspective. It is to dismantle the current model of bioethics and reconstitute it. Roberts's work suggests the depth of the challenges we are starting to see to the old bioethics paradigm.

II. THE SHIFT IN HEALTH LAW

The paradigm shift in health law is subtler and less obvious. There is no single statement of the old paradigm in health law comparable to Beauchamp and Childress's *Principles*, a book that became the dominant statement of bioethics' approach. Nor is there a unified methodology debate now in health law comparable to the bioethics debate about whether to dethrone principlism and what to embrace instead. Moreover, as I noted above, health law has been less given to philosophical abstraction and more prone to empiricism, at least in some areas.[85] Consequently, while I analyzed above the shift under way in bioethics, here I have to argue that there is any discernible shift at all.

The shift is to be found in a much increased tendency to evaluate health law less in terms of doctrinal elegance and the coherence of middle-level rules, and more in terms of its good, bad, or negligible effects in clinical settings. Accepted doctrinal approaches to surrogate decision-making and the use of advance direc-

[82] *See* Nancy E. Kass, *Reproductive Decision Making in the Context of HIV: The Case for Nondirective Counseling*, *in* AIDS, WOMEN AND THE NEXT GENERATION: TOWARDS A MORALLY ACCEPTABLE PUBLIC POLICY FOR HIV TESTING OF PREGNANT WOMEN AND NEWBORNS 308 (Ruth R. Faden et al. eds., 1991).

[83] *See supra* note 38.

[84] *See* Roberts, *supra* note 41. As Roberts' title suggests, she abjures the common strategy of developing an analysis of medicine's mistreatment of women and then as a near afterthought extending the analysis to women of color or people of color. Instead, her starting point is the experiences of women of color, a perspectival shift of tremendous consequence, she argues.

[85] *See supra* note 6 and accompanying text.

tives, for example, are now undergoing fundamental challenge in light of empirical data on each. The middle-level rules our courts and legislatures developed casting surrogates as agents enunciating the views of incapacitated patients and advance treatment directives as a way to extend patient autonomy past loss of decisional capacity, are unsettled by discovering that surrogates do little better than chance in replicating patients' views[86] and that the few people who use directives vary in how strictly they wish them construed.[87] In other words, the rise of empiricism and challenge to deductivism in bioethics is mirrored by an intensified empirical investigation of health law's effects. It is also mirrored by an intensified conviction that good health law will be developed out of intimate knowledge of how health care settings work, and how law effects different actors in those settings. Sound health law will be cultivated from the ground up.

A number of studies demonstrate the newly intensified empiricism and indicate that there may be fundamental problems with accepted legal doctrines and mechanisms. Advance directives have provoked a substantial amount of empirical study, especially since Congressional enactment of the Patient Self-Determination Act (PSDA) requiring all health care facilities that accept Medicaid and Medicare reimbursement to inquire routinely whether patients have directives and to honor those directives.[88] Indeed, all states now formally recognize at least some kinds of directives for health care, by statute, judicial decision, or both.[89] And directives have been one of the great hopes for solving the problems that surround end-of-life decision-making: if people would only specify what treatment they want later after loss of decisional capacity, or would only designate a proxy decision maker to take over for them, we could confidently rely on those choices as an exercise of patient self-determination.

Yet there are serious problems in the clinic. The great majority of patients do not execute directives, in part it seems because their physicians are reluctant to broach the topic.[90] Even when patients do execute directives, it is unclear how the documents should be construed; one study suggests that only thirty-nine percent wish them construed strictly.[91] In any case, another study suggests that one-quarter of directives are ignored or overridden in the clinic, sometimes to provide more treatment than specified in the document, and sometimes to provide less.[92]

As discussed above, surrogate decision-making is another area in which previously settled legal and ethical standards are now under fire due to empirical investigation.[93] If surrogates do little better than chance in replicating patients' choices[94]

[86] On surrogates research, see *infra* notes 93-94 and accompanying text.

[87] On directives research, see *infra* notes 88-92 and accompanying text.

[88] *See, e.g.*, Joan M. Teno et al., *The Impact of the Patient Self-Determination Act's Requirement that States Describe Law Concerning Patients' Rights*, 21 J. L. MED. & ETHICS 102 (1993); Joanne Lynn & Joan M. Teno, *After the Patient Self-Determination Act: The Need for Empirical Research on Formal Advance Directives*, HASTINGS CTR. REP., Jan.-Feb. 1993, at 20. On the PSDA generally, see Susan M. Wolf et al., *Sources of Concern About the Patient Self-Determination Act*, 325 NEW ENG. J. MED. 1666 (1991).

[89] *See* ALAN MEISEL, THE RIGHT TO DIE § 10.7 (1989 & Supp. 1993).

[90] *See* Wolf et al., *supra* note 88, at 1666-67 and studies cited therein.

[91] *See* Ashwini Sehgal et al., *How Strictly Do Dialysis Patients Want Their Advance Directives Followed?*, 267 JAMA 59 (1992).

[92] *See* Marion Danis et al., *A Prospective Study of Advance Directives for Life-Sustaining Care*, 324 NEW ENG. J. MED. 882, 884-85 (1991).

[93] *See supra* page 404 .

[94] *See* Allison B. Seckler et al., *Substituted Judgment: How Accurate Are Proxy Predictions?*,

then it is hard to maintain that the surrogate is acting as the patient's agent and choosing as the patient probably would.

There are still other studies showing how law can precipitate problems in the clinic. A Texas study of physicians' attitudes and knowledge about the law and their reported practices shows that most of the physicians surveyed hold inaccurate beliefs, making them reluctant to honor refusals of life-sustaining treatment.[95]

As noted above, this burgeoning empiricism in health law is not without earlier precedents. Among the most important is work from the University of Pittsburgh published in the 1980s examining how informed consent took place in a psychiatric hospital.[96] That study showed serious problems with the informed consent process. The skepticism that study provoked about the process echoes such earlier writings as Jay Katz's *Informed Consent—A Fairy Tale?*[97]

Yet what is new and, I am claiming, a paradigm shift is a deepened skepticism about all sorts of health law, and the demand that health law be evaluated empirically to see how it works or does not work in the clinic.[98] We see health law now as a process only one part of which is middle-level rules and nicely drafted documents, statutes, and judicial decisions. That part is health law on paper. But all of that paper will be perceived, misperceived, or ignored by actors in health care settings. Further pressures will be brought to bear on how legal dictates and documents are understood. At the end of this long Rube Goldberg–like process will be a patient in a bed whose care will be influenced (or whose care will fail to be influenced) by the written law.[99] Health law as a field is now more interested than ever in this entire process, the entire Rube Goldberg machine. The bottom line is not pretty documents or elegant opinions, but what happens to the patient in the bed. What we are learning now about what happens to that patient is destabilizing established legal approaches. That is the paradigm shift.

As in the case of the bioethics paradigm shift, here too the rise of the new

---

115 ANNALS INTERNAL MED. 92 (1991); Tom Tomlinson et al., *An Empirical Study of Proxy Consent for Elderly Persons*, 30 GERONTOLOGIST 54 (1990); Nancy R. Zweibel, *Treatment Choices at the End of Life: A Comparison of Decisions by Older Patients and Their Physician-Selected Proxies*, 29 GERONTOLOGIST 615 (1989); Joseph G. Ouslander et al., *Health Care Decisions Among Elderly Long-Term Care Residents and Their Potential Proxies*, 149 ARCHIVES INTERNAL MED. 1367 (1989); Richard F. Uhlmann et al., *Physicians' and Spouses' Predictions of Elderly Patients' Resuscitation Preferences*, 43 J. GERONTOLOGY M115 (1988).

[95] S. Van McCrary et al., *Treatment Decisions for Terminally Ill Patients: Physicians' Legal Defensiveness and Knowledge of Medical Law*, 20 L. MED. & HEALTH CARE 364 (1992). For additional analysis of physicians' perceptions of law see, for example, Henry S. Perkins et al., *Impact of Legal Liability, Family Wishes, and Other "External Factors" on Physicians' Life-Support Decisions*, 89 AM. J. MED. 185 (1990); Marshall B. Kapp & Bernard Lo, *Legal Perceptions and Medical Decision Making*, 64 MILBANK Q. (Supp. 2) 163 (1986). There is a significant literature on physicians practicing "defensive medicine" to minimize perceived legal exposure. *See, e.g.*, Barry M. Manuel, *Professional Liability: A No-Fault Solution*, 322 NEW ENG. J. MED. 627 (1990).

[96] *See* CHARLES W. LIDZ ET AL., INFORMED CONSENT: A STUDY OF DECISIONMAKING IN PSYCHIATRY (1984). *See also* PAUL S. APPELBAUM ET AL., INFORMED CONSENT: LEGAL THEORY AND CLINICAL PRACTICE (1987); Meisel & Roth, *supra* note 7. An important recent contribution on informed consent is Peter H. Schuck, *Rethinking Informed Consent*, 103 YALE L.J. 899 (1994). *See also* Marjorie Maguire Shultz, *From Informed Consent to Patient Choice: A New Protected Interest*, 95 YALE L.J. 219 (1985).

[97] Jay Katz, *Informed Consent—A Fairy Tale? Law's Vision*, 39 U. PITT. L. REV. 137 (1977).

[98] That deepened skepticism is apparent even in the informed consent area. *See, e.g.*, *With a Human Face*, *supra* note 4.

[99] The Rube Goldberg analogy risks making the process sound linear, but that process may, of course, be full of loops and feedback.

empiricism is bolstered by concern that we know too little about differences of gender, race, and insurance status. Many of the patient's rights that have been victoriously secured by health law innovations over the last couple of decades may work best for insured nonminority individuals. Indeed, Dorothy Roberts argues that the legal requirements of informed consent and patient confidentiality erode significantly when the patient is a poor woman of color receiving her care in a public clinic or facility.[100] Similarly, some researchers examining the use of advance directives have found African American and Hispanic individuals less likely to complete them,[101] suggesting that this legal innovation too may not work as well for members of certain racial and ethnic groups. In addition, the outpouring of data showing poorer health status and lesser access to health care among African Americans has provoked proposals for legal reform.[102]

This suggests that empirical evaluation of how health law works or fails in the clinic must pay attention to differences of gender, race, and insurance status. Indeed, because those crafting law—lawyers, judges, and legislators—will most typically be insured and from majority racial and ethnic groups, their own experience and introspection will be a systematically flawed basis for forming and evaluating health law.[103] Empirical work to surface the experience of others will be essential.

As in the case of the bioethics paradigm shift, the health law shift is guaranteed to provoke anxiety. When previously accepted rules and mechanisms seem not to work well in the clinic, perhaps particularly for some more vulnerable patients, it is not clear whether to abandon those rules and mechanisms or to cleave to them and simply work harder to make them function in the clinic. This is no idle concern: there are renewed challenges now to the very notion of patients' rights in the face of clinical realities.[104] This is the advantage of turning to pragmatism to understand what is going on in bioethics and health law. The pragmatism debates can show how to salvage a progressive vision of clinical change, and how to rescue patients' rights.

III. THE NEW PRAGMATISM

The turn toward empiricism, rejection of theoretical elegance as the measure of good bioethics and health law, and insistence instead on evaluating what meets the needs of individuals in clinical settings is a diagnostically pragmatist move. Pragmatism, the one distinctively American philosophy,[105] is associated with the work of Charles Sanders Peirce,[106] William James,[107] and John Dewey.[108] "For

[100] *See* Roberts, *supra* note 41.

[101] *See, e.g.*, Rubin et al., *supra* note 39.

[102] *See, e.g.*, Randall, *supra* note 79.

[103] *Cf.* Miles & August, *supra* note 59, at 91 (finding gender bias among judges construing evidence of women's treatment preferences).

[104] *See, e.g.*, *Language of the Law*, *supra* note 2; *With a Human Face*, *supra* note 4. Challenges to patients' rights have been frequent in the history of bioethics, though less so in health law. *See, e.g.*, John Ladd, *Legalism and Medical Ethics*, *in* CONTEMPORARY ISSUES IN BIOMEDICAL ETHICS 1 (John W. Davis et al. eds., 1978).

[105] *See* WEST, *supra* note 12, at 182 ("American pragmatism is widely regarded as *the* distinctive American philosophy . . . .").

[106] *See, e.g.*, PHILOSOPHICAL WRITINGS OF PEIRCE (J. Buchler ed., 1955).

[107] *See, e.g.*, WILLIAM JAMES, PRAGMATISM (1975).

[108] *See, e.g.*, JOHN DEWEY, ART AS EXPERIENCE (1934); JOHN DEWEY, EXPERIENCE AND NATURE (1925).

them, philosophy should be committed to examining the consequences and practical effects of conceptions when exploring truth, meaning, and action."[109] "The heart of pragmatist thought is the view that the ultimate test is always experience."[110]

Cornel West and others credit Richard Rorty with championing a pragmatist revival starting in the 1960s but gathering steam in the 1970s and 1980s.[111] Among legal scholars Rorty has succeeded. Minow and Spelman enumerate several examples of Rorty's influence in the work of Thomas Grey, Joseph Singer, and Spelman herself.[112] Others have also embraced pragmatism in recent times.[113] Probably the surest indication of pragmatism's revival is highly visible debate about its merits.[114]

Oddly, there has been no comparable discussion of pragmatism in bioethics. The Beauchamp and Childress text lacks even an index heading for pragmatism.[115] Very few articles use the term.[116]

Yet pragmatism seems the right rubric under which to group a host of the new trends in bioethics as well as health law. This is not to erase the variety in what is emerging; even those scholars writing on pragmatism acknowledge a plurality of pragmatisms with important distinctions among them.[117] But the exhortations now being heard in the interlocked fields of bioethics and health law—to return to the clinic, to investigate empirically what is going on there as a basis for devising interventions, to evaluate legal and ethical innovations in terms of their actual effects on patients and others, and to be skeptical of abstract approaches devised far from the patient's bedside—seem to be part of the neopragmatist revival.

The great advantage of regarding them as such is the immediate applicability of recent debates about pragmatism. To situate our bioethics and health law developments in the broader pragmatist revival may save us from having to reinvent the wheel, introduce important cautions, and throw our own debates into new relief. In turn, it may make developments in our domain useful to others outside bioethics and health law who are already debating pragmatism.[118]

---

[109] Minow & Spelman, *supra* note 70, at 1610.

[110] Farber, *supra* note 12, at 1341 (citation omitted).

[111] *See* WEST, *supra* note 12, at 3, 196-97; Minow & Spelman, *supra* note 70, at 1610-11.

[112] Minow & Spelman, *supra* note 70, at 1611 n.52.

[113] *See, e.g.*, Margaret Jane Radin, *The Pragmatist and the Feminist*, 63 S. CAL. L. REV. 1699 (1990); Farber, *supra* note 12.

[114] See, for example, *Symposium on the Renaissance of Pragmatism in American Legal Thought*, *supra* note 12, and criticism of pragmatism by Judge Richard A. Posner in that symposium and Ronald Dworkin in LAW'S EMPIRE (1986).

[115] *See* BEAUCHAMP & CHILDRESS, *supra* note 4, at 541. Nor does their chapter on "Types of Ethical Theory," where they canvass a wide array of alternatives, some inductivist, include pragmatism. *Id.* at 44-119. The closest they come there is in explaining that casuistry "focuses on practical decisionmaking in particular cases." *Id.* at 92.

[116] One that does is Williams, *supra* note 12, at 1021. *See also* William J. Winslade, *Ethics Consultation: Cases in Context*, 57 ALB. L. REV. 679, 683 (1994) (acknowledging his study of pragmatism); Leonard M. Fleck, *Just Health Care Rationing: A Democratic Decisionmaking Approach*, 140 U. PA. L. REV. 1597, 1600 (1992); Sharron Dalton, *What Are the Sources and Standards of Ethical Judgment in Dietetics?*, 91 J. AM. DIETETIC ASS'N 545 (1991). Jonsen and Toulmin include a discussion of pragmatism in THE ABUSE OF CASUISTRY, *supra* note 9, at 281-83. Mary Briody Mahowald does as well in WOMEN AND CHILDREN IN HEALTH CARE: AN UNEQUAL MAJORITY 264-65 (1993).

[117] *See, e.g.*, WEST, *supra* note 12; Radin, *supra* note 113, at 1705.

[118] Some of those already debating pragmatism have actually ventured into bioethics and health law domains. *See, e.g.*, MARTHA MINOW, MAKING ALL THE DIFFERENCE: INCLUSION, EXCLUSION, AND AMERICAN

If the shift in bioethics and health law paradigms is indeed part of a new pragmatism, three lessons from the pragmatism literature are important. First, a central debate about pragmatism, and certainly the recent pragmatism revival, has been whether its emphasis on real world experience and consequences indicates that it is anti-theory.[119] This echoes the methodology debate in bioethics, where some defend the continuing need for some kind of higher-order theory or at least principles even as they endorse greater attention to particulars and the individual case.[120]

Even adherents of pragmatism have acknowledged that there is danger in theory-less attention to particulars. It risks what has been called "complacent pragmatism."[121] This is pragmatism that becomes mired in understanding what is, at the expense of being able to formulate a vision of what ought to be.

Clearly this is a danger both bioethics and health law court in embracing empiricism and inductivism. Both fields need an additional orienting notion to shape the questions asked in investigating what is, the evaluation of what is discovered, and prescriptions for change. Here it is salutary to heed Martha Minow and Elizabeth Spelman in their analysis of pragmatism's demand for careful attention to context: "the call to context reflects a critical argument . . . that prevailing legal and political norms have used the form of abstract, general, and universal prescriptions while neglecting the experiences and needs of women of all races and classes, people of color, and people without wealth."[122] Similarly, Cornel West advocates a "prophetic pragmatism" that would "give prominence to the plight of those people who embody and enact the 'postmodern' themes of degraded otherness, subjected alienness, and subaltern marginality, that is, the wretched of the earth . . . ."[123] In other words, pragmatist empiricism, far from being the enemy of progressive change, is motivated by the realization that the needs of those historically most vulnerable and wronged must be brought to the fore to take priority.

Not all empiricism and inductivism in bioethics and health law seems borne of this vision. Careful attention to the experiences of physicians uncomfortable with patients' and surrogates' affirmative demands for treatment, for example, could ground prescriptions for resolving the current futility debate that would only exacerbate historical wrongs done to patients.[124] Linking the bioethics and health

---

LAW 312-49 (1990) (on forgoing life-sustaining treatment); Margaret Jane Radin, *Market-Inalienability*, 100 HARV. L. REV. 1849 (1987) (discussing *inter alia* surrogate motherhood and blood donation).

[119] *See* Cornel West, *The Limits of Neopragmatism*, 63 S. CAL. L. REV. 1747, 1748 (1990); Singer, *supra* note 15, at 1823-26.

[120] *See* Jonsen, *supra* note 9; Arras, *supra* note 9.

[121] *See, e.g.*, Radin, *supra* note 113, at 1708-09 n.26, 1720-22. Radin further quotes William James: "One misunderstanding of pragmatism is . . . that it loves intellectual anarchy as such and prefers a sort of wolf-world absolutely unpent and wild and without a master or a collar to any philosophical class-room product, whatsoever." *Id.* at 1715 (quoting WILLIAM JAMES, PRAGMATISM 128 (1975)).

[122] Minow & Spelman, *supra* note 70, at 1632-33.

[123] WEST, *supra* note 12, at 237.

[124] On the futility debate, see, for example, Robert D. Truog et al., *The Problem with Futility*, 326 NEW ENG. J. MED. 1560 (1992); Daniel Callahan, *Medical Futility, Medical Necessity: The-Problem-Without-A-Name*, HASTINGS CTR. REP., July-Aug. 1991, at 30; Lawrence J. Schneiderman et al., *Medical Futility: Its Meaning and Ethical Implications*, 112 ANNALS INTERNAL MED. 949 (1990); John D. Lantos et al., *The Illusion of Futility in Clinical Practice*, 87 AM. J. MED. 81 (1989); Susan M. Wolf, *Conflict Between Doctor and Patient*, 16 LAW MED. & HEALTH CARE 197 (1988); Stuart J. Youngner, *Who Defines Futility?*, 260 JAMA 2094 (1988).

law shifts to pragmatism thus reveals that current ferment in these fields should be about more than the merits of empiricism or questions of methodology per se; it should be about the vision we ought to pursue and whether that vision is ultimately progressive.

A second relevant debate about pragmatism is whether it is incompatible with a strong concept of rights.[125] Ronald Dworkin claims that pragmatism gives judges and others license to ignore or override rights and the documents from which they spring in our culture, preeminently the Constitution.[126] Rights become merely instrumental means to some other end.

This too is an important caution for bioethics and health law—the ascendancy of empiricism and inductivism may suggest that all features of a situation under study, including the rights involved, are equally malleable and should be regarded in equally instrumental terms. That would be a large step backward for bioethics and health law. The most progressive aspirations of each have often been framed as work to secure moral and legal rights for those people historically without them—patients and research subjects.

Moreover, as Daniel Farber argues, viewing rights in instrumental terms would be a misunderstanding and misuse of pragmatism. "[L]iving in a society that does recognize the existence of legal rights, the American pragmatist need not view those rights as purely instrumental means of acquiring other goods. . . . [P]ragmatism is consistent with a true commitment to rights . . . ."[127] At the same time, pragmatism highlights a significant feature of rights: that merely proclaiming or even legislating them does not make rights real for those who need them. Thus, pragmatism will urge bioethics and health law to undertake study and work in clinical settings to see how pronounced rights can be made to function for patients and research subjects.

Finally, pragmatism's emphasis on the importance of dialogue as a means of understanding the real world and the needs to be met[128] has implications for bioethics and health law. It suggests that both fields, in scrutinizing specific problems, must always ask whether the views of those people who have most at risk are being heard. Thus I have advocated the need for "patient-centered process" in the workings of hospital ethics committees and more broadly, to ensure that patients themselves are heard when their cases are considered.[129] Similarly, a potent criticism of Oregon's proposed plan for health care rationing was that it focused on children receiving Medicaid, those people least likely to wield political clout and so be able to protest and discipline the program.[130]

---

[125] *See* Farber, *supra* note 12, at 1343-48.

[126] *See* DWORKIN, *supra* note 114, at 95, 151, 378.

[127] Farber, *supra* note 12, at 1347-48.

[128] *See, e.g.*, Steven D. Smith, *The Pursuit of Pragmatism*, 100 YALE L.J. 409, 434 (1990) ("[p]ragmatists . . . stress the importance of 'dialogue' in evaluating experience and in constructing and criticizing theories" (footnote omitted)).

[129] *See* Susan M. Wolf, *Toward a Theory of Process*, 20 LAW MED. & HEALTH CARE 278 (1992); Susan M. Wolf, *Ethics Committees and Due Process: Nesting Rights in a Community of Caring*, 50 MD. L. REV. 798 (1991).

[130] *See* Arthur Caplan, *Rationing Medicaid Would Hurt Kids Most*, ST. PAUL PIONEER PRESS, Sept. 9, 1990, at G3; Arthur Caplan, *The Unkindest Cut Goes to the Kids*, ST. PAUL PIONEER PRESS, Oct. 23, 1989, at 1E.

IV. CONCLUSION

Neither the paradigm shift in bioethics nor the one in health law is secure. Both are controversial and embattled. That should be no surprise. As Jay Healey taught, both fields are about the struggle between patients and physicians, and increasingly insurers, health plans, and governmental authorities. These are struggles over power, enormous amounts of money, and, finally, the lives and health of individuals.

Bioethics and health law are at a crossroads. I am arguing that it is worth fighting about which way they turn. After all, these fields are supposed to be a way to deliberate about the future of health care and health care reform, biomedical science, genetics, disability, reproduction, death—matters of great moment.

We can continue in both fields down the well trod road of conversations among experts, governed by top-down theory and the elegance of abstract pronouncements, largely inattentive to differences of race, ethnicity, gender, and insurance status. Or we can head down a different path, one more winding and complex. This is a path shaped by the twists and turns of empiricist investigation, with detailed attention to context. It will be wide enough to accommodate multiple proposals and critiques as to method, with full attention to feminist, race-attentive, and other contributions. It will be teeming with people, the patients and research subjects whose fates are most at stake in clinical settings.

Following a path marked by the early pragmatists, emboldened by the progressive vision of neopragmatists such as Cornel West, bioethics and health law can now head out over truly new ground.

[2]

The Empire of Death: How Culture and Economics Affect Informed Consent in the U.S., the U.K., and Japan

George J. Annas[†] and Frances H. Miller[‡]

I. INTRODUCTION

American culture reflects a paradox: the more openly we discuss death and its inevitability, the more money we spend to postpone and deny it. Sherwin Nuland's book *How We Die*,[1] a frank description of the way our bodies deteriorate with and without medical intervention, topped the *New York Times* best seller list in the spring of 1994. At the same time, Jack Kevorkian, arguably the world's best known physician, was being acquitted of violating Michigan's law against assisted suicide, while a Michigan commission was debating legislative changes to permit physicians to help their terminally ill patients kill themselves. Despite such open discussion of death and expansion of the informed consent doctrine, U.S. medical expenditures at the end of life remain astronomically high.[2] Most of this elevated spending is attributable to new medical technology.

In J.G. Ballard's *Empire of the Sun*,[3] the United States, British and Japanese cultures are contrasted through the eyes of a young British boy incarcerated by the Japanese army in China during World War II. Ballard describes "the emergence of a particularly American world out of the failures of two traditionally dominant forms of social authority."[4] British society was organized according to rigid social class structure and Japanese society was based on the cult of the emperor, but as the war progressed, Japan and the United Kingdom found their traditional power relationships undermined. On the other hand, the more egalitarian United States attained world dominance through the use of death-producing atomic technology. The British boy learned not only that power is arbitrary, but also that his survival required "absolute submission to the conditions of power."[5]

---

† J.D., M.P.H., Edward R. Utley Professor of Health Law, Boston University Schools of Law, Medicine, and Public Health; Director, Law, Medicine & Ethics Program, Boston University.

‡ J.D., Professor of Law, Boston University School of Law and Professor of Public Health, Boston University School of Public Health.

Troyen Brennan, Peter Davis, Leonard Glantz, Dean Hashimoto, David Hughes, Wendy Mariner, Naoko Miyaji, and the members of the University of Texas and Boston University Law Schools' faculty colloquia made valuable comments on earlier drafts.

1 SHERWIN NULAND, HOW WE DIE (1993).

2 *See generally* A.A. Scitovsky, *"The High Cost of Dying" Revisited*, 72 MILBANK Q. 561 (1994); A.A. Scitovsky, *The High Cost of Dying: What do the Data Show?*, 62 MILBANK Q. 591 (1984).

3 J.G. BALLARD, EMPIRE OF THE SUN (1984).

4 Dennis A. Foster, *J.G. Ballard's Empire of the Senses: Perversion and the Failure of Authority*, 108 PUBLICATIONS MOD. LANGUAGE ASS'N AM. 519, 527 (1993).

5 *Id.* at 528.

Death and technology still remain linked in all three cultures, but this link now appears more evident in medicine than in the military where it was historically central. Medicine has even adopted military metaphors as its own. Physicians speak of fighting invaders with a massive armamentarium, of giving orders, and of practicing medicine on the front lines.[6] The U.S.'s Human Genome Project now splits the gene to forge links to life, much as science once split the atom and forged links to death.

The United States now concentrates its research efforts on this death-defying technology rather than on the death-producing technology that drove so much of our economy during the Cold War era. The United Kingdom and Japan, by way of contrast, use death-defying technology much less frequently. In the British and Japanese cultures, people seem to fear end of life less, yet the idea of death is hidden from public discourse. Preoccupation with the manner of death and with the use of ever-improving medical technology to postpone death is not apparent. In part as a consequence, their health care costs are less than half of ours, and are relatively stable, while those of the United States continue to escalate.

It may not be surprising that medical power—the authority of physicians and the potency of medicine—appears arbitrary to many patients. But U.S. patients no longer necessarily accept that their survival depends on their submission to medical technology. The law's doctrine of informed consent seeks to tame both death and arbitrary medical intervention to the will of the individual. Nonetheless, many Americans spend much of their time and many of their health care dollars attempting to prevent death by unproven means.

Historically, most Americans have treated health care as a private commodity whose price, and therefore availability, is primarily determined by market forces. In such a context, the law not unsurprisingly places a high premium on information disclosure by physicians. Personal autonomy—an individual's power to choose among medical options—enjoys its most zealous protection under U.S. jurisprudence.[7] The dominant U.S. version of informed consent is grounded on principles of patient/consumer autonomy, and seems to enhance market choice. But a strong theme of collectivism now runs through some discussions of U.S. health policy.[8] President Clinton was elected at least in part because he promised Americans universal health insurance coverage, but that promise has been all but abandoned, at least for the short-run. Moreover, unless health care funding increases dramatically, universal coverage would force limits on services that insured Americans are accustomed to receiving. This raises the politically charged specter of rationing.[9] The

[6] *See* George J. Annas, *Reframing the Debate on Health Care Reform by Replacing Our Metaphors*, 332 NEW ENG. J. MED. 744 (1995); SUSAN SONTAG, ILLNESS AS A METAPHOR, 57 (1978); SUSAN SONTAG, AIDS AND ITS METAPHORS (1989).

[7] *See, e.g.*, PAUL STARR, THE SOCIAL TRANSFORMATION OF AMERICAN MEDICINE 445 (1982). *Cf.* Lawrence J. Schneiderman et al., *Medical Futility: Its Meaning and Ethical Implications*, 112 ANNALS INTERNAL MED. 949, 953 (1990) (patient autonomy has highest value in hierarchy of principles of medical ethics).

[8] *See, e.g.*, TROYEN BRENNAN, JUST DOCTORING, MEDICAL ETHICS IN THE LIBERAL STATE (1991); Symposium, *The "Oregon Plan"*, 1 HEALTH MATRIX 135 (1991); H. Denman Scott et al., *Universal Insurance for American Health Care: A Proposal of the American College of Physicians*, ANNALS INTERNAL MED. 511 (1992). *See also* Symposium, *Managed Competition: Health Reform American Style?*, HEALTH AFF., Supp. 1993.

[9] The term *rationing* is used in this article in its popular sense to denote care which could conceivably confer medical benefit, but which is withheld for economic rather than clinical reasons. In fact, the U.S. has always rationed health services, but we do so by relegating the uninsured to the margins of health care delivery systems, rather than by

rationing theme may also be detected in a handful of reported legal opinions.[10] The patient sovereignty central to informed consent doctrine in the U.S.'s death-denying society poses serious obstacles to this collective trend. In countries where health care is publicly financed, disclosure requirements are much less explicit, and local law may actually discourage doctors from revealing information about diagnosis, prognosis, and alternative forms of treatment.

We theorize in this Article that the content and the style of imparting medical information can profoundly affect a country's total health expenditures.[11] We believe a society's general attitude toward death (as well as other cultural influences), will shape the type and amount of information that individual patients receive. In this Article we explore the cultural role and the economic impact of telling patients the truth about what doctors actually know—or don't know—about their medical conditions, and about therapy that might help (but could also harm) them. We concentrate particularly on truth-telling concerning prognosis when life-threatening illness has been diagnosed, because this dramatic case most clearly reveals systemic values.[12] The analysis focuses on the United States, with comparisons to informed consent law in the United Kingdom[13] and Japan.[14] We look specifically at the cultural determinants of medical practice in each country in Part II, and at the law which affects physician–patient interaction in Part III. We believe that a society's cultural attitude toward death strongly affects its approach to health sector finance, and we explore that interplay in Parts IV and V. These factors in turn influence the information the law requires doctors to provide their patients/consumers.

Finally, we conclude in Part VI that what doctors truthfully tell U.S. patients about prognosis and treatment alternatives, and about the degree of scientific uncertainty associated with their illnesses, will affect the way health service allocation takes place in the future. We suggest that when U.S. patients are more honestly

withholding specific services from insureds. *Cf.* NORMAN DANIELS, JUST HEALTH CARE (1985) (past experience makes it easier for us to tolerate excessive services than to limit providing them).

[10] *See, e.g.*, Harris v. McRae, 448 U.S. 297 (1980) (Stevens, J., dissenting):

> There are some especially costly forms of treatment that may reasonably be excluded from the [Medicaid] program in order to preserve the assets in the pool and extend its benefits to the maximum number of needy persons. Fiscal considerations may compel certain difficult choices in order to improve the protection afforded to the entire benefited class.

Id. at 355. *Cf.* Julia Field Costich, Note, *Denial of Coverage for "Experimental" Medical Procedures: The Problem of De Novo Review Under ERISA*, 79 KY. L.J. 801 (1990-91).

[11] For example, patient treatment choices vary when the same information is presented in terms of probability of death, rather than possibility of survival. Barbara J. McNeil et al., *On the Elicitation of Preferences for Alternative Therapies*, 306 NEW ENG. J. MED. 1259 (1982).

[12] This article will not directly examine the ramifications of informing patients when the financial or technical resources required to provide treatment that might benefit them are unavailable, but see generally, Mark Hall, *Informed Consent to Rationing Decisions*, 71 MILBANK Q. 645 (1993); Frances H. Miller, *Denial of Care and Informed Consent in English and American Law*, 18 AM. J.L. & MED. 37 (1992).

[13] On recent health sector reorganization in the U.K., see Patricia Day & Rudolf Klein, *Britain's Health Care Experiment*, HEALTH AFF., Fall 1991, at 39.

[14] On health sector organization in Japan, see MILTON I. ROEMER, NATIONAL HEALTH SYSTEMS OF THE WORLD, VOL. 1: THE COUNTRIES 153-61 (1991). *See also*, John K. Iglehart, *Japan's Medical Care System* (pts. 1 & 2), 319 NEW ENG. J. MED. 807, 1166 (1988); Naoki Ikegami, *Japanese Health Care: Low Costs Through Regulated Fees*, 10 HEALTH AFF. 87 (1991); Aki Yoshikawa, et al., *How Does Japan Do It? Doctors and Hospitals in a Universal Health Care System*, STAN. L. & POL'Y REV., Fall 1991, at 111.

informed about prognosis, and about the negative aspects of many aggressive therapies, public perceptions about the definition and desirability of limiting health services—particularly, but not only, for terminal illness—will change. We also examine the implications for Japan and the U.K. should they adopt U.S. technology and informed consent rules.

II. CULTURE AND MEDICAL SCIENCE

The definition of good medical care varies enormously from country to country.[15] For example, German and French physicians for decades routinely prescribed government-financed "spa cures" for their patients.[16] Such therapy choices would invite professional scorn, not to mention malpractice litigation, and would not be covered by insurance if prescribed by U.S. doctors. The international medical community often disagrees significantly about appropriate diagnosis and treatment.[17] Most physicians are relatively ignorant, if not openly skeptical, about scientific findings reported from foreign countries.[18]

At a more fundamental level, medical experts often frankly disagree about what constitutes disease.[19] Many physical states defined and treated as worthy of medical intervention in the U.S., such as moderately elevated blood pressure, are considered unremarkable variations of the human condition elsewhere in the world.[20] By way of contrast, low blood pressure is treated as a medical disorder in Germany[21] while at the same time it is welcomed as a longevity indicator in both the U.S. and the U.K.[22] American travelers becoming ill in foreign countries are often surprised to learn that 98.6° is not necessarily the gold standard for normal body temperature, notwithstanding what they have been led since childhood to believe.[23] Far from

[15] LYNN PAYER, MEDICINE & CULTURE (1988) [hereinafter MEDICINE & CULTURE]; *cf.* THE RELEVANCE OF SOCIAL SCIENCE FOR MEDICINE (Leon Eisenberg & Arthur Kleinman eds., 1981); E. Phelps, *Diffusion of Information in Medical Care*, J. ECON. PERSP., Summer 1992, at 23.

[16] German patients have been entitled to six-week insurance-paid stays at health spas every three years. Richard A. Knox, *Germany's Health Care: A Model*, BOSTON GLOBE, October 25, 1992, at 71, 73. German health reforms recently eliminated spa coverage, however. *Health Budget Using European Models Promising for United States, ProPAC Told*, PENS. & BEN. DAILY (BNA), April 14, 1993. For a general description of the German system, see MICHAEL ARNOLD, HEALTH CARE IN THE FEDERAL REPUBLIC OF GERMANY (1991).

[17] MEDICINE & CULTURE, *supra* note 15, at 96, reports neurosis as the leading diagnosis by British GPs. Neurosis was not even mentioned in the top twenty diagnoses in Germany for the same time period, presumably stemming from German cultural hostility to psychiatry.

[18] A.M.W. Porter, *Three Threats to Standards of Medical Practice*, 1 LANCET 1071, 1071 (interviews with French and British doctors reveal that they rarely read each others' medical journals). British doctors tend to be empiricists distrustful of theory *per se*, while French doctors are trained as Cartesian thinkers, tending to dismiss empiricism as riskily anecdotal. *See* MEDICINE & CULTURE, *supra* note 15, at 37-44.

[19] *See* LYNN PAYER, DISEASE MONGERS: HOW DOCTORS, DRUG COMPANIES, AND INSURERS ARE MAKING YOU FEEL SICK 1-100 (1992) (how the U.S. "creates" disease).

[20] *See, e.g.*, Lawrence K. Altman, *U.S. Seeks Attack on Hypertension*, N.Y. TIMES, October 31, 1992, at 5.

[21] MEDICINE & CULTURE, *supra* note 15, at 25 ("low blood pressure [is] treated with eighty-five drugs as well as hydrotherapy and spa treatments in Germany").

[22] *See* James M. Robbins et al., *Treatment for a Nondisease: The Case of Low Blood Pressure*, 16 SOC. SCI. & MED. 27 (1982).

[23] In the U.K. for example, thermometers are calibrated to show 96.4° as normal body temperature. *Cf.*, *Should Physicians Abandon 98.6° as a Standard of Normal Body Temperature?*, INTERNAL MED. WORLD REP., October 15-31 1992, at 1.

being an "exact" science with commonly acknowledged definitional, diagnostic, and treatment principles, scientific uncertainty permeates medicine.[24]

Professional cultural values also both overtly and subliminally prejudice medical practice, as do the cultural values imbedded in the particular society in which physicians practice their skills.[25] Moreover, patients have culturally influenced attitudes of their own that affect their willingness to accept—as well as their response to receiving—medical therapy.[26] The Jehovah's Witness[27] and Christian Science[28] cases, as well as the abortion controversy,[29] have spotlighted religion's powerful influence on receptiveness to medical intervention in the U.S. and elsewhere. Less immediately obvious cultural influences can have an equally strong impact on patient perception of medical risks and benefits.[30]

The U.S. public has always been culturally predisposed toward action in the face of threatened adversity, medical or otherwise.[31] Lynn Payer's masterful book *Medicine & Culture*,[32] quoting such odd bedfellows as Oliver Wendell Holmes and Luigi Barzini, links the aggressive American approach toward medicine to the frontier spirit,[33] and to Americans' deeply ingrained belief that "the main purpose of a

---

[24] David M. Eddy, *Variations in Physician Practice: The Role of Uncertainty*, HEALTH AFF., Summer 1984, at 74. *Cf.*, Franz Inglefinger, *Arrogance*, 303 NEW ENG. J. MED. 1507 (1980).

[25] For example, the Gallic ideal of the (slim) feminine form prompts French plastic surgeons to counsel breast reduction for the same patients who could—at least until the recent controversy over silicone implant safety—be plausible candidates for breast augmentation in the U.S.'s more curvaceously inclined cultural milieu. *Cf. Fashion World Should Look at Real Women; the Surgeon's Version*, N.Y. TIMES, Feb. 26, 1992, at A20; Robert M. Veatch, *Consensus of Expertise: The Role of Consensus of Experts in Formulating Public Policy and Estimating Facts*, 16 J. MED. & PHIL. 427 (1991) (values of medical experts differ from values of lay people). *See generally* MEDICINE & CULTURE, *supra* note 15; Klim McPherson, *International Differences in Medical Care Practices*, *in* OECD SOCIAL POLICY STUDIES NO. 7, HEALTH CARE SYSTEMS IN TRANSITION: THE SEARCH FOR EFFICIENCY 17 (Organization for Economic Co-Operation and Development ed., 1990).

[26] ARTHUR KLEINMAN, PATIENTS AND HEALERS IN THE CONTEXT OF CULTURE, (1980). *Cf.* Nancy Scheper-Hughes, *Social Indifference to Child Death*, 337 LANCET 1144, 1145 (1991) ("Parents and public officials throughout the world have often failed to see infant and child [illness or] death as either a personal tragedy or an important social issue.").

[27] *In re* Osborne, 294 A.2d 372 (D.C. 1972) (competent patient may refuse life-saving blood transfusion where no compelling state interest involved); *cf. In re* President & Directors of Georgetown College, 331 F.2d 1000, 1008 (D.C. Cir. 1964) (blood transfusion ordered despite patient's religious refusal to consent, because "[t]he state, as parens patriae, will not allow a parent to abandon a [seven month-old] child . . . .").

[28] Winters v. Miller, 446 F.2d 65 (2d Cir. 1971) (Christian Scientist mental patient challenged forced administration of tranquilizers, citing constitutionally protected religious beliefs).

[29] *Cf.* ROEMER, *supra* note 14, at 90.

[30] Mary DOUGLAS, RISK ACCEPTABILITY AND SOCIAL SCIENCES (1985).

[31] Kerr L. White, *Foreword* to MEDICINE & CULTURE, *supra* note 15, at 10, 11; Rudolf Klein, *Rationing Health Care*, 289 BRIT. MED. J. 143, 144 (1984) ("America is a perfectibility of man society in which illness and debility are seen as challenges to action and patients tend to be demanding consumers.").

[32] MEDICINE & CULTURE, *supra* note 15.

[33] "How could a people which . . . has contrived the Bowie knife and the revolver . . . which insists in sending out yachts and horses and boys to outsail, outrun, outfight and checkmate all the rest of creation; how could such a people be content with any but 'heroic' practice? What wonder that the stars and stripes wave over doses of ninety grains of sulfate of quinine and that the American eagle screams with delight to see three drachms of calomel [a potent purge] given at a single mouthful?" 9 OLIVER WENDELL HOLMES, THE WRIT-

man's life is to solve problems."[34] For decades Americans have tolerated—if not encouraged—the delivery of superfluous medical services under the rubric of medical necessity, financed by cost-pass-through health insurance.[35] However, escalating health care costs, a sometimes stagnating economy, increased patient awareness of the hazards of medical intervention, and the dubious success of modern technology in prolonging dying have prompted at least some reevaluation of an indiscriminately aggressive approach to medical care.

Cost containment pressures are bringing home the lesson that medical necessity is actually a fluid notion, continually reconceived as scientific understanding, payment incentives, and culture evolve.[36] Containing costs necessarily implies setting limits on health care expenditures, and cultural values are critical to determining where those limits will lie.[37] When the 70,000-member American College of Physicians advocated caps on national health expenditures in September of 1992, a sea-change in professional values (at least among primary care physicians) gained public visibility.[38] When an ultimately successful presidential candidate ventured to include spending caps in his pre-election agenda for health sector reform, one can be sure that at least he tested the political winds before proposing such a radical change in the *status quo*.[39] Those winds shifted dramatically in the interim, but while the opposition was mobilizing, the candidate was elected.

III. CULTURE AND INFORMED CONSENT

In this section we examine the legal doctrine of informed consent in three widely differing national cultures: the United States, the United Kingdom, and Japan. We analyze the theory and function of informed consent through the lens of death in each country, to understand why the amount of information physicians give their patients/consumers can affect the way health resource allocation takes place. While we concentrate on these three countries, we believe the analysis can be applied to other industrialized nations as well.

Although we focus here on choice involving treatment alternatives, choice in medicine occurs at two preliminary stages as well. First, health "insurance plans" are selected either by or for patients. Second, patients pick their personal physi-

---

INGS OF OLIVER WENDELL HOLMES, MEDICAL ESSAYS (1888), quoted in MEDICINE & CULTURE, *supra* note 15, at 127.

[34] LUIGI BARZINI, THE EUROPEANS 239 (1983).

[35] STARR, *supra* note 7, at 434; HENRY J. AARON & WILLIAM B. SCHWARTZ, THE PAINFUL PRESCRIPTION: RATIONING HOSPITAL CARE 4 (1984).

[36] For general background, see generally BRUNO LATOUR & STEVE WOOLGAR, LABORATORY LIFE: THE CONSTRUCTION OF SCIENTIFIC FACTS (1979); John B. McKinley, *From "Promising Report" to "Standard Medical Procedure": Seven Stages in the Career of a Medical Innovation*, 59 MILBANK Q. 374 (1981); MICHAEL WALZER, SPHERES OF JUSTICE 86-91 (1983). Moreover, many Americans may be beginning to perceive that cost containment is the price they must pay for broader—or even continued—access to health insurance coverage.

[37] Daniel Callahan, *The Oregon Initiative: Ethics and Priority Setting*, 1 HEALTH MATRIX 157 (1991); Leslie Pickering Francis, *Consumer Expectations and Access to Health Care*, 140 U. PA. L. REV. 1881 (1992); Michael J. Garland, *Setting Health Care Priorities in Oregon*, 1 HEALTH MATRIX 139 (1991); David C. Hadorn, *The Problem of Discrimination in Health Care Priority Setting*, 268 JAMA 1454 (1992); Paul T. Menzel, *Consumer Expectations and Access to Health Care: A Commentary*, 140 U. PA. L. REV. 1919 (1992).

[38] Scott et al., *supra* note 8, at 511.

[39] Bill Clinton, *The Clinton Health Care Plan*, 327 NEW ENG. J. MED. 804, 805, (1992).

cians from among those sanctioned by their plan. Each of these decisions is subject to cultural influences, which may determine the range of alternatives available. In countries with single-payer systems, the government controls the total budget for health services, thereby limiting those services that can be supplied to everyone. Under the U.K.'s National Health Service (NHS), for example, the patient's primary care physician is expected to function as gatekeeper to medical specialists, who generally will treat patients only on referral.[40]

In insurance-based systems like those in the U.S. and Japan, citizens can usually go directly to the doctor of their own choosing, although in the U.S. that range of choice is now commonly limited by the patient's managed care insurance contract. In all systems the specific treatment decision itself, however, including the decision to refuse treatment, is made within the confines of the particular physician-patient relationship. We concentrate on the amount of information each country's law requires doctors to convey within this relationship, especially when life-threatening illness occurs, as a vehicle for examining the interplay among financing, cultural attitudes toward death, and choice.

A. The United States

A British physician has described the United States as "the land of freedom, democracy, self-reliance, and market competition."[41] This description is reflected in the modern U.S. version of informed consent, which itself can be traced to the early part of the twentieth century. As an Illinois court put it in 1906:

> Under a free government at least, the free citizen's first and greatest right which underlies all others—the right to the inviolability of his person, in other words his right to be himself, is the subject of universal acquiescence, and this right necessarily forbids a physician . . . to violate without permission the bodily integrity of his patient by a major or capital operation.[42]

Initially, United States judicial opinions described the requirement of consent to medical treatment as necessary to avoid the intentional tort of battery. By the 1970s, however, courts had begun to reformulate the physician's duty to inform as a negligence concept, required by the fiduciary nature of the doctor-patient relationship. Doctors had been telling patients relatively little, and *informed* consent became recognized as necessary to promote "shared decision-making."[43] It soon became not only a legal doctrine promoting self-determination, but a core ethical principle as

---

[40] The U.K. General Medical Council's principles of professional conduct state, "a specialist should not usually accept a patient without reference from the patient's general practitioner." (UK) General Medical Council, Professional Conduct And Discipline: Fitness To Practice 22 (1991). For a description of the NHS internal market reforms initiated in 1991, see Frances H. Miller, *Competition Law and Anticompetitive Professional Behavior Affecting Health Care*, 55 Mod. L. Rev. 453, 460 (1992).

[41] John Fay, *The Mouse and the Elephant: Can Primary Care Save the U.S. Health System?*, 340 Lancet 594 (1992).

[42] Pratt v. Davis, 118 Ill. App. 161, 166 (1905), *aff'd*, 244 Ill. 30, 79 N.E. 562 (1906).

[43] Not so coincidentally, the Medicare and Medicaid programs, initiated pursuant to the Social Security Act of 1965, Pub. L. No. 89-97, 79 Stat. 286 (1965) (codified as amended at 42 U.S.C. §§ 1395-1396v (1988 & Supp. V 1993)), made the issue of choice meaningful to a large segment of the population which previously had limited access to health services.

well.[44] Informed consent requirements implement the fundamental principle that "adults are entitled to accept or reject health care interventions on the basis of their own personal values and in furtherance of their own personal goals."[45]

California courts, especially the California Supreme Court, have been the nation's most influential in shaping the U.S. doctrine of informed consent. The California Supreme Court decided the case of *Cobbs v. Grant*[46] in the wake of the consumer, civil rights, and women's movements of the 1960s. In *Cobbs* a patient had sued his physician for failure to disclose the inherent risks of ulcer surgery: a splenectomy and the development of an additional ulcer later occurred. The court abandoned the battery theory, and replaced it with a negligence cause of action, holding that the physician owed the patient an affirmative *duty* to disclose certain information. This duty could not be derived from practices customarily engaged in by other reasonably prudent physicians, since few surgeons then disclosed this type of risk information to their patients. Rather, the court found the duty inherent in the fiduciary nature of the doctor-patient relationship.[47]

Under the *Cobbs* rule, the ultimate choice among alternative treatments, like all other marketplace decisions, rests with the patient-consumer. Just as banks must disclose annual percentage interest rates to depositors and borrowers, and used car salesmen must disclose actual mileage to buyers, so physicians must disclose risks and alternatives of proposed medical procedures to patients. A market system presumes that individual decisions will be based on consumer information. Informed consent doctrine assumes that the patient's doctor is the appropriate person to provide this information, and requires disclosure so that the patient can be a knowledgeable consumer of the medical product.[48]

Most recently, the California Supreme Court refused to redefine the required content of informed consent, and its opinion in *Arato v. Avedon*[49] underlines the

---

[44] PRESIDENT'S COMMISSION FOR THE STUDY OF ETHICAL PROBLEMS IN MEDICINE AND BIOMEDICAL AND BEHAVIORAL RESEARCH, MAKING HEALTH CARE DECISIONS 2-3 (1982).

[45] *Id. See also* GEORGE J. ANNAS, THE RIGHTS OF PATIENTS 83-85 (2d ed. 1989).

[46] 502 P.2d 1 (Cal. 1972). The other candidate for leading U.S. case is Canterbury v. Spence, 464 F.2d 772 (D.C. Cir. 1972). We prefer *Cobbs* because the California courts have continued to refine it.

[47] In supporting the patient's right to decision-making authority, the court noted the patient's "abject dependence" on the doctor for medical information. This dependency, coupled with the trust the patient must have in their doctors, generated the physician's duty to disclose. *Cobbs*, 502 P.2d at 9. The hospital settled, but the case against physician was never retried because the plaintiff's lawyer believed that his client could not meet the objective "reasonable person" causation standard. The court also used the concept of materiality to identify the information that physicians must disclose; *material* information is that which might lead a reasonable person to reject the recommended therapy (and opt for an alternative or no treatment at all). The California Supreme Court specifically required the following pieces of information to be disclosed (others would be added later): a description of the proposed procedure, its risks (of death and bodily harm) and benefits (including probability of success), alternative treatments (including no treatment) with their risks and benefits, and problems associated with recuperation. *Id.* at 10-11.

[48] Since 1972 the California Supreme Court has also required physicians to inform patients of the risks of refusing screening tests such as Pap smears. Truman v. Thomas, 611 P.2d 902 (Cal. 1980). It has also mandated that doctors inform patients about potential financial conflicts of interest which might influence them to make recommendations influenced by personal reasons unrelated to their patients' best interests. Moore v. Regents of Univ. of Cal., 793 P.2d 479 (Cal. 1990).

[49] 858 P.2d 598 (Cal. 1993).

difficulty we still have in dealing with death. Miklos Arato, a forty-three-year-old electrical contractor, was operated on to remove a nonfunctioning kidney on July 21, 1980. During surgery a tumor was found in the tail of his pancreas, and doctors removed the tumor along with the surrounding tissue and lymph nodes. Several days later, the surgeon met with Mr. Arato and his wife. He told them that he thought he had excised all of the tumor and referred them to an oncologist. The surgeon did not tell them that only about five percent of patients with pancreatic cancer survive for five years, nor did he give Mr. Arato a reasonable estimate of his life expectancy. The oncologist told the Aratos that there was a substantial chance of a recurrence, and that a recurrence would mean that the disease was incurable. He recommended experimental chemotherapy and radiation treatment, acknowledging that this might produce no benefit. The oncologist was not asked for, and did not volunteer, a prognosis.

In the following April, while the chemotherapy and radiation treatment were continuing, the cancer recurred. Even though the physicians believed Mr. Arato's life expectancy could then be measured in months, they did not tell him so. Mr. Arato died on July 25, 1981, approximately one year after doctors diagnosed his disease. His wife and two adult children then brought suit against the surgeons and oncologist, alleging that they had an obligation under California's informed consent doctrine to tell Mr. Arato, before asking him to consent to chemotherapy, that approximately ninety-five percent of people diagnosed with pancreatic cancer die within five years.[50] The plaintiffs argued that the statistical prognosis should have been disclosed because it indicated that even with successful treatment Mr. Arato would probably have lived only a short time.[51] If Mr. Arato had known the facts, the plaintiffs believed, he would not have undergone the rigors of the experimental treatment. He would instead have chosen to live out his last days at peace with his wife and family, and would have made final arrangements for his financial and business affairs. As a result of his ignorance he was induced not to so plan; his contracting business had gone bankrupt, and his estate incurred substantial tax losses.

On the basis of standard California jury instructions on informed consent requirements, the jury returned a verdict in favor of the physicians.[52] A California

[50] At trial it was shown that at the first meeting with his oncologist, Mr. Arato had filled out an eighteen-page questionnaire in which he answered "yes" to the question: "If you are seriously ill now or in the future, do you want to be told the truth about it?" The physicians who treated Mr. Arato justified their nondisclosure of the statistical prognosis on a variety of grounds, most based on traditional medical paternalism. His surgeon, for example, thought Mr. Arato had shown such great anxiety about his cancer that it was "medically inappropriate" to disclose specific mortality rates. The chief oncologist said he understood that patients like Mr. Arato "wanted to be told, but did not want a cold shower." He thought that reporting extremely high mortality rates might "deprive a patient of any hope of a cure," and that this was medically inadvisable. His physicians also said that during his seventy visits with them over a one-year period, Mr. Arato had avoided ever specifically asking about his own life expectancy and that this indicated that he did not want to know the information. In addition, all the physicians testified that the statistical life expectancy of a group of patients had little predictive value when applied to a particular patient. *See*, George J. Annas, *Informed Consent, Cancer, and Truth in Prognosis*, 330 NEW ENG. J. MED. 223 (1994).

[51] The physicians measured success in terms of added *months* of survival. Arato v. Avedon, 11 Cal. Rptr. 2d 169, 172 (Cal. Ct. App. 1992).

[52] The instructions read by the trial judge stated:

> Except as hereinafter explained, it is the duty of the physician to disclose to the patient all material information to enable the patient to make an informed

court of appeals reversed the decision in a two-to-one opinion, stating that physicians have an obligation to disclose life expectancy statistics to patients so that they may take timely action to plan the financial and other aspects of their deaths.[53] The defendant-physicians then appealed.

Instead of taking the opportunity to resolve what the California Supreme Court described as a "critical standoff" in the development of informed consent doctrine between the extremes of absolute patient sovereignty and medical paternalism, the court focused on one very narrow question, and upheld the trial court. It analyzed whether California's standard jury instructions should be revised to require the specific disclosure of a patient's life expectancy, as predicted by mortality statistics.[54] Framing the question so narrowly made answering it relatively easy. The court described the physician-patient relationship as "an intimate and irreducibly judgment-laden one" that had to be judged within "the overall medical context." As for general statistics on life expectancy, the court found them of little use to individual patients. The court thought, for example, that "statistical morbidity values derived from the experience of population groups are inherently unreliable and offer little assurance regarding the fate of the individual patient."[55]

> decision regarding proposed treatment.
>
> Material information is information which the physician knows or should know would be regarded as significant by a reasonable person in the patient's position when deciding to accept or reject a recommended medical procedure. To be material a fact must also be one which is not commonly appreciated.
>
> A physician has no duty of disclosure beyond that required of physicians of good standing in the same or similar locality when he or she relied upon facts which would demonstrate to a reasonable person that the disclosure would so seriously upset the patient that the patient would not have been able to rationally weigh the risks of refusing to undergo the recommended treatment.
>
> Even though the patient has consented to a proposed treatment or operation, the failure of the physician to inform the patient as stated in this instruction before obtaining such consent is negligence and renders the physician subject to liability for any damage legally resulting from the failure to disclose or for any injury legally resulting from the treatment if a reasonably prudent person in the patient's position would not have consented to the treatment if he or she had been adequately informed of the likelihood of his [sic] premature death.

Arato, 858 P.2d at 602 n.3.

[53] *Arato*, 11 Cal. Rptr. 2d at 169.

[54] *Arato*, 858 P.2d at 598.

[55] Perhaps most important, the court described this case as one that was "fairly litigated" and properly put in the hands of "the venerable American jury," which had rendered a reasonable verdict that it was not prepared to second-guess. The court concluded:

> Rather than mandate the disclosure of specific information as a matter of law, the better rule is to instruct the jury that a physician is under a legal duty to disclose to the patient all material information—that is, "information which . . . would be regarding as significant by a reasonable person in the patient's position when deciding to accept or reject a recommended medical procedure"—needed to make an informed decision regarding a proposed treatment.

Id. at 607. The patient's desire to be told the truth, as evidenced by his answer on the questionnaire, was found to be irrelevant, since the physician has an independent legal duty to tell the "truth" (although a patient can waive the right to information). The court also dealt with the issue of expert testimony, noting that in addition to the information required to be disclosed by *Cobbs* (the nature and benefits of the proposed treatment, its risks of death or serious harm, reasonable alternatives and their risks, and problems of recuperation), physicians must also disclose any other information which another skilled practitioner would disclose. The court ruled that specific data on life expectancy fell within this standard. Thus, the defendant physicians were properly permitted to call expert medical

If the only issue is whether the law should require physicians always to disclose statistical life-expectancy data to critically ill patients as part of the informed consent process, the court's conclusion is defensible and perhaps unavoidable. But this issue is much too narrow a basis for refining the informed consent decision. Standing alone, statistical probabilities of survival may indeed not be material for an individual patient. Statistical probabilities become material, however, if they indicate whether the particular patient is likely to survive, or predict that patient's probable quality of life with and without treatment. The informed consent issue thus centers on disclosure of proposed treatment success rates concerning both survival prospects and quality of life for the specific individual. This is the type of material information patients have a right to know under *Cobbs*—not only because it concerns their bodies, but, more importantly, because it concerns their lives.[56]

Unfortunately, the plaintiffs in *Arato* did not argue the necessity for explaining success rates, because then the result could have (and should have) been different. In *Cobbs*, which *Arato* affirms, the California Supreme Court had said:

> A medical doctor, being the expert, appreciates the risks inherent in the procedure he is prescribing, the risks of a decision not to undergo the treatment, and the probability of a successful outcome of the treatment . . . . The weighing of these risks against the individual subjective fears and hopes of the patient is not an expert skill. Such evaluation and decision is a nonmedical judgment reserved to the patient alone.[57]

This language explicitly requires physicians to explain the probability that a proposed treatment will be successful, and implicitly requires the physician to tell the patient what the physician means by "success." In *Arato*, the court correctly concluded that the disclosure of a statistical life-expectancy profile of all pancreatic cancer patients, by itself, was not required to inform Mr. Arato properly of his prognosis. However, such information can be invaluable when coupled with an explanation of why the physician thinks the patient's case is or is not typical. Group data are the basis for predictions in individual cases, including both treatment recommendations and statements about probable risks and benefits. Mr. Arato's physicians relied on group data, for example, when they told him that if his cancer recurred it would be incurable. The court should have made clear that a reasonable person would consider it material to know not only the probability of success of a proposed treatment, but what the doctor means by success. Without this information the physician, not the patient, really makes the treatment decision. This result is precisely what the doctrine of informed consent is designed to prevent.

End-of-life care will come under increasing scrutiny as expanded health insurance coverage makes cost control an even more dominant concern of U.S. medical policy. Approximately thirty percent of the Medicare budget is now spent on treatment during the last year of its beneficiaries' lives. Significant savings could be achieved by decreasing utilization within that period.[58] Congress had both cost

---

witnesses to testify that it was not standard practice in the medical community in 1980 to disclose specific life-expectancy data.

[56] Alexander M. Capron, *Duty, Truth and Whole Human Beings*, HASTINGS CTR. REP., Aug. 1993, at 13-14. *See also*, ANATOLE BROYARD, INTOXICATED BY MY ILLNESS (1992); PETER NOLL, IN THE FACE OF DEATH (1989).

[57] Cobbs v. Grant, 502 P.2d 1, 10 (Cal. 1972).

[58] *See* Peter A. Singer & Frederick H. Lowy, *Rationing, Patient Preferences, and Cost*

containment and autonomy objectives in mind when it passed the Patient Self-Determination Act[59] in 1990, which requires health facilities receiving Medicare and Medicaid funding to give patients written information about their rights to refuse treatment under state law. Subjecting people to expensive and unwanted treatment at the end of life makes no economic sense, and undermines patient sovereignty.[60] Pressure to disclose both prognosis and the negative side-effects of treatment for terminal conditions should increase for these reasons alone.[61]

Organ transplantation policy illustrates the potential for informed consent doctrine to enhance patient autonomy *and* save money where extreme and expensive medical interventions are involved.[62] The Massachusetts Organ Transplantation Task Force recognized this explicitly in its 1984 Report. It noted that only three ways to reduce deaths among patients on organ transplantation waiting lists exist, at least so long as organ shortage remains a problem. These are (1) to increase resources devoted to organ procurement; (2) to make medical criteria more strict; and (3) to persuade individuals not to join waiting lists at all.[63] In the Task Force's words:

> Of these three options, only number 3 has the promise of both conserving resources and promoting individual autonomy. While we assume that most persons medically eligible for a transplant would want one, we also assume . . . some would not—at least if they understood all that was involved, including the need for a lifetime commitment to daily immunosuppression medications and periodic medical monitoring for rejection symptoms. Accordingly, it makes policy sense to publicize the risks and side-effects of transplantation, and to require careful explanations of the procedure to be given to prospective patients *before* they undergo medical screening.[64]

This strategy of providing accurate information in the hope of dissuading people from seeking medical intervention also underlies legislative "informed consent" requirements for disclosure prior to abortion.[65] These statutes require physicians to discuss fetal development and related issues before obtaining consent for pregnancy termination.[66] Mandatory disclosure regarding the effects of abortion on fetuses is frankly designed to decrease demand for it.[67]

---

of Care at the End of Life, 152 ARCHIVES INTERNAL MED. 478 (1992); Ezekiel J. Emanuel & Linda L. Emanuel, *The Economics of Dying—The Illusion of Cost Savings at the End of Life*, 330 NEW ENG. J. MED. 540 (1994).

[59] 42 U.S.C. § 1395cc (f)(1)(A)(i) (Supp. V 1993).

[60] George J. Annas, *The Health Care Proxy and the Living Will*, 324 NEW ENG. J. MED. 1210 (1991).

[61] *Id.*

[62] *Cf.* RENÉE C. FOX & JUDITH P. SWAZEY, SPARE PARTS 208 (1992).

> One of the most urgent value questions is whether, as poverty, homelessness, and lack of access to health care increase in our affluent country, it is justifiable for American society to be devoting so much of its intellectual energy and human and financial resources to the replacement of human organs.

Id.

[63] DEPT. OF PUBLIC HEALTH, COMMONWEALTH OF MASSACHUSETTS, REPORT OF THE MASSACHUSETTS TASK FORCE ON ORGAN TRANSPLANTATION (Oct. 1984) (George J. Annas, Chairman, Oct. 1984).

[64] *Id.* at 83.

[65] *See generally* Paula Berg, *Toward a First Amendment Theory of Doctor-Patient Discourse and the Right to Receive Unbiased Medical Advice*, 74 B.U. L. REV. 201 (1994).

[66] *See, e.g.*, Planned Parenthood v. Casey, 112 S. Ct. 2791 (1992) (plurality opinion).

[67] *See* Pub. Act 81-1078, § 3.5(2), 1979 Ill. Laws 4108, 4115 (repealed 1984) which

In the U.S., informed consent is well entrenched in theory, but in practice patient autonomy continues to be elusive for many reasons.[68] First, patients (particularly seriously ill ones) remain abjectly dependent on their physicians, who still make most choices *for* them because of the information inequality between doctor and patient.[69] Arnold Relman estimates that in the U.S. "probably more than 70 percent of all expenditures for personal health care are the result of decisions of physicians."[70] Moreover, the *way* physicians impart information influences patient choice. For example, patients tend to go along with therapy their physicians recommend when probable outcomes are discussed in terms of survival percentages, but reject it when those very same outcomes are presented in terms of death statistics.[71]

Secondly, although the United States has a capitalistic, market-driven economy and views medicine as a private good, public expenditures on health care account for more than forty percent of the approximately one trillion dollars that Americans will spend on health care in 1995.[72] The public sector will be *the* major payer within a few years, even in the absence of major structural change. Finally, financial incentives in our system may simply overwhelm the legal pressure to inform patients adequately. In commenting on his study suggesting that fully half of the coronary angiograms now done in the U.S. are unnecessary,[73] Thomas B. Graboys recently explained the difficulties cardiologists have in exploring diagnostic and treatment options with their patients. He concluded, "It is [just] easier to say we will do the angiogram and other invasive studies, and we will get paid five times as much."[74]

B. The United Kingdom

In the U.K., medical care has long been viewed as a publicly provided good, and choices are constrained by, among other things, the total budget government commits to medical services.[75] Informed consent doctrine therefore downplays patient choice in comparison with the U.S. In Britain's leading informed consent case,[76] Amy

required doctors performing abortions to hand patients the following written statement: "The State of Illinois wants you to know that in its view the child you are carrying is a living human being whose life should be preserved. Illinois strongly encourages you not to have an abortion but to go through to childbirth."

[68] Jay Katz, The Silent World Of Doctor And Patient (1984).

[69] Kenneth Arrow, *Uncertainty and the Welfare Economics of Medical Care*, 53 Am. Econ. Rev. 941 (1963). *See also* Stanley J. Reiser, *Consumer Competence and the Reform of American Health Care*, 267 JAMA 1511 (1992) (physicians and managers make most health care decisions; consumer competence must be developed to bring about a consumer-determined health care system).

[70] Arnold Relman, *The New Medical-Industrial Complex*, 303 New Eng. J. Med. 963, 966 (1980).

[71] McNeil et al., *supra* note 11, at 1261.

[72] Michael Meier, *These Economic Experts Advocate Higher Taxes*, Star Tribune, Jan. 7 1995, at 1.

[73] Thomas Graboys et al., *Results of a Second Opinion Trial Among Patients Recommended for Coronary Angiography*, 268 JAMA 2537, 2537 (1992).

[74] Lawrence K. Altman, *Study Sees Excess in X-Rays*, N.Y. Times, Nov. 11, 1992, at 16. *See generally* Arnold S. Relman, *Self-Referral—What's at Stake?*, 327 New Eng. J. Med. 1522 (1992).

[75] *See generally* Rudolph Klein, The Politics Of The NHS (2d ed. 1989). For a summary of informed consent rules in European countries, see Kenk Leenen et al., The Rights Of Patients In Europe (1993).

[76] Sidaway v. Bethlem Royal Hosp. Governors, 1 All E.R. 643, 646 (1985).

Doris Sidaway underwent a laminectomy (her second) which had an inherent risk of one to two percent of paralysis. The surgery left her paralyzed on her right side. The trial court ruled that her physician was under no legal obligation to disclose those inherent surgical risks; the appeals panel affirmed, as did the House of Lords.

The primary question before the five Law Lords hearing the case was the source of the physician's duty to disclose information. As in the U.S., English malpractice law is based on the proposition that a physician "is not guilty of negligence if he has acted in accordance with a practice accepted as proper by a responsible body of medical men skilled in that particular art."[77] This is known as the *Bolam* test. While many U.S. courts have abandoned this physician-oriented rule for informed consent cases, the House of Lords did not. Four of five Law Lords accepted a physician-centered standard of disclosure, although with differing emphases.

Lord Diplock's speech held that the *Bolam* test determined the physician's duty to disclose, noting that its merit consisted in permitting physicians to base practice on that "accepted as proper by a body of responsible and skilled medical opinion."[78] Lord Templeman believed that physicians fulfill their duty of disclosure when they provide patients with sufficient information to make a "balanced judgment."[79] In his view, the decision of what precise information to impart is for the doctor, so long as the goal is honoring "the patient's right to information which will enable the patient to make a balanced judgment."[80]

Lord Bridge, joined by Lord Keith, generally agreed that *Bolam* governed disclosure, but would reserve judicial authority to overrule medical custom in certain instances:

> I am of the opinion that the judge might in certain circumstances come to the conclusion that disclosure of a particular risk was so obviously necessary to an informed choice on the part of the patient that no reasonably prudent medical man would fail to make it.[81]

Lord Scarman alone would have altered the *Bolam* rule in informed consent cases in favor of a patient-centered standard of disclosure, since he considered self-determination a basic human right.[82]

---

[77] Bolam v. Friern Hosp. Management Comm., 1 W.L.R. 582, 582 (1957).

[78] Sidaway, 1 All ER at 657.

[79] *Id.* at 666.

[80] *Id.*

[81] *Id.* at 663. As an example, Lord Bridge cited the Canadian case of *Reibl v. Hughes*, 114 D.L.R. 1 (1980), which involved a ten percent risk of stroke from an operation. He characterized this as "[a] substantial risk of grave consequences," which "[i]n the absence of some cogent clinical reason why the patient should not be informed" would require disclosure. In addition, Lord Bridge noted that "when questioned specifically by a patient of apparently sound mind about risks involved in a particular proposed treatment, the doctor's duty must . . . be to answer both truthfully and as fully as the questioner requires." *Id.* at 661.

[82] *Id.* at 649. In Lord Scarman's view, the doctor's duty to disclose material risks "[a]rises from his patient's rights." The duty in any case should depend upon "[t]he degree of probability of the risk materializing and the seriousness of possible injury if it does." On the other hand, Lord Scarman held that the one percent risk of paralysis involved in Amy Sidaway's case was "slight." It was sufficiently remote to require the plaintiff "[t]o establish that the risk was so great that the doctor should have appreciated that it would be considered a significant fact by a prudent patient . . . ." Since Mrs. Sidaway had not demonstrated this, Lord Scarman voted with the other four Law Lords to dismiss the appeal. *Id.* at 654-55.

What *Sidaway* actually stands for is a matter of some dispute. David Meyers has argued that Lord Bridge's speech giving judges the right to second-guess the sufficiency of the information doctors disclose, "may well lead to a modified version of the 'informed consent' doctrine the Lords apparently were so anxious, for policy reasons, to avoid."[83] He does, however, offer the trite caution that "only time will tell."[84] So far, time has not been particularly kind to an expansive informed consent doctrine in England. As Meyers and others have noted, a post-*Sidaway* court of appeals decision, *Gold v. Haringey Area Health Authority*, wrongly concluded that *Sidaway* stood for the proposition that the *Bolam* test was decisive on informed consent.[85] Other commentators have, properly we think, suggested that *Gold* misinterpreted *Sidaway*:

> [Under *Sidaway*] the Judge was "free" to form his own view if he regarded the information which was lacking as "obviously necessary for an informed choice" or a "balanced judgment." The problem with the Court of Appeals approach in *Gold* was that their reading of *Sidaway* failed to look beyond the strict limits of Lord Diplock's speech. Had they done so, this backward step, giving conclusive force to medical evidence, could have been avoided.[86]

Consumer advocates in Britain have not been silent in the wake of *Sidaway*, or persuaded that physicians alone should set disclosure rules.[87] Sarah Boston and Jill Louw are advocates for full disclosure when breast cancer has been diagnosed. They disapprove of surgeon Michael Baum's statement in *Breast Cancer: The Facts*: "Women should trust the medical profession that they are working for the benefit of womankind; once this trust is lost there is no hope at all."[88] Boston and Louw counter that "trust is a two-way relationship based on mutual respect," and go on to say that "[b]etter-informed patients can no longer be treated in the paternalis-

---

[83] DAVID W. MEYERS, THE HUMAN BODY AND THE LAW 131 (2d ed. 1990).

[84] *Id.*

[85] [1988] Q.B. 481, 3 W.L.R. 649 (1987) (failed sterilization procedure where alternative forms of contraception were not disclosed). *See also* Andrew Grubb, *Contraceptive Advice and Doctors—A Law Unto Themselves?*, 47 CAMBRIDGE L.J. 12 (1988).

[86] Dieter Giesen & John Hayes, *The Patient's Right to Know—A Comparative View*, 21 ANGLO-AM. L. REV. 101, 106 (1992).

[87] *Cf.* JULIA NEUBERGER, ETHICS AND HEALTH CARE: THE ROLE OF RESEARCH ETHICS COMMITTEES IN THE UNITED KINGDOM (1992).

[88] SARAH BOSTON & JILL LOUW, DISORDERLY BREASTS 31 (1987). More recently, Professor Baum has suggested a new way to conduct randomized clinical trials (RCTs) of treatment for "ladylike cancers." In his words, "Since women, unlike men, enjoy a natural generosity of spirit, it should not be too difficult to establish an organization of women, committed to fight cancer on all fronts . . . . If we were to establish a Europe-wide organization with a membership of a million women over the age of 35, 1 in 1,000 of these will get breast cancer each year, about 1 in 2,000 will get ovarian cancer, and one in 4,000 cervical cancer." In Professor Baum's scheme, all one million women will have been kept informed of ongoing cancer research, "and thus they will not only expect to be offered entry into a controlled trial, but perhaps even demand it." Most important is Baum's continuing view that informed consent is a "charade," and that his plan (which rests on the unlikely proposition that both arms of all RCTs of female cancer are always better than currently accepted treatment) will advance science and let women fulfill their moral (if uninformed, or misinformed) obligation to take part in his research. Michael Baum, *New Approach for Recruitment into Randomised Controlled Trials*, 341 LANCET 812, 813 (1993).

tic and autocratic manner of the past."[89] As we will see evidenced more starkly in Japan, cancer is often a loaded term in British medical practice,[90] and Boston and Louw observe:

> Our society regards the word cancer as a taboo word and its usage is still evaded, particularly by doctors in talking to their patients.... It is often the patient herself who wants and needs the word spelled out clearly to grasp the reality.[91]

Consumer complaints about continuing medical paternalism have had some effect. For example, the NHS took Lord Bridge's *Sidaway* statement seriously and issued *Patient Consent to Examination or Treatment*, and a *Guide to Consent for Examination or Treatment*, to all NHS doctors in September of 1990.[92] NHS intended these documents to govern NHS practice, and included the statement, "where treatment carries substantial risks the patient must be advised of this by the doctor so that consent may be well-informed." Christopher Heneghan, a surgeon at Ealing Hospital, subsequently responded in *The Lancet* with a textbook example of persisting medical paternalism. He argued that the Department's advice is "clearly wrong," and puts patients "at risk by giving them so much information that they refuse *necessary* treatment."[93] It hardly needs pointing out that what a doctor views as necessary treatment for a particular patient may not be what that patient considers necessary in the context of his or her particular life circumstances. A recent study suggests that British doctors and not their patients are the ones who really fear that imparting information unnecessarily raises patient anxiety.[94]

C. Japan

As an island nation with a homogeneous population enjoying universal access to reasonably priced medical care, Japan resembles the United Kingdom. But while Japan has borrowed many aspects of Western culture during this century, it has retained its unique cultural identity. For example, its universal health insurance is patterned on the German model organized around employment,[95] but other aspects of the German system have been rejected.[96] Although it is impossible to encapsulate a culture in one person's works, Japan's great writer, Yukio Mishima, probably spoke for the Japanese people and their culture as articulately as anyone can. In *Temple of Dawn*, the lawyer Honda contemplates death at the same time he contemplates taking a mistress:

> If Honda had been so inclined, he could have selected the most beautiful of the young geishas and become her patron. It could be a pleasure to buy her

[89] *Id. Cf.* Thurstan Brewin, *Truth, Trust and Paternalism*, 2 LANCET 490 (1985).

[90] *Cf.* Clive Seale, *Communication and Awareness About Death: A Study of a Random Sample of Dying People*, 32 SOC. SCI. MED. 943 (1991).

[91] BOSTOW & LOUW, *supra* note 88, at 32.

[92] National Health Service management documents (1990) (issued by the Department of Health).

[93] Christopher Heneghan, *Medicine and the Law: Consent to Medical Treatment*, 337 LANCET 421 (1991) (emphasis added).

[94] D.D. Kerrigan et al., *Who's Afraid of Informed Consent?*, 306 BRIT. MED. J. 298 (1993).

[95] *See* sources cited *supra* note 14.

[96] *See* Naoki Ikegami, *The Economics of Health Care in Japan*, 258 SCI. 614 (1992) (describing the Japanese health care system). *See also* sources cited *supra* note 14.

> anything she requested and enjoy her coquetry, tenuous as a spring cloud . . . those tiny feet so neatly clad in white custom-made *tabi*. She would be a perfectly dressed doll in her kimono. All this could belong to him. But he could at once foresee the conclusion. *Boiling water of passion would overflow and the dancing ashes of death would fly up to blind him.*[97]

The Japanese people may seem to deny death in daily life as much as Americans do, but, as this passage reflects, their literature express its inevitability without romance.

Japan has yet to accept the doctrine of informed consent. "Nonetheless ever since Professor Koichi Bai introduced the West German legal concept of informed consent into Japanese academic legal theory in 1970, the number of medical malpractice suits alleging the physician's breach of duty to obtain informed consent has increased steadily."[98] However, "the right of the patient to take part in the decision-making process to a large extent remains ignored."[99]

Japan's leading informed consent decision, *Makino v. The Red Cross Hospital*, involves the information disclosed to a cancer patient.[100] In January of 1983, Makino went to a major hospital in Nagoya complaining of stomach pain. Her doctors told her that they suspected a gall bladder condition and asked her to return in a week for more tests. At that time they had made a preliminary diagnosis of cholecystic cancer, a diagnosis which they reaffirmed on three additional visits within the month. However, they never communicated their suspicions to the patient. Her physicians wanted a biopsy to make a definitive diagnosis, but they did not tell her the real reason for wanting her to return for surgery. Instead they simply told her she had "a rather bad gall bladder."

Makino had planned a trip to Singapore in March, and made an appointment to return to the hospital in April. She later canceled the appointment, and never returned because she felt quite well. In June, however, she collapsed and was treated for cancer at another hospital. She died in December. The lawsuit filed by her husband and children alleged that the hospital should have informed her (or her husband) of the preliminary cancer diagnosis in January or February, and that their failure to do so induced the patient to make a mistaken and fatal judgment to postpone treatment.

The district court ruled that physicians have a duty to make diagnoses and to provide adequate treatment. Physicians must also inform patients *or* their families about the nature of the illness, the expected course of therapy, and its anticipated effects, "'since the patient has a right to self-determination on his own therapy.' How such information should be given is in the discretion of the doctor to the extent that the patient's right of self-determination is not infringed."[101] Except for the

---

[97] YUKIO MISHIMA, THE TEMPLE OF DAWN 195 (1973) (emphasis added).

[98] Hiroyuki Hattori et al., *The Patient's Right to Information in Japan—Legal Rules and Doctor's Opinions*, 32 SCI. MED. 1007, 1009 (1991) [hereinafter *Patient's Right in Japan*].

[99] *Id.* at 1007.

[100] Our description of this case is taken entirely from Norio Higuchi, *The Patient's Right to Know of a Cancer Diagnosis: A Comparison of Japanese Paternalism and American Self-Determination*, 31 WASHBURN L.J. 455, 458-61 (1992) (citing Judgment of May 29, 1989 (Makino v. The Red Cross Hospital), Chisai [Nagoya District Court], 1325 Hanji 103 (Japan)). *See also* Fred Hiatt, *Japan Court Ruling Backs Doctors; Judge Says That Patients May Be Kept Ignorant of Their Illnesses*, WASH. POST, May 30, 1989, at A9.

[101] Higuchi, *supra* note 100, at 460 (quoting Makino).

family's involvement, to this point the opinion is fairly consistent with those of most U.S. courts. However, the right enunciated was quickly gutted. The decision articulated a wide-open therapeutic privilege which permits doctors to decide, in their discretion, when, to whom, and in how much detail information shall be conveyed.

The court concluded in *Makino* that since the physicians had never confirmed their diagnosis of cholecystic cancer by biopsy, they had no duty to disclose their suspicions. Moreover, even if such a final diagnosis had been made, "it would be unreasonable" to require physicians to disclose the diagnosis of a virtually incurable disease to a patient.[102] Finally, such a diagnosis is most properly disclosed to the family, *not* the patient. The *Makino* court found that the defendant-physicians' plan to disclose only upon the subsequent hospital admission, which the patient canceled, was reasonable. Further, the court held that the doctors had no duty to do anything more than they had done.[103]

Japanese commentator Norio Higuchi found this case very helpful, noting that:

> [T]he decision takes a step forward at the least, even though, I admit, it is only a small step, from the previous rulings by courts. While the prior decisions have held it depends upon the doctor's discretion whether he should inform or not, the court says that the discretion in the doctor is limited to the questions as to whom, when and in how much detail he should inform.[104]

Professor Higuchi also argues that to conclude that the court found a duty to disclose and a right to self-determination only after a definitive diagnosis has been made oversimplifies the opinion. Instead Higuchi believes that the physician had a duty to inform under the facts of this case, but properly exercised his discretion about how to inform the patient within the confines of that duty.[105]

A Westerner is struck not so much with the amount of discretion ceded to physicians (essentially the state of U.S. law prior to the 1970s, and of British law today), but by the accepted concept that informing the patient's family is equivalent to informing the patient herself. The Japanese concept of dependency may best explain the failure of informed consent to be adopted.[106] Professor Rihito Kimura explains:

> Autonomy . . . is out of keeping with the Japanese cultural tradition. Our culture, nurtured in Buddhist and Confucian teaching, has developed the idea of suppressing the egoistic self. To be autonomous and independent is sometimes regarded as egocentric. Thus, in Japan each human being is dependent on others in the family, and the social, economic and political communities.[107]

---

[102] *Id.*

[103] *Id.* at 461.

[104] *Id.* at 462 (footnote omitted).

[105] *Id.* at 463. Other commentators have not been so kind. *See, e.g.*, Noritoshi Tanida, *Patients' Rights in Japan*, 337 LANCET 242, 243 (1991).

[106] *See, e.g.*, RUTH BENEDICT, THE CHRYSANTHEMUM AND THE SWORD (1946); TAKEO DOI, THE ANATOMY OF DEPENDENCE (1971). Takeo Doi is unimpressed by individualism in America, however. As he observes about American conformity, "even in a society in which individuals stand out, the appearance of real individuals is strangely absent." TAKEO DOI, THE ANATOMY OF SELF 57 (1985).

[107] Rhito Kimura, *In Japan, Parents Participate but Doctors Decide*, HASTINGS CTR. REP., Aug. 1986, at 22, 23.

Stephan Salzberg argues in his study of Japan's mental health laws that in the Japanese world view, "autonomy, to a lesser or greater extent, yields to the nurturance and security provided by one's group, and especially one's family."[108] He notes that obtaining consent from family members instead of from the patient "is a common practice... especially when patients themselves are kept in the dark regarding their own cancerous or other life-threatening conditions."[109] Other Japanese observers concur:

> Even in cases where the patient is competent to give his or her individual consent, substitute consent by the family or close relatives is a common practice in order to avoid disturbing the patient emotionally . . . the Japanese favor being indirect and do not like complete information about a serious condition to be stated explicitly.[110]

Japan's failure to embrace Western notions of informed consent reflects the alternatives available in its health care system, which downplays the individual and hence de-emphasizes high-cost, low-yield technology. While the health sector emphasizes universal access and cost control, the general quality of care in Japan is lower than Western standards.[111] Medical training in Japan is relatively weak and classroom-based only, and little medical specialty certification exists. Physicians on average spend less than five minutes with each patient per visit, and all physicians are paid on the same tightly regulated fee-for-service schedule, regardless of individual experience or training. Doctors increase their incomes by seeing patients repeatedly, and by directly selling to them the average of five drugs that are prescribed at each clinical encounter. Moreover, drug retailing accounts for as much as forty percent of the average physician's income.[112] Doctors also tend to hospitalize most of their patients in private solo-practice office-based clinics which they own,[113] and where the average patient stay is fifty-two days.[114] Physicians resist sending patients to the relatively few Japanese hospitals offering sophisticated care, because patients tend not to return thereafter for the lower-technology services they offer.

These entrepreneurial aspects of medical practice explain why the citizens of Japan spend a larger percentage of their health care expenditures (thirty percent) on drugs than do the citizens of any other country.[115] The comparable U.S. figure, for

[108] Stephan M. Salzberg, *Japan's New Mental Health Law: More Light Shed on Dark Places?*, 14 INT'L J.L. & PSYCHIATRY 137, 153 (1991) (footnote omitted).

[109] *Id.*

[110] Tanida, *supra* note 105, at 1014.

[111] *See generally* Naoki Ikegami, *Japanese Health Care: Low Cost Through Regulated Fees*, 10 HEALTH AFF. 87 (1991).

[112] M. POWELL & M. ANESAKI, HEALTH CARE IN JAPAN (1990). *See also* Theodore R. Marmor, *Japan: A Sobering Lesson*, 14 HEALTH MGMT. Q. 10, 12 (1992).

[113] Japan had about 200,000 physicians in 1988; doctors are permitted to run their own nineteen-bed or smaller clinics—anything larger is classified as a hospital. About 30 percent of all Japanese physicians, called *Kaigyo-i*, or clinic doctors, own their own clinics. Their monthly income is approximately four times higher than that of hospital-based doctors. Aki Yoshikawa et al., *How Does Japan Do It? Doctors and Hospitals in a Universal Health Care System*, 3 STAN. L. & POL'Y REV. 111, 124 (1991). *See also* Martatoshi Abe, *Japan's Clinic Physicians and Their Behavior*, 20 SOC. SCI. MED. 335 (1985).

[114] Ikegami, *supra* note 111, at 89-90.

[115] *Id.*; Marmor, *supra* note 112, at 10 (quoting a 1980 figure of 38 percent).

example, is approximately five percent.[116] Not only do Japanese doctors prescribe (and sell) many drugs, but many of these drugs appear useless from a scientific perspective. For example Krestin, an anti-cancer drug with no proven efficacy anywhere else in the world, is one of the most popular drugs in Japan.[117] Physicians apparently feel less guilty about failing to inform patients that they have cancer when they can prescribe the ineffective Krestin, because it produces no debilitating side-effects.

In short, the Japanese health care system "works" at a comparatively low level of expenditure in large part because patients are rarely informed about diagnoses or about the relatively few available alternative forms of treatment. Major changes in the Japanese health care system will require doctors to give patients more information. Pressure is mounting to develop more specialty referral hospitals, but patients must be persuaded to utilize them. As the *Makino* case illustrates, more candid disclosures about diagnosis and treatment may be required in order to secure patient compliance with the therapy physicians do recommend.[118]

Japan also remains the only industrial society to reject brain death criteria, thus rendering heart transplantation currently impossible in Japanese hospitals. Some observers contend that difficult interpersonal relationships among families and physicians at the time of death generate this resistance.[119] Others believe it results from general religious or societal views about the innate meaning of death.[120] However, Japanese physicians must give families far more detailed explanations and much fuller disclosure—at a time when such discussions are not currently held—in order for Japan to implement brain death criteria. Perhaps as a portent of change, the Japanese Ministry of Health and Welfare has recently argued for modifications in traditional physician practices of nondisclosure.[121] The Ministry has concluded that even in the case of terminally ill cancer patients, the diagnosis should be revealed.[122]

---

[116] Gale Eisenstadt, *The Doctor's Margin*, FORBES, Nov. 23, 1992, at 44. The Japanese are the largest per capita consumers of drugs in the world, at $1,668 per capita in 1989, as compared with $1,098 in the United States. Mitsuru Mabuchi, *Doctor Criticizes Overdose of Ineffective Drugs in Japan*, JAPAN ECON. NEWSWIRE, Aug. 1, 1990. *See also Blaming Someone Else: Japan Needs Better Arrangements for Conducting Clinical Trials of New Therapeutic Drugs*, 371 NATURE 89 (1994).

[117] *A Shot in the Arm*, BUS. TOKYO, April 1992, at 40. Japanese doctors like to prescribe Krestin to "treat" a variety of cancer-related symptoms in order to avoid telling terminal patients the difficult truth. Though harmless, the drug has never been proven effective, and the Japanese Ministry of Health and Welfare recently warned doctors to reduce the number of prescriptions they write. *See also* Nicholas Kristof, *When Doctor Won't Tell Cancer Patient The Truth*, N.Y. TIMES, Feb. 25, 1995, at 2.

[118] *See* Ikegami, *supra* note 111.

[119] *See* Kate Brown, *Death and Access: Ethics in Cross-Cultural Health Care*, in CHOICES AND CONFLICT: EXPLORATIONS IN HEALTH CARE ETHICS 85, 87 (E. Friedman ed. 1992); *see also* Kazumasa Hoshino, *Legal Status of Brain Death in Japan: Why Many Japanese Do Not Accept "Brain Death" as a Definition of Death*, 7 BIOETHICS 234 (1993). Terminating treatment in persistent vegetative states has only recently even been discussed. *See Japanese Panel Backs 'Death With Dignity'*, AM. MED. NEWS, July 11, 1994, at 23.

[120] Brown, *supra* note 119, at 85; Hoshino, *supra* note 119, at 234; *Japanese Panel Backs 'Death With Dignity'*, *supra* note 119, at 23.

[121] N. Ianida, *Patients' Rights in Japan* (letter), 337 LANCET 242 (1991); *see* MELVIN KONNER, MEDICINE AT THE CROSSROADS 3-27 (1993).

[122] Ianida, *supra* note 121, at 242; *see* KONNER, *supra* note 121, at 3-27.

IV. CULTURE, CHOICE, AND HEALTH RESOURCE ALLOCATION

Patient knowledge advances personal autonomy; it elevates consent to medical treatment from a flak jacket merely protecting doctors from battery liability to an enhancement of patient sovereignty.[123] But as the foregoing discussion demonstrates, not all cultures place the same value on truth-telling and on an individual's ability to make fully informed choices, nor do they share the same fear of death.[124] Informed consent legal doctrine reflects and shapes societal value choices, and thus it varies from country to country, and from time to time within countries.

Total expenditures on health care vary considerably across national borders as well.[125] It is not a coincidence that the U.S., which treats health care as a market good, spends far more money on the health sector than does any other country in the world.[126] Moreover, it does so while approximately fourteen percent of its population remains uninsured. Three years ago, the U.S. spent 131 percent more per capita on health care than did Japan, and almost 200 percent more than did the U.K.[127] For all that expenditure, however, the U.S. trails behind the U.K., Japan, and many other industrialized nations in such basic health-outcome measurements as infant mortality, perinatal mortality, and male life expectancy.[128]

The U.S. accords the highest status in the world to informed consent in part because we engage in the fiction that patients actually exercise economic choice when they purchase medical services. However, individuals usually are better situated to exercise economic choice when they buy health insurance, or at least when choosing among competing insurance plans that their employers subsidize.[129] The luxury of choice is conspicuously curtailed for the approximately forty million of Americans who are still uninsured.

Health care markets have traditionally deviated significantly from the competitive ideal, propelled by a variety of forces.[130] Chief among these forces are information problems and purchasing subsidies. Medical information is often difficult for

---

[123] *Cf.*, L.J. Donaldson's description of consent in *Re J*, UK Court of Appeal (July 10, 1992), focusing on protection for the physician rather than for the patient.

[124] *See* AARON & SCHWARTZ, *supra* note 35 at 16-17.

[125] *See, e.g.*, U.S. GENERAL ACCOUNTING OFFICE, GOA/HRD-92-9, HEALTH CARE SPENDING CONTROL: THE EXPERIENCE OF FRANCE, GERMANY AND JAPAN (1991) [hereinafter HEALTH CARE SPENDING CONTROL]; George J. Schieber & Jean-Pierre Poullier, *International Health Spending and Utilization Trends*, 7 HEALTH AFF. 105 (1988).

[126] *See* U.S. DEPT. OF COMMERCE, STATISTICAL ABSTRACT OF THE UNITED STATES 1992, tbl. no. 1368, *Health Expenditures—Selected Countries: 1980-1990* 829 (1992). This is true whether one measures such expenditures in absolute terms, as a percentage of national GNP, or as a per capita expenditure. *Id.* Nor is it merely a fluke that the world's highest medical malpractice litigation rates, and its highest percentage of specialist physicians as compared with primary care doctors (family practitioners, internists and pediatricians), are found in the U.S. as well. Steven A. Schroeder, *Physician Supply and the U.S. Medical Marketplace*, 11 HEALTH AFF. 235 (1992). *Cf.* Basil S. Markesinis, *Litigation Mania in England, Germany and the USA: Are We So Very Different?*, 49 CAMB. L.J. 233 (1990).

[127] Leslie M. Greenwald, *Meaning in Numbers*, HEALTH MGMT. Q. 6, 7, tbl. 1 (Third Quarter 1992).

[128] *Id.* at 7, 9, tbl. 6.

[129] *Cf.* Clark Havighurst, *Prospective Self-Denial: Can Consumers Contract Today to Accept Health Care Rationing Tomorrow?*, 140 U. PA. L. REV. 1755 (1992).

[130] *See generally* Mark V. Pauly, *Is Medical Care Different? Old Questions, New Answers*, 13 J. HEALTH POL. POL'Y & L. 227, 233 (1988); *Competition in the Health Sector*, 1977 F. T. C. CONF. PROC.

patients to assimilate,[131] sometimes emotionally painful,[132] and in rare cases even potentially harmful[133] for them to absorb. Moreover, the financial ramifications of patients' treatment choices are usually obscured by health insurance and tax subsidies for medical and insurance purchases, if not by forthright governmental provision of care.[134] Defensive medicine[135] and the technological imperative[136] further skew health markets toward unnecessary services, particularly in the United States. Regulatory supply restrictions such as certificate of need programs make unsuccessful attempts to redress this imbalance.[137]

Different cultures take differing official approaches to health resource allocation. Some countries rely primarily on governmental price and spending controls that affect everything from technology acquisition to hospital and physician reimbursement rates. For example, in the circumstances of tightly managed supply that exist in the U.K., primary care physicians assume powerful gatekeeping functions. These general practitioners must filter patient demand for medical services from clinical "need" for limited specialist and high technology care. This filter entails correspondingly narrower scope for individual choice.[138] When medical choice is constrained by supply limitations, telling patients about potentially beneficial but economically unattainable therapy can be criticized as inhumane.[139] However, such

---

[131] Cathy J. Jones, *Autonomy and Informed Consent in Medical Decisionmaking: Toward a New Self-Fulfilling Prophecy*, 47 WASH. & LEE L. REV. 379, 428 (1990).

[132] Margaret A. Drickamer & Mark S. Lachs, *Should Patients with Alzheimer's Disease be Told Their Diagnosis?*, 326 NEW ENG. J. MED. 947 (1992). As diagnostic markers and therapy improve, doctors will be compelled to disclose painful information in order to secure informed consent for initiating therapy.

[133] *See* Elizabeth G. Patterson, *The Therapeutic Justification for Withholding Medical Information: What You Don't Know Can't Hurt You, or Can It?*, 64 NEB. L. REV. 721 (1985); Margaret A. Somerville, *Therapeutic Privilege: Variation on the Theme of Informed Consent*, 12 L. MED. & HEALTH CARE 4 (1984).

[134] The government itself furnishes health care under Great Britain's National Health Service. In the U.S., where approximately 41 percent of medical services are government-funded, government provides some services directly through institutions such as Veterans Administration, city, state and county hospitals, etc.

[135] *See* Kirk B. Johnson et al., *A Fault-Based Administrative Alternative for Resolving Medical Malpractice Claims*, 42 VAND. L. REV. 1365, 1394-95 (1989); E. Haavi Morreim, *Cost Containment and the Standard of Medical Care*, 75 CAL. L. REV. 1719, 1731 (1987). *But see* GEORGE J. ANNAS, STANDARD OF CARE: THE LAW OF AMERICAN BIOETHICS 4 (1993) [hereinafter STANDARD OF CARE]. ("[A]ny medical treatment done primarily to protect the physician from potential lawsuits [rather than to benefit the patient], although sometimes legal, is by definition unethical.").

[136] AARON & SCHWARTZ, *supra* note 35, at 66.

[137] *See generally* Frank A. Sloan et al., COST, QUALITY AND ACCESS IN HEALTH CARE: NEW ROLES FOR HEALTH PLANNING IN A COMPETITIVE ENVIRONMENT (1988). *Cf.* David A. Grimes, *Technology Follies: The Uncritical Acceptance of Medical Innovation*, 269 JAMA 3030 (1993). There is little doubt, however, that supply in large measure determines demand in medical care. This helps explain the paradox that the more organs become available for kidney, liver, and heart transplants in the United States, the longer the waiting lines for these transplants have grown. George J. Annas, *The Paradoxes of Organ Transplantation*, 78 AM. J. PUB. HEALTH 621 (1988).

[138] *See* Robert G. Lee & Frances H. Miller, *The Doctor's Changing Role in Allocating U.S. and British Medical Services*, 18 L. MED. & HEALTH CARE 69 (1990); Robert Schwartz & Andrew Grubb, *Why Britain Can't Afford Informed Consent*, HASTINGS CTR. REP., Aug. 1985, at 19.

[139] "The key to turning down the patient 'is not to get eyeball to eyeball with him because if you do there is no way you can actually say no.'" AARON & SCHWARTZ, *supra* note 35, at 107 (commenting on how British physicians cope with scarce medical resources).

disclosure can also mobilize public opinion to challenge resource allocation inconsistent with societal values.[140]

The General Medical Council (which licenses British doctors) explicitly reinforces the gatekeeping function by warning in its principles of professional conduct: "a specialist should not usually accept a patient without reference from the patient's general practitioner."[141] Violation of this "ethical" rule could at least theoretically result in licensure sanctions. However, the British Medical Association surely contemplates political activism on the part of the medical profession when its own ethical principles state, "the doctor may decide to tell the patient that [specialist] treatment is not available because of lack of funds," suggesting that "patients may complain to politicians."[142]

In countries officially dependent on gatekeeping like the U.K., informed consent doctrine not unsurprisingly favors professional rather than patient-oriented standards of disclosure, particularly with regard to treatment alternatives.[143] Other cultures—most prominently the U.S.—prefer to let a more entrepreneurial market set the basic dimensions for health sector investment.[144] U.S. informed consent law generally reflects support for market allocation mechanisms, and thus tends to expand the possibilities for patient choice through more thoroughgoing informed consent requirements.[145]

But how can we explain Japan, where physicians are highly entrepreneurial and most hospitals and all clinics are privately owned, yet where the law supports keeping patients in the dark about diagnoses of serious illness?[146] First, Japan does not impose the same budgetary controls that cap total health care spending in the U.K., although it regulates physician fees tightly and capped the number of hospital beds in 1985.[147] It is dangerous for outsiders to generalize about any society, but cultural analysts from both Japan and America agree that in Japan individuality is deemed subservient to group needs and ideals. As a consequence, the proper role of the patient is to follow the instructions of the physician, who presumably has a superior

[140] Miller, *supra* note 12, at 56-57.

[141] GENERAL MEDICAL COUNCIL (UK), PROFESSIONAL CONDUCT AND DISCIPLINE: FITNESS TO PRACTICE 22 (1991).

[142] BRITISH MEDICAL ASSOCIATION, PHILOSOPHY & PRACTICE OF MEDICAL ETHICS 73 (1988).

[143] On the U.K., see Schwartz and Grubb, *supra* note 138, at 19 (commenting on Sidaway v. Royal Bethlem Hospital, [1985] 2 W.L.R 483). *See generally* Frances H. Miller, *Informed Consent for the Man on the Clapham Omnibus: A British Cure for the "American Disease?"*, 9 W. NEW ENG. L. REV. 169 (1987).

[144] Successful health sector competition requires informed medical service purchasers; patients—or their surrogate purchasers—must understand diagnosis probabilities, treatment alternatives, risks, and personal costs of all kinds before making choices about consuming services. Such information traditionally emanates from providers, whose position on treatment issues may be entirely patient-centered, but could also be compromised for reasons ranging from altruistic paternalism, to scientific elitism, to direct conflict of economic interest.

[145] In the U.S., see Canterbury v. Spence, 464 F.2d 772 (D.C. Cir. 1972); Cobbs v. Grant, 502 P.2d 1 (Cal. 1972). Although the states are more or less split on patient-centered versus physician-dominated standards of disclosure, the trend is toward a patient-centered standard. Even though tort reform legislation in some states has modified patient-centered standards of disclosure, cultural expectations push toward disclosure of more complete information than is required in other countries.

[146] *See* James Sterngold, *Japan's Health Care: Cradle, Grave and No Frills*, N.Y. TIMES, Dec. 28, 1992, at A1.

[147] Ikegami, *supra* note 111, at 614.

understanding of the patient's illness and its significance.[148]

Regardless of official government policy concerning health sector resource allocation, more or less flexibility concerning that policy usually exists within any society in practice. This flexibility is strongly influenced by the general cultural attitude toward death, and by what patients, health policy experts, and financiers actually know or believe about the availability and efficacy of medical services.[149] In the majority of industrialized nations, where health care is considered a public good essentially guaranteed by government, spending caps, regulated fees, and central planning for capital expenditures are philosophically *de rigueur.*[150]

This tradition is under severe challenge. Even the U.K., a long-standing and successful showcase for socialized medicine, in 1991 introduced competitive forces to boost efficiency in the National Health Service.[151] By separating the government's provider function from its purchaser role, the NHS now forces health care institutions to compete for explicitly capped government funds.[152] On the other hand, the U.S., which treats health care as a private good and espouses health sector competition as the primary allocation device, has elected a President committed on record (at least at one time) to collectivist ideas about spending caps.[153] Anyone with a good imagination can visualize American and European ships of state steaming right past one another in mid-Atlantic, each vainly searching the other's shores for solutions to the woes besetting domestic health systems.

Perfect health sector efficiency and equity are unattainable goals for any society. Neither scientific truth nor the human condition remain static,[154] and economic resources are never infinite. Setting limits on medical expenditures seems related to a society's view of mortality, but it begins with a recognition that limits are *necessary*. British Minister of Health Enoch Powell once aptly described the demand for medical care as potentially infinite:

---

[148] *See* Tanida, *supra* note 105, at 1014.

[149] Providers have been deliberately omitted here, although their treatment recommendations give them a particularly powerful position in decision-making at the micro level, because they "sell" rather than buy medical services.

[150] *See* Brian Abel-Smith, *Cost Containment and New Priorities in the European Community*, 70 MILBANK Q. 393 (1992); HEALTH CARE SPENDING CONTROL, supra note 125. However, European countries such as the Netherlands, which ensures residents virtually universal access to basic health services though a mix of mandatory and voluntary health insurance, are currently exploring reforms to increase health sector competition. CHRIS HAM ET AL., HEALTH CHECK: HEALTH CARE REFORMS IN AN INTERNATIONAL CONTEXT (1990); J. Van Londen, *Netherlands: Rational Choices In Health Care*, 340 LANCET 228 (1992).

[151] National Health Service and Community Care Act, 1990, ch. 19 (Eng.).

[152] Frances H. Miller, *Competition Law and Anticompetitive Physician Behavior*, 55 MOD. L. REV. 453, 455-63 (1992). Sweden is also contemplating competition initiatives to improve state-provided medical services. Richard B. Saltman, *Competition and Reform in the Swedish Health System*, 64 MILBANK Q. 597 (1990).

[153] Paul Cotton, *Less is More and More is Less in Health Care: Proposals Offered in '92 Campaign*, 268 JAMA 1635-39 (1992). Moreover, the state of Oregon has implemented overt rationing for its Medicaid patients, after the Clinton Administration waived Medicaid conditions of participation to enable Oregon to limit treatment for certain medical conditions.

[154] P. B. Beeson, *Changes in Medical Therapy During the Past Half Century, in* MEDICINE 59, 79-99 (1980) (value of 60 percent of remedies in first edition of Cecil's Textbook of Medicine rated as harmful, dubious or merely symptomatic by the time the 14th edition was published; only 3 percent offered fully effective prevention or treatment by then-current standards).

> There is virtually no limit to the amount of medical care an individual is capable of absorbing . . . not only is the range of treatable conditions huge and rapidly growing; there is also a vast range of quality in the treatment of these conditions . . . . There is hardly a type of condition from the most trivial to the gravest which is not susceptible of alternative treatments under conditions affording a wide range of skill, care, comfort, privacy, efficiency [etc.] . . . there is a multiplier effect of successful medical treatment. Improvement in expectation of survival results in lives that demand further medical care. The poorer (medically speaking) the quality of the lives preserved by advancing medical science, the more intense are the demands they continue to make. In short, the appetite for medical treatment *vient en mangeant.*[155]

Any country's health policy must continuously grapple with economic scarcity and with scientific, political, and cultural change. The successes and failures of other systems can be illuminating, but cultural attitudes toward medical information and other medical issues as well must be unearthed and understood if reform imported from other countries can succeed in new environments.[156] Of course, societies and medical practitioners must grapple with the role of malpractice litigation in setting standards of care.

Customary medical practice, the standard against which a doctor's conduct is usually measured in a medical malpractice action, reflects the way resources are spent on care for individual patients in every culture.[157] Since patients rarely refuse their doctors' recommendations for therapy, physician treatment preferences strongly influence the way societies allocate total health resources. But the concept of customary medical practice defies precise definition. What doctors actually *do* develops gradually over time as physicians adapt treatment to scientific advance, economic rewards and penalties, and more generalized legal and cultural incentives, especially a society's attitude toward death.[158] In most countries the evolution of medical custom over the past few decades can be diagrammed as shown in Figure 1, revealing a generally upward trajectory in the direction of more intensive—and expensive—medical services. In the U.S., the managed care initiatives of the past decade have somewhat tempered the ascent of that curve. However, some fear that more universal health insurance will usher in an era of more Draconian cost containment, in which we will begin rationing necessary services instead of merely reducing superfluous care.[159]

In reality, customary medical practice does not conform to the precisely defined concept pictured abstractly as a single line in Figure 1.[160] John Wennberg and

[155] KLEIN, *supra* note 75, at 67-68; *see also*, STANDARD OF CARE, *supra* note 135.

[156] Lawrence H. Thompson, *Observations on "Cost Containment and New Priorities in the European Community" by Brian Abel-Smith*, 70 MILBANK Q. 417 (1992).

[157] Richard E. Leahy, *Rational Health Policy and the Legal Standard of Care: A Call for Judicial Deference to Medical Practice Guidelines*, 77 CAL. L. REV. 1483, 1484 (1989).

[158] For a detailed look at U.S. financial incentives, see STEVEN R. EASTAUGH, HEALTH CARE FINANCE: ECONOMIC INCENTIVES AND PRODUCTIVITY ENHANCEMENT (1992).

[159] *See generally* Symposium, *Rationing Health Care: Social, Political and Legal Perspectives*, 18 AM. J. L. & MED. 1 (1992); Symposium, *The Law and Policy of Health Care Rationing: Models and Accountability*, 140 U. PA. L. REV. 1505 (1992).

[160] In the U.S., the practice guidelines and total quality improvement initiatives have sensitized many health professionals and policy makers to the broad range of physician

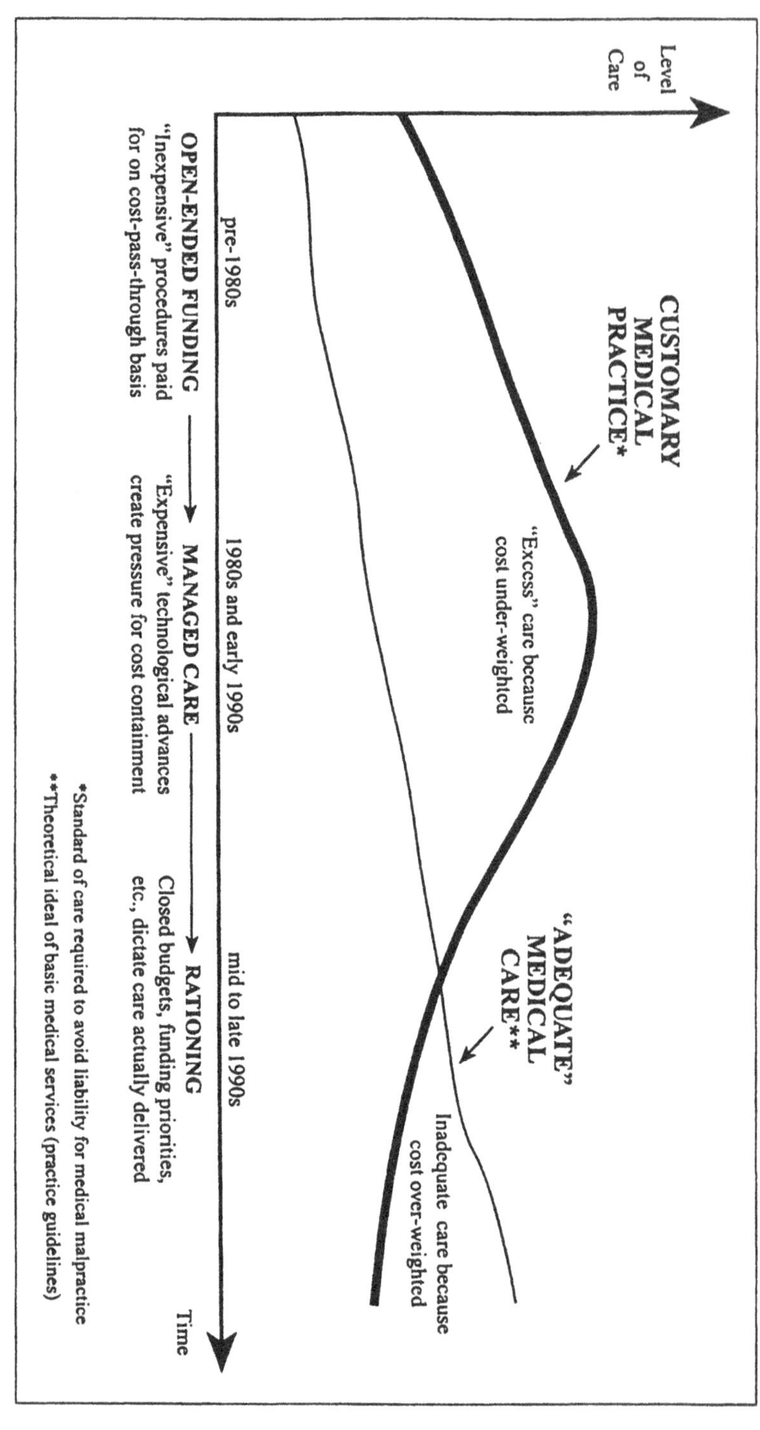

FIGURE 1. CUSTOMARY MEDICAL PRACTICE OVER TIME.

others have convincingly demonstrated that physicians' treatment choices vary widely, and are often influenced as much by individual training as by scientific evidence.[161] The medical literature also documents persuasively that when physicians receive additional income from their diagnostic methods or their treatment recommendations, utilization increases dramatically.[162] Similar physicians thus often do completely dissimilar things for identically situated patients for widely varying reasons.

Rather than the single line depicted in the foregoing diagram, customary practice actually constitutes a wide band of professional behavior, whose outer borders reflect the extremes of individual physicians' practice preferences. At any given moment, doctors employing a wide variety of treatments and skills for identical conditions may be practicing nonnegligently in the eyes of the law.[163] Nonetheless, they might also be providing superfluous or deficient care from the viewpoint of scientifically demonstrable safety and efficacy.[164] The concept of customary medical care can simultaneously embrace both completely useless medical services and downright dangerous dereliction of duty, because it is ordinarily derived from what physicians actually *do*, not from what they *should* do. This reality is depicted in the following refinement of the first diagram (see Figure 2).

Well-documented evidence of unwarranted treatment variations gave rise to U.S. practice guidelines and total quality improvement movements. These U.S. variations prepare the uninitiated for the startlingly expansive spectrum of diagnostic and therapeutic strategies conventionally utilized for identical medical conditions in other industrialized nations.[165] These sometimes radically different approaches produce nearly identical or even better results than our own as measured by standard morbidity and mortality indices.[166] Surgical intervention rates adjusted for population difference illustrate this point. U.S. surgeons performed more than six times as many hysterectomies as did their Japanese counterparts in 1980, and twice as many

---

treatment preferences parading under the banner of customary practice. *See generally* Peter G. Goldschmidt, *Can Practice Guidelines Reduce Malpractice Claims?*, 267 JAMA 2602 (1992); Leahy, *supra* note 157; Morreim, *supra* note 135, at 1731-36.

[161] John E. Wennberg, *Dealing with Medical Practice Variations: A Proposal for Action*, 3 HEALTH AFF. 6 (1984); John E. Wennberg, *Variations in Medical Care Among Small Areas*, 126 SCI. AM. 120 (1984).

[162] *See, e.g.*, Thomas S. Crane, *The Problem of Physician Self-Referral under the Medicare and Medicaid Antikickback Statute*, 268 JAMA 85 (1992); Bruce Hillman et al., *Physicians' Utilization and Charges for Outpatient Diagnostic Imaging in a Medicare Population*, 268 JAMA 2050 (1992); Jean Mitchell et al., *Physician Ownership of Physical Therapy Services: Effects on Charges, Utilization, Profits, and Service Characteristics*, 268 JAMA 2055 (1992). *See generally* MARC A. RODWIN, MEDICINE, MONEY & MORALS (1993).

[163] Barry R. Furrow, *Medical Malpractice and Cost Containment: Tightening the Screws*, 36 CASE W. RES. L. REV. 985, 1008-10 (1986).

[164] *See* Gordon Guyat et al., *Evidence-Based Medicine: A New Approach to Teaching the Practice of Medicine*, 268 JAMA 2420 (1992) (advocating a de-emphasis on "intuition, unsystematic clinical experience, and pathologic rationale as sufficient grounds for clinical decision-making").

[165] *See generally* MEDICINE & CULTURE, *supra* note 15.

[166] Of the three countries compared in this article, in 1988 the U.S. spent the most per capita and had the worst statistics with regard to infant mortality, perinatal mortality and male life expectancy. Japan spent less per capita than any other of the three countries except the U.K. and had the best statistics in these areas. Leslie M. Greenwald, *Meaning in Numbers*, HEALTH MGMT. Q., Third Quarter, 1992, at 9, tbl. 6.

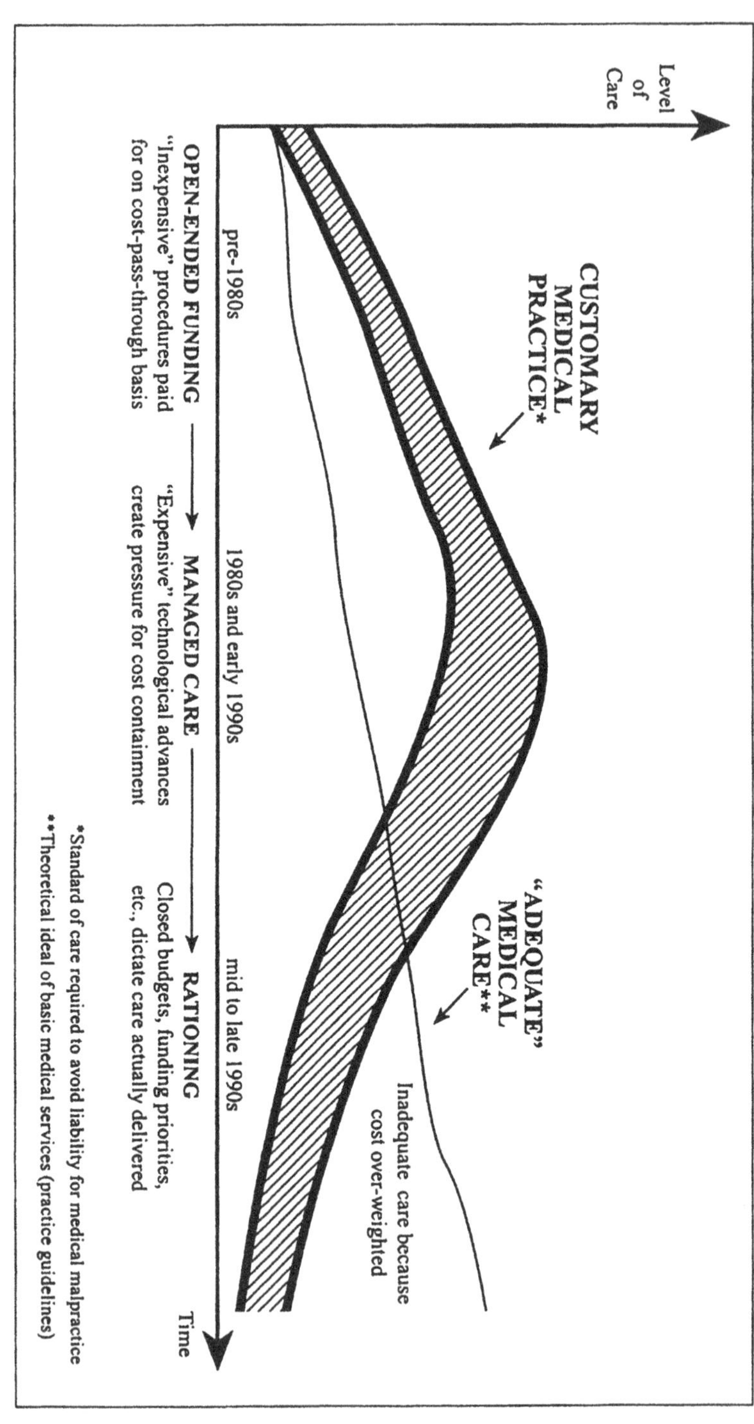

FIGURE 2. RANGE OF CUSTOMARY MEDICAL PRACTICE OVER TIME.

as doctors performed in the U.K.[167] They carried out ten times as many coronary artery bypass operations as did U.K. physicians, and *sixty* times as many as were done in Japan.[168] On the other hand, Japanese physicians performed almost twice as many appendectomies in that same year as did doctors in the U.S. or the U.K.[169]

Although environmental and demographic factors may explain some of these variations, cultural expectations and reimbursement patterns in each country play a central role in the frequency of surgical procedures.[170] If we had depicted customary medical practice in the world's industrialized nations on the foregoing diagram, the width of the customary practice band would be so wide as to render the term "customary" meaningless.

V. CULTURE AND DEATH

How can we account for the continuing formal differences in informed consent doctrine in the U.S., Britain, and Japan, notwithstanding burgeoning respect for autonomy in the latter countries and a new appreciation for setting limits in the U.S.? Perhaps even though the governing legal theories are different and reflect different cultural expectations, physician disclosure practices are actually quite similar. Japan's most famous case of nondisclosure involved the late Emperor Hirohito, who died in 1989 without ever having being told that he was suffering from intestinal cancer.[171] Although Americans tend to react smugly when told about the Hirohito case, on further reflection one might conclude that we may treat our own "emperors" in somewhat the same way.

In 1991 Paul Tsongas was a strong contender for the Democratic Presidential nomination, and one of the centerpieces of his campaign concerned his successful fight against cancer. After the election it was revealed that his illness had recurred in 1987, and he suffered an additional recurrence in late 1992. How much Tsongas knew about his prognosis remains unclear, as is how much his physicians told him after his initial bone marrow transplant. Tsongas may sincerely have believed that the operation "cured" him of cancer, and if so his physicians apparently did nothing to dissuade him or the American public from that belief. As physician-reporter Lawrence Altman put it, "No less than the outcome of the 1992 Presidential primaries, and thus the election itself, could have been influenced by . . . [Tsongas' treating physicians'] withholding of critical information."[172] Even after his second recurrence Tsongas told a press conference that he "had not discussed his progno-

[167] McPherson, *supra* note 25, at 22.

[168] *Id.* Japan has relatively few sophisticated tertiary care hospitals; open heart surgery is for that reason alone relatively rare. Only two percent of hospital beds are designated for intensive care of medical and surgical patients (compared with more than six percent in the U.S.). C.A. Sirio et al., *An Initial Comparison of Intensive Care in Japan and the United States*, 20 CRITICAL CARE MED. 1207 (1992).

[169] McPherson, *supra* note 25. Japanese doctors are paid fee-for-service, and many are thought to perform unnecessary routine surgery to generate higher incomes. Pathology reports on excised appendixes reveal that approximately sixty percent were not diseased. ROEMER, *supra* note 14, at 160.

[170] *See generally* McPherson, *supra* note 25.

[171] Susan Chira, *Hirohito, 124th Emperor of Japan, is Dead at 87*, N.Y. TIMES, Jan. 7, 1989, at 1.

[172] Lawrence K. Altman, *Tsongas's Health: Privacy and the Public's Right*, N.Y. TIMES, Jan. 17, 1993, at 26.

sis in detail with his doctors."[173]

The cases of Hirohito and Tsongas support the view that complete physician candor with patients is not universally observed in any culture, at least not when dealing with cancer or other life-threatening illness. Surveys of American physicians also support the hypothesis that while physicians recognize their legal obligation to inform patients about diagnosis and the risks of recommended treatment, they are much less forthcoming about prognosis. For example, a major 1982 survey of Americans and their physicians performed for the President's Commission for the Study of Ethical Problems in Medicine and Biomedical and Behavioral Research found that eighty-five percent of Americans would want their physicians to give them a "realistic estimate of how long" they had to live if they had "a type of cancer that usually leads to death in less then a year."[174] On the other hand, more than half of all U.S. physicians would either refuse to speculate on how long a patient "with a fully confirmed diagnosis of lung cancer in an advanced stage" would live, or would say that "you can't tell how long he might live, but stress that it could be for a substantial period of time."[175]

In a more recent but smaller study, Japanese researcher Naoko Miyaji conducted structured interviews with thirty-two east coast physicians in various specialties. She found that while physicians routinely told patients about their diagnosis, when dealing with prognosis "many physicians try to give patients very vague information."[176] Statistically, her results were virtually identical to those found by the President's Commission: half of the physicians would not explicitly tell patients they were dying. Physicians often justify their evasion by explaining that patients usually know this anyway, but as Miyaji observes, there may be "a significant gap between the patient's perception and the physician's."[177] Miyaji notes that information-giving can be used by physicians to control the situation as much as information-withholding. Regarding prognosis information she concludes:

> physicians' focusing on treatment options and leaving out prognosis (the worse part of the information) is the key to understanding the coexistence of information control with patient-centered ethical norms in the context of current American medicine.[178]

These studies and the facts in *Arato*[179] support the proposition that U.S. doctors behave similarly to those Japanese physicians who will not tell patients they have cancer because they believe patients see cancer as a death sentence and will be unnecessarily depressed. They also behave as do British doctors, who are able to rationalize economic limits on their ability to offer cancer patients every kind of sophisticated therapy so long as they can avoid getting "eyeball to eyeball," where

---

[173] Lawrence K. Altman, *Tsongas Says He Mishandled Issue of His Cancer*, N.Y. TIMES, Dec. 1, 1991, at A1.

[174] PRESIDENT'S COMMISSION FOR THE STUDY OF ETHICAL PROBLEMS IN MEDICINE AND BIOMEDICAL AND BEHAVIORAL RESEARCH, MAKING HEALTH CARE DECISIONS, VOL. TWO: APPENDICES, EMPIRICAL STUDIES OF INFORMED CONSENT 221-24, 245 (1982).

[175] *Id.* at 246.

[176] Naoko T. Miyaji, *The Power of Compassion: Truth-Telling Among American Doctors in the Care of Dying Patients*, 36 SOC. SCI. MED. 249, 257 (1993).

[177] *Id.*

[178] *Id.* at 262.

[179] *See supra* text accompanying notes 49-58.

frank conversation might have to ensue.[180] Not surprisingly, the hospice movement, which rejects heroic medical treatment and is openly designed to ease the natural transition to death, first flowered in England.[181]

We hypothesize that a culture's general attitude toward death dictates what prognosis information physicians will provide to patients, as well as how both physicians and patients view reasonable medical interventions throughout their adult lives. Where cultures are more homogeneous than the U.S., such as those of Japan and England, we would expect more cultural agreement on treatment recommendations. Prognosis disclosure may therefore be less important. Moreover, the closer the physician and patient are in terms of economic class and attitudes toward death, the less likely explicit disclosure will be seen as necessary or appropriate. In the U.S., because cultural diversity is more pronounced and a wider gulf between the economic and spiritual belief systems of physicians and their patients may exist, the law may be more needed to enforce disclosures because patients cannot "trust" their doctors to act based on shared values. Even legal sanctions, however, will often be insufficient to make candid disclosure a reality.

Ultimately a culture's view of death, and the role of medicine in preventing or postponing it, is at work when unpleasant or uncertain medical facts are not communicated to patients. In the U.S., for example, we usually seem to accept that prolonging life (at virtually any price) is a reasonable goal for medicine. Thus, procedures are introduced and utilized that offer hope of extending life without regard to cost, or even to the quality of the life prolonged. As two physician commentators describe it, "The medical profession in the United States has reflected our society's unwillingness to accept death as part of life and to face it with some humility . . . how sterile and technological our profession has become."[182]

Our seemingly automatic use of technology to protract the dying process has spawned development of a clearly articulated legal right to refuse treatment. More than fifty state appeals court decisions and an opinion of the U.S. Supreme Court have affirmed this patient prerogative.[183] In a country where still no right of access to basic health services exists, and where the major problem for approximately forty million Americans is obtaining any medical care outside hospital emergency departments, the development of such a right seems remarkable. The rallying cry of U.S. medical ethics has been focused more on the "right to die" than on the right to health care.[184] We continue to debate physician-assisted suicide and euthanasia far more passionately than we debate the appropriate minimum benefit package.[185] Ameri-

---

[180] AARON & SCHWARTZ, *supra* note 35, at 107.

[181] *See* Cicely Saunders, *Dying They Live: St. Christopher's Hospice*, *in* NEW MEANINGS OF DEATH 153-79 (H. Feifel ed., 1977). Recently, the House of Lords specifically articulated that not only may competent patients decline medical treatment, but artificial feeding may also be withheld from patients in a persistent vegetative state. Airedale NHS Trust v. Bland, 2 WLR 316 (1993) (Eng.).

[182] C. Cassel & D. Meier, *Morals and Moralism in the Debate over Euthanasia and Assisted Suicide*, 323 NEW ENG. J. MED. 750, 751 (1990).

[183] *See, e.g.*, Cruzan v. Director, Mo. Dep't Health, 497 U.S. 490 (1989). *See also* ALAN MEISEL, THE RIGHT TO DIE (1989).

[184] *See* STANDARD OF CARE, *supra* note 135, at 85-118.

[185] *See* NEW YORK STATE TASK FORCE ON LIFE AND THE LAW, WHEN DEATH IS SOUGHT (1994); MARGARET BATTIN, THE LEAST WORST DEATH (1994); Michigan v. Kevorkian, No. 9951, 1994 Mich. LEXIS 3033 (Dec. 13, 1994). In November, 1994, Oregon passed its Ballot Measure 16, which gives legal immunity to physicians prescribing lethal drugs to their competent, terminally ill patients who request them. *See* George J. Annas, *Prescribing Death: The*

cans rightly fear that doctors often ignore their wishes to refuse treatment, and to have proper medication for pain control near the end of life. Physician surveys consistently indicate that doctors routinely ignore patient wishes to end treatment, undermedicate for pain, and continue to see death as professional failure.[186]

Jay Katz made many of these points more than a decade ago in his insightful book *The Silent World of Doctor and Patient*.[187] Katz noted that American physicians may fear death even more than their patients. They use silence to protect themselves from their own fears and to avoid discussing the uncertainties of medical treatments with their patients. But, as Katz notes, such silence amounts to abandoning the patient, who may suffer more from "premortem loneliness" and isolation than from the prospect of dying itself.[188] If patients and physicians are to communicate effectively with one another, Katz argues that physicians must learn to share uncertainty with their patients, especially near death. He also argued, as we do, that honest disclosures "about the elective nature of many treatments—about the benefits of their employment or delay, and about the risks of intervention or delay" could play a vital role in helping to contain medical costs.[189]

Daniel Callahan has gone even further, and seems correct in asserting that the U.S. health care system is ultimately driven by an attempt to cope with our own mortality.[190] Illness is seen not as leading to inevitable death, but as a challenge to be overcome. Callahan has compared improvements in medical care with space exploration, noting that, "No matter how far you go, there's always farther you can go."[191] He believes U.S. society will never accept limits on either medical expenditures or personal autonomy until we learn to accept our own mortality. In his words:

> To me, the great question is: How are we going to think about progress in the future? What kind of progress is genuinely of benefit to people? . . . I think the answer has to be something more complex than the fact that people get sick and die. For me, the fundamental reality underlying progress is that *no matter how far we go, people are still going to get sick and they are still going to die.* No matter how much money we throw into progress, that fundamental human reality will remain.[192]

Callahan has also said that there are no *acceptable* causes of death in the U.S. We set up national institutes of health designed to prevent death from all its leading causes.[193] Ivan Illich argues that in "every society the dominant image of death determines the prevalent concept of health . . . . A society's image of death reveals the level of independence of its people, their personal relatedness, self-reliance and aliveness."[194] Illich traces Western civilization's view of death as it has evolved from "God's call,"

Oregon Initiative, 33 NEW ENG. J. MED. 1240 (1994) [hereinafter *Prescribing Death*].

[186] *See, e.g.* M. Z. Solomon et al., *Decisions Near the End of Life: Professional Views on Life-Sustaining Treatments*, 83 AM. J. PUB. HEALTH 14 (1993).

[187] JAY KATZ, THE SILENT WORLD OF DOCTOR AND PATIENT 219 (1984).

[188] *Id.* at 223, citing Avery D. Weisman & Thomas P. Hackett, *Predilection to Death: Death and Dying as a Psychiatric Problem*, 23 PSYCHOSOMATIC MEDICINE 232, 250-51 (1961).

[189] *Id.* at 228.

[190] Daniel Callahan, *Living Within Limits: The Future of Health Care*, 7 TRENDS HEALTH CARE L. & ETHICS 15, 16 (1992).

[191] *Id.* at 16.

[192] *Id.* (emphasis added).

[193] D. CALLAHAN, THE TROUBLED DREAM OF LIFE: LIVING WITH MORTALITY (1993).

[194] IVAN ILLICH, MEDICAL NEMESIS 122 (1975).

to a natural occurrence, to a force of nature, to an untimely event, to "the outcome of a specific disease certified by the doctor." In his view, "The hope of doctors to control the outcome of specific diseases gave rise to the myth that they had power over death."[195] It also fueled their patients' hopes that death could be overcome.

In a market-driven economy, where physicians are producers and patients are consumers, Illich argues that society permits people to die only when their bodies "refuse any further input of treatment," after which they "become useless not only as a producer but also as a consumer . . . [and] must finally be written off as a total loss."[196] In this ICU-maximal-treatment model, "[d]eath has become the ultimate form of consumer resistance."[197] Nor is this irrelevant to health care finance. A young physician who could not prevent the medical brutalization of his dying doctor-father by other U.S. physicians laments: "Our health care system is structured to meet reimbursement rather than patients' needs. Tremendous amounts of money are spent prolonging death, not life."[198]

Cancer, again, provides a useful example. Even in the United States, effective standard treatments for most cancers simply do not exist.[199] A 1990 survey, for example, found that fully one-third of all drugs used on cancer patients are of unproven safety and efficacy for the purpose for which they are administered.[200] Unapproved use is even more prevalent for malignancies that have metastasized than for cancers at earlier stages. Oncologist Charles Moertel, commenting on the study, noted that the major beneficiaries of such unproven and futile approaches are the "appointment book of the oncologist" and "the pharmaceutical companies and their stockholders."[201] In short, business concerns appear to supplant both medical ethics and patient interests. As to the argument that oncologists are just responding to the demands of dying patients, Moertel rejoins: "This argument abandons the scientific basis for medical practice and could just as well be used to justify quackery. Also, one wonders how many patients with advanced pancreatic cancer, for example, would really demand cytotoxic drugs if the sheer futility of such therapy was honestly explained."[202]

In countries like Japan and the U.K., which do not spend inordinate amounts of money on health care at the end of life, failure to discuss prognosis seems to be societally acceptable because death is not viewed as professional defeat. It is accepted as both natural and necessary by physicians and their patients alike.[203]

---

[195] *Id.* at 140; *see also* KATZ, *supra* note 187, at 1-79.

[196] ILLICH, *supra* note 194, at 149.

[197] *Id.*

[198] Norman Paradis, *Making a Living Off the Dying*, N.Y. TIMES, April 25, 1992, at 23.

[199] *See* John C. Bailar III & Elaine M. Smith, *Progress Against Cancer?*, 314 NEW ENG. J. MED. 1226 (1986); Tim Beardsley, *A Way Not Won*, SCI. AM., Jan., 1994, at 130.

[200] Thomas Laetz & George Silberman, *Reimbursement Policies Constrain the Practice of Oncology*, 266 JAMA 2996 (1991).

[201] Charles G. Moertel, *Off-Label Drug Use for Cancer Therapy and National Health Care Priorities*, 266 JAMA 3031 (1991). *See also* David V. Schapira et al., *Intensive Care, Survival, and Expenses of Treating Critically Ill Cancer Patients*, 269 JAMA 783 (1993); Cornelius O. Granai, *Ovarian Cancer—Unrealistic Expectations*, 327 NEW ENG. J. MED. 197 (1992).

[202] Moertel, *supra* note 201, at 3031. On end-of-life medical experiments, see generally George J. Annas, *The Changing Landscape of Human Experimentation: From Nuremberg to Helsinki and Beyond*, 2 HEALTH MATRIX 119 (1992); George J. Annas, *Faith (Healing), Hope and Charity at the FDA: The Politics of AIDS Drug Trials*, 34 VILL. L. REV. 771 (1989).

[203] Not all Japanese observers agree with this position. Moreover, a culture's view of

As Rihito Kamura has explained of Japan, "Death is an integral part of the Japanese cultural tradition. Most Japanese people resist the modern, technological death in which machines can supplant important rituals surrounding death and dying."[204] Because members of these relatively more homogeneous societies share common perceptions about how much medical intervention is appropriate at the end of life, comprehensive discussion of treatment alternatives between doctor and patient seems less necessary.

In the more pluralistic U.S. society, however, there is less social consensus on the role of medicine toward the end of life, and physician biases toward more aggressive treatment may offend the value systems of many Americans. These people are going to great lengths, such as executing living wills, petitioning courts to terminate treatment, and committing suicide, to assert that merely prolonging the dying process is unacceptable to them.[205]

Physicians often tend to treat patients with terminal illness aggressively for a variety of motives, including misplaced fear of civil (or even criminal) litigation if they do not.[206] Their heroic efforts to ward off the inevitable often compromise the quality of their patients' remaining lives in ways that doctors would rarely elect for themselves. When physicians impart straightforward information about prognosis, their patients are enabled to exercise the same degree of informed choice about end-of-life care as the doctors would. In such situations, the right to refuse treatment may be more important to patient self-determination than the ability to demand such treatment or even to choose among treatment options. Accurate information about prognosis thus promotes patient autonomy *and* can save significant health care expenditures on treatment that patients would decline were they "truly" informed.[207]

---

death may change radically over a short period of time. For example, Naokao Miyaji, *see supra* note 176, was kind enough to comment on an early draft of this article. She doubts that our view of the Japanese attitude towards death is correct and thinks at least in the post-World War II period "the notion that death should be avoided at all costs is very prevalent" in Japan. Letter from Naokoa Miyaji to George J. Annas & Frances Miller (June 2, 1993) (on file with authors). If she is correct, we are likely to see an enormous increase in medical care expenditures in Japan as its physicians adopt the expensive technological interventions used so freely in the U.S. and encourage their use. *See infra* Figure 3 at page 392.

[204] Rihito Kimura, *Anencephalic Organ Donation: A Japanese Case*, 14 J. MED. & PHIL. 97, 100 (1989). Kimura cites the Japanese text of EMIKO NAMIHIRA, CULTURE OF ILLNESS AND DEATH (1990) to support his conclusions.

[205] *See Prescribing Death*, *supra* note 185. It also seems fair to conclude that physicians are at least as afraid of death as their patients are, and much more likely to view death as a professional defeat. *See supra* note 202 and sources cited therein; *see also* P.C. Thauberger & E.M. Thauberger, *A Consideration of Death and a Sociological Perspective of the Quality of the Dying Patient's Care*, 8 SOC. SCI. & MED. 437 (1974). In one study where twenty-four severely burned patients were told that survival with their degree of burns was unprecedented, twenty-one of them and/or their families chose nonheroic treatment. Sharon H. Imbus & Bruce E. Zawacki, *Autonomy for Burned Patients When Survival Is Unprecedented*, 297 NEW ENG. J. MED. 308 (1977).

[206] Physicians' economic self-interest often reinforces this preference for heroic treatment. *See generally* RODWIN, *supra* note 162.

[207] The amount that could be saved is not known, has been variously calculated, and is dependent upon one's assumptions. *See* Singer & Lowy, *supra* note 58, at 478 (arguing, based on study showing 70 percent of people would refuse life sustaining treatment if incompetent and with poor prognosis, that up to $109 billion of medical care could be saved each year if everyone in U.S. executed a living will expressing that preference, and these requests were honored.) Others put possible savings much more modestly, at about $20 billion annually. Emanuel & Emanuel, *supra* note 58, at 540.

If we are correct, a country's overall health care expenditures can be strongly influenced by the amount of honest prognosis information made available to patients. Assuming that sophisticated and expensive medical technology is available, Figure 3 impressionistically summarizes the relationship between prognosis information and health care expenditures.

The U.S. is now at the point marked A on this chart, but we hypothesize that, with more open and honest prognostic information, it could move back down to A′. Japan, with increasing emphasis on technology and more openness about treatment alternatives, could move up from B to B′. The U.K., now at C, could stay constant (point C′) notwithstanding more prognosis information because of global budgeting constraints. The U.K. could also shift its entire curve upward to C″ if more information about prognosis and alternatives generates pressure for more government investment in health service delivery, particularly high technology.

The recent United States emphasis on outcomes data could produce both better informed patients and savings in medical expenditures, so long as outcomes research is carried out with scientific integrity.[208] These studies identify treatments and procedures falling into a variety of efficacy categories, and can also pinpoint those providers delivering substandard or unduly expensive care. They also can evaluate patient satisfaction with medical care and its results. "Never beneficial" or futile treatments, or those delivered by providers deficient in skills or cost effectiveness, will—or arguably should if insurance subsidy is involved—be simply eliminated from the medical care system.

John Wennberg has correctly suggested that *patients* are the ones who should make the real final treatment choices, based in large measure on a personal evaluation of outcomes and other prognosis data, as applied to the length and quality of their own lives.[209] An early Wennberg study showed that many Maine urologists did prostate surgery primarily to relieve symptoms (such as having to get up in the middle of the night to urinate), rather than to prevent progression When patients themselves were queried, however, their attitudes toward their symptoms varied. Some patients were not bothered much by the symptoms at all. Patients also differed from their doctors in assessing the significance of treatment risks, "particularly surgery-induced impotence and operative mortality."[210]

The key to reducing variations, in Wennberg's opinion, thus depends not on learning more from laboratory findings or clinical exams, but rather "depends on learning what patients want, and this can only be ascertained by asking patients . . . [who should be informed] that they indeed have a choice and that their choice should depend on their own preferences . . . ."[211] When fully informed of the risks and benefits, only one of five severely symptomatic men actually chose the prostate surgery their doctors recommended.[212]

---

[208] On outcomes research generally, see J. Jarrett Clinton, *Outcomes Research—A Way to Improve Medical Practice*, 266 JAMA 2057 (1991); John E. Wennberg, *Outcomes Research, Cost Containment, and the Fear of Health Care Rationing*, 323 New Eng. J. Med. 1202 (1990).

[209] John A. Wennberg, *AHCPR and the Strategy for Health Care Reform*, Health Aff., Winter 1992, at 67, 68 [hereinafter *Strategy for Health Care Reform*]. *See also* Craig Fleming et al., *A Decision Analysis of Alternative Treatment Strategies for Clinically Localized Prostate Cancer*, 269 JAMA 2650 (1993).

[210] *Strategy for Health Care Reform*, *supra* note 209, at 69.

[211] *Id.*

[212] *Id.* Studies of patient preferences regarding quality of life versus increased changes

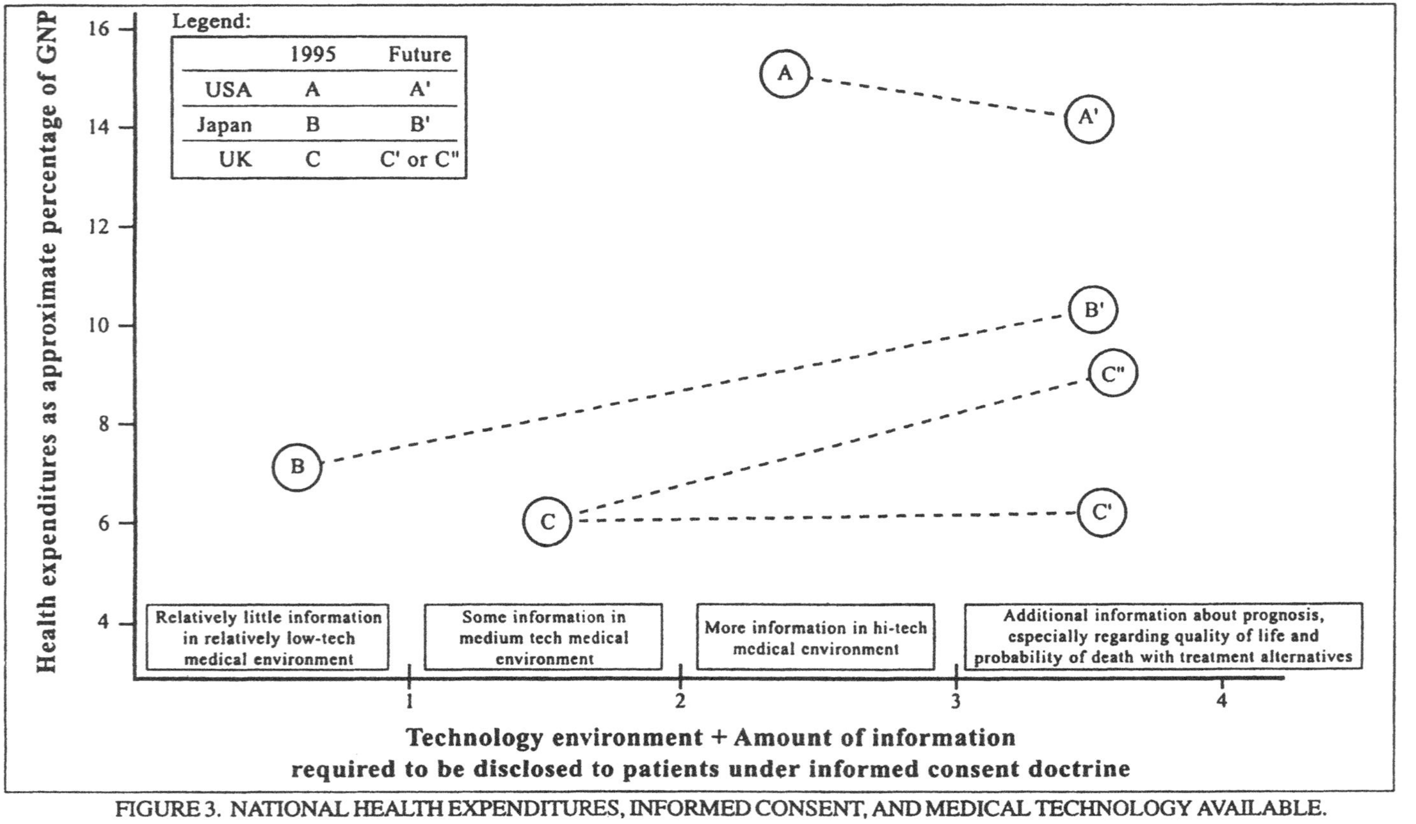

FIGURE 3. NATIONAL HEALTH EXPENDITURES, INFORMED CONSENT, AND MEDICAL TECHNOLOGY AVAILABLE.

VI. CONCLUSION

Our cover story in the U.S. is autonomy. But the payment system, reinforced by fear of death, is actually the dominant force driving the American health sector.[213] The United States is said to have the best health care system in the world, but only the wealthy and well-insured can afford to have access to all that modern medicine can provide. As we have seen, enjoying such access in ignorance of likely outcomes is at best a mixed blessing. Because of the crushing costs and our almost unique preoccupation with avoiding (or at least delaying) death, this "best" system is not sought after by any other country in the world. Our system is nonexportable precisely because of its expense. Although the payment system for medical services and attitudes toward death also drive the health care systems of Japan and the U.K., they have driven them in different directions.

A society's cultural beliefs concerning death influence health resource allocation, and will be reflected in a country's informed consent laws. Where individualism is highly prized and medical care is seen as a market good, legal doctrine will place a high premium on information disclosure to facilitate patient/consumer choices, especially among treatment alternatives. Countries like the U.K. and Japan with more collective notions about health care, and where citizens are more likely to defer to authority, will be less interested in choice and thus less inclined to emphasize full disclosure or truth-telling. Instead the content of disclosure will generally be discretionary with physicians.

Nonetheless, informed consent probably gets more attention than it deserves with regard to treatment alternatives. Physicians everywhere in fact usually make decisions about therapy *for* their patients rather than with them. This may be inevitable given information asymmetry and patient dependence, and may be what even American courts mean when they designate the doctor-patient relationship as a "trust" or fiduciary relationship.[214] The medical profession does get to set its own standards for practice in the last analysis, and for most diseases physician treatment preferences affect the manner in which information is conveyed to their patients. The doctor's ability to shade information may be as or more important than the

---

of longer term survival also support the proposition that patients value quality of life more than quantity. *See, e.g.*, Barbara J. McNeil et al., *Speech and Survival: Tradeoffs Between Quality and Quantity of Life in Laryngeal Cancer*, 305 NEW ENG. J. MED. 982 (1981); Barbara J. McNeil et al., *Fallacy of the Five-Year Survival in Lung Cancer*, 299 NEW ENG. J. MED. 1397 (1978).

[213] The most egregious example of this point is set forth in Grace Plaza v. Elbaum, 588 N.Y.S.2d 853 (N.Y. App. Div. 1992), *aff'd and certified question answered*, 623 N.E.2d 513 (N.Y. 1993). A New York Court of Appeals, which had previously ruled that Jean Elbaum had left clear and convincing evidence that she never wanted tube feeding if she were in a persistent vegetative state, nonetheless required her husband to pay for more than a year of such treatment (in excess of $100,000) even though her nursing home had informed him (before he sued to enjoin treatment) that "'even if irrefutable evidence of the patient's wishes were forthcoming, Grace Plaza is not willing to undertake removal of the gastrostomy tube . . . .'" 588 N.Y.S.2d at 863. With such outrageous medical and judicial acts, no form of national health insurance can be affordable. *See* George J. Annas, *Adding Injustice to Injury: Compulsory Payment for Unwanted Treatment*, 327 NEW ENG. J. MED. 1885 (1992).

[214] Lambert v. Park, 597 F.2d 236 (10th Cir. 1976). *See generally* Maxwell J. Mehlman, *Fiduciary Contracting: Limitations on Bargaining Between Patients and Health Care Providers*, 51 U. PITT. L. REV. 365 (1990).

content of the disclosure itself. Thus, patients may end up with little real choice among treatment alternatives.

Choice, at least the choice to forgo treatment altogether, seems to be most contested and most necessary at the end of life. In Japan, where few or no heroic efforts are made to prolong the life of dying patients, there is little interest in the right to die movement. In the U.S., however, following cases like those of Karen Ann Quinlan and Nancy Cruzan, the right to refuse treatment is central to the self-determination debate, and is likely to be dominant in future resource allocation controversies as well.[215] With this in mind, taking informed consent more seriously with regard to prognosis should help to make health systems more responsive to the true preferences of their respective patient populations.

There is no justification for forcing unwanted, expensive, and useless treatment on citizens at life's end. Nor will most patients demand futile, painful and expensive therapy once they are fully informed of the consequences. Thus, informed consent, especially regarding the truth about prognosis, may be the only way the U.S. can limit the use of expensive and ineffective treatment at the end of life consistent with cultural expectations about patient autonomy. It may also be one of the few ways we can avoid massive new expenditures and still underwrite universal health insurance.

We opened this Article with some thoughts from a British writer. We close with the views of an American one. John Updike has observed, America is a victim not of limits, but of dreams: "There is no enough. That's one of the words Americans have a very hard time learning: the word enough."[216] This is probably why Updike ends his Rabbit books with Rabbit, responding to his son's cries of "Don't *die*, Dad, don't," by saying, "'Well, Nelson . . . all I can tell you is, it isn't so bad.' Rabbit thinks he should maybe say more, the kid looks so wildly expectant, but enough. Maybe. Enough."[217]

---

[215] Given the differences between Japan and the U.S., it is striking that, concerning incompetent patients, the two most important U.S. decisions upholding the right to refuse treatment, *In re* Quinlan, 355 A.2d 647 (N.J. 1976) and Cruzan v. Director, Mo. Dept. Health, 497 U.S. 490 (1989), both center on attempts to give the patient's *family* ultimate decision-making authority. One can see U.S. jurisprudence—at least where incompetent patients are involved—reaching for the Japanese family-centered model of health care decision making. Regardless of the law, however, U.S. physicians have traditionally made decisions for incompetent patients in conjunction with their families, with no court proceedings whatsoever.

[216] *Quoted in* Dennis Farney, *Novelist Updike Sees a Nation Frustrated by its Own Dreams*, WALL ST. J., Sept. 16, 1992, at A1, A8.

[217] JOHN UPDIKE, RABBIT AT REST 512 (1990). See also Christopher Ricks, BECKETT'S DYING WORDS 1 (1995): "Most people most of the time want to live for ever. This truth is acknowledged in literature . . . . But like many a truth, it is a half-truth . . . . For, after all, most people some of the time, and some people most of the time, do not want to live for ever."; and WILLIAM S. BURROUGHS, THE WESTERN LANDS 257 (1987), who ends his book on our search for immortality by asking, "How long does it take a man to learn that he does not, cannot want what he 'wants'?"

Part II
Patient Rights

Informed Consent

[3]

Bye-Bye Bolam: A Medical Litigation Revolution?

MARGARET BRAZIER* AND JOSÉ MIOLA**

I. INTRODUCTION

When McNair J. delivered his direction to the jury in *Bolam* v. *Friern Hospital Management Committee*[1] just over forty years ago, it can only be a matter of speculation whether he ever appreciated how famous, or infamous, the *Bolam* test would become. For defendants in medical malpractice claims, and for health professionals generally, *Bolam* may be viewed as no more than simple justice requiring that they, like other professionals, be judged by their peers. Many academic commentators[2] and organisations campaigning for victims of medical accidents perceive the *Bolam* test very differently. *Bolam*, in their judgment, has been used by the courts to abdicate responsibility for defining and enforcing patients' rights. In its original context, actions for medical negligence, *Bolam* ran out of control. The test became no more than a requirement to find some other expert(s) who would declare that they would have done as the defendant did. More disturbingly, *Bolam* infiltrated all sorts of other areas of medical law, being utilised to prevent development of any doctrine of informed consent this side of the Atlantic, and allowed to become the standard for judging the welfare interests of patients lacking the requisite mental capacity to make their own treatment decisions. *Bolam*, out of control and out of context, came close to acquiring demonic status in some quarters.

Late in 1997, Lord Browne-Wilkinson in *Bolitho* v. *City & Hackney Health Authority*[3] sought to correct what he believed had been a misinterpretation of *Bolam*. His Lordship reiterated that ultimately the courts, and only the courts, are the arbiters of what constitutes reasonable care. Doctors cannot be judges in their own cause. *Bolitho* struck

---

* Professor of Law, Institute of Medicine, Law and Bioethics, University of Manchester.

**Lecturer in Law, Faculty of Law, University of Leicester. We would like to thank Jean McHale, Giorgio Monti and Sara Fovargue for their helpful comments on earlier drafts of this paper.

[1] [1957] 1 W.L.R. 582.

[2] See, *e.g.* M. Khan and M. Robson, '*Bolam* Rides Again', (1995) 2(2) P.I.L.M.R. 105; N.H. Harris, 'Standards of Practice', (1997) 141 S.J. Supp. Exp. 38; D.K. Feenan, 'Beyond *Bolam*: Responding to the Patient', (1994) 1 Med. L. Int. 177; and J. Keown, 'Burying *Bolam*: Informed Consent Down Under', (1994) 53 C.L.J. 16.

[3] [1998] A.C. 232, (H.L.).

fear into medical hearts. The past twenty years has seen numbers of claims for medical malpractice rise dramatically,[4] levels of damages have rocketed; yet the proportion of successful claims remains low. Undermining judgment by their peers might remove even this latter crumb of comfort. Does *Bolitho* herald a medical litigation revolution at which health professionals should tremble?

Lord Browne-Wilkinson's speech and the decision in *Bolitho* have now been elegantly analysed by a number of medical lawyers.[5] This paper attempts a rather broader view of the potential impact of a series of developments, including the decision in *Bolitho*, which we argue are likely to change the face of health care law in this country. *Bolitho*, recent case-law on informed consent, the establishment of the National Institute of Clinical Excellence and the Law Commission's proposals relating to treatment of mentally incapacitated patients are just some of the factors which we contend will in many cases ensure that the courts no longer blindly accept assertions of good medical practice, but evaluate that practice. Substance will be given to patients' interests in welfare and autonomy. However, we shall also seek to demonstrate that such developments should not cause doctors or other health professionals to fear for their professional integrity or independence. Returning the *Bolam* test to its proper limits and appropriate context will be beneficial, rather than detrimental, to medicine and to medical litigation. The revolution, if it can be so styled, will be a velvet revolution, not a bloodbath.

II. BOLAM REVISITED

We need first to revisit *Bolam* itself. The facts are well-known so we rehearse them only briefly. The plaintiff had undergone electro-convulsive therapy (ECT). No relaxant drug was administered to him nor was any restraint used to control the convulsive movements which happen during ECT. He suffered a fractured hip. At that time professional practice varied widely about the use of drugs and physical restraint, and in relation to whether patients should be warned of the

---

[4] Accurate figures are difficult to find. Answers to parliamentary questions suggests that payments in medical negligence claims cost the NHS £179 million in 1993–4; £160 million in 1994–5; £149.1 million in 1995–6; see V. Harpwood, *Medical Negligence and Clinical Risk: Trends and Developments 1998* (Monitor Press, 1998) at vii. The Secretary of State for Health claimed that in 1996–7 the cost of litigation approached £300 million yet only 17 per cent of claims succeeded; see *Hansard* (H.C.) 24.3.98, Cols. 165–6.

[5] N. Glover, '*Bolam* in the House of Lords', (1999) 15 P.N. 42; A. Grubb, 'Negligence Causation and *Bolam*', (1998) 6 Med. L. Rev. 378. M.A. Jones, 'The *Bolam* Test and the Responsible Expert', (1999) *Tort Law Review* 226; H. Teff, 'The Standard of Care in Medical Negligence—Moving on from Bolam', (1998) 18 O.J.L.S. 473.

risk of fractures. Experts disagreed. McNair J. saw the issue as quite simply one of professional negligence. He formulated what might be described as a two-part test. Part I may be seen as uncontroversial: 'The test is the standard of the ordinary skilled man exercising and professing to have that special skill.'[6] The defendant need not attain the 'highest expert skill' but must achieve the ordinary level of competence expected of a person in his profession and practising in a particular specialty of that profession.

Part II is more problematic and the source of later misunderstanding of *Bolam* itself. The core dispute in professional negligence cases which are defended often centres on just what does constitute 'proper practice' or 'ordinary competence' in relation to the procedure in dispute. The profession itself cannot agree whether or not a particular practice amounts to adequate care of the patient's, or client's, interests. In such cases, McNair J. held:

> A doctor is not guilty of negligence if he has acted in accordance with a practice accepted as proper by a *responsible* body of medical men skilled in that particular act . . . a doctor is not if he is acting in accordance with such a practice, *merely* because there is *a* body of opinion taking a contrary view.[7]

Once again, in context, *Bolam* Part II is unexceptionable and governs all forms of professional liability. It is not special pleading for doctors. The very nature of professional services involves the exercise of skills, and the possession of a body of knowledge, not shared by the public at large. Judges are not qualified to make professional judgments on the practices of other learned professions. *If*, in a claim against an architect, the dispute concerns either whether her original design plans recognised and dealt with risks posed by subsidence, or whether, in delegating certain responsibilities to a quantity surveyor she acted properly, only her peers can identify to the judge what amounts to appropriate and safe practice. When those peers disagree and the disagreement illustrates genuine and well founded debate within a profession on good practice, judges are not generally equipped to adjudicate in such a dispute. A professional should not be penalised, and be held to be incompetent, just because a judge fancies 'playing' at being architect, solicitor or doctor.

In particular, judges will have difficulty in dealing with cases of disputed practice in the following instances: where practice is evolving rapidly in a new specialty or sub-specialty of a profession, identifying *responsible* practice will be demanding. Where exceptionally complex scientific or technical issues are moot, the lawyer-judge may be some-

[6] *Op. cit.*, n. 1 at 586.
[7] *Ibid.* at 587.

what out of his or her depth. When either evolving practice or highly technical issues, or both, pose delicate questions of risk assessment, judges may quite properly be hesitant to intervene to second-guess the opinion held, and reasonably held, by one body of opinion within a profession. All these considerations apply (or should apply) to all professions. Yet only in relation to medicine has the *Bolam* test of professional negligence been so excoriated.

III. BOLAM OUT OF CONTROL

What distinguishes medical litigation from other areas of professional liability is in part that a series of judgments (or maybe a gloss on those judgments) have given rise to a perception that all *Bolam* requires is that the defendant fields experts from his or her medical specialty prepared to testify that they would have followed the same course of management of the patient-plaintiff as did the defendant. If such experts can be identified, are patently honest and stand by their testimony vigorously, neither they nor the defendant will be asked to justify their practice. The judge will play no role in evaluating that expert evidence. As Michael Jones notes, it may be that judges find it difficult to find against members of the medical profession on questions of negligence, or, doctors' lawyers may just be better players of the litigation game.[8] The result however, as Jones points out, is that out of six medical negligence claims before the House of Lords in 16 years the 'score' was *Plaintiffs 0; Defendants 6*! Yet in other professional negligence claims, time after time, judges have made it clear that expert opinion must be demonstrably responsible and reasonable.

In *Edward Wong Finance Co. Ltd.* v. *Johnson Stokes and Master*[9] a practice nearly universally endorsed by solicitors in Hong Kong was nonetheless found to be negligent. Hong Kong practice on mortgage completion provided for the money to be handed over to the borrowers on receipt of an undertaking from the borrowers' solicitors to hand over the requisite deeds. A dishonest solicitor absconded with the money never having provided the documents which constituted security to the loans. The lenders sued their own solicitors. The Privy Council held that the solicitors were negligent despite having conformed to the general practice of the profession in Hong Kong. The risk of fraud was obvious and inherent in the practice. It could have been prevented with ease. Evidence that other respected professionals followed the same 'unsafe' practice was not sufficient to amount to conclusive evidence

---

[8] *Op. cit.* at 236.

[9] [1984] A.C. 296, P.C.

that that practice was responsible. It self-evidently was not. In relation to many professions, other than medicine, the courts have on a number of occasions adopted an equally robust approach to ensure that peer evidence cannot be used simply to sanction negligence.[10] Judges have declared that the principles governing medical negligence are no different from those applying to other professions, that doctors and surgeons fall into no special category, but reality has not met the rhetoric.

In *Maynard* v. *West Midlands Regional Health Authority*[11] the trial judge who heard and evaluated the expert evidence found for the plaintiff declaring honestly that he had weighed the evidence and 'preferred' the opinion of the plaintiff's expert. The House of Lords in no uncertain terms declared that 'a judge's preference for one body of distinguished professional opinion to another is not sufficient to establish negligence in a practitioner whose actions have received the approval of those whose opinions, truthfully held, honestly expressed, were not preferred'.[12] Lord Scarman continued 'in the realm of diagnoses and treatment negligence is not established by preferring one respectable body of professional opinion to another'.[13] In similar vein, it mattered not in *De Freitas* v. *O'Brien*[14] that the disputed procedure was one only a tiny minority of neurosurgeons (four or five out of two hundred and fifty consultants) would consider safe. The ethos of medical litigation came to be seen as sanctioning a modern form of trial by battle. Line up your champion expert in sober garb and with letters after his name and the defendant could not fail. In its most grisly form, the trial by expert reached its nadir in *Whitehouse* v. *Jordan*[15] where it appeared that obstetricians had unbridgeable divisions on relatively simple issues of management of trial of labour.

If our attack on *Bolam* out of control seems too highly coloured, consider the argument advanced by counsel for the defendant in *Bolitho* itself and (to a limited extent) conceded by the trial judge. If the evidence advanced by expert witnesses is truthful the judge cannot question its logical force. *Bolam*, in suits for medical malpractice, was interpreted, whatever the judges might say, to allow judgment by colleagues to substitute for judgment by the courts.

---

[10] See, *e.g. Lloyds Bank Ltd.* v. *E.B. Savory & Co.* [1933] A.C. 201; *Stokes* v. *Guest, Keen & Nettlefold (Bolts and Nuts) Ltd.* [1968] 1 W.L.R. 1176; *Roberge* v. *Bolduc* (1991) 78 D.L.R. (4th) 666; *Re The Herald of Free Enterprise: Appeal by Captain Lowry, Independent*, 18.12.87.

[11] [1984] 1 W.L.R. 634, (H.L.).

[12] At 639.

[13] *Ibid.*

[14] [1993] 4 Med. L.R. 281.

[15] [1981] 1 W.L.R. 246, (H.L.).

IV. BOLAM OUT OF CONTEXT

However unsatisfactory *Bolam* may have become in its original context, what is much more disturbing is that the *Bolam* test has been allowed to become the litmus test not just of clinical practice but of medical ethics. Davies eloquently argues that the dominant judicial approach in medical law has become '[w]hen in doubt "Bolamise"'.[16] Three key areas of ethical judgment have in turn effectively been 'Bolamised'. 'Informed consent' was hustled into a *Bolam* straight-jacket. The criteria for determining the legality of the treatment of mentally incapacitated patients, even whether such patients live or die, was subjected to *Bolam*. In both of the above areas the *Bolam* test is invoked overtly. In our third example the *Gillick*, and post-*Gillick*, debacle, we contend that Bolam crept in by the back door.

A. *Overt Bolamisation*

Lord Scarman, that stalwart defender of *Bolam* in *Maynard* v. *West Midlands Regional Health Authority*, took a different view in *Sidaway* v. *Royal Bethlem Hospital*.[17] Addressing the doctor's duty to disclose information about the risks of proposed treatment he adopted the 'prudent patient' standard. The majority voted for *Bolam*. A patient was prima facie entitled to be told only so much as a responsible body of medical opinion judged prudent. Lord Bridge did declare that there might be circumstances where a judge would come to the conclusion '... that disclosure of a particular risk was so obviously necessary to an informed choice on the part of the patient that no reasonably prudent medical man would fail to make it'.[18] He appeared to re-enforce the words of Sir John Donaldson M.R. in the Court of Appeal who had said:

> [The courts] cannot stand idly by if the profession, by an excess of paternalism, denies its patients real choice. In a word, the law will not allow the medical profession to play God ... I think that, in an appropriate case, a judge would be entitled to reject a unanimous medical view if he were satisfied that it was manifestly wrong and that the doctors must have been misdirecting themselves as to their duty in law.[19]

---

[16] M. Davies, 'The "New *Bolam*" Another False Dawn for Medical Negligence?', (1996) 12 P.N. 10.

[17] [1985] 1 All E.R. 643, (H.L.).

[18] *Ibid.* at 663.

[19] [1984] 1 All E.R. 1018 at 1028.

Yet subsequent judgments of the Court of Appeal in *Blyth* v. *Bloomsbury Health Authority*[20] and *Gold* v. *Haringey Health Authority*[21] effectively limited patient choices to what their doctor thinks good for them. The Court of Appeal in *Blyth* and *Gold* operated on a strong preference for Lord Diplock's approach in *Sidaway*. Failure to give a patient adequate advice on the merits and demerits of proposed treatment was simply an issue relating to breach of duty of care to be judged identically (i.e. in conformity to *Bolam*) to any other alleged breach of duty.[22]

B. Widening the Bolamite Spectrum

In re F (Mental Patient: Sterilisation)[23] marked yet a further step in the process of *Bolamisation*. *Re F* addressed the lawfulness of medical treatment of adults incapable of consenting to on their own behalf. F was a 36-year-old woman, an informal patient in a mental hospital, who was believed to have entered into a sexual relationship with a male patient. She was said to have a mental age of five and the verbal capacity of a two-year-old. The House of Lords concurred in the findings of the trial judge and the Court of Appeal that the common law neither provided for any form of proxy consent on behalf of mentally incapacitated adults nor did the *parens patriae* power of the courts survive to sanction treatment.[24] Given the lacuna in the law, all the judges involved in *Re F* agreed on the following principle: treatment of a person unable to consent to treatment (temporarily or permanently) was justified on a principle of necessity:

> [A] doctor can lawfully operate on, or give other treatment to, adult patients who are incapable, for one reason or another, of consenting to his going so, provided that operation or other treatment concerned is in the best interests of such patients.[25]

Where the Law Lords disagreed with the Court of Appeal, however, was as to how 'best interests' might be judged. All three judges in the Court of Appeal argued that *Bolam* was insufficiently stringent to determine whether proposed treatment was in the patient's best interests.

---

20 [1993] 4 Med. L.R. 151, (C.A.).

21 [1987] 2 All E.R. 888, (C.A.).

22 See Kerr L.J.'s judgment in *Blyth*, *op. cit.*, n. 20, particularly at 155.

23 [1990] 2 A.C. 1, (C.A. and H.L.).

24 See generally, P. Fennell, *Treatment Without Consent: Law, Psychiatry and the Treatment of Mentally Disordered People Since 1845* (Routledge & Kegan Paul 1996); B.M. Hoggett, 'The Royal Prerogative in Relation to the Mentally Disordered: Resurrection, Resuscitation or Rejection' in M.D.A. Freeman (ed.), *Medicine, Ethics and Law* (Stevens 1988).

25 At 55 *per* Lord Brandon.

The Court of Appeal had rejected Scott Baker J.'s view that the test of what was in the interests of an incapacitated patient was little different from that for negligence. Neill L.J. said of *Bolam* in this context:

> But to say that it is not negligent to carry out a particular form of treatment does not mean that that treatment is necessary. I would define necessary in this context as that which the *general body of medical opinion* in the particular speciality would consider to be in the best interests of the patient in order to maintain the health and service the well-being of the patient[26] (our emphasis).

The House of Lords rejected any suggestion that a *Bolam-plus* test was called for. Conformity to *a* reasonable and responsible body of medical opinion sufficed.[27] Lord Goff acknowledged that decisions about the welfare of a mentally incapacitated person are not exclusively within medical expertise. He declared:

> No doubt, in practice, a decision may involve others besides the doctor. It must surely be good practice to consult relatives and others who are concerned with the care of the patient. Sometimes, of course, consultation with a specialist or specialists will be required; and in others, especially where the decision involves more than purely medical opinion, an inter-disciplinary team will in practice participate in the decision.[28]

Note that his words are permissive. The decision *may* involve others. Good practice would entail *consultation* with relatives. The ultimate arbiter remains the doctor. Best interests is judged by *Bolam* alone. That the pros and cons of sterilising women unable to consent themselves to loss of their reproductive capacity ' . . . involved principles of law, ethics and medical practice' had been openly acknowledged in *Re B (A Minor) (Wardship: Sterilisation)*[29] when the Law Lords had two years earlier considered the sterilisation of minors. The pervading influence of *Bolam* granted medical practitioners control not just of their own practice but of matters of medical ethics and law as well,[30] extending in *Airedale N.H.S. Trust* v. *Bland*[31] to the ethics of withdrawal of life-sustaining treatment.

---

[26] At 32; and see *per* Lord Donaldson M.R. at 18.
[27] At 560 *per* Lord Brandon; at 567 *per* Lord Goff.
[28] *Ibid.* at 567.
[29] [1988] A.C. 199 at 205–6 *per* Lord Templeman.
[30] Graphically illustrated in *Re P (A Minor) Wardship: Sterilisation* [1989] 1 F.L.R. 182 where the expert opinion of one gynaecologist appeared to determine the fate of 17-year-old mentally incapacitated girl: see M Brazier, 'Down the Slippery Slope', (1990) 6 P.N. 25.
[31] [1993] 1 All E.R. 821 (H.L.) at 861 *per* Lord Keith; 871 *per* Lord Goff.

In cases which have followed *Bland*, judges have on several occasions simply deferred to the doctors. In *Frenchay N.H.S. Trust* v. *S*,[32] Sir Thomas Bingham M.R. first said that it would be wrong to assume that '... what the doctor says is the patient's best interest is the patient's best interest'.[33] However, he continued by noting that to question such a medical opinion would leave the doctor in an extremely difficult and unsatisfactory position, into which 'one should be reluctant to lead doctors'.[34] It seems that a court will only depart from the medical practitioner's definition of the patient's best interests in rare cases. Perhaps unsurprisingly, there is little evidence of such questioning of medical authority. In *Re G*,[35] Sir Stephen Brown P. was faced with a conflict where the doctors and the patient's wife supported the withdrawal of treatment, but G's mother did not. He stated that while the views of relatives should be considered, they were not determinative, and the views of the doctors should be followed.[36]

C. *Covert Bolamisation*

In the context of informed consent and treatment of mentally incapacitated patients, *Bolam* appears centre stage. In *Gillick* v. *West Norfolk and Wisbech Area Health Authority*,[37] *Bolam* is never expressly invoked, or even cited in any of their Lordships' speeches. Yet a similar judicial policy of handing over sensitive issues of ethics to the doctors surfaces again. Girls under 16 can be prescribed 'the Pill' if judged to be '*Gillick* competent' by a doctor and his clinical judgment endorses such treatment as in their interests.[38] Lord Fraser is quite open about this process of 'medicalising' ethics:

> The medical profession have in modern times become entrusted with very wide discretionary powers going beyond the strict limits of clinical judgments and, in my opinion, there is nothing strange about entrusting them with this further responsibility *which they alone are in a position to discharge satisfactorily*[39] (our emphasis).

If *Gillick* may be understood as covertly applying the *Bolam* test to mature minors, just as *F* openly applies it to mentally incapacitated

---

[32] [1994] 2 All E.R. 403.

[33] *Ibid.* at 411.

[34] *Ibid.* at 411–2.

[35] [1995] 2 F.L.R. 528.

[36] See A. Grubb, 'Incompetent Patient in PVS: Views of Relatives; Best Interests', (1995) 3 Med. L. Rev. 80.

[37] [1985] 3 All E.R. 402 (H.L.).

[38] See J. Eekelaar, 'The Emergence of Children's Rights', (1986) 6 O.J.L.S. 161, and J. Montgomery, 'Children as Property', (1988) 51 M.L.R. 323.

[39] *Op. cit.*, n. 37 at 413.

adults, the subsequent judgments on minors' incapacity to refuse treatment become more comprehensible. The Court of Appeal in *Re R (A Minor) (Wardship Medical Treatment)*[40] and *Re W (A Minor) (Wardship: Medical Treatment)*[41] effectively denies either parents or older children decision-making powers. The 'reasonable doctor' determines whether or not to override the adolescent's refusal of treatment, regardless of whether or not the young person is *Gillick*-competent. The doctor is free to act on consent to treat granted by either parent or by the minor. Lord Donaldson in *Re W* describes consent as a flak-jacket. Where the patient is a mentally competent adult, only the patient can provide the doctor with a flak-jacket to protect her doctor from the fire of litigation. When the patient is a minor, that patient and her parents are all empowered to proffer the requisite protection to the doctor.[42] And if no flak-jacket is forthcoming from the parents or the minor, the doctor can apply to the court to sanction treatment which responsible medical practice judges necessary to protect the minor's welfare.[43]

In *Re R*, Lord Donaldson had used a different, if equally colourful, metaphor. He likened consent to a key. A *Gillick*-competent minor acquired a key to consent to treatment, but his parents retained all their separate rights as keyholders, as did the court. His Lordship abandoned 'keys' for 'flak-jackets' in *Re W* because, he acknowledged, keys can lock, as well as unlock doors. The impact of *Re W* is to grant the power to decide disputes about the treatment of a minor to the medical profession. *Bolam* may not be cited in either *Gillick* itself or the hotly disputed judgments which came later and abrogated any substantive claim to adolescent autonomy,[44] nonetheless a Bolamite philosophy prevails. A body of responsible medical opinion is presumed to be the best arbiter of disagreements about treatment, whether those disagreements be between doctors and young patients, doctors and the patient's parents, or amongst doctors themselves.

Where the *Bolam* philosophy enters the legal arena surreptitiously, it may be disguised by the use of terms such as 'clinical judgment' or 'best

---

[40] [1991] 4 All E.R. 177 (C.A.).

[41] [1992] 4 All E.R. 627 (C.A.).

[42] See M. Brazier and C. Bridge, 'Coercion or Caring', (1996) 16 L.S. 84. Also see G. Douglas, 'The Retreat from *Gillick*', (1992) 55 M.L.R. 569; and J. Eekelaar, 'White Coats or Flack-Jackets? Doctors, Children and the Courts—Again', (1993) 109 L.Q.R. 182.

[43] *Re E (A Minor) (Wardship: Medical Treatment)* [1992] 1 F.L.R. 386. See, *e.g.* C. Bridge, 'Adolescents and Mental Disorders: Who Consents to Treatment?', (1997) 3 Med. L. Int. 51; and C. Bridge, 'Religious Beliefs and Teenage Refusal of Treatment', (1999) 62 M.L.R. 585.

[44] Ian Kennedy, *e.g.* sees Lord Donaldson as 'Driving a coach and horses through *Gillick*': I. Kennedy, 'Consent to Treatment: The Capable Person' in C. Dyer (ed.), *Doctors, Patients and the Law* (Blackwell 1992) at 60.

interests', as in *Re F.* In *Re W*, 'medical ethics' is the chosen disguise. Lord Donaldson accepts that doctors must take account of a minor's objections to treatment. He says:[45]

> . . . [m]edical ethics also enter into the question. The doctor has a professional duty to act in the best interests of his patient and advise accordingly . . . [and in the event of disagreement] he will need to seek the opinion of other doctors and may well be advised to apply to the court for guidance.

The wise doctor will heed his Lordship's words. Assuming he does so, is it likely that a court will reject the body of opinion advanced by the doctor and his colleagues? Is the outcome not all too often *Bolam* under another name? The extension of a Bolamite philosophy, way beyond the original context of *Bolam*, has led many commentators to charge that the courts (and the legislature) have allowed social and moral questions surrounding individual rights to become "medicalised"[46]. Human rights have been squeezed out of health care law.[47] What we must now address is whether the process of Bolamisation may be about to be reversed.

V. BOLITHO: NEW DAWN OR FALSE DAWN?

The medical malpractice claim brought on behalf of Patrick Bolitho, which culminated in the judgment of the House of Lords in *Bolitho* v. *City & Hackney Health Authority*,[48] is at first glance an unlikely candidate to become a landmark case in medical litigation. The central issue in dispute is a problem of causation rather than breach of duty. Our focus is on the potential impact of Lord Browne-Wilkinson's

---

[45] *Re W, op. cit.*, n. 41 at 635.

[46] Sally Sheldon, *e.g.* highlights the way in which the issue of abortion has been medicalised: S. Sheldon, 'Subject only to the Attitude of the Surgeon Concerned: The Judicial Protection of Medical Discretion', (1996) 5 *Social and Legal Studies* 95. For a more general discussion of this point, see E. Ginzberg (ed.), *Medicine and Society—Clinical Decisions and Societal Values* (Westview 1987); or, for a highly polemic and extreme view, T. Szasz, *The Theology of Medicine* (Oxford University Press 1979). Szasz argues that we have allowed the medical profession to become as much a force for social control as the church in previous centuries, and attributes this to our human desire to abrogate responsibility to others. Although controversial, this view may explain, for some, the *Bolam* explosion. The introductory chapter of the book sets out his position.

[47] See I. Kennedy, 'Consent to Treatment: The Capable Person' in C. Dyer (ed.), *Doctors, Patients and the Law*, *op. cit.*, n. 44.

[48] [1998] A.C. 232, (H.L.).

review of the *Bolam* test so we explore the facts of the case itself and the intricacies of the causation debate only briefly.[49]

Patrick Bolitho, aged two-years-old, was admitted to the defendants' hospital suffering from respiratory difficulties. A couple of days earlier he had been treated in the same hospital for croup. The day after his readmission to hospital, Patrick's breathing deteriorated and a nurse summoned the paediatric registrar, Dr Horn. The registrar said that she would attend as soon as possible, but did not do so. Patrick, however, recovered, quickly regaining his colour and energy. At 2.00 pm Patrick suffered a second episode of breathing difficulties. The doctor was again summoned and failed to attend. Patrick recovered briefly. Unhappily at 2.30 pm he collapsed, his respiratory system failed, and he suffered a cardiac arrest resulting in catastrophic brain damage. Patrick subsequently died and the proceedings were continued by the administratrix of his estate. The essence of the claim was whether the defendants were responsible for the brain damage caused by the cardiac arrest. The hospital admitted negligence on the part of Dr Horn in failing either to attend Patrick or arrange for a suitable deputy to examine the child. They denied liability on the grounds that, even had she attended Patrick, Dr Horn would not have intubated him. To prevent the cardiac arrest which caused his brain damage, Patrick would have to have been intubated prior to 2.30 pm.

The trial judge accepted Dr Horn's evidence that she would not have intubated Patrick before 2.30 pm.[50] He went on to examine expert evidence as to whether or not a competent doctor who had attended Patrick *should* have intubated the child. The plaintiffs' five experts all testified that the evidence of respiratory distress was such that a respiratory collapse should have been contemplated and Patrick should have been intubated immediately to prevent such a catastrophe. The defendants' three experts contended that the evidence suggested that, apart from the two acute episodes of breathing problems, Patrick seemed quite well, and intubation itself was not a risk free process in such a young child. A responsible doctor would not have intubated before 2.30 pm. The trial judge found that the views of the two leading experts, Dr Heaf for the plaintiff, and Dr Dinwiddie for the defendants, were diametrically opposed. Dr Dinwiddie was an especially impressive

---

[49] For literature on causation in *Bolitho* see: M.A. Jones, *op. cit.*, n. 5; or more generally, C. Foster, 'Causation in Medical Negligence Cases: Recent Developments', (1996) 140 S.J. 1098; J. Finch, 'Medical Negligence: Liability and Causation', (1998) 14 P. & M.I.L.L. 9.

[50] The judge found as a fact that she would have made preparations for speedy intubation if later required but that such preparations would have made no difference to the ultimate outcome.

witness. Both represented a responsible body of professional opinion, espoused by distinguished and truthful experts. Accordingly, applying the *Bolam* test, as he interpreted it, the judge was obliged to conclude that Patrick's injury did not result from the defendants' admitted negligence. The judge placed great weight on Lord Scarman's speech in *Maynard* v. *West Midlands Regional Health Authority*[51] stressing it was not for him to prefer one *respectable* body of professional opinion to another. The Court of Appeal upheld the first instance judgment.[52]

Two questions were central to the appeal before the Law Lords. (1) Did the *Bolam* test have any application at all in deciding issues of causation? (2) Does the *Bolam* test require a judge to accept without question truthful evidence from eminent experts? The House of Lords answered the first question in the affirmative. Generally where the only question relevant to causation is simply 'what would have happened but for the defendants' negligence?' the *Bolam* test has no part to play in causation. Exceptionally, as on the facts of this case, an answer to the question 'what *would* have happened *if* . . . ?' simply prompts the further question of 'what *should* have happened?' Having found as a fact that Dr Horn would not have intubated Patrick, whether or not her negligence caused his injury depended on what she *should have done*—what the competent doctor attending the child would have done. Hence the *Bolam* test was inevitably central to that second question of causation.[53]

As to the second issue before their Lordships, does *Bolam* require that a judge accept the views of one truthful body or experts, even if unpersuaded of its logical force, Lord Browne-Wilkinson (with whom his brethren agreed) forcefully rejected any such proposition. The court is not bound to find for a defendant *simply* because he leads evidence from a body of experts who genuinely believe that the defendant's practice conformed to sound medical practice. As McNair J. had stressed in *Bolam* itself the practice must be one endorsed by *responsible* opinion, 'a standard of practice recognised as proper by a *reasonably* competent body of opinion'.[54] These adjectives, Lord Browne-Wilkinson ruled, ' . . . all show that the court has to be satisfied that the exponents of the body of opinion relied upon can demonstrate that such opinion has a logical basis'.[55] Analysing earlier case-law on professional negligence, especially the opinion of the Privy Council in *Edward Wong Finance*

---

[51] [1984] 1 W.L.R. 634, (H.L.) discussed *supra* at Section III.
[52] [1994] 1 Med. L.R. 381; note the dissenting judgment of Simon Brown L.J.
[53] See A. Grubb, 'Negligence: Causation and *Bolam*', (1998) 6 Med. L. Rev. 378.
[54] *Op. cit.*, n. 1 at 586.
[55] *Op. cit.*, n. 3 at 241–2.

Co. Ltd. v. *Johnson Stokes & Master*,[56] he went on to declare that in the vast majority of cases the fact that distinguished experts hold a particular opinion will demonstrate the responsibility of that opinion. Nonetheless '. . . if, in a rare case, it can be demonstrated that the professional opinion is not capable of withstanding logical analysis, the judge is entitled to hold that the body of opinion is not reasonable or responsible.'[57]

Doctors, like all other professionals, cannot be judges in their own cause. The judge in a malpractice claim is free to, must be ready to, scrutinise the basis of opinion professed to him as representing responsible practice. *Bolitho* must not be oversold. Lord Browne-Wilkinson speaks of *rare* cases and emphasises later in his judgment that it will 'very seldom' be right for a judge to reach a conclusion that views genuinely held by competent experts are unreasonable. On the facts of the claim before him he concluded that there was no basis for dismissing the defendants' expert evidence (especially that of Dr Dinwiddie) as illogical. There were sound reasons not to intubate. Lord Browne-Wilkinson does no more than seek to restore *Bolam* to its original limits. McNair J.'s full judgment is crystal clear that he did not intend to give doctors *carte blanche* to clothe inadequate practice with some sort of official blessing, thereby effectively sanctioning negligent practice. McNair J. makes it clear that negligence is not proven merely because a doctor conforms to one school of thought and practice rather than another but says forcefully that:

> . . . that does not mean a medical man can obstinately and pig-headedly carry on with some old technique if it has been proved contrary to what is really substantially the whole of informed medical opinion.[58]

Before looking at what restoring *Bolam* to its original limits might mean in practice, we need first to consider whether the attempt to do so in *Bolitho* will actually take root. For *Bolitho* is not the first judgment which seeks to correct misperceptions of the *Bolam* test. In *Hucks* v. *Cole*,[59] decided in 1968, albeit not reported until 1993, Sachs L.J. used language almost identical to that of Lord Browne-Wilkinson in *Bolitho*.

---

[56] [1984] A.C. 296; discussed *supra* in section III.

[57] *Ibid.* at 243.

[58] [1957] 1 W.L.R. 582 at 587. It would appear, therefore, that Bolamisation for over 40 years has been based on an erroneous interpretation of the case. As Grubb exclaims in his casenote on *Bolitho*: 'Eureka! The courts have got it at last. Expert evidence, whether of professional practice or otherwise, is not conclusive in a medical negligence case that the defendant has not been careless.' A. Grubb, 'Negligence: Causation and *Bolam*', *op. cit.* at 380.

[59] [1993] 4 Med. L.R. 393, (C.A.).

In *Joyce* v. *Merton, Sutton & Wandsworth Health Authority*,[60] the Court of Appeal had asserted an authority to scrutinise expert evidence to determine whether that evidence represented a responsible judgment of good practice.[61] Yet none of these judgments were hailed as reining in *Bolam* or altering the face of malpractice litigation. Will *Bolitho* really make a difference? We believe it will.

Self-evidently, *Bolitho* is a decision from the House of Lords, the highest court in the land. Lord Browne-Wilkinson's words carry ultimate authority. *Bolitho* has already made a difference. *Bolitho* has been applied by the Court of Appeal to uphold a judgment against a defendant general practitioner. In *Marriott* v. *West Midlands Health Authority*[62] the judges concluded that the expert opinion advanced in the doctor's favour was not defensible. Most importantly *Bolitho* has been decided at a time when other developments also point to a revolution in the way medical malpractice is judged. Medicine itself is changing with practitioners increasingly evaluating their own practice and seeking to develop evidence-based medicine.[63] The traditional guardians of clinical standards, the Royal Colleges of Medicine, have over the last decade become more and more proactive, issuing guidelines about good practice with reference to treatment and procedures. The government in its White Paper, *The New NHS*,[64] stated its intention to establish national standards and guidelines for services and treatments. To give substance to that intention, the National Institute of Clinical Excellence (NICE) has been established to develop guidelines for good practice, not just in the context of new drug treatments, but in a much wider sphere of reviewing all forms of therapies and procedures.[65] The Commission for Health Improvement will oversee clinical services and tackle shortcomings.[66] The day of the unfettered autonomy of the individual consultant is over. The profession in partnership with govern-

[60] [1996] 7 Med. L.R. 1 (C.A.), and see *Clarke* v. *Adams* (1950) S.J. 599; *Jones* v. *Manchester Corp.* [1952] 2 All E.R. 125; *Wisznieski* v. *Central Manchester Health Authority* [1996] 7 Med. L.R. 245.

[61] The action failed on grounds of causation: see A. Grubb, 'Medical Negligence, Breach of Duty and Causation', (1996) 4 Med. L. Rev. 86.

[62] [1999] Lloyd's Rep. Med. 23.

[63] See generally, T. Felton and G. Lister, *Consider the Evidence: The NHS on the Move Towards Evidence Based Medicine* (Coopers and Lybrand 1996).

[64] *The New NHS* (Cmd. 3807, 1997). Analysed by V. Harpwood, *op. cit.*, n. 4 at 114–16.

[65] See, *A First Class Service: Quality in the New NHS* (DoH 1999) which states at para. 2.27 that NICE will provide '[c]lear, authoritative, *guidance* on clinical and cost effectiveness . . . to front line clinicians' (our emphasis). Similarly, in a speech on 31 March 1999, the Secretary of State for Health said that 'NICE will give *advice* on the clinical and cost effectiveness of both new and existing technologies'. The full text of this speech can be found in the NICE website at http://www.nice.org.uk.

[66] See ss.19–24 Health Act 1999.

ment[67] is moving to set transparent standards for increasing numbers of treatment. The judge confronted by individual experts who disagree about good practice will in certain cases be able to refer to something approaching a 'gold standard'.

One other factor combines with *Bolitho* to make it more likely that *Bolam* in the context of malpractice litigation can be returned to its original limits. Doctors have (rightly or wrongly) had a 'bad press' lately,[68] so that in June 1998, *The Guardian*[69] declared '. . . secrecy and clubbiness are still the prevailing attitudes at the top of a profession, where the main concern often seems to be protect doctors, not patients'. The events in Bristol,[70] which resulted in Professor Ian Kennedy being asked to review circumstances surrounding the deaths of several infants after cardiac surgery, are perhaps the worst of a number of tragic cases where gross medical error has had disastrous results. Moreover, the effect of the trial of the GP, Harold Shipman, on the public's automatic presumption of beneficence on the part of the medical practitioner is likely to be severe and long lasting. Blind acquiescence on the part of the judiciary to any plausible opinion expressed by an apparently exalted medical practitioner no longer looks like a viable policy.

VI. HOW WILL BOLITHO WORK THEN?

If *Bolitho* is to make a difference to medical litigation, some clear view on how Lord Browne-Wilkinson's revision of *Bolam* will work is needed. He declares that the court must be satisfied that expert opinion has 'logical force'; that it is capable of withstanding 'logical analysis'. Yet later he acknowledges that assessment of medical risks and benefits is a matter of clinical judgment which a judge would not normally be able to make without expert evidence. Nor may a judge simply operate on his 'preference' for one set of opinion over another. We almost seem to come full circle. While the medical experts are to be required, in rare cases, to justify their opinions on logical grounds, there still appears to be a prima facie presumption that non-doctors will not be able fully to comprehend the evidence. This leads inexorably to a conclusion that the evidence cannot, after all, be critically evaluated by a judge. Put another

---

[67] Or even, on occasion in partnership with lawyers? The BMA and Law Society produced a joint document regarding capacity to consent in 1996: *Assessment of Mental Capacity: Guidance for Doctors and Lawyers* (BMA and Law Society 1996).

[68] See, 'Struck-off Doctors Risk Merit Pay Cut', *The Guardian*, 11.8.98, at 6; 'Senior Doctors Lose Right to Draw Huge Bonuses', *The Observer*, 9.8.98, at 3.

[69] *The Guardian*, 25.6.98, at 12.

[70] See A. Treasure, 'Lessons from the Bristol Case', (1998) 316 *B.M.J.* 1685; R. Smith, 'All Changed, Changed Utterly', (1998) 316 *B.M.J.* 1917.

way, the difficulty in establishing the logic or otherwise of medical evidence lies in an argument that laypersons may not be capable of understanding the merits of such logic. It becomes easier to see how the *Bolam* has metamorphosed in the way it did, appearing to grant doctors something close to immunity from suit.

The judgment of *Hucks* v. *Cole*,[71] cited with unqualified approval in *Bolitho*, may assist in breaking the circle. In *Hucks* v. *Cole* the facts were as follows. Dr Cole, a general practitioner, was treating a woman in the final weeks of her pregnancy for a septic finger. He was well aware that the area was infected with *streptococcus pyrogenes* capable of developing into puerperal (childbirth) fever. Yet he continued to prescribe tetracycline rather than penicillin. After giving birth Mrs Hucks succumbed to puerperal fever. All the medical experts acknowledged that penicillin would have prevented the puerperal fever. Four defence experts nonetheless testified that they, like Dr Cole, would not have prescribed penicillin. Tetracycline was a slightly cheaper drug and they would have regarded the risk of puerperal fever as low. By 1968 cases of puerperal fever were rarely seen in the United Kingdom. The Court of Appeal upheld the trial judge's findings of negligence. Sachs L.J. said:

> When the evidence shows that a lacuna in professional practice exists by which risks of grave danger are *knowingly* taken, however small the risk, the court must anxiously examine the lacuna—particularly if the risk can be *easily* and *inexpensively* avoided.[72]

Sachs L.J. acknowledged that the evidence indicated that other doctors would have done as the defendant did was 'a very weighty matter'. But such evidence could not be conclusive. The experts agreed about the risk of harm to the patient. They agreed that there was an obvious means of eliminating risk. The defendants' experts failed to provide any convincing explanation for rejecting that obvious means of protecting the patient. *Hucks* v. *Cole* required that experts explain the grounds for adopting a course of treatment clearly contrary to at least a significant body of opinion among their peers. In *Bolitho* itself, Lord Browne-Wilkinson says that in weighing risks and benefits the judge must assure himself that ' . . . experts have directed their minds to the question of comparative risks and benefits and have reached a defendable conclusion on the matter'.[73]

That approach is exactly the approach taken by the Court of Appeal

---

[71] [1993] 4 Med. L.R. 393 (C.A.).
[72] *Ibid.* at 397.
[73] *Op. cit.*, n. 3 at 243.

in *Marriott* v. *West Midlands Health Authority*[74] in finding against the defendant doctor. The plaintiff fell and suffered head injuries. He was unconscious for about half an hour. He was taken to hospital for X-rays and investigation but discharged the next day. Once home, he remained unwell. He had headaches. He was lethargic and had no appetite. Eight days after his fall he was visited by his general practitioner, the second defendant. The defendant carried out certain neurological tests at the plaintiff's home. He found no abnormalities on the basis of those tests. He advised the plaintiff's wife to telephone him again if her husband's condition deteriorated and suggested painkillers. Four days later the plaintiff's condition worsened. He was re-admitted to hospital and a large extradural haematoma was operated on. The surgery revealed a skull fracture and internal bleeding. The plaintiff was left paralysed and suffering from a speech disorder.

The plaintiff claimed both that the hospital was negligent in discharging him prematurely on the first occasion, and that his general practitioner was negligent in not referring him back to hospital when he visited him at home. It is this latter claim against the general practitioner with which we are concerned. The plaintiff alleged that his general practitioner should have perceived the seriousness of his injury and subsequent symptoms, and that further investigation at that stage would have prevented the catastrophic deterioration in this condition. The key question was whether a responsible general practitioner should have judged that a full neurological investigation was necessary. Should he have done more than the simple tests he carried out at the plaintiff's home? Such tests, all agreed, were insufficient to exclude an intracranial lesion.

The plaintiff's experts testified that, given the patient's history (in particular that he had been unconscious for a period of time after the fall), and in the light of his symptoms and failure to improve after coming home, the doctor ought to have sent him back to hospital. The defendant's expert argued that she would support a decision to leave the plaintiff at home as the risk of an intracranial lesion causing a sudden collapse was very small. The trial judge held first that the defendant's expert's view of the plaintiff's condition was over-optimistic being based largely on the defendant's witness statement. She went on to say that, although the risk of an intracranial lesion was very small, '. . . the consequences, if things go wrong, are disastrous to the patient. In such circumstances, it is my view that the only reasonably prudent course . . . is to re-admit for further testing and observation'.[75]

[74] [1999] Lloyd's Rep. Med. 23; analysed in M.A. Jones, 'The Illogical Expert', (1999) 15 P.N. 117.

[75] *Ibid.* at 27.

In the appeal court, the judge's exercise in risk assessment was upheld at least by Beldam L.J.[76] She was entitled to weigh the admittedly small risk of something going wrong against the seriousness of the consequences. Facilities to carry out a comprehensive neurological examination were readily available in local hospitals. Given the devastating nature of the consequences of the risk of an intracranial lesion, no reasonable or responsible general practitioner would have exposed the plaintiff to that risk.

Marriott is no doubt an extreme case and one where the defendant's own expert witness offered him less than whole-hearted support. Beldam L.J. noted that to some extent both parties' experts tended to focus on what their individual approach might have been, rather than what would have constituted responsible practice. It is a judgment which provoked from Michael Jones[77] the following pertinent question:

> In five or ten years time will *Marriott* mark the beginning of a sea-change in judicial attitudes to medical negligence actions, or will it stand out as an isolated, and comparatively rare, example of a case in which logical analysis ruled?

We hope and believe that the former is the case, that *Marriott* will mark the beginning of a revolution in judicial attitudes to medical negligence claims.

Bolitho has set in train a process whereby judges scrutinise medical evidence, using the same mixture of common sense and logical analysis that they use to scrutinise other expert evidence in negligence claims against professionals such as architects and accountants. That process of scrutiny will be aided and enhanced by the revolution within medicine itself. Where clinical guidelines have been developed in relation to a disputed treatment, the judge will be enabled to judge the individual expert testimony in context of the profession's considered judgment.

A simple example can be drawn from claims relating to failure to warn patients of the risks that both male and female sterilisation occasionally fail.[78] Nature triumphs over medical science and the relevant 'tubes' reconnect themselves. A spate of cases on failed sterilisation surfaced from the 1970's onwards. Practice clearly varied widely as to whether patients were warned of the risk of failure. The outcome of consequent medical negligence claims also varied widely. That outcome depended on the skill of the defendants' lawyers in finding eminent

[76] With whom Swinton Thomas L.J. agreed; Pill L.J. considered it unnecessary to resort to *Bolitho*.
[77] *Op. cit.*, n. 74 at 120.
[78] See *e.g. Thake* v. *Maurice* [1984] 2 All E.R. 513, (C.A.); *Eyre* v. *Measday* [1986] 1 All E.R. 488, (C.A.); *Gold* v. *Haringey Health Authority* [1987] 2. All E.R. 888 (C.A.).

doctors to testify that they did not consider that proper practice required them to warn of the risk of failure.[79] Today the position different. In the context of female sterilisation, the Royal College of Obstetricians and Gynaecologists advises on a practice of full and frank disclosure. Department of Health guidelines, supported by a special consent form, require disclosure. Any doctors still not warning their patients of the risks of failed sterilisation will be hard pressed to establish the logic of rejecting a case endorsed by the leaders of the profession. Failure to warn of the risk of sterilisation failing will be condemned as neither reasonable nor responsible. Ironically, a defendant who fails to warn a patient of the risk of sterilisation reversing itself may still escape any substantial liability. For while he or she is unlikely to avoid a finding of negligence, the House of Lords in *McFarlane* v. *Tayside Health Board*[80] controversially ruled that damages may not be awarded in respect of the costs of caring for and bringing up a healthy child. The House of Lords upheld an award of £10,000 damages for the mother in compensation for the pain and discomfort of pregnancy and childbirth,[81] but rejected the much larger claim of £100,000 in relation to the costs of the child's upbringing as irrecoverable economic loss.

Failed sterilisation is an exceptionally easy target. The profession *and* the Department of Health have promulgated clear guidance in a case where the possibility of arguing justification for departing from that guidance looks remote. However a commitment has been made to develop similar sorts of guidelines over a wide spectrum of medicine, especially through the National Institute of Clinical Excellence. The Institute's central purpose is to rationalise and co-ordinate clinical guidance on effective treatment, in appropriate cases developing something close to protocols on disease-management. Presumably such guidance will be written lucidly, in terms intelligible to judges in medical malpractice claims. The judge will have access to material, independent of the particular dispute before him, enabling him to assess the logic of the parties' cases. *Bolitho*, plus more ready access to clinical guidelines, suggests a more proactive role for judges assessing expert evidence. Nor will clinical guidelines necessarily be the only source of judicial guidance on the logic of the evidence presented by the parties.[82] The burgeoning literature on medical developments, often presented in a style

[79] See, *e.g. Gold*. The case concerned a failed sterilisation carried out in 1979. The Court of Appeal held that as at the time of the procedure there was a responsible body of medical opinion that would not have given such a warning, then the plaintiff's case must fail.

[80] [1999] 4 All E.R. 961.

[81] Note Lord Millett's dissent denying damages to the mother too.

[82] See Harpwood *op. cit.*, n. 4 at 100–21; and see V. Harpwood, 'NHS Reform, Audit, Protocol and Standards of Care', (1994) 1 Med. L. Int. 241.

comprehensible to lay people, may also be resorted to much more frequently in litigation.[83] *Bolitho* demands that doctors explain their practice. Doctors themselves are developing tools which will enable judges to review those explanations.

There will be those who have doubts whether judges will be ready to use those tools. Reluctance to engage in an exercise some judges perceive as 'meddling' in clinical autonomy is starkly demonstrated in *R.* v. *Cambridge Health Authority ex parte B*[84] where Sir Thomas Bingham M.R. declared that:

> the courts are not, contrary to what is sometimes believed, arbiters as to the merits of cases . . . Were we to express opinions as to the likelihood of the effectiveness of medical treatment, or as to the merits of medical judgment, then we should be straying far from the sphere which under our constitution is accorded to us. We have one function only, which is to rule upon the lawfulness of decisions. That is a function to which we should strictly confine ourselves.

In the Court of Appeal[85] in *Bolitho* itself, Dillon L.J., while affirming that expert evidence was not immune from judicial scrutiny, set the burden of proof to justify rejection of such evidence at an almost impossibly high level. To question the defendant's evidence a court must be ' . . . clearly satisfied that the views of that group of doctors were *Wednesbury* reasonable *i.e.* views such as no reasonable doctor could have held'. He went on to say ' . . . that would be an impossibly strong thing to say of the honest views of experts'.[86] Were Lord Browne-Wilkinson's 'rare' cases to be judged by this 'Dillon' benchmark, they may prove to be so rare as to be almost invisible. The opportunity to develop what Harpwood[87] describes as 'a more objective approach to the standard of care required of doctors' would have been squandered.

There are those who view the development of guidelines and their use as dire for both patients and doctors. They argue that centrally directed standards will undermine the *art* of medicine, especially if courts judging malpractice claims do treat such standards as a gold standard. The distinguished physician, Sir Douglas Black,[88] has said of guidelines

---

[83] See *e.g.* J. Collier (ed.), *Guidelines for Management of Common Medical Emergencies.*

[84] [1995] 2 All E.R. 129 at 136.

[85] [1993] 4 Med. L.R. 381.

[86] *Ibid.* at 392.

[87] *Op. cit.*, n. 4 at 107.

[88] See D. Black, 'Guidelines or Gumption? The Role of Medical Responsibility: A View from the Profession' in S.R. Hirsch and J. Harris (eds.), *Consent and the Incompetent Patient: Ethics, Law and Medicine* (Royal College of Psychiatrists 1988). See also J. Warden, 'NICE to Sort out Clinical Wheat from Chaff', (1999) 318 *B.M.J.* 416 expressing similar fears.

'... they can become ossified and too rigid for the flexibility required in the heterogeneous circumstances of clinical practice'. Commentators, such as Sir Douglas Black, fear that doctors, to avoid litigation, will cease to treat the individual and concentrate on ticking the relevant boxes. We argue that such an outcome should not result from either the process of setting standards or the use of standards in litigation.

We attempt an example to illustrate our optimism, acknowledging that our knowledge of obstetrics may well be flawed. Obstetricians hold radically different opinions on good practice in relation to delivery of a premature breech baby. A number strongly argue that such an infant should be delivered by caesarean section. Others allow labour to proceed. Assume that after clinical trials and reviews of the evidence, NICE issued *guidance* recommending delivery by caesarean. Does it follow that any obstetrician who nonetheless allows trial of labour will *inevitably* be found liable in negligence? Not at all. Several factors might logically justify departing from that guidance. First, the patient's own wishes and feelings must be taken into account. Second, her circumstances will be relevant. It may be that for most women the ratio of risk to benefit of a caesarean delivery points in favour of such surgery. But were the woman likely to return to a part of the world where in a subsequent pregnancy she would be at risk of a ruptured uterus[89] or if she planned a large family that ratio would itself alter radically. Even her own size and obstetric history could alter advice designed for the generality of labouring women. All the guidance would require is that once again the defendant justifies, and *explains*, the management of the particular case.[90]

Doctors may also fear that *Bolitho* will have adverse effects on the litigation process itself. The pessimistic medical observer of malpractice litigation may reason as follows: More claimants will now try it on. Even when confronted by substantial evidence of a body of expert opinion supporting the defendant, claimants will play the *Bolitho* card. They, and their lawyers, will contend that that opinion lacks any logical basis. Cases will be dragged out for even longer periods of time. Further expert evidence will be required to counter allegations of illogicality. Costs will spiral. The bitterness of litigation will increase when the defendant is attacked, not just as a doctor who has made a mistake, but as one whose practice *lacks any rational basis*.

Such a catastrophic scenario ignores several factors. *Bolitho* speaks of rare cases. One would at least wish to assume that most practice does have a rational basis? Perhaps it may be the case that there are medical

---

[89] See W. Savage, *A Savage Enquiry: Who Controls Childbirth* (Virago 1986).

[90] In his speech launching NICE (*op. cit.*, n. 65), the Secretary of State assured doctors that clinical judgment in relation to individual patients would continue to be respected.

experts a little too willing to testify in support of practices any of their peers no longer consider sound. *Bolitho* may simply result in cases which should not be contested being settled more swiftly and economically. Moreover, contemporaneously with the advent of a post-*Bolitho* era, the civil justice system is undergoing radical change as a result of Lord Woolf's review.[91] The full extent of Woolf's proposals and their implementation in the new Civil Procedure Rules is beyond the scope of this paper. However, some points are worthy of note here. Case-management is designed to restrain the worst excesses of adversarial litigation. Most importantly, reforms relating to expert evidence ought to reduce both delay and confrontation in the system. Judges are empowered to appoint a single expert in straightforward cases.[92] When each party continues to call their own experts, the judge can require the use of experts' meetings.[93] The experts will be directed to ascertain which matters they can agree together and submit a joint report where possible. Better training for experts is urged by Woolf and the creation of a pool of experts was recommended in his Interim Report. The aim of reforming the civil justice system is to achieve easier access to, and a higher quality of, expert evidence.[94] Misuse of expert evidence which renders litigation akin to trial by battle should become much rarer, countering fears that *Bolitho* itself will become a new battleground for experts. Woolf appears to emphasise conciliation and common ground among, rather than confrontation between, the experts in trials.

VII. INFORMATION DISCLOSURE—*BOLAM* RESTRAINED

In the context of straightforward claims for medical negligence, *Bolitho* simply restores *Bolam* to its proper limits and treats claims for medical negligence like other claims for professional negligence. *Bolitho* does not undermine either the role of clinical judgment or peer review of professional practice. Medical competence remains for the most part a medical matter. De-Bolamisation is not in this context *de-medicalisation*. As Teff has noted, '[judicial] involvement is not the same as encroachment, or even engagement' in clinical freedom.[95] It is in other sorts of dispute between patients and their doctors that the *Bolam* test may well either be substantially diluted or abandoned altogether.

We would suggest that information disclosure and the supremacy of

[91] *Access to Justice: Final Report* (HMSO 1996).

[92] Para. 35.7.

[93] Para. 35.12.

[94] See Harpwood's reference about how effective reforms in relation to expert evidence will be; *op. cit.*, n. 4 at 96–100.

[95] H. Teff, *Reasonable Care* (OUP 1994) at 16.

the 'reasonable doctor test' may be the first *Bolitho* casualty. The nature of the issue before the court in claims that the defendant doctor failed to give her patient sufficient information about the risks and side-effects, and alternatives to the treatment proposed, involve questions which judges can much more easily assess than the issues arising in claims relating to, say, diagnoses or modes of treatment. Attempting to analyse whether or not the doctors' justification for non-disclosure is logical and rational will not be a task bedevilled by too much technical or scientific detail.

However, one reading of *Bolitho* might suggest that Lord Browne-Wilkinson excluded information disclosure from his efforts to restore *Bolam* to its proper context. His Lordship declares that 'in cases of diagnoses and treatment there are cases where, despite a body of professional opinion sanctioning the defendant's conduct, the defendant can properly be held liable in negligence'.[96] Then appears in brackets the following cryptic phrase: '(I am not here considering questions of disclosure of risk).'[97] An interpretation of that throwaway phrase as meaning that information disclosure disputes were to be judged on the basis of what his Lordship had declared to be a misinterpretation of *Bolam* would be itself illogical and irrational. Either, his Lordship was simply and correctly flagging up the fact that questions of information disclosure were simply not relevant on the *facts* of *Bolitho*, or, more probably, Lord Browne-Wilkinson considered that restraining *Bolam* in the context of information disclosure had already been achieved.

In *Sidaway* itself, we have already noted that Lord Bridge made it clear that there might be cases where '... disclosure of a particular risk was so obviously necessary to an informed choice on the part of the patient that no reasonably prudent medical man would fail to make it'.[98] Many years in advance of *Bolitho*, Lord Bridge had sought to clarify the point that expert opinion to negate negligence must be *responsible*. Again as we have seen earlier, subsequent judgments in *Blyth* v. *Bloomsbury Health Authority* and *Gold* v. *Haringey Health Authority* appeared to endorse an unrestrained Bolamite interpretation of *Sidaway*. Other more recent case-law breathes new life into Lord Bridge's words.

Prior to *Bolitho* in the House of Lords, in *Smith* v. *Tunbridge Wells Health Authority*,[99] Morland J. condemned the expert evidence offered on behalf of the defendant as 'neither reasonable nor responsible'.

---

[96] *Op. cit.*, n. 3 at 243.
[97] *Ibid.*
[98] *Op. cit.*, n. 17 at 663. Lord Templeman's speech can also be interpreted in this way (see A. Grubb, 'Negligence: Causation and *Bolam*', (*op. cit.*, n. 5) at 382–3).
[99] [1994] 5 Med. L.R. 334.

Failure to warn a young man of the risk of impotence inherent in rectal surgery deprived the plaintiff of an informed choice in relation to that surgery. In finding the defendants negligent, Morland J. described himself as ' . . . applying the *Bolam* test as elucidated in *Sidaway*'.[100] That *Bolam* was already restrained in the context of information disclosure is an opinion re-enforced by the judgment of the Court of Appeal in *Pearce* v. *United Bristol Healthcare N.H.S. Trust*,[101] a case decided subsequent to the decision of the House of Lords in *Bolitho.* Lord Woolf M.R. had no doubts that *Bolitho* applied to claims concerning information disclosure and appeared to perceive Lord Browne-Wilkinson's general approach in *Bolitho* as essentially in the same vein as Lord Bridge's more restricted qualification of the *Bolam* test in *Sidaway.*

The facts of the case, briefly, are as follows. Mrs Pearce was pregnant with her sixth child. The child was two weeks overdue. She was seen by her obstetrician who told her that medical intervention (in the form of an induction or a caesarean), was inappropriate. He warned her of the risks to the foetus of an induction, and the inherent risks to herself of a caesarean, but did not tell her of the increased risk of stillbirth associated with non-intervention, estimated at 0.1–0.2 per cent. Reluctantly, she agreed to non-intervention. Sadly the child was stillborn. Mrs Pearce alleged that failure to advise her of the risk of stillbirth was negligent.

Lord Woolf's judgment concludes in the defendant's favour. In the circumstances of the case, the 'very, very small additional risk' to the child was not a sufficiently 'significant risk' to render the doctor negligent in failing to advise Mrs Pearce of that risk, especially given her distressed condition at the time of the consultation. His reasoning, however, departs significantly from an unrestrained application of the *Bolam* test. He cites both Lord Bridge in *Sidaway*, and Lord Browne-Wilkinson in *Bolitho*, to support a proposition capable of effecting a radical departure from a 'reasonable doctor' test. Lord Woolf declares that the law requires that ' . . . if there is a significant risk which would affect the judgment of a *reasonable patient*, then in the normal course it is the responsibility of a doctor to inform the patient of that significant risk, if the information is needed so that the patient can determine for him or herself as to what course she should adopt'[102] (our emphases).

The cynic will of course respond that whatever his Lordship's language, the Court of Appeal rejected Mrs Pearce's claim finding it not to ' . . . be proper for the courts to interfere with the clinical opinion of the

[100] *Ibid.* at 339.

[101] [1999] P.I.Q.R. 53.

[102] *Ibid.* at 59.

medical man responsible for treating Mrs Pearce'.[103] Even the cynic must concede that, whatever the outcome on the facts, the 'reasonable doctor' test received a body blow in *Pearce*.[104] It survives only if the 'reasonable doctor' understands that he must offer the patient what the 'reasonable patient' would be likely to need to exercise his right to make informed decisions about his care. The recent guidance to doctors from the General Medical Council re-enforces that message.[105] Patients must be given the information they want or ought to know. Judges evaluating information disclosure practices will be encouraged to take a more pro-patient stance not just by the higher courts but by the medical profession itself.

VIII. THE LAW COMMISSION—*BOLAM* ABANDONED?

In the context of claims for medical negligence, including claims relating to information disclosure, all that can be said at this stage is that the courts *appear* to be prepared to reign in the worst excesses of the *Bolam* test. It is in relation to the principles governing the treatment of mentally incapacitated adults that *Bolam* may literally be abandoned. Nearly five years after the Law Commission published its report[106] on reforming the law relating to decision-making on behalf of mentally incapacitated persons, the government announced its intention to implement a number of those proposals.[107] Among the proposals to be included in legislation[108] is the Law Commission's recommendation that while a "best interests" test should continue to govern what treatment be provided for those unable to consent to treatment on their own behalf, statutory guidance should define 'best interests'. The Law Commission vigorously condemned resort to *Bolam* to define the "best interests" of a vulnerable patient. Its Report declares:

> [I]t should be made clear beyond any shadow of a doubt that acting in a person's best interests amount to something more than

[103] *Ibid.* at 60.

[104] Grubb ('Negligence: Causation and *Bolam*'), *e.g.* argues that in *Pearce* the Court of Appeal has 'shown a renewed appetite to set the standard of disclosure' (at 384).

[105] *Seeking Patients' Consent: The Ethical Considerations* (GMC 1999).

[106] Law Commission Report No.231, *Mental Incapacity*. In December 1997 the Lord Chancellor's Department issued a further consultation paper *Who Decides? Making Decisions on Behalf of Mentally Incapacitated Adults* (Cmd. 1803). That consultation paper solicited further views on the proposals made by the Law commission, albeit that the Law Commission's Report was itself based on several years of consultation and three prior consultation papers.

[107] *Making Decisions* (Cmd. 4465) (LCD 1999).

[108] No timetable for introducing such legislation into Parliament has been set.

> not treating a person in a negligent manner. Decisions taken on behalf of a person lacking capacity require a careful, focused consideration of that person *as an individual.* Judgments as to whether a professional has acted negligently, on the other hand, require a careful, focused consideration of how that particular professional acted as compared with the way which other reasonable professionals would have acted.[109]

Judgments about the welfare of mentally incapacitated patients are no longer to be classified as primarily clinical judgments. The spotlight shifts from the doctor to the patient. In its original proposals the Law Commission suggested that regard must be had to the following four matters in assessing a patient's best interests:[110]

(1) The ascertainable past and present wishes and feelings of the person concerned, and the factors that person would consider it able to do so;
(2) the need to permit and encourage the person to participate, or improve his or her ability to participate, as fully as possible in anything done for and any decision affecting him or her;
(3) the views of other people whom it is appropriate and practicable to consult about the person's wishes and feelings and what would be in his or her best interests;
(4) whether the purpose for which any action or decision is required can be as effectively achieved in a manner less restrictive of the person's freedom of action.

Subsequent consultation led the government to propose a further two factors to be included in legislation:[111]

(5) whether there is a reasonable expectation of the person recovering capacity to make the decision in the reasonably foreseeable future;

(6) the need to be satisfied that the wishes of the person without capacity were not the result of under influence.

The Law Commission's approach demands a focus on the patient as an individual and rejects the notion that doctors should be able to hide behind some cloak of professional opinion. The doctor caring for a

---

[109] Law Commission Report No.231, *op. cit.*, n. 106 at para. 3.27.

[110] See paras. 3.26–3.37.

[111] *Making Decisions, supra*, n. 107 at para. 1.12. The following paragraph sensibly provides that that the statutory list of factors to be taken into account in assessing best interests '. . . should not be applied too rigidly' and should not exclude consideration of any relevant factor in a particular case.

mentally incapacitated person will be required to exercise *her* judgment to meet the needs of that person. In determining what the person's medical needs might be, the opinion of other doctors may well be relevant, but the doctor must give equal weight to her patient's social needs and individual characteristics. Assessing which treatment options meet the patient's overall welfare, professional opinion takes a back seat. Such an approach does more than simply reject the *Bolam* test as the arbiter of patients' best interests. It rejects a Bolamite philosophy. In the opening paragraph of its Report, the Law Commission notes[112] that the law is out of date, and does not rest on clear or modern foundations of principle. It has failed to keep up with social changes. It has also failed to keep up with developments in our understanding of the rights and needs of those with mental disability.

The whole tenor of the Law Commission Report, in so far as it concerns medical decision-making, reflects a change of emphasis from professional responsibilities to patients' *rights*. The Law Commission explicitly recognises that the medical profession has failed certain groups of patients, that there has been unacceptable discrimination against people with ' . . . mental disabilities (and especially mental illness) in the past by *medical practitioners;* the law and society as a whole'.[113] They highlight the growth of a 'rights culture' and the proliferation of documents emphasising the 'obligation of providers to consumers of services'.[114] Such language is inconsistent with a philosophy which allows the providers, the doctors, to dictate what those services will comprise. Rather, the law, in whatever context, must seek to ascertain what the patient is entitled to and what her needs demand.

Legislation effectively overruling that part of the judgment in *Re F*, which applied the *Bolam* test to determine 'best interests', will constitute only a relatively minor exercise in *de*-Bolamisation. What will be of equal interest will be whether legislative reform in one area of health care law will prompt the judiciary too to embark on a retreat from *Bolam* more generally. We sought to argue earlier that even in judgments which do not overtly invoke the *Bolam* test, a Bolamite philosophy prevailed. In *Gillick*, and subsequent cases concerning disputes about the treatment of minors, the judiciary once again regarded professional opinion as the best arbiter of any dispute and showed reluctance to investigate the validity of such professional judgments. Rooting out *covert*, possibly unintentional, resort to *Bolam* will not be an easy process. It will take place if, and only if, the courts acknowledge that past deference to medical opinion has been somewhat misguided and

[112] *Op. cit.*, n. 106 at para. 1.1.

[113] At para. 2.40, emphasis added.

[114] *Ibid.*

are prepared to struggle to give substance to rhetoric surrounding patients' rights, whatever their age or mental capacity. Predicting which way the courts will jump is nigh on impossible.

IX. *BOLAM*—IN RETREAT

If the judgment in *Bolitho* stood alone, as the only indicator of a medical litigation revolution, we would have had substantial doubts whether any change, even change well short of revolution, might be expected in health care law. Lord Browne-Wilkinson's words might go as much unheeded as those of Sachs L.J.'s in *Hucks* v. *Cole*. However, we have sought to demonstrate that the timing of the decision, amidst a host of other relevant developments affecting the provision of health care, suggests that in several contexts medical professional opinion will be subjected to rigorous scrutiny. *An* expert opinion, be it one on allegations of professional negligence, disclosure of risks, or the appropriate care of certain groups of patients, will no longer be determinative of professional obligations.

In claims for medical negligence the emergence of sources of neutral and independent guidance on good practice will empower judges to utilise *Bolitho* and assess whether the opinion advanced by each party's experts is logical and defensible. No flood of judgments ruling expert evidence to be illogical and indefensible should be expected. Nonetheless the swift resort to *Bolitho* in *Marriott* show that courts may now be ready to restore *Bolam* to its original limits.

The Court of Appeal in *Pearce* applied *Bolitho* in the context of an information disclosure claim. Read together with the first instance judgment in *Smith* v. *Tunbridge Wells Health Authority*, *Pearce* signals that announcements of the stillbirth of 'informed consent' in England were premature. The era of unquestioning acceptance of Lord Diplock's application of the *Bolam* test expressed as by him in *Sidaway* is over. Lord Scarman's extra-judicial injunction[115] to 'ignore Lord Diplock's opinion' may be (belatedly) about to enter into force. An obligation to disclose any significant risk which would affect the judgment of a reasonable patient can never be defined by reference to a body of professional opinion alone. In an era when the General Medical Council directs clinicians that they ' . . . must take appropriate steps to find out what patients want to know and ought to know about their condition and its treatment'[116] blind adherence to *Bolam* in its unrestrained, and much misunderstood, form should no longer be possible.

---

[115] See 'Consent, Communication and Responsibility', (1986) 79 *J. Roy. Soc. Med.* 697.
[116] *Seeking Patients' Consent: The Ethical Considerations*, *op. cit.*, n. 105.

Returning *Bolam* to its original limits does not exclude expert medical opinion about what should have been done for, or said to, the patient. It simply treats that opinion as evidence, whose weight will depend on the circumstances of particular cases. Professional opinion advanced by doctors will be evaluated on a par with professional opinion advanced by other kinds of professionals. In many instances, professional opinion will remain highly, and rightly, influential.

The prospect of the English courts suddenly revising the tradition of decades and actively seeking to arrogate to themselves the making of clinical judgments is remote. Neither the decision in *Bolitho* nor the other developments outlined in our paper threaten the *proper* boundaries of medical judgment. Doctors themselves are now partners in a process which should strive to ensure that medical practice is soundly based on evidence and reason. The leaders of the profession have moved to acknowledge the importance of working in partnership with patients. *Bolitho* is a decision delivered in the midst of an era when the common law itself is immersed in change. The entry into force of the Human Rights Act 1998, in October 2000, will require that judges pay much more attention generally to claimants' rights. The Law Commission's emphasis on identifying the rights of mentally incapacitated patients and defining the obligations of doctors in the context of those rights will have relevance to all patients.

If there is to be a 'revolution' in health care law, as with all revolutions, it will have many causes and *Bolitho* may prove to be of less significance than others. The decision does, however, signal judicial will, at the highest level, to return *Bolam* to its proper context. Together with the many other factors prompting change, inappropriate deference to medical opinion should be replaced by legal principles which recognise the imperative to listen to both doctors and patients and which acknowledge that the medical professional is just as much required to justify his or her practice as the architect or solicitor.

[4]

ROGERS V. *WHITAKER* AND INFORMED CONSENT IN AUSTRALIA: A FAIR DINKUM DUTY OF DISCLOSURE

DON CHALMERS* and ROBERT SCHWARTZ**

In *Rogers* v. *Whitaker*[1] the High Court of Australia squarely faced the conflict between the patient-oriented "American" rule of informed consent that was recognised in *Canterbury* v. *Spence*[2] and the doctor-oriented British rule articulated in *Sidaway* v. *Governors of Bethlem Royal Hospital.*[3] The High Court determined that the law of informed consent was a species of the law of professional negligence, and that it was to be evaluated by applying ordinary principles of negligence. While formally rejecting parts of both *Canterbury* and *Sidaway*, the unanimous six justices[4] of the High Court effectively endorsed the patient-oriented "American" rule of liability while leaving open the question of whether the narrow American principle of causation, which has virtually eliminated informed consent actions in the United States, would be applied in Australia. Thus, the High Court has presented Australia with the strongest and most patient-oriented (and, consequently, most plaintiff-oriented) doctrine of informed consent among the common law jurisdictions.

In addressing the issue, however, the High Court did not resolve some of the most significant questions surrounding informed consent actions. First, the High Court was not given an opportunity to decide the question of whether causation would be evaluated subjectively, as is the usual practice in negligence cases, or by the much narrower objective standard, as is the practice in most American jurisdictions. Secondly, the High Court left open a number of questions about who decides how much information must be provided to patients—the judge or the jury, what constitutes relevant evidence on the issue of what a physician

---

* Professor of Law and Head of Department, University of Tasmania.

** Professor of Law, University of New Mexico and Visiting Professor of Law, University of Tasmania.

[1] *Rogers* v. *Whitaker* (1992) 67 A.L.J.R. 47 (High Court of Australia).

[2] *Canterbury* v. *Spence* 464 F. 2d 772 (1972) (D.C. Cir.).

[3] *Sidaway* v. *Governors of Bethlem Royal Hospital* [1985] A.C. 871 (H.L.).

[4] The seventh member of the full court, Justice Deane, did not participate in this case. Justice Deane has been a vigorous advocate of reform of the tort law to make it a rational, coherent, and unified body of law. It seems likely that he would be pleased with the rule enunciated in this case.

should have disclosed to a patient, and how far the potentially very broad duty of patient education might extend. In any case, a cautious note should be sounded about structural attributes of the Australian legal system (most significantly, the absence of contingent fee contracts) and the existence of a strong Australian social welfare safety net (which provides substantial security to those injured through medical misadventure—or otherwise, for that matter), which makes it unlikely that informed consent cases will flood the Australian courts, even with the adoption of this liberal rule in *Rogers* v. *Whitaker*.

I. FACTS

Maree Lynette Whitaker lost virtually all sight in her right eye as a consequence of a penetrating injury from a piece of wood when she was nine years old, in 1946. Despite this disability, she led a normal life. She had a happy marriage, raised four children, became employed in several different occupations (including that of a nurses' aide), actively participated in sporting activities, worked in her garden, and collected stamps, coins, and antiques. When she was in her late forties and preparing to re-enter the paid work force after three years spent in the care of her injured son, she saw her general practitioner to arrange for an eye examination. She was referred to an ophthalmic surgeon, who referred her on to Mr Rogers. Mr Rogers had good news for Ms Whitaker: surgery could both improve the appearance of her right eye and, most likely, bring back sight to that eye. Ms Whitaker, however, was not an easy patient. The trial judge found that Ms Whitaker "incessantly questioned [Mr Rogers] as to, amongst other things, the possible complications, to the point of irritating him",[5] and that she was, to Mr Rogers's knowledge, "keenly interested in the outcome of the suggested procedures including any complications as far as they affected her eyes ..."[6] Indeed, the doctor said that "no one who had ever walked through his door had asked so many questions".[7] Ms Whitaker was so concerned about the possibility that a medical error could result in the surgery being performed on the wrong eye that this worry was noted in the medical record. Despite her misgivings about the surgery generally, and her extraordinarily high sensitivity to the condition of her eyes, after two discussions with Mr Rogers, Ms Whitaker consented to the surgery.

The surgery was performed on Ms Whitaker by Mr Rogers in a professionally competent way, although it was not successful in restoring

---

[5] *Rogers* v. *Whitaker* (1991) 23 N.S.W.L.R. 600 at 610F *per* Handley J.A.

[6] *Ibid.*, at 610E.

[7] *Ibid.*, at 610D.

any vision to her right eye. What is worse, Ms Whitaker suffered an extremely rare complication of the surgery, sympathetic ophthalmia, which resulted in the deterioration of her previously sighted left eye, and she lost virtually all sight in that eye within the next eighteen months. She was, thus, left virtually blind. As a consequence of her blindness she was forced to give up almost all of the leisure activities in which she had engaged. She also was placed on a steroid regimen which resulted in her gain of over thirty kilograms and the breakdown of her happy relationship with her husband. She was unable to re-enter the paid job market, and unable to concentrate on other activities. As Handley J.A. in the Court of Appeal recognised, "[t]here can be no doubt that her blindness has had a devastating impact on her previous way of life."[8]

Ms Whitaker commenced a negligence action against Mr Rogers, and she based her claims for negligence on the plaintiff's usual catalogue of possible errors. The trial judge found that "the diagnosis, the operation, and the post-operative care and treatment of the respondent were carried out without negligence".[9] The only claim supported by the evidence was the claim that Mr Rogers had failed to inform Ms Whitaker adequately of the risk of sympathetic ophthalmia. Mr Rogers knew of the possibility of sympathetic ophthalmia, and he knew that it could render Ms Whitaker blind, as it ultimately did. He also knew that the risk of sympathetic ophthalmia was about one in 14,000, and that it might be slightly higher for those who had suffered eye trauma in the past. He had no particular reason for failing to mention it, and there was no therapeutic reason for failing to mention it; indeed, he considered sympathetic ophthalmia the "worst possible ophthalmic result" of the surgery.[10] The only justification he could offer for his failure to mention it was that it "did not come to mind".[11] Evidence accepted at the trial[12] showed that a substantial number of ophthalmic surgeons in Australia in 1984 did not provide information on sympathetic ophthalmia to patients undergoing this surgery in the absence of a specific inquiry about whether surgery on one eye could affect the sight in the other eye, an inquiry Ms Whitaker never put in those words.

The trial judge, Campbell J., sitting without a jury, found that Mr Rogers was negligent in failing to inform Ms Whitaker of the risk of sympathetic ophthalmia, and he found that this negligence caused her

---

[8] *Ibid.*, at 621.
[9] *Ibid.*, at 611.
[10] *Ibid.*, at 610.
[11] *Ibid.*
[12] *Whitaker* v. *Rogers* (1990) Aust. Torts Reports 81-062.

injury; *i.e.* if she had known of the risk she would not have undergone the treatment. He assessed damages at $808,564.38. Mr Rogers appealed on the grounds that the trial court applied the wrong substantive rule of informed consent, and both sides appealed on the issue of damages; Mr Rogers claimed they were excessive and Ms Whitaker claimed that they were manifestly inadequate. The New South Wales Court of Appeals rejected all the grounds of appeal, and the High Court of Australia considered only the question of the substantive principle to be applied in informed consent cases.[13]

II. INFORMED CONSENT AS AN ACTION IN NEGLIGENCE

The Australian courts properly treated the action as one sounding in negligence, not the intentional tort of battery. In the earliest days of the development of the doctrine of informed consent, it was perceived as a species of battery.[14] If a physician were to trespass upon another's body (by cutting into it with a surgical appliance, for example) without that person's consent, that would constitute battery just as any other person's trespass upon another in the same way (by wielding a knife against the other in the perpetration of a robbery, for example) would constitute battery. If the "consenting" patient were not informed of the nature, purpose, risks, and alternatives of the proposed medical treatment, it was argued, the consent was thus vitiated and the subsequent performance of the medical procedure became a battery. The courts were uncomfortable treating informed consent actions as intentional torts because a doctor's failure to explain a remote and hypothetical risk to a frightened patient seems very different from a violent knife-wielding robber's attack on a stranger. The kind of culpability normally associated with battery is absent in the vast majority of doctor–patient encounters, even when the doctor does not fully and

---

[13] The NSW Court of Appeals' decision is reported and commented upon at (1993) 1 Med. L. Rev. 115 where the English Court of Appeal decision in *Blyth* v. *Bloomsbury H.A.* (1987) *Times*, February 11, is discussed.

[14] There are several good histories of the doctrine of informed consent. The basic history is laid out particularly well in I. Kennedy and A. Grubb, *Medical Law: Text and Materials* (Butterworths 1989) at 216–29. See also D. Louisell and H. Williams, *Medical Malpractice* (1987) at s. 22.04. See also S. McLean, *A Patient's Right to Know* (Dartmouth 1989) chs. 5–7; M. Powers and N. Harris, *Medical Negligence* (Butterworths 1990) ch. 10; P. D. G. Skegg, *Law Ethics and Medicine* (Oxford, Clarendon Press 1984) ch. 4; E. Picard, "Consent to Medical Treatment in Canada" (1981) 19 *Osgoode Hall Law Journal* 140; and B. Bromberger, "Patient Participation in Decision Making: Are the Courts the Answer?" (1983) 6 *University of New South Wales Law Journal* 1.

adequately inform the patient of all risks, benefits, and alternatives of treatment.[15]

While a patient may still be able to bring a battery action against a physician when the physician proceeds without any arguable claim that the patient consented to the treatment provided,[16] there is now agreement throughout common law jurisdictions that the failure adequately to inform a patient of the risks, benefits, and alternatives to treatment (as distinguished from the complete failure to seek any patient consent for the treatment rendered) is a species of the law of negligence, not a part of the law of battery.[17] To be liable in negligence the defendant must be the subject of a duty established by law, breach that duty, and, by that breach, cause the plaintiff to suffer damages.[18] While the determination of the nature and extent of a duty is ordinarily a matter of law, the question of whether that duty has been breached in a particular case is ordinarily a matter of fact.[19]

III. THE QUESTION FOR THE HIGH COURT: WHICH NEGLIGENCE STANDARD?

Rogers v. *Whitaker* neatly presented the High Court with a choice between the two prevailing negligence theories of informed consent. On the one hand, the patient-oriented theory provides that a physician has breached his legal duty to the patient if he fails to provide the information that a reasonable patient in the position of this patient would want to know under the circumstances—*i.e.* information that such a patient

---

[15] See I. Kennedy and A. Grubb, *supra*, at 223–5, which discusses the criminal law background of this notion of consent. An excellent discussion of the difference between the law of battery and the law of negligence as it applies to informed consent can be found in M. Somerville, "Structuring the Issues in Informed Consent" (1981) 26 *McGill Law Journal* 740.

[16] See *Perna* v. *Pirozi* 457 A.2d 431 (1983) (N.J. Sup. Ct.) ("ghost surgery", where a patient consents to surgery by one surgeon and it is then performed by another); *Choinard* v. *Marjani* 575 A.2d 238 (1990) (Conn. App.) (bilateral breast surgery after consent to surgery on only one breast); *Bommareddy* v. *Superior Court* 222 Cal. App. 3d 1017 (1990) (surgery on the right eye after patient consented only to surgery on the left eye).

[17] This agreement is noted in virtually every source. See I. Kennedy and A. Grubb, *supra*; and Justice Laskin's oft-cited opinion for the Supreme Court of Canada in *Reibl* v. *Hughes* (1980) 114 D.L.R. 3d 1. Informed consent is based in negligence in Canada, see *Reibl*, *supra*, the United Kingdom, see *Sidaway*, *supra* and forty-nine of the fifty United States. See B. Furrow *et al.*, *Health Law*, (2nd edn. 1991) at 327, n. 7. The negligence basis of informed consent law has also been recognised in Australia. See *F.* v. *R.* (1983) 33 S.A.S.R. 189 (South Australia Sup. Ct.)

[18] These are the elements of all negligence actions. See J. Fleming, *Law of Torts*, (7th edn. *Law Book Co.* 1987) chs. 7 and 8.

[19] *Ibid.*

would find material to make a decision about treatment.[20] On the other hand, the physician-oriented theory provides that a physician has breached his legal duty to the patient if he fails to provide information that reasonable physicians do, in fact, disclose under the circumstances. Under this theory, a physician has breached a duty and thus may be liable in negligence only if the physician fails to give the patient information that would be provided by *all* other reasonable physicians.[21]

There is no question that the risk of sympathetic ophthalmia would be a material risk to a reasonable person in the position of Ms Whitaker, who was extremely concerned about maintaining the vision in her good eye, and continuously questioned Mr Rogers about that. Similarly, there is no question that some otherwise reasonable ophthalmic surgeons in Australia in 1984 did not inform their patients of this risk, and there was credible and unrebutted testimony from responsible ophthalmic surgeons who said they would not have informed Ms Whitaker of this risk under the circumstances of this case. Thus, if the Court were to adopt the patient-oriented rule, Mr Rogers would be in breach of the duty recognised in law to provide material information to patients. If the Court were to adopt the physician-oriented rule, Mr Rogers would not be in breach of the duty because he acted in accord with the standard set by his professional peers. Under the American rule, Mr Rogers is liable; under the English rule, he is not liable.

IV. THE DECISION OF THE HIGH COURT

In affirming the decision of the trial court and the New South Wales Court of Appeal, the High Court of Australia clearly and explicitly

[20] This theory was first explicitly accepted in *Canterbury* v. *Spence* 464 F.2d 772 (1972) (D.C.Cir.). Perhaps for this reason it is sometimes called the "American" rule, although only about half of the American jurisdictions have actually accepted it; the other half apply the doctor-oriented test. See B. Furrow *et al.*, *Health Law*, (2nd edn.) *supra*, at 336–7 n. 1. Of course, there are many variations on this patient-oriented rule; for example, some jurisdictions apply a subjective test (asking what this patient would want to know), some apply an objective test (asking what the hypothetical reasonable patient would want to know), and most apply the combination of those two that formed the basis of the test in *Canterbury* itself (asking what a reasonable patient in the position of this patient would want to know). Different jurisdictions also interpret the word "material" in different ways.

[21] This theory was adopted by the House of Lords in *Sidaway* v. *Governors of Bethlem Royal Hospital* [1985] A.C. 871, applying the general rule of medical liability expressed in *Bolam* v. *Friern Hospital Management Committee* [1957] 1 W.L.R. 582. Perhaps for this reason it is sometimes called the "English" rule. When combined with the "responsible minority" principle which holds that a physician may live up to the standards of any responsible portion of the profession, this rule is extremely tolerant of physician behaviour.

chose the patient-oriented "American" rule, even if the High Court felt obliged to distance itself from the considerations that make the rule so well accepted in the American jurisdictions. Although the High Court now regularly distinguishes and departs from the British precedent[22] which would have been binding less than a decade ago when appeals to the Privy Council were still permitted,[23] in *Rogers* the High Court also takes pains to point out that it will not slavishly accept American precedent. Over the past decade the High Court has spent a great deal of collective energy reforming and rationalising the law of torts and creating a distinctive Australian law, not dependent on any other common law approach, and it has found that its thoughtful and restrained view of tort liability has strongly influenced other common law courts, including the House of Lords, which have adopted many of the tort law arguments first advanced in High Court judgments.[24]

In developing the Australian law of informed consent, the High Court first attempts to simplify the law and justify the application of ordinary negligence principles by establishing the existence of a consistent, unitary principle of negligence law that applies to all facets of the health care provider's work. The Court then explains why it rejects the British physician-oriented approach to informed consent and why it finds the American basis for the development of informed consent law (or, at least, the language used in the American cases) unsatisfactory. Finally, while supporting its holding on non-binding Australian precedent, the High Court adopts a carefully and simply articulated version of the "American" rule, with all of the problems and uncertainties (and, presumably, all of the advantages) that rule has brought to those American jurisdictions which have adopted it.

A. The Unitary Duty

In a relatively unusual joint judgment, five members of the High Court[25] begin by pointing out that the physician's duty to diagnose, treat, and provide information are each part of "a single comprehensive

---

[22] See Sir Anthony Mason C.J., "An Australian Law for Australia?", Address to the Law Council of Australia Convention, Adelaide, September 1991 26 *Law Notes* No. 10 at 14. There was an unsuccessful effort at first instance to submit that *Sidaway* was in fact binding on the Supreme Court of New South Wales, see *Whitaker* v. *Rogers* (1990) Aust. Torts Reports 81-062 at 68, 316–17.

[23] Appeals from the High Court of Australia to the Privy Council were abolished in 1975 by the Privy Council (Appeals from the High Court) Act 1975 (Cth.). However appeals from the State Supreme Courts were still possible until the Australia Act 1986. In fact leave was granted until 21 February 1985 for appeals from New South Wales.

[24] See *Jaensch* v. *Coffey* (1984) 155 C.L.R. 549, *Sutherland Shire Council* v. *Heyman* (1985) 157 C.L.R. 424.

[25] Mason C.J. and Brennan, Dawson, Toohey and McHugh JJ.

duty covering all the ways in which a doctor is to exercise his skill and judgment".[26] This single comprehensive duty is that of "the ordinary skilled person exercising and professing the special skill" of the defendant.[27] As Justice Gaudron points out in her concurring opinion,

> There is no difficulty in analysing the duty of care of medical practitioners on the basis of a "single comprehensive duty" covering diagnosis, treatment and the provision of information and advice, provided that it is stated in terms of sufficient generality. Thus, the general duty may be stated as a duty to exercise reasonable professional skill and judgment. But the difficulty with that approach is that a statement of that kind says practically nothing—certainly, nothing worthwhile—as to the content of the duty.[28]

The question, as Justice Gaudron's comment makes clear, is not what general duty of care is applicable to every act of every physician, or every act of every professional, or to all actors of all kinds: that duty—the general duty to exercise due care—is perfectly well established and equally perfectly void of meaning. The question is how that duty is to be applied to a doctor's obligation to provide information to a patient. After all, if providing information is simply another part of a doctor's professional work—like diagnosing and treating illness—then the doctor should be measured in the same way that she is measured when diagnosing and treating illness; she should be measured by comparing her conduct with that of other reasonable professionals in like circumstances.

The Court points out that even though the question of whether a physician carries out diagnosis or treatment competently is to be measured in just this way, the question of whether a physician has given the patient all of the "relevant information to choose between undergoing and not undergoing the treatment is a question of a different order".[29] Thus, while "[t]he duty of a medical practitioner to exercise reasonable care and skill in the provision of professional advice and treatment is a single comprehensive duty .... the factors according to which a court determines whether a medical practitioner is in breach of the requisite standard of care will vary according to whether it is a case involving diagnosis, treatment or the provision of information or advice; the different cases raise varying difficulties which require considerations of different factors".[30] In other words, whether, on the one hand, the physician's legal duty with regard to diagnosis and treatment is the

---

[26] (1992) 67 A.L.J.R. 47 at 48, quoting Lord Diplock in *Sidaway*, *supra*, at 893.
[27] *Ibid.*
[28] *Ibid.*, at 53 (footnotes omitted).
[29] *Ibid.*, at 52.
[30] *Ibid.*, at 51, citing *F.* v *R.* (1983) 33 S.A.S.R. 189 at 191.

same as the legal duty with regard to the provision of advice, and it is merely the breach of those duties which are measured in different ways, or whether, on the other hand, the duties themselves are different, is a semantic quibble. In either case, Australian courts now treat the physician's obligation to provide diagnosis and treatment quite differently from the physician's obligation to provide advice.

B. Rejecting the British Rule

The House of Lords considered this same issue in the *Sidaway* case, and a majority did determine that the breach of the duty of care as it applies to diagnosis, treatment, and the provision of advice should be measured in the exactly the same way, in each case by asking what other similarly situated professionals would do. The Law Lords reached this result by applying the general principle of malpractice law, which was articulated in *Bolam* v. *Friern Hospital Management Committee*[31] and summarised by Lord Scarman in his (effectively) dissenting speech in *Sidaway*:

> The *Bolam* principle may be formulated as a rule that a doctor is not negligent if he acts in accordance with a practice accepted at the time as proper by a responsible body of medical opinion even though other doctors adopt a different practice. In short, the law imposes the duty of care: but the standard of care is a matter of medical judgment.[32]

The High Court rejected this standard for several reasons. First, in *Sidaway* the Law Lords were divided themselves about the way the *Bolam* test should be applied to evaluate the provision of medical advice; three of the Law Lords would give some authority to the judiciary to find liability for the failure to warn of some risk of a medical procedure even against unrebutted expert testimony that some otherwise responsible physicians would not have warned the patient of the risk in question.[33] Secondly, as the High Court points out, the *Bolam* test "has invariably been applied in English courts",[34] but has not been so well accepted in Australia, "even in the sphere of diagnosis and treatment, the heartland of the skilled medical practitioner".[35]

Most significantly, though, the High Court concluded that the *Bolam* test was inappropriate because it did not attach any significance to the

---

[31] [1957] 1 W.L.R. 582.

[32] [1985] A.C. 871 at 881, quoted in the joint judgment, *supra*, at 48–9.

[33] The position of the Law Lords is summarised by the High Court, *supra*, at 49–50. Only Lord Diplock would apply the language of *Bolam* to informed consent cases in an inflexible manner.

[34] *Supra*, at 49 (footnote omitted).

[35] *Supra*, at 50.

patients' questions to their physicians. If expert testimony were to show that some reasonable physicians would not answer a question (or answer it dishonestly, for that matter), the *Bolam* test would not impose liability for failure to answer that question (or for answering it dishonestly). Indeed, the facts of *Rogers* v. *Whitaker* itself suggest the unfairness of such a standard. While Ms Whitaker did not specifically ask about sympathetic ophthalmia, she certainly communicated her concern about her sighted eye to Mr Rogers; it would be terribly arbitrary and unfair to her to allow Mr Rogers to ignore her obvious and clearly manifested concern because she did not use the proper magic words when she put her questions. As the High Court points out in dicta, "the opinion that the respondent should have been told of the dangers of sympathic ophthalmia only if she had been sufficiently learned to ask the question seems curious ...[36] Even if she had asked, though, under the British rule Mr Rogers would not have had to answer her questions honestly if other members of the ophthalmic surgeon brotherhood would not have done so. Unlike the House of Lords, the High Court of Australia is not willing to delegate essentially unreviewable authority to determine how patients should be advised, and whether their questions should be answered, to the physicians who are responsible for advising those patients.

C. Rejecting the American Language: "Informed Consent" and "Self Determination"

Perhaps overzealous to distinguish itself from the American courts and the "American" approach to informed consent, the High Court draws a distinction between its position and the "American" position: it argues that the American phrases such as "the patient's right of self-determination", and, for that matter, the term "informed consent" itself, are "of little assistance in the balancing process that is involved in the determination of whether there has been a breach of the duty of disclosure" and thus are not relevant to a determination of the duty of physicians to disclose information.[37] As the High Court joint judgment correctly points out, the term "informed consent" is an "amorphous phrase" that can be misleading to those not familiar with this area of the law.[38] Despite that, though, it is now a well accepted legal term that

[36] *Supra*, at 53.

[37] *Supra*, at 52.

[38] *Supra*, at 52. The High Court is not the first to object to the term, of course, although not all objections are based in the same analysis of the problem. Kennedy and Grubb argue that the "aphorism" of "informed consent", which "has entered the language as being synonymous with valid consent", is misleading and unhelpful. I. Kennedy and A. Grubb, *supra* at 215. For another compelling criticism of the term, see *Reibl* v. *Hughes* (1980) 14 D.L.R. (3d) 1.

describes an area of law with at least as much precision and honesty as other tort law terms such as "products liability," "strict liability," or "mass torts". While the Court's decision to eliminate that Americanism does no harm to the law, it does not really help much either.

On the other hand, the High Court's insistence that "the right of self-determination" is "of little assistance in the balancing process that is involved in the determination of whether there has been a breach of the duty of disclosure"[39] is inconsistent with its own evaluation of the purpose of the duty of disclosure. Why is the duty any different in the area of disclosure than in the area of diagnosis and treatment? Quoting more congenial and highly significant local Australian precedent,[40] the High Court concludes that courts must determine the standard of care in disclosure cases "after giving weight to 'the paramount consideration that a person is entitled to make his own decisions about his life' ".[41] This paramount consideration is identical to the "right of self determination", of course, and it is exactly the reason that the High Court refuses to delegate to physicians the opportunity to set their own standards for disclosure. The Australian law would stand on a firmer foundation if this purpose for the law of informed consent (or physician disclosure, or patient advertisement, as the High Court may please to call it) were formally acknowledged.

D. The Holding of the High Court

Despite its attempt to distinguish its approach from that taken by the American courts, and in particular from the approach in *Canterbury* v. *Spence*, the legal duty described in *Rogers* v *Whitaker* is virtually identical to the patient-disclosure-oriented rule announced in *Canterbury* and its American progeny. The High Court clearly announced its holding:

> The law should recognise that a doctor has a duty to warn a patient of a material risk inherent in the proposed treatment; a risk is material if, in the circumstances of the particular case, a reasonable person in the patient's position, if warned of the risk, would be likely to attach significance to it or if the medical practitioner is or should reasonably be aware that the particular patient, if warned of the risk, would be likely to attach significance to it.[42]

---

[39] *Supra*, at 52. The Court cites *Canterbury* v. *Spence* as an example of the use of this phrase. *Ibid.*, n. 35.

[40] *F.* v. *R.* has been recognised as a significant case by a few overseas commentators. See comments on this case by D. Giesen, *International Medical Malpractice Law* (Martinus Nijhoff London 1988).

[41] *Supra*, at 51, quoting *F.* v. *R.* (1983) 33 S.A.S.R. 189 at 193.

[42] *Supra*, at 52.

This is an exceptionally broad rule, imposing a duty on health care professionals to provide all information to which a reasonable person in the patient's position would be likely to attach significance—whatever that may mean.[43] Justice Gaudron would adopt an even broader principle and require the revelation of all information "that is relevant to a decision or course of action ... that would, in other cases, found a duty to warn".[44] She would treat the physician's duty to warn patients of risks much as she would treat any other duty to warn; indeed, she relied upon *Wyong Shire Council* v. *Shirt*,[45] which imposed a duty properly to warn of shallow water in a water skiing area upon a shire council, to support her general statement of the duty to warn.

The High Court correctly notes that it is accepting the approach that was adopted by the highly respected South Australian Chief Justice King in *F.* v. *R.*, which itself depended upon the Canadian Supreme Court opinion in *Reibl* v. *Hughes*, and that was recommended by Lord Scarman, dissenting in *Sidaway*. The High Court does not mention that it is adopting the language of *Canterbury* v. *Spence*, which provided that "the test for determining whether a particular peril must be divulged is its materiality to the patient's decision: all risks potentially affecting the decision must be unmasked".[46] This extraordinarily broad requirement of disclosure is leavened by language that now sounds very familiar:

> a risk is thus material when a reasonable person, in what the physician knows or should know to be the patient's position, would be likely to attach significance to the risk or cluster of risks in deciding whether or not to forego the proposed therapy.[47]

Indeed, the broad holding of *Rogers* v. *Whitaker* is virtually identical to the holding of *Canterbury* v. *Spence*, and it defines the physician's duty

---

43 The rule is an amalgam of one that would view the patient objectively (referring to "a reasonable person in the patient's position") and one that would view the patient subjectively (referring to "the particular patient") in establishing just what information the physician must disclose in each case. Of course, to the extent that a patient's known interests, desires, fears, and concerns must be taken into account to determine what a reasonable person "in the patient's position" would consider significant, the objective rule is reduced to the subjective rule; a "reasonable person" with all of the attributes and thoughts of the patient would have to evaluate a proposed treatment in the same way that that particular patient would evaluate it.

44 *Supra*, at 54.

45 (1980) 146 C.L.R. 40.

46 *Canterbury* v. *Spence*, *supra*, at 786.

47 *Canterbury* v. *Spence*, *supra*, at 787, quoting Waltz and Scheuneman, "Informed Consent to Therapy" (1970) 64 *Northwestern University Law Review* 628 at 640.

to disclose in language that is almost identical to what has become known as the "American" rule.[48]

The implications of this principle of law are just as uncertain in Australia as they have proved to be in the American jurisdictions that have adopted the same rule. The duty of care is to be defined as a matter of law, and not by the professional peers of the defendant—that much is clearly established. But how does the law go about making that definition and determining whether a duty has been breached in any particular case? What are the respective roles of the judge and the jury? The High Court adopts the position of *F.* v. *R.* that what must be disclosed by the physician in any particular case "depends upon a complex of factors: the nature of the matter to be disclosed; the nature of the treatment; the desire of the patient for information; the temperament and health of the patient; and the general surrounding circumstances".[49] But how are these factors to be weighed, and who is to weigh them? If the law is truly defining the duty itself, then it is an issue for the court. On the other hand, if there is a unitary duty of care that applies to diagnosis, treatment, and disclosure of information (as the High Court at first suggests) and the issue is whether that duty was breached in a particular case, the evaluation of these factors must be left to the jury, or in the absence of a jury, to the judge as fact finder. Perhaps the fact-based nature of this inquiry makes it particularly appropriate for jury determination: this is the kind of finding that cannot be justified by a reasoned opinion, but depends upon the community conscience and the sense of fairness and propriety that jurors possess in their roles as representatives of the community. The inability of the High Court, or any of the American courts, to explain how these factors are to be

---

[48] The holding of *Rogers* v. *Whitaker* is similar to the holding in *Canterbury* v. *Spence* in one other way also; both recognise the doctrine of "therapeutic privilege" as an exception to the general rule of informed consent. *Canterbury* would permit the use of the "therapeutic privilege" if a physician's communication of a risk would "present a threat to the patient's well-being". *Canterbury*, *supra*, at 789. *Canterbury* suggests that such a threat would occur when a patient would become "so ill or emotionally distraught" at hearing the information that the patient could not make a rational decision, or the treatment would be "complicate[d] or hinder[ed]", or the patient would suffer "psychological damage". *Ibid.* The joint judgment of the High Court formally announces that the "duty [to provide information to patients] is subject to the therapeutic privilege", *supra*, at 52, and it suggests that the privilege is applicable where "there is a particular danger that the provision of all relevant information will harm an unusually nervous, disturbed or volatile patient ..." *Ibid.* In her separate opinion, Justice Gaudron casts doubt on an independent doctrine of "therapeutic privilege", arguing that the factors that give rise to this defence are adequately treated as parts of elements of the underlying *prima facie* negligence action *supra*, at 54–5.

[49] *Supra*, at 51, citing *F.* v. *R.* (1983) 33 S.A.S.R. 189 at 192–3.

evaluated and weighed against each other effectively hand-balls[50] the issue on to those whose findings need not be explained and are not reviewable on appeal.[51]

The ambiguity over which legal institution—the judge or the jury—is to be given the significant task in informed consent cases is reflected in the ambiguity over what constitutes evidence relevant to the issue of what that duty is, and whether it has been breached. It is obvious what constitutes relevant evidence under the physician-oriented English approach; the testimony of physicians is both necessary and sufficient because the factual question does not extend beyond what other professionals would do under similar circumstances. It is not at all obvious what constitutes relevant evidence under the patient-oriented approach. The High Court does recognise some role for expert medical testimony, accepting the language from the Supreme Court of Canada, quoted in *F.* v. *R.*, that "expert medical evidence is, of course, relevant to findings as to the risks that reside in or are a result of recommended surgery".[52] Several American cases have also found that medical testimony is relevant, and, perhaps, necessary, to prove: "(1) the risks involved concerning a particular method of treatment, (2) alternative methods of treatment, (3) the risks relating to such alternative methods of treatment, and (4) the results likely to occur if the patient remains untreated."[53] Unlike the expert medical testimony in all other medical malpractice cases, though, and unlike the expert medical testimony offered in informed consent cases under the British rule, the expert testimony in Australia could not address the ultimate question of what information should have been provided to the patient. Indeed, the extremely broad doctrine of *res ipsa loquitur* in Australia, where that doctrine is viewed as nothing more than permission to the fact finder to make reasonable inferences based on common sense,[54] may make it a

---

[50] *I.e.* 'passes the buck'. An Australian footballer caught in a crowd and unable effectively to run or kick the ball may hand-ball it to a team mate. Sometimes such a move is part of a clever strategy that advances the ball, and sometimes it is a result of cowardice.

[51] A wide variety of courts have handled different issues in different ways. A one per cent risk of paralysis, as in *Canterbury*, may be sufficient to require revelation, while a similar risk of lengthy recovery may not. See Furrow *et al., supra*, at 338, for more examples.

[52] *Supra*, at 51, citing *F.* v. *R.* quoting *Reibl* v. *Hughes* (1980) 114 D.L.R. (3d) 1 at 13.

[53] *Cross* v. *Trapp* (1982) 294 S.E. 2d 446 at 455 (W. Va.). See also *Sard* v. *Hardy* (1977) 379 A. 2d 1014 (Md.) and *Festa* v. *Greenberg* (1986) 511 A. 2d 1371 (Pa. Super.).

[54] See, for example, *Kilgannon* v. *Sharpe Bros. Pty. Ltd.* (1986) 4 N.S.W.L.R. 600 per Kirby J. For a general account of *res ipsa loquitur* in Australia, see Fleming, *Torts* (7th ed.) at 291–301 and Morison, Phegan, and Sappideen, *Cases on Torts*, (6th edn.), at 416–35.

useful evidentiary tool in informed consent cases after *Rogers* v. *Whitaker*.

There is, finally, uncertainty over the extent of the duty to disclose. The High Court recognises that physicians perform many tasks, including the diagnosis and treatment of illness and the disclosure of information relevant to their patients' health status. Once the doctrine of informed consent is disentangled from the tort of battery, under which the liability technically resulted from the subsequent touching rather than the failure to inform, there is no reason to believe that the health education function of the physician must be particularly closely related to the diagnosis and treatment functions; a physician's duty to educate her patient is independent of her duty to diagnose and treat her patient, and, perhaps, just as important. Thus, a physician may be liable for failure to provide information even when a patient decides against a proposed treatment, or even when there is no treatment that has been proposed.

For example, the High Court has not foreclosed an action against a physician who fails to obtain an adequately "informed refusal", like the action recognised in California in *Truman* v. *Thomas*,[55] where a physician was found negligent for failing to explain to an impecunious patient the risk that was a consequence of deciding not to have a pap smear and who subsequently died of a cancer that would have been discovered earlier had she undergone this recommended procedure. Does the independent health education function of the physician that is recognised, at least implicitly, by the High Court require a physician to tell his patients generally about the ills caused by cigarette smoking, eating too much fat, having unprotected sex, possessing a firearm, working in a mine, walking in the sun, and, generally, engaging in any other seriously risky behaviour that he knows (or should know) is a kind of behaviour undertaken by the patient? Does a primary care physician, at the least, have a duty to assure that her patients have a good general health education—under penalty of a malpractice action? Such a duty would recognise the extraordinary importance of obtaining a good medical history, and of developing a thoughtful and sensitive relationship with patients. It would also encourage preventive medicine and attention to health maintenance by making those physicians who negligently fail to provide their patients with information necessary to keep themselves healthy liable for their patients' subsequent illnesses and injuries. While the High Court does not go so far as to formally recognise this kind of action in *Rogers* v. *Whitaker*, the case depends upon a rationale that would seem to require it.

---

[55] (1980) 611 P. 2d 902 (Cal. Sup. Ct.).

E. Causation and Liability for Failure to Disclose

The existence of a duty and the breach of that duty are but two elements of a negligence action. In order for a patient successfully to argue that a physician is liable in negligence for failure to disclose information to the patient, the patient must also show that the breach of the duty by the physician actually (and proximately) caused some damage to the patient. Indeed, the causation requirement is the reason that American jurisdictions, with such patient-oriented substantive law on disclosure, see so few successful informed consent actions. In the seminal case of *Canterbury* v. *Spence* the court faced the question of whether the causation test should be the subjective standard applied in all other negligence actions—would this patient have foregone this procedure if she were provided with the withheld information?—or an objective one—would a reasonable patient have foregone this procedure if she were provided with the withheld information? Concerned that the subjective view would "place the physician in jeopardy of the patient's hindsight and bitterness",[56] and that in hindsight every person injured during a medical procedure would testify that she would have foregone the procedure if only she had access to whatever information was withheld, the court concluded that the objective rule would "ease the fact-finding process and better assure the truth as its product".[57]

This objective rule, which has been adopted in most American jurisdictions,[58] eliminates the possibility of informed consent actions arising out of most medical procedures. For example, no reasonable person with appendicitis would choose to forego an appendectomy if fully informed about the risks, benefits, and alternatives of the appendectomy; the choice to forego the treatment simply would not be a reasonable one. Thus, an appendectomy cannot give rise to a negligence-based informed consent action (in the American jurisdictions that have adopted the objective causation rule, anyway), no matter what that person is (or is not) told about the procedure, because the patient will not be able to show that a reasonable person would have foregone the appendectomy under any circumstances, with all the information. Thus, virtually all necessary medical procedures are effectively exempt from informed consent actions under the American rule. Indeed, in American jurisdictions which adopt the objective causation

---

[56] *Canterbury*, *supra*, at 790. See also submission of counsel for Mr Rogers, Mr Sackar Q.C. at the trial in *Whitaker* v. *Rogers* (1990) Aust. Torts Reports 81–062 at 68, 307.

[57] *Canterbury*, *supra*, at 791.

[58] F. Rozovsky, *Consent to Treatment* s. 1.13.4 (1984). For an account of the rules adopted in different American jurisdictions, see *Fain* v. *Smith* (1985) 479 So. 2d 1150 (Ala.).

test, only truly elective procedures can give rise to successful informed consent actions. What American jurisdictions give to patient-plaintiffs with a broad substantive rule of duty, they take back with their very narrow rule of causation.

The causation issue was raised in *Rogers* v *Whitaker*, of course. Mr Rogers argued that Ms Whitaker would have undergone the procedure even if she were told that there were a one in 14,000 chance of sympathetic ophthalmia, while Ms Whitaker testified that "if someone had said one in a million chance, there would be no operation".[59] Ultimately, the High Court was not faced with the question of what standard to apply in analysing causation in an informed consent case because Mr Rogers's counsel made no submission on that issue and was thus deemed to have waived the issue in the High Court.[60] However, both the trial court and the Court of Appeal applied the subjective causation standard ordinarily applied in tort cases,[61] and that was the standard applied by the full court of the South Australia Supreme Court in *F.* v. *R.*, which formed the basis of the *Rogers* opinion. In the trial court, Campbell J. held that:

> ... it was for the Plaintiff to show on a *subjective* basis that she would not have undergone the operation had she been warned of the risk of sympathetic ophthalmia.[62] (emphasis added)

In the Court of Appeal Mahoney J.A. did not consider the question of whether the test was a subjective or an objective one, although he did address the question of causation.[63] He found that although the failure to warn did not *physically* cause the sympathetic ophthalmia of the defendant, the Court was concerned with a causal relationship of a different kind. It was the breach of the duty by Mr Rogers to give sound advice when asked questions that was the cause of the plaintiff's decision to undergo the surgery, and therefore, the cause of the harm.[64] Handley J.A. considered the issue of causation[65] and held that the causative link was provided in this case by the reliance Ms Whitaker placed on the advice of Mr Rogers. While Handley J.A. does not formally announce that he has chosen the subjective, rather than objective, standard for causation, he refers to a number of subjective considerations that suggest that he presumed the test

---

59 (1991) 23 N.S.W.L.R. 600 at 611.

60 *Supra*, at 53.

61 See (1991) 23 N.S.W.L.R. 600 at 618.

62 *Whitaker* v. *Rogers*, (1990) Aust. Torts Reports 81–462 at 68,308, citing *Ellis* v. *Wallsend District Hospital* (1989) Aust. Torts Reports 80–259.

63 *Rogers* v. *Whitaker* (1991) 23 N.S.W.L.R. 600 at 608.

64 Citing *Barnes* v. *Hay* (1988) 12 N.S.W.L.R. 337. See also the decision of the High Court in *March* v. *E. and M. H. Stramare Pty. Ltd.* (1991) 65 A.L.J.R. 334.

65 (1991) 23 N.S.W.L.R. 600 at 618–19.

would be the subjective one usual in negligence cases.

If the High Court applies the traditional subjective rule of causation, the Court will have adopted the disclosure-oriented pro-plaintiff substantive duty without imposing the objective rule of causation used in American jurisdictions to protect doctors from the consequences of that broad substantive principle. In other words, if Australia maintains the subjective causation principle applied in virtually all negligence cases, Australian law will be more favourable to plaintiffs in informed consent actions than the law of any other jurisdiction.

V. CONSEQUENCES OF THE HIGH COURT DECISION

Despite its plaintiff-oriented approach, the High Court's decision in *Rogers* v. *Whitaker* is unlikely to open the floodgates of informed consent litigation in Australia for three reasons: (1) Australia is yet to permit contingent fees in tort litigation, (2) the Australian social safety net assures that those injured in medical accidents do not become impoverished and desperate, and (3) the Australian health care system could not afford it. First, and most significantly, the vast majority of potential medical malpractice (and, thus, informed consent) plaintiffs cannot take the financial risk that their actions will be unsuccessful. Under the American system of compensation of legal counsel, a medical malpractice plaintiff bears little economic risk. If the action is successful, the plaintiff collects less than the full judgment—a portion of the judgment goes to pay the fees of the plaintiff's counsel—but if the plaintiff is unsuccessful, she bears only the formal court costs of the actions. She is not responsible for any fees for her own counsel, and, under the prevailing American rule, she will not be responsible for any fees of the successful defendant's counsel. An American malpractice plaintiff faces the potential for tremendous gain, and virtually no potential for loss and these incentives act to encourage malpractice litigation. Under the current Australian scheme for financing litigation, use of the contingent fee is not permitted in any state[66] and a potential medical

[66] There are several pending proposals that would allow contingent fees in limited cases, and under some judicial supervision. If any of these proposals become effective, they may alter the incentives to bring medical malpractice (and other tort) actions. These proposals are part of a major review of professional indemnity arrangements in relation to the medical profession which is being conducted by the Commonwealth Department of Health, Housing and Community Services for which a discussion paper was issued in February 1992. This discussion paper, *Compensation and Professional Indemnity in Health Care*, broaches a number of options for reform including introduction of no-fault compensation schemes and the introduction of structured common law damages to replace lump sum payments and other ways to contain defendants' costs; these options for reform are proposed against the back drop of the present unsatisfactory conduct of medical negligence litigation.

malpractice plaintiff thus faces the economic hurdle of paying her own legal counsel, and, if she loses the action, paying her adversary's as well. The Australian malpractice plaintiff faces the same potential gain that an American plaintiff faces, but a much more substantial potential loss, and there is a much reduced incentive to bring a malpractice action.[67] Indeed, the cost of litigation of an average malpractice case—probably over $50,000 when both sides total their fees and other expenses—is enough to push a middle class Australian into poverty. It is the very unusual case where such a great risk is worth the potential gain.

Secondly, the Australian social safety net, which protects Australians who have become unemployed, disabled, or otherwise disadvantaged makes it less important for Australians to have access to the medical malpractice system. As the *Canterbury* court recognised, plaintiffs in informed consent cases are likely to possess both hindsight and bitterness,[68] and the bitterness of Americans who have been injured is likely to turn into desperation as well. Americans injured through an act of the health care system, whether a result of negligence or bad luck, may lose their ability to work, their income, their health care, their very ability to survive. It is hardly surprising that the medical malpractice system has been substituted for the social welfare system that does not exist, and that courts stretch to find some form of compensation for those who will slip into poverty unless they receive something from the health care system itself. Indeed, the malpractice system thus becomes a kind of *de facto* social insurance scheme, albeit a very inefficient one, spreading the cost of injuries suffered by one patient on to others receiving treatment in the system through the collection of malpractice insurance premiums from health care providers. In a country with a real social welfare system, like Australia or the United Kingdom,[69] this is

[67] The incentives in Australia are similar to those in the United Kingdom, where the contingent fee is also currently banned (but see Courts and Legal Services Act 1990, s.58). One study showed that the vast majority of medical malpractice actions commenced under this system were brought by the very wealthy (who could afford the potential loss) or the very poor (who were not exposed to that loss because they qualified for legal aid). The middle class was essentially excluded from bringing such actions. See A. Grubb and R. Schwartz, "Why Britain Can't Afford Informed Consent" (1986) 16 *Hastings Center Report* 22. See also F. Miller, "Informed Consent for the Man on the Clapham Omnibus: An English Cure for the 'American Disease'?" (1987) 9 *Western New England Law Review* 169. Of course, there is also a positive incentive in the contingent fee system: the plaintiff's counsel, who is not paid unless the action is successful, has a strong incentive to screen cases carefully, and there is a powerful incentive not to proceed with cases unless the plaintiff's counsel believes that they have substantial merit.

[68] See n. 56, *supra*.

[69] See A. Grubb and R. Schwartz, "Why Britain Can't Afford Informed Consent", *supra* n. 67.

simply unnecessary. With a lower desperation level among potential plaintiffs, and a less immediate need for resources to maintain one's life style, there is less incentive among those potential plaintiffs actually to file legal actions against health care providers.[70]

Finally, the limited resources spent on health care in Australia necessarily will provide a limit on actions in informed consent, because the health care system simply cannot offer a very large range of health care choices to all Australians.[71] No court could require a physician to inform patients of a treatment that is unavailable in Australia, or unavailable to a person in that patient's position; if patients were given this range of choices, they would bankrupt the system. The limit on the choices actually available to patients within the government-financed Medicare system (and the heavily government-subsidised private system) in Australia provides a natural limit on the information that must be provided to patients in the system.[72]

VI. CONCLUSION

This arguably simple case[73] has resolved the question of the applicable test of informed consent in Australia. The High Court followed a rather sparse line of highly persuasive Australian Supreme Court authority which has consistently rejected the English physician-oriented test.[74] While rejecting the American justification for a patient-oriented test, the High Court ultimately adopted the principle, and, almost verbatim, the substantive language of *Canterbury* v. *Spence*, the seminal case which first articulated the "American" patient-oriented approach. The Court applied this test both to determine the scope of the doctor's *to volunteer*

[70] Litigation is unpleasant under any circumstances, and, cost aside, most people would rather avoid being a party to a law suit.

[71] For example, Australia spends about half what the United States does, per capita, on health care. If a treatment modality is available anywhere in the world, it is likely to be available to anyone who desires it (and can pay for it, or convince a third party to do so) in the United States. That is not true in Australia where some kinds of treatments—new and very expensive antibiotics and antihypertensives, for example—are simply not available, or not available without some form of central review. It would make no sense to provide a patient with information on a treatment modality thus unavailable.

[72] The same is true in the United Kingdom, where the narrow rule on informed consent has been attributed to the need to limit choices available to patients. See A. Grubb and R. Schwartz, *supra* n. 67.

[73] In fact Handley J.A. in *Rogers* v. *Whitaker* (1991) 23 N.S.W.L.R. 600 at 615 described it as "... a simple case which is not governed, and which ought not to be governed, by the *Bolam* test".

[74] *Goode* v. *Nash* (1979) 21 S.A.S.R. 419 at 422; *Albrighton* v. *Royal Prince Alfred Hospital* [1980] 2 N.S.W.L.R. 542 at 562–3; *F.* v. *R.* (1983) 33 S.A.S.R. 189 at 193; and *Rogers* v. *Whitaker* (1991) 23 N.S.W.L.R. 600 at 608, 618, 619.

information and *to answer questions* even though only the latter was directly before the Court.

The absence of contingent fees in tort litigation, the existence of a high quality and universally accessible health care system, and the presence of a strong social safety net in Australia combine to suggest that the broad principle of informed consent now applicable in Australia—arguably the most patient- and plaintiff-oriented in any common law jurisdiction—will not result in an avalanche of informed consent litigation. Although for these reasons *Rogers* v. *Whitaker* may not substantially alter legal practice, in this case the High Court does formally articulate something many physicians have been arguing for a long time: the practice of medicine is not limited to the mechanistic diagnosis and treatment of physical and mental conditions. Rather, physicians have a duty to provide information to their patients—information that extends beyond the risks, benefits, and alternatives of proposed courses of treatment—and this duty independent of the duty competently to diagnose and treat. Just as it is within the duty of physicians to figure out carefully and cleverly how to diagnose and treat defined ailments, it is within the duty of physicians to figure out carefully and sensitively how to educate patients about the medical procedures those patients are offered, and, by logical extension, about other health matters as well.

Even though, as has been seen, the High Court's decision does leave a number of questions unanswered, the decision is consistent with some important extracurial proposals in favour of greater disclosure to patients by medical practitioners. These proposals are aimed towards a cooperative model of informed decision making involving both the patient and the medical practitioner. In a combined report, the Australian, Victorian, and New South Wales Law Reform Commissions recommended that the prestigious National Health and Medical Research Council of Australia be invited to develop guidelines for the medical profession to assist in the provision of information about proposed treatment and procedures.[75] These are now being developed as a basis for the establishment of new professional standards.[76]

---

[75] Law Reform Commission of Victoria Report No. 24; Australian Law Reform Commission Report No. 50, New South Wales Law Reform Commission Report No. 62, *Informed Decisions About Medical Procedures* (June 1989).

[76] National Health and Medical Research Council Working Party, *General Guidelines for Medical Practitioners on Providing Information to Patients*: Preliminary Discussion Paper, Australian Government Pub. Service 1991. The joint report of the Australian, Victorian and New South Wales Law Reform Commissions recommended that once these guidelines are settled, legislation should be enacted in the different states requiring that the guidelines be admissible as evidence in all appropriate professional negligence actions, and that the courts consider them in deciding whether a doctor has acted reasonably in relation to providing a patient with information.

Reproductive Rights

Frozen Embryos

[5]

DISPUTING OVER EMBRYOS: Of Contracts and Consents

Ellen A. Waldman*

I. INTRODUCTION

Divorce courts are all too familiar with the wrenching questions of who gets what when a married couple separates. A complex body of family law exists to guide determinations of how communally owned property should be divvied up.[1] In the last few years, however, advances in the high-tech field of fertility medicine—particularly the ability to cryopreserve embryos[2] and store them indefinitely[3]—have begun to pose perplexing questions of post-divorce rights of ownership.[4] When a married couple jointly donate gametes

---

* Associate professor at Thomas Jefferson School of Law. I gratefully acknowledge the excellent research assistance of Jane Conners as well as the helpful comments of colleagues Mary Beth Herald, Kenneth Vandevelde and Colin Crawford. I would also like to thank my mother Lois Waldman, whose dutiful readings are but a small part of the support and encouragement she provides.

1. To illustrate, one practice guide to California Family Law devotes over 370 pages to a discussion of property division issues. WILLIAM P. HOGOBOOM & DONALD B. KING, *Marital Property*, 1 CAL. PRAC. GUIDE FAMILY L. 8-1 to 8-366.6 (2000).

2. Some courts and commentators, when referring to the fertilized egg at the developmental stage when cryopreservation takes place, use the term pre-embryo or pre-zygote. *See infra* note 47 and accompanying text. A pre-embryo or pre-zygote refers to the morula and blastocyst stages, which occur in the fourteen days following fertilization. Continued cell differentiation and the development of the ectoderm, mesoderm, and endoderm layers mark the emergence of the embryo proper. TABER'S CYCLOPEDIC MEDICAL DICTIONARY 621, 1543 (18th ed. 1997) [hereinafter TABER'S]. For the sake of simplicity, this paper will use the term embryo, except when quoting courts or commentators who use the term pre-embryo or pre-zygote.

3. D. Summers et al., *Pregnancy Rates Following the Transfer of Thawed Embryos that Had Been Cryopreserved for Long Intervals Using a Simplified Freezing and Thawing Technique*, 10TH WORLD CONGRESS ON IN VITRO FERTILIZATION AND ASSISTED REPRODUCTION 71, 72 (1997) (Evaluation of the pregnancy and implantation rates of embryos transferred after being frozen for periods ranging from 2 to 4.8 years reveals rates comparable to transfers of embryos cryopreserved for shorter periods of time. Available data indicate that survival and implantation of cryopreserved embryos are not affected by the duration of cryostorage in liquid nitrogen.); *cf.* David Colker, *It's a Boy: Embryo is Viable after 1990 Freezing Pregnancy*, L.A. TIMES, Feb. 17, 1998, at B1 (reporting successful delivery of baby from embryo cryopreserved for eight years).

4. The problem of determining embryo disposition may arise out of the divorce context. An unmarried couple who have jointly contributed to the creation of cryopreserved embryos may solicit the courts in sorting out post-separation claims. To date, however, the cases have involved married couples whose dispositional dilemmas have accompanied divorce proceedings. *See infra* note 6.

to create a fertilized embryo, whose post-divorce claims for dispositional authority should trump?[5] This question has already been the subject of a number of cases.[6] As similar litigation percolates through the courts,[7] all signs indicate that disputes over embryos will grow in both number and complexity.

5. One initial question raised by embryo ownership claims is whether embryos should be treated as children or property. If embryos are in fact budding children, arguably a best-interest standard should prevail. In fact, one trial court characterized a couple's frozen embryos as children and applied a best interests standard in awarding custody to the mother seeking implantation. Davis v. Davis, No. E-14496, 1989 WL 140495, at *11 (Tenn. Cir. Ct. Sept. 21, 1989). This holding, however, was soundly rejected by the appellate and supreme courts of that state, and does not reflect the regnant view. Davis v. Davis, No. 180, 1990 WL 13087, at *1-3 (Tenn. App. Sept. 13, 1990), *aff'd.* 842 S.W.2d 588, 594-597 (Tenn. 1992). Generally, a consensus is emerging that embryos are neither persons nor property, but entities that should be accorded special respect due to their potential for human life. Ethical Committee of the American Fertility Society, *Ethical Considerations of Assisted Reproductive Technologies*, 62 FERTILITY & STERILITY No. 5, (Supp. Nov. 1994) [hereinafter *Ethical Considerations*] ("[W]e find a widespread consensus that the preembryo is not a person but is to be treated with special respect because it is a genetically unique, living human entity that might become a person."). This consensus view is not universal, however. *See* LA. REV. STAT. ANN. §§ 9:124, 9:126-27, 9:129 (West 1999) (defining in vitro fertilized human ovum as a juridical person, with all attendant rights and protections). Moreover, it is not at all clear what according embryos special respect entails. The state supreme court in *Davis* went out of its way to specify that embryos deserve greater respect than other types of human tissue due to their potential for human life and the symbolic meaning they hold for people. *Davis*, 842 S.W.2d at 596. The court then decided the case looking solely at the gamete donors' interests, disregarding entirely any interests the embryos, as entities deserving of special respect, might have. *Id.* at 602.

6. *See generally* A.Z. v. B.Z., No. 95-D-1683-DV (Mass. Prob. & Fam. Ct. Mar. 25, 1996), *aff'd*, 725 N.E.2d 1051 (Mass. 2000); J.B. v. M.B., No. FM-04-95-97 (N.J. Super. Ct. Sept. 28, 1998) (letter opinion granting summary judgment) (on file with author), *aff'd*, 751 A.2d 613 (N.J. Super. Ct. App. Div. 2000); Bohn v. Ann Arbor Reprod. Med. Assocs., No. 97-16310-CK (Mich. Cir. Ct. Jun. 24, 1998); Kass v. Kass, 663 N.Y.S.2d 581 (N.Y. App. Div. 1997), *aff'd*, 696 N.E.2d 174 (N.Y. 1998); Wendel v. Wendel, No. D 191962 (Ohio C.P. Dom. Rel. Ct. filed July 21, 1989); Davis v. Davis, 842 S.W.2d 588 (Tenn. 1992); C.A. 5587/93, Nachmani v. Nachmani, 49(1) P.D. 485 (Isr.).

7. *See* Nathan Koppel, *A Tangled Web We Weave When In Vitro We Conceive*, NAT'L L.J., March 15, 1999, at A9 (discussing In the Interest of O.G.M., 988 S.W.2d 473 (Tex. App. 1999), which raises questions of parental status where an embryo cryopreserved during marriage is implanted post-divorce. Plaintiff father in that case claimed parental privileges, despite the fact that the embryo was implanted several months after his divorce from the mother. Defendant mother contended that her ex-husband should assume the status of a sperm donor, with no parental rights or responsibilities toward the child. The Texas court of appeals affirmed the trial court's grant of paternity to the former husband, holding that statutes addressing parental rights as to children conceived with donor sperm or eggs, did not control the issue of paternity for a child of a known donor); *see also* Laurence M. Cruz, *Frozen Human Embryos in Dispute*, AP ONLINE, May 5, 2000 (discussing dispute over embryos created from divorcing husband's sperm and donor eggs). The wife, while bearing no biological connection to the embryos, seeks custody of the embryos to raise herself. The husband seeks to donate the embryos to a two-parent family. *Id.* The case is currently being considered by the Washington state appeals court. *Id.*

To date, American courts facing embryo disputes have taken one of two tacks. Under the first and more longstanding approach, courts presume that prior agreements regarding disposition of frozen embryos should be enforced.[8] Most scholarly commentary supports this approach.[9] In two recent decisions, however, courts have refused to enforce dispositional agreements that would allow implantation of frozen embryos over the objection of one parent. According to these courts, contracts that foist parenthood on an unwilling individual violate public policy.[10]

This paper considers cases decided under the first approach. Where courts have determined that dispositional agreements are valid and enforceable, they have been unconcerned with the location and manner in which these agreements are signed. They have endorsed the use of dispositional agreements, even where the agreements are embedded in informed consent documents provided by fertility clinics as a precursor to obtaining treatment.[11] Faced with the unsavory task of determining embryo ownership, most courts have treated the fertility clinics' informed consent documents as reliable transcriptions of each signatory's intent.[12] Despite

---

8. *Davis*, 842 S.W.2d at 597. In discussing the validity of the agreement, the *Davis* court stated:

> We believe, as a starting point, that an agreement regarding disposition of any untransferred preembryos in the event of contingencies (such as the death of one or more of the parties, divorce, financial reversals, or abandonment of the program) should be presumed valid and should be enforced as between the progenitors.

Id.; *see also A.Z. v. B.Z.*, Docket No. 95-D-1683-DV, at 22.

> Where the gamete-providers have made a knowing agreement regarding the disposition of the preembryos, the agreement should be enforced. . . . The enforcement of a dispositional contract allows all parties involved, to wit, the gamete-providers, the doctors and the clinicians, to rely on the agreement as a fundamental mean[s] [sic] for resolving disputes which may arrive.

Id. at 22-23 (citing *Davis*, 842 S.W.2d at 597); *Kass*, 696 N.E.2d at 180 ("Agreements between progenitors, or gamete donors, regarding disposition of their pre-zygotes should generally be presumed valid and binding, and enforced in any dispute between them." (citing *Davis*, 842 S.W.2d at 597)).

9. *See infra* note 127.

10. *A.Z. v. B.Z.*, 725 N.E.2d at 1057-58; *J.B. v. M.B.*, 751 A.2d at 619-20.

11. *Kass*, 696 N.E.2d at 180 (noting that the dispositional "agreement" at issue was contained in informed consent documents provided by the IVF program, but nevertheless concluding that the agreements should be enforced).

12. The Massachusetts Supreme Court, in its *A.Z. v. B.Z.* opinion, constitutes a striking exception. In that case, the court, in dicta, expressed concern over the procedural irregularities that plagued the dispositional agreement at issue in that case. The court made special mention of the fact that the agreement was located in the fertility clinic's consent form and was likely not intended by the parties to govern in a dispute between them. *See infra* notes 111-123 and accompanying text. That court, however, stated that even if the parties had entered into an unambiguous dispositional agreement through impeccably fair procedures, the court would still not enforce a

ample evidence that patients often sign such documents with little or no appreciation of their content, judicial inquiry into the validity of these "agreements" has been limited.

This paucity of judicial scrutiny is surprising given the courts' and legislatures' treatment of reproductive decisions reached in other contexts. In adoption proceedings or surrogate mother contracts, where parties seek to waive important reproductive opportunities, courts and legislative bodies generally either preclude enforcement or require procedural safeguards to ensure such waivers are knowing and thoughtful. In disputes involving frozen embryos, however, the courts have largely dispensed with any meaningful review of the contracting process by which dispositional terms are established. While lawmakers have proposed legislation that offers some protections, these initiatives fall short of the type of requirements that would ensure couples' awareness of the significance of the dispositional agreements they sign.

Although the enforcement of contracts that limit procreative opportunities remains controversial,[13] this paper does not take issue with the intrusion of market principles into the intimacies of reproduction. Contracts, when properly conceived and executed, can play a valuable role in clarifying the rights and obligations of all providers and purchasers of aid in reproduction.[14] Couples seeking infertility treatment should have the opportunity to consider how they want their embryos to be handled in the event of death, disability, or divorce, and to have their articulated wishes carried out. These dispositional agreements, however, should not be tucked into informed consent agreements; considered as an adjunct to the main event of obtaining treatment. As in adoption or surrogate motherhood agreements,

contract that required a party to unwillingly enter into an intimate family relationship. Consequently, the court's procedural criticisms are dicta and may have limited impact on the way in which dispositional agreements are devised.

13. Scholars initially critiqued the limits dispositional agreements place on the procreational rights of an individual who agrees to discard or donate the embryos, but later seeks their implantation. *See* Judith Daar, *Contract Does Not Override a Woman's Right to Use Fertilized Eggs*, L.A. DAILY J., May 22, 1998, at 6; Ellen H. Moskowitz, *Some Things Don't Belong in Contracts*, NAT'L L.J., June 8, 1998, at A25. Recently, however, a different type of criticism has emerged. This critique focuses on the party who initially sought to bring a child into the world, and now wishes to avoid a parental relationship with the product of those efforts. According to this critique, the danger is not the thwarting of procreational opportunities, but their coerced actualization. Carl Coleman, *Procreative Liberty and Contemporaneous Choice: An Inalienable Rights Approach to Frozen Embryo Disputes*, 84 MINN. L. REV. 55, 80-88 (1999); *see generally A.Z. v. B.Z.*, 725 N.E.2d 1051 (Mass. 2000); *J.B. v. M.B.*, 751 A.2d 613 (N.J. Super. Ct. App. Div. 2000).

14. John A. Robertson, *Prior Agreements for Disposition of Frozen Embryos*, 51 OHIO ST. L.J. 407, 414 (1990) [hereinafter Robertson, *Prior Agreements*].

dispositional agreements should be thoughtfully crafted—the product of a separate contracting process in which the parties are prompted to seriously consider the contingencies at issue and the options available.

To provide background, Part II briefly discusses the advances in fertility medicine that have spawned this new species of dispute. Part III introduces the major cases involving frozen embryo disputes that either endorse or discuss how dispositional agreements should be interpreted. Part IV reviews the informed consent literature and argues that the consent documents generated by fertility clinics constitute unreliable indicators of patient dispositional intent and unsatisfactory fodder for contract construction. Further assessing the courts' embrace of contract concepts in the frozen embryo setting, Part V tests the robustness of dispositional agreements according to unconscionability doctrine and suggests that they are doctrinally infirm and in need of procedural reform. Part VI surveys legislative and judicial treatment of waivers of reproductive opportunities in adoption and surrogacy contracts. It suggests that the flippancy with which courts are allowing the waiver of rights in the embryo disposition context represents an inappropriate divergence from the courts' and legislatures' normally protective stance toward procreative liberty. This part concludes that only embryo disposition agreements that have been taken out of informed consent documents and located in a separate agreement, devised through procedures designed to ensure full patient participation, deliberation and choice, deserve judicial endorsement. Part VII considers several legislative responses to the problems of contested embryos—a Florida statute enacted in 1997, and three bills currently being considered in the New York and New Jersey legislatures. This part highlights the salutary aspects of these bills, and suggests modifications and additions that might further improve the quality of dispositional agreements and better facilitate patient autonomy and choice.

II. ADVANCES IN ASSISTED REPRODUCTIVE TECHNOLOGY AND EMBRYO CRYOPRESERVATION

Given the number of couples seeking aid in reproduction, it is perhaps not surprising that custody battles now include claims to jointly created embryos. Approximately three million married couples are considered infertile.[15] Of

15. Infertility is defined as a failure to conceive after at least twelve months of unprotected intercourse. Bryan D. Cowan, *Infertility Evaluation*, *in* CLINICAL REPRODUCTIVE MEDICINE 168 (Bryan D. Cowan & David B. Seifer eds., 1997). *See* American Society for Reproductive Medicine (ASRM), *Fact Sheet: Infertility*, *at* http://www.asrm.org/fact/patients/FactSheets/

this group, increasing numbers are seeking the assistance of medical technology in their quest for a child.[16]

Infertility may be a function of male or female anatomical difficulties.[17] Male factor infertility typically involves problems in sperm production or delivery.[18] Female factor infertility typically stems from ovulation defects as well as fallopian tube and uterine abnormalities.[19] Certain infertility factors may be successfully treated by medication, lifestyle changes, or surgery such as a vasovasostomy[20] or a myomectomy.[21] Where these interventions are ineffective to cure the anatomical or hormonal impediments to fertilization and passage of the egg from ovaries to uterus, Assisted Reproductive Technologies ("ART")[22] may be used to achieve a union of egg and sperm. In vitro fertilization ("IVF"),[23] the oldest and most well-known of these

infertility-Fact.pdf (last visited Sept. 9, 2000) (reporting that over six million American women and their partners suffer from infertility).

16. The latest data on infertility available at CDC are from the 1995 National Survey of Family Growth. Of the approximately 60 million women of reproductive age in 1995, about 1.2 million . . . had had an infertility-related medical appointment within the previous year, and an additional [9.3 million] had received infertility services at some time in their lives. (Infertility services include medical tests to diagnose infertility, medical advice and treatments to help a woman become pregnant . . . .

CENTERS FOR DISEASE CONTROL AND PREVENTION, 1997 ASSISTED REPRODUCTIVE TECHNOLOGY SUCCESS RATES 3 (1999) [hereinafter 1997 ART SUCCESS RATES]. The American Fertility Society's membership has grown exponentially, from 3,600 in 1974, see U.S. CONGRESS, OFFICE OF TECHNOLOGY ASSESSMENT, *Infertility: Medical and Social Choices* 5 (U.S. Govt. Printing Office, May 1988), to 10,500 in 1999. ASRM, *Services Offered to Health Professionals*, *at* http://www.asrm.org/Professionals/mainprof.html (last visited Sept. 9, 2000). In 1997, 335 fertility clinics reported to the Centers for Disease Control that they carried out a total of 71,826 ART cycles resulting in deliveries of 24,582 babies. 1997 ART SUCCESS RATES, at 9-10.

17. Cowan, *supra* note 15, at 168.

18. ROBERT R. FRANKLIN & DOROTHY KAY BROCKMAN, IN PURSUIT OF FERTILITY 153-69 (2d ed. 1995) (discussing importance of sperm volume, motility and morphology and problems generated by tubal obstructions and obstructions in the testes).

19. Cowan, *supra* note 15, at 168-69; *see also* FRANKLIN & BROCKMAN, *supra* note 18, at 26-30, 79-81, 88-92, 114-22 (discussing endometriosis, tubal diseases, and ovulatory disorders resulting from hormonal imbalances, dietary factors and stress).

20. A vasovasotomy is surgery designed to reverse a vasectomy and reopen an occluded vas deferens. TABER'S, *supra* note 2, at 2067.

21. A myomectomy is surgery to remove uterine fibroids. *Id.* at 1260.

22. "ART are techniques designed to assist infertile women to conceive and give birth." *Id.* at 162. Another slightly more poetic explication defines assisted reproductive technology as the "art and science of getting gametes together." Earl P. Steinberg et al., *Profiling Assisted Reproductive Technology: Outcomes and Quality of Infertility Management*, 69 FERTILITY & STERILITY 617, 618 (1998).

23. In Vitro Fertilization ("IVF") "is the mixing of an egg and sperm in a dish 'in vitro' followed by incubation in a temperature-controlled, CO_2-enriched environment . . . . Embryogenesis is followed by the transfer of some or all of these freshly generated embryos

technologies, involves medically stimulating the ovaries to produce eggs. These eggs are then removed from the woman's ovaries where they are placed in a culture, fertilized with sperm, incubated for several days, and then transferred into the uterus.[24]

The process of retrieving eggs from a woman's ovaries poses significant risks. In most instances, drugs are administered to stimulate egg production so that several eggs can be retrieved.[25] These drugs pose an increased risk of multiple births[26] and ovarian hyperstimulation syndrome, a condition that may result in abnormal blood clotting, major organ damage, respiratory distress, or stroke.[27] Additionally, some studies suggest a correlation between fertility drugs and ovarian cancer.[28] The egg extraction process is

---

directly to the patient's uterus through the cervix." Alan S. Penzias, *Gamete Technologies*, *in* CLINICAL REPRODUCTIVE MEDICINE 214 (Bryan D. Cowan & David B. Seifer eds., 1997).

24. Additional ART techniques continue to proliferate. In addition to IVF, infertile couples may avail themselves of a varied menu of surgical procedures. These include: Gamete Intra-fallopian Transfer ("GIFT"), in which the eggs are removed from the ovaries, placed in a catheter with sperm and deposited in the fallopian tubes, where, it is hoped, fertilization and implantation will occur. *Id.* TABER'S, *supra* note 2, at 769. Zygote Intra-fallopian Transfer ("ZIFT"), in which the one-celled egg, a zygote, is fertilized with sperm extra-corporeally and the resulting embryo is placed in the fallopian tube the day after fertilization. Penzias, *supra* note 23, at 214; TABER'S, *supra* note 2, at 1982. Tubal Embryo Transfer ("TET"), in which eggs at the 2-cell to 4-cell stage are fertilized extra-corporeally with the resulting embryos transferred to the fallopian tube two days after fertilization. Penzias, *supra* note 23, at 214. Zona Drilling and Partial Zona Dissection, in which small holes are drilled into the outer covering (the zona pellucida) of the egg to assist sperm penetration. *Id.* at 218. Microsurgical Epididymal Sperm Aspiration ("MESA"), in which sperm are extracted directly from the epididymis and placed in contact with the egg. AMERICAN SOCIETY FOR REPRODUCTIVE MEDICINE, PRACTICE COMMITTEE REPORT, NEW TECHNIQUES FOR SPERM ACQUISITION IN OBSTRUCTIVE AZOOSPERMIA 4 (Aug. 1999). Intracytoplasmic sperm injection ("ICSI"), in which a single sperm is injected into the egg's cytoplasm. Penzias, *supra* note 23, at 219. Subzonal Insemination ("SUZI"), in which several sperm are injected underneath the outer covering of the egg, but not directly into the egg's cellular fluid. *Id.* at 218; *see also* Advanced Fertility Center of Chicago, *Infertility Education Pages*, *at* http://www.advancedfertility.com/infer.edu.htm (last visited Sept. 9, 2000).

25. The drugs most commonly used to spur ovulation of multiple eggs are clomiphene citrate, pituitary gonadotropins, ("FSH" and "LH"), human chrorionic gonadotropin ("hCG"), human menopausal gonadotropins ("hMG"), and gonadoptropin-releasing hormone ("GnRH"). Diane K. Wysowski, *Use of Fertility Drugs in the United States, 1973 through 1991*, 60 FERTILITY & STERILITY 1096, 1097 (1993); Penzias, *supra* note 23, at 216 ("The most common stimulation protocols include combinations of gonadotropin-releasing hormone agonist (GnRH-a) and human menopausal gonadotropins (hMGs)."); *see also* FRANKLIN & BROCKMAN, *supra* note 18, at 237.

26. Joyce A. Martin & Milissa M. Park, *Trends in Twin and Triplet Births: 1980-97*, 47 NAT'L VITAL STATISTICS REPORTS No. 24 1, 5 (Sept. 14, 1999) (noting that triplet and higher order multiple births increased by 404 percent from 1980 to 1997, and attributing two-thirds of the increase to fertility enhancing therapies).

27. ASRM, *Fact Sheet: Side Effects of Gonadoptropins*, *at* http://www.asrm.org/factsheets/gonadoptropins-Fact.pdf (last visited Sept. 9, 2000).

28. *See generally* Mary Ann Rossing et al., *Ovarian Tumors in a Cohort of Infertile Women*, 331 NEW ENGLAND JOURNAL OF MEDICINE 771 (1994). *But see* Gad Potashnik et al., *Fertility*

also burdensome. Extraction is accomplished by inserting a needle through the vaginal wall and into an ovarian follicle. Follicle fluid and the eggs contained within are then suctioned out. Clinics generally provide some sedation, but most women report moderate or severe pain despite the provision of analgesic.[29] Common side effects following the procedure include abdominal or vaginal discomfort and bleeding from the vaginal puncture site. Less commonly, some women have required major surgery to repair damage caused by needle puncture of nearby organs.[30] Additionally, some practitioners report severe infections following approximately one in 400 extractions.[31]

Cryopreservation, the freezing of untransferred embryos, allows women undergoing IVF to minimize these risks and burdens. Transfer of fertilized eggs following a stimulated cycle may, if unsuccessful, be followed by transfer of cryopreserved eggs in a later cycle.[32] Cryopreservation thus reduces the number of cycles of egg retrieval necessary to achieve pregnancy, which lessens the physical risks associated with ovarian stimulation and the process of egg extraction.[33] Because each cycle of egg

Drugs and the Risk of Breast and Ovarian Cancers: Results of a Long-term Follow-up Study, 71 FERTILITY & STERILITY 853, 857 (1999) (reporting data that fails to support linkage between fertility drug usage and increased risk of breast cancer).

29. S. Bhattacharya et al., *How Effective is Patient-Controlled Analgesia? A Randomized Comparison of Two Protocols for Pain Relief During Oocyte Recovery*, 12 HUMAN REPRODUCTION 1440, 1442 (1997) ("What this study shows clearly is that we have yet to achieve a safe and effective technique for abolition of pain during outpatient oocyte recovery . . . .").

30. AMERICAN SOCIETY FOR REPRODUCTIVE MEDICINE, IVF AND GIFT: A GUIDE TO ASSISTED REPRODUCTIVE TECHNOLOGY 13 (1995).

31. D. Dicker et al., *Severe Abdominal Complications after Transvaginal Ultrasonographically Guided Retrieval of Oocytes for In Vitro Fertilization and Embryo Transfer*, 59 FERTILITY & STERILITY 1313, 1315 (1993) (reporting on life-threatening complications resulting from ultrasonically guided transvaginal aspiration—of 3,656 aspiration procedures, 14 patients developed severe complications requiring remedial surgery).

32. 1997 ART SUCCESS RATES, *supra* note 16, at 39 ("Frozen (cryopreserved) cycles are those in which previously frozen embryos are thawed and then transferred.").

33. *Id.*

> Because frozen cycles use embryos formed from a previous stimulated cycle, no stimulation or retrieval is involved. As a result, these cycles are usually less expensive and less invasive than cycles using fresh embryos. In addition, freezing some of the embryos from a retrieval procedure may increase a woman's overall chances of having a child from a single retrieval.

Id.; *see also* William N. Burns et al., *Survival of Cryopreservation and Thawing with all Blastomeres Intact Identifies Multicell Embryos with Superior Frozen Embryo Transfer Outcome*, 72 FERTILITY & STERILITY 527, 527 (1999)

> The cryopreservation of human embryos provides many clinical benefits, including a reduction in the risk of major multiple pregnancy, an increase in the number of ETs [embryo transfers] and hence pregnancies per stimulation and retrieval cycle, the avoidance of ovarian hyperstimulation syndrome in

retrieval costs several thousand dollars,[34] cryopreservation significantly lowers the costs of achieving pregnancy.[35] Additionally, the availability of frozen embryos lessens the incentives to transfer large numbers of eggs in each stimulated cycle, a practice linked to multiple gestation[36] and poor outcomes for mother and children.[37] These benefits, among others, have led the ethics committee for the American Society of Reproductive Medicine to conclude that cryopreservation is an "essential component of all programs offering IVF."[38]

Fertility consumers have not been blind to the many advantages cryopreservation offers. The rate of use for this procedure continues to grow

---

> high-risk settings, the preservation of future childbearing capability in women facing ovarian surgery or cancer therapy, and a reduction in patient expense and risk from additional stimulation and retrieval cycles.

Id. Cryopreservation may also enhance the likelihood of pregnancy because it allows the woman to delay implantation and transfer frozen embryos during an unstimulated menstrual cycle, when her body is drug-free and unstressed by surgical intrusion. Robertson, *Prior Agreements, supra* note 14, at 408.

34. Infertility, Gynecology & Obstetrics, Medical Group of San Diego, AMC., Fee Information for IVF/Gift: Overview (1996) [*hereinafter* IGO Medical Group] (listing costs associated with ovulation induction, retrieval, fertilization and implantation as ranging between $9,000 and $10,000 dollars) (form on file with author).

35. *Id.* (listing costs to thaw and implant cryopreserved embryos as ranging between $3,000 and $3,500). The cost of a regular IVF cycle is approximately four times that of a cycle using cryopreserved eggs. Telephone Interview with Sheila Dimarzo, Lab Director, IGO Medical Group (July 18, 2000). Bradley J. Van Voorhis et al., *The Efficacy and Cost Effectiveness of Embryo Cryopreservation Compared with Other Assisted Reproductive Techniques*, 64 FERTILITY & STERILITY 647, 649 (1995) ("The overall cost per delivery for all of the 'fresh' ART procedures was decreased by nearly $6,000 by the addition of cryopreserved ETs [embryo transfers].").

36. New York State Task Force on Life and the Law, Executive Summary of Assisted Reproductive Technologies: Analysis and Recommendations for Public Policy, April 1998, at http://www.health.state.ny.us/nysdoh/taskfce/index.htm (last visited Sept. 9, 2000) ("Infertility treatment is the major factor that has been implicated in the nationwide surge in the number of multiple births."); Burns, *supra* note 33, at 527.

37. *See generally* Laura A. Schieve et al., *Live-Birth Rates and Multiple-Birth Risk Using In Vitro Fertilization*, 282 J. AM. MED. ASSOC. 1832 (1999)

> One common practice that aims to increase the likelihood of pregnancy is to transfer multiple embryos (often more than 3) into the uterine cavity. This treatment approach also presents an important drawback, however, because it increases the risk for multiple birth. Multiple-birth infants are at significant risk for a number of adverse outcomes including preterm delivery, low birth weight, congenital malformation, fetal and infant death, and long-term morbidity and disability among survivors. Twins are 5 times as likely, and triplet and higher-order infants 13 times as likely, as singleton infants to die during the first year of life.

Id. at 1832 (footnotes omitted).

38. *Ethical Considerations, supra* note 5, at 58S-59S.

exponentially. In 1988, 14,657 embryos were frozen.[39] That number climbed to 23,865 in 1990.[40] Today, individual centers boast of freezing over 2,000 embryos annually, and there are over 300 medical centers that offer assistance in embryo creation or implantation.[41] It is estimated that there are approximately one million embryos stored worldwide, including at least 100,000 in the United States.[42]

As the divorce rate remains steady at between 40-50%,[43] it is inevitable that some divorcing couples will have embryos in storage and disagree as to their fate. The first state supreme court case to address this issue, *Davis v. Davis*,[44] adumbrated themes that would later be repeated and elaborated in the New York appellate and high court opinions in *Kass v. Kass*,[45] and the lower court opinion in *A.Z. v. B.Z.*[46] In each case, the court embraced contract law as the preferred paradigm for resolving embryo disposition disputes. The next section reviews these cases.

---

39. JOHN A. ROBERTSON, CHILDREN OF CHOICE: FREEDOM AND THE NEW REPRODUCTIVE TECHNOLOGIES 98, 109 (1994) [hereinafter ROBERTSON, CHILDREN OF CHOICE].

40. *Id.*

41. Genetics and IVF Institute, *Human Embryo Cryopreservation (Embryo Freezing) and Frozen Embryo Transfer Cycles*, *at* http://www.givf.com/embryov.html (last visited Sept. 9, 2000). The Centers for Disease Control identified 356 programs that use some form of ART embryology procedures. CENTERS FOR DISEASE CONTROL, FINAL REPORT: SURVEY OF ASSISTED REPRODUCTIVE TECHNOLOGY: EMBRYO LABORATORY PROCEDURES AND PRACTICES 10 (1999).

42. Gina Maranto, *Embryo Overpopulation*, SCIENTIFIC AMERICAN, Apr. 1996, at 16.

43. Provisional data for the twelve-month period ending June, 1999, show that roughly half of all marriages end in divorce. CENTERS FOR DISEASE CONTROL AND PREVENTION, BIRTHS, MARRIAGES, DIVORCES, AND DEATHS: PROVISIONAL DATA FOR JUNE 1999, 48 NAT'L VITAL STATISTICS REPORTS 8 (June 8, 2000). The current divorce rate is calculated at somewhere between 40-50% for young first-time marrieds. Scott Stanley, *What Really is the Divorce Rate?*, Divorce Support, *at* http://divorcesupport.about.com/library/weekly/aa061699.htm (last visited Sept. 9, 2000).

44. 842 S.W.2d 588 (Tenn. 1992).

45. 663 N.Y.S.2d 581 (N.Y. App. Div. 1997).

46. No. 95-D-1683-DV (Mass. Prob. & Fam. Ct. Mar. 25, 1996).

III. JUDICIAL AND SCHOLARLY TREATMENT OF FROZEN EMBRYO DISPUTES

A. The Major Cases[47]

47. The cases discussed below in no way represent the universe of litigation involving custody claims over cryopreserved embryos. Other cases exist; however, they either did not result in judicial opinions, or are not directly relevant to the issues discussed in this paper. For example, *Wendel v. Wendel*, No. D 191962 (Ohio C.P. Dom. Rel. Ct. filed July 21, 1989), involved a wife's claim for custody over a cryopreserved embryo stored at the Cleveland Clinic. Robertson, *Prior Agreements*, *supra* note 14, at 411-14. The husband wanted the embryo destroyed and argued that the wife had signed an agreement prior to the fertilization treatments authorizing destruction in the event the couple divorced. *Id.* While the court granted a temporary injunction prohibiting the clinic from destroying the embryo prior to a divorce court ruling, the court never issued a definitive ruling on custody because the parties eventually agreed that the embryos had been stored for such a lengthy period of time that they were no longer viable for implant. Interview with John V. Heutsche, counsel for Mary Wendel (Oct. 1, 1998).

Bohn v. Mobley, (No. 97-26334-DC, *consolidated with* Bohn v. Ann Arbor Reprod. Med. Assocs., No. 97-16310-CK (Mich. Cir. Ct. Jun. 24, 1998)) is not directly relevant because it does not involve judicial interpretation of a dispositional agreement contained in fertility clinic informed consent forms. *See generally* Bohn v. Ann Arbor Reprod. Med. Assocs., No. 97-16319-CK (Mich. Cir. Ct. Jun. 24, 1998). However, the court's opinion is illuminating in its eagerness to interpret the consent forms as the written portion of a part-oral, part-written contract between the couple to only implant the embryos if both parties agree. *Id.* at 7. Ms. Bohn, the former Mrs. Mobley, filed a breach of contract claim against the fertility clinic based on the clinic's refusal to transfer the remaining cryopreserved embryos to her on demand. *Id.* The court held that the consent forms signed by Mr. and Mrs. Mobley, along with oral conversations with her husband, constituted a contract between Mrs. Mobley and her husband, and the clinic to transfer the embryos for implantation only upon the request of both Mr. and Mrs. Mobley. *Id.* at 8.

J.B. v. M.B, 751 A.2d 613 (N.J. Super. Ct. App. Div. 2000), is also not directly relevant because the New Jersey appellate court chose not to enforce the couple's dispositional agreement on public policy grounds. The court's concern, however, was unrelated to the location of the agreement or the process by which it was constructed. Rather, the court was troubled by the consequences of enforcing the agreement, which would require the wife to become a parent against her will.

In that case, J.B., the wife, sought destruction of the embryos she had created with her ex-husband, while M.B, the divorcing husband, sought custody of the embryos in order to implant them in a future partner or donate them to a childless couple. The parties had signed a consent form which included the following language:

> I, J.B. (patient) and M.B (partner) agree that all control, direction and ownership of our tissues will be relinquished to the IVF Program under the following circumstances:
>
> 1. A dissolution of our marriage by court order, unless the court specifies who takes control and direction of the tissues . . . .

Id. at 616. Additionally, M.B. argued that J.B. had orally agreed that, in the event of divorce, the embryos would be donated to an infertile couple. *Id.*

The lower court ignored the existence of the written consent form language and the husband's arguments that the couple's oral agreement should be enforced. Rather, the court held that the *raison d'etre* for the IVF procedure was to conceive a child within the marriage. J.B. v. M.B., FM-04-95-97, at 6-7 (N.J. Super. Ct. Sept. 28, 1998) (letter opinion granting summary judgment)

1. *Davis v. Davis*[48]

Mary Sue Davis endured five ectopic pregnancies and six IVF attempts before her last ART procedure on December 8, 1988.[49] On that date, nine ova were retrieved and fertilized, two were implanted, and seven were frozen for possible future transfer.[50] No pregnancy resulted from that procedure, and three months later her husband, Junior Davis, filed for divorce.[51] Significantly, the Davises had neither signed a written agreement, nor orally discussed what should be done with the embryos in the event of a divorce.[52] When the divorce negotiations began, the couple found they were able to negotiate a settlement about everything except the embryos. Mary Sue wanted to implant them; Junior wanted them destroyed.[53]

(on file with author). Because the couple "did not go through the IVF process with the idea in mind to begin an enterprise of selling or donating embryos to other couples" the court held in favor of the wife. *Id.* at 6.

On appeal, the Appellate Division of the Superior Court, affirmed the lower court ruling, though on different grounds. J.B. v. M.B., 751 A.2d at 620. Rejecting the superior court's *raison d'etre* analysis, the appellate court explicitly acknowledged the existence of the written agreement contained in the clinic consent form, as well as the couple's alleged oral agreement to donate the embryos in the event of divorce. The court, however, declined to enforce either contract on public policy grounds. Noting that M.B. could still produce sperm and did not need to use the frozen embryos in order to procreate, the court observed, "enforcement of the alleged contract to create a child would impair the wife's constitutional right not to procreate, whereas permitting destruction of the embryos would not effectively impair the husband's reproductive rights." *Id.* at 619. Noting that New Jersey recognizes neither surrogacy contracts, nor actions seeking to enforce a promise to marry or surrender a child for adoption, the court determined that the state's public policy forbid enforcement of contracts "to enter into familial relationships" where one individual has experienced a change of heart. *Id.* at 620. ("Thus, the observation of the Supreme Judicial Court of Massachusetts that 'agreements to enter into familial relationships (marriage or parenthood) should not be enforced against individuals who subsequently reconsider their decisions' is as apposite in New York as it is in Massachusetts.") *Id.* Because the New Jersey court is unwilling to enforce a contract where doing so will create unwanted genetic ties, it is clear that no contracting process will cure what the court considers to be a fatal substantive defect. There is much one could say about the New Jersey court's approach, but such commentary is beyond the scope of this paper. It is enough to note that the reasoning of this case, as well as that of the Massachusetts Supreme Court's opinion in *A.Z. v. B.Z.*, require responses outside the ambit of the reforms suggested here.

48. 842 S.W.2d 588 (Tenn. 1992).

49. *Id.* at 591.

50. *Id.* at 592.

51. *Id.*

52. Apparently, the clinic, like most fertility clinics, had a consent form that couples were required to sign before initiating cryopreservation. No consent form was presented to the Davises, however, because "the clinic was in the process of moving," and the consent forms could not be located. *Id.* at 592 n.9.

53. *Id.* at 604.

The Tennessee Supreme Court, in ruling in favor of Junior Davis,[54] initiated the judicial presumption favoring a contractual approach to these issues. Although no party contended that a prior agreement existed regarding disposition of the embryos in the event of divorce, the court went out of its way to endorse the validity and enforceability of such agreements. The court said in dicta "that an agreement regarding disposition of any untransferred preembryos in the event of contingencies (such as the death of one or more of the parties, divorce, financial reversals, or abandonment of the program) should be presumed valid and should be enforced as between the progenitors."[55] The court acknowledged that dispositional agreements might be signed before the parties can truly understand the nature of the physical and emotional journey upon which they have embarked. Nevertheless, the court maintained that such agreements should be modified only through joint agreement.[56] In the absence of jointly agreed upon modifications, the court suggested that previously-signed dispositional "agreements should be considered binding."[57] Because the Davises had not entered into a dispositional agreement, the court conducted a balancing test, weighing Mary Sue's interests in procreation versus Junior's interests in avoiding procreation. After balancing these countervailing rights in the case before it, the court announced a presumption in favor of the right to avoid procreation,[58] and denied Mary Sue's request for control over the embryos.[59]

54. The trial court's finding that the seven frozen embryos were human beings and that the state had an interest in these smallest of citizens, led them to award Mary Sue temporary custody so that she could proceed with implantation. Davis v. Davis, 1989 WL 140495, at *8-10 (Tenn. Cir. Ct. Sept. 21, 1989). The Tennessee court of appeal reversed, holding that the embryos were not children and that Junior's constitutional right to avoid procreation should be granted equal weight vis-a-vis Mary Sue's right to implant. Concluding that the parties shared an interest in the embryos, Mary Sue and Junior were awarded "joint control" with "equal voice over their disposition." Davis v. Davis, 1990 WL 13087, at *3 (Tenn. Ct. App. Sept. 13, 1990).

55. *Davis*, 842 S.W.2d at 597.

56. *Id.*

57. *Id.*

58. The court determined that the burdens that would be imposed on Junior if he were to become an unwilling parent were considerable. Junior had testified that after his parents' divorce he rarely saw his father, and suffered severe problems as a result. Consequently, he stated he was "vehemently opposed to fathering a child" he would not live with. *Id.* at 603-04. Mary Sue Davis's interest in implantation was characterized as somewhat tertiary. By the time the Supreme Court of Tennessee heard the case, Mary Sue no longer sought to implant the embryos herself, but to donate them to another couple. *Id.* at 590. Her interest was limited to seeing the embryos she had borne hardships to harvest attain personhood. The court held:

> Refusal to permit donation of the preembryos would impose on her the burden of knowing that the lengthy IVF procedures she underwent were futile, and that the preembryos to which she contributed genetic material would never become children. While this is not an insubstantial emotional burden, we can

2. *Kass v. Kass*[60]

Steven and Maureen Kass suffered many long, expensive years of fertility treatment before divorcing. Maureen Kass "underwent the egg retrieval process five times and fertilized eggs were transferred to her nine times."[61] During the final procedure, sixteen eggs were retrieved, resulting in nine pre-zygotes.[62] Four pre-zygotes were transferred to her sister for implantation, and five were cryogenically preserved.[63] When Mrs. Kass's sister did not become pregnant and expressed an unwillingness to continue to participate in the fertility program, the marriage crumbled.[64] Mrs. Kass subsequently filed for divorce. Like many other divorcing couples who had sought fertility treatment, the Kasses were able to agree on everything except what should be done with the embryos.[65]

The Kass' effort to secure fertility services involved considerable paperwork. The Kasses signed four consent forms.[66] The first two explained the risks and benefits of in vitro fertilization and embryo transfer.[67] The third consent form entitled "Informed Consent Form No. 2: Cryopreservation of Human Pre-zygotes" was a seven page single-spaced form relating specifically to cryopreservation.[68] Page three of this form expressly addressed what should be done with the embryos in the event of divorce: "In the event of divorce, we understand that legal ownership of any stored pre-zygotes must be determined in a property settlement and will be released as directed by order of a court of competent jurisdiction."[69]

In the next paragraph, the form required the couple to consider "[t]he possibility of . . . death or any other unforeseen circumstances that may result in neither of us being able to determine the disposition of any stored frozen pre-zygotes"[70] and directed the couple to select one of three options set out in Addendum 2-1. Addendum 2-1 stated: "In the event that we no

> only conclude that Mary Sue Davis' interest in donation is not as significant as the interest Junior Davis has in avoiding parenthood.

Id. at 604.

59. *Id.*
60. 696 N.E.2d 174 (N.Y. 1998).
61. *Id.* at 175-76.
62. *Id.* at 177.
63. *Id.*
64. *Id.*
65. *Id.*
66. *Id.* at 176.
67. *Id.*
68. *Id.*
69. *Id.*
70. *Id.*

longer wish to initiate a pregnancy or are unable to make a decision regarding the disposition of our stored, frozen pre-zygotes, we now indicate our desire for the disposition of our pre-zygotes . . . ."[71]

The form allowed for three possibilities: donation of the embryos to a childless couple; use of the embryos for research purposes; and thawing and disposal of the embryos with no research performed upon them.[72] The Kasses initialed the second option.[73]

The trial court, relying on the abortion cases for the proposition that a husband cannot force a woman to either terminate or bring her pregnancy to term, held that Mrs. Kass's right to control the embryos was sovereign.[74] Having concluded that Mrs. Kass had exclusive right to the embryos, the court then considered whether she had waived that right in agreeing to the dispositional provisions in the fertility clinic's consent form. The court found no waiver had occurred.[75]

The appellate court reversed, roundly rejecting the trial court's conclusions.[76] While the trial court dismissed the contractual angle of the case, finding constitutional doctrine more apposite, the appellate court reversed the analysis.[77] The court attacked as "fundamental error" the trial court's assumption that a woman's right to dictate the course of an in vivo pregnancy implies an equal prerogative to control unilaterally the outcome of

71. *Id.* at 176-177.

72. Exhibit A—Informed Consent Form No. 2 Annexed to *Kass* Answer 41-49 (Long Island IVF Program, Informed Consent Form No. 2, Cryopreservation of Human Pre-zygotes (Feb. 1990) (on file with author) [hereinafter *Kass* Informed Consent Form No. 2] (seven page consent form used by the Long Island IVF Program at John T. Mather Memorial Hospital). The form is signed, initialed, and dated May 12, 1993 by Mr. and Mrs. Kass. *Id.* at 48.

73. *Id.* at 47.

74. Kass v. Kass, 1995 WL 110368, at *2 (N.Y. Sup. Ct. Jan. 18, 1995) (citing Roe v. Wade, 410 U.S. 113 (1973), and Planned Parenthood of Missouri v. Danforth, 428 U.S. 52 (1976)). The trial court noted that "[i]t cannot seriously be argued that a husband has a right to procreate or avoid procreation following an in vivo fertilization." *Id.* Finding "no legal, ethical or logical reason why an in vitro fertilization should give rise to additional rights on the part of the husband," the court held that an in vitro husband's right to avoid procreation terminates "after his participation in an in vitro program." *Id.* at *3.

75. The court held that the proviso stating that, "in the event of divorce, legal ownership of any pre-stored pre-zygotes must be determined in a property settlement and will be released by an order of a Court of competent jurisdiction" simply records an agreement that distribution "would be subject to the directives of the divorce court." *Id.* at *4. Addendum 2-1, which is contingent upon neither party being able to determine disposition of the embryos, was, according to the court, inapplicable to the divorce dispute. The court held, "there is nothing before me . . .which would compel a conclusion that plaintiff has waived her right to determine the future of the subject zygotes." *Id.* at *5.

76. Kass v. Kass, 663 N.Y.S.2d 581, 585 (N.Y. App. Div. 1997).

77. *Id.* at 583.

an in vitro fertilization.[78] The error, the appellate court noted, was failing to see that a pregnant woman's right to control her pregnancy is based on a right to bodily integrity not implicated in IVF until implantation occurs.[79] The court rejected *Roe v. Wade* as binding authority in the Kass' dispute.[80]

Finding that constitutional doctrine yielded no clear winner, the appellate court seized upon contract law for its analytical compass.[81] Contrary to the trial court's reading, this court determined that the informed consent documents signed by the Kasses reflected their mutual intent to turn the embryos over for research should they divorce.[82] Reading the informed consent documents as a contract between the couple, the court resurrected the *Davis* language that "an agreement regarding disposition of any untransferred preembryos in the event of contingencies . . . should be presumed valid and should be enforced . . . ."[83] The appellate court interpreted the informed consent documents as constituting such an agreement, and thus denied Mrs. Kass custody of the embryos.[84]

The court of appeals, in affirming the appellate court's opinion, also cited the *Davis* dicta with approval and highlighted the benefits that accrue when progenitors specify in advance what they want done with frozen embryos should contingencies arise.[85] According to the court, parties can achieve enhanced procreative liberty and efficient dispute resolution when, "before embarking on IVF and cryopreservation," they "think through possible contingencies and carefully specify their wishes in writing."[86] Not only do the hopeful parents benefit from advance dispositional directives, so too do the clinics. The court noted, "[w]ritten agreements also provide the certainty needed for effective operation of IVF programs."[87] The court considered the fertility clinic's authorship and provision of the forms irrelevant because, while each party advanced a different interpretation of the dispositional intent embodied in the forms, neither party argued that the intent manifest on the documents' face differed from their actual intentions when signing.[88] Further, neither party argued that they were coerced or otherwise misled into

78. *Id.* at 585.
79. *Id.* at 585-86.
80. *Id.*
81. *Id.* at 586.
82. *Id.* at 587-88.
83. *Id.* at 587.
84. *Id.* at 590.
85. *Id.* at 587.
86. Kass v. Kass, 696 N.E.2d 174, 180 (N.Y. 1998).
87. *Id.* (citations omitted).
88. *Id.* at 180.

signing the forms.[89] The court of appeals found, as did the appellate court, that "the informed consents signed by the parties unequivocally manifest their mutual intention that in the present circumstances the pre-zygotes be donated for research to the IVF program."[90] In so doing, the court of appeals shut the door on Mrs. Kass' last chance at genetic motherhood.

The New York intermediate and court of appeals, like the *Davis* court before them, latched onto contract doctrine as the appropriate mode of resolving embryo disposition disagreements, without considering either the content or process by which the dispositional agreement at issue was reached.[91] These courts were untroubled by the fact that the agreement they were construing was drafted by the fertility clinic, presented to the parties on a take it or leave it basis, contained a highly constricted range of dispositional choices,[92] and was signed without any formal counseling or dialogue sensitizing the parties to the implications of their decisions.[93]

3. *A.Z. v. B. Z.*[94]

A.Z and B.Z pursued fertility treatment, first in Virginia, then in Massachusetts, for three years.[95] The wife, B.Z., underwent six in vitro procedures and endured two ectopic pregnancies.[96] Each time eggs were retrieved from B.Z. and fertilized, the couple signed a consent form authorizing removal and cryopreservation of excess embryos. Over the three years, the couple signed seven separate informed consent forms. Each form contained a dispositional provision listing six options available in the event of divorce. Each form also allowed the couple to write in alternative

89. *Id.* ("While these documents were technically provided by the IVF program, neither party disputes that they are an expression of their own intent regarding disposition of their pre-zygotes. Nor do the parties contest the legality of those agreements, or that they were freely and knowingly made.").

90. *Id.* at 181.

91. *See, e.g.*, Janet L. Dolgin, *An Emerging Consensus: Reproductive Technology and the Law*, 23 VT. L. REV. 225, 260-281 (1998) (noting that *Kass*, and its progenitor, *Davis*, represent the judiciary's strongest commitment to contract law in reproductive disputes, in contrast to cases that employ more traditional notions of family and parenthood).

92. In the *Kass* case, for example, neither member of the couple was provided the option of keeping the embryos, arranging for implantation and raising the resulting child as a single or remarried parent. *See supra* note 70. The same is true in the *Wendel* case. *Supra* note 47, and *infra* notes 181-82 and accompanying text.

93. Kass v. Kass, 696 N.E.2d 174, 176 (N.Y. 1998).

94. A.Z. v. B.Z., No. 95-D-1683-DV (Mass. Prob. & Fam. Ct. Mar. 25, 1996).

95. *Id.* at 4-5.

96. *Id.* at 15.

mechanisms for disposing of the embryos otherwise not listed as options on the form.[97]

Each of the seven cryopreservation informed consent forms signed by A.Z. and B.Z. contained identical dispositional language. In each form, the couple bypassed the pre-printed options for disposition, electing instead to fashion their own contingency plan. In the blank lines provided, B.Z. wrote that in the event the couple should become separated, the embryos should be returned to her for implantation.[98]

In the first of the cryopreservation consent forms, completed in the fall of 1988, both A.Z. and B.Z. were present and signed the forms at the same time.[99] A.Z. watched B.Z. write in the tailored dispositional language granting B.Z. custody over the embryos in the event of separation.[100] A.Z. then signed the form after discussing with his wife the dispositional language and its ramifications.[101] The form was witnessed by a third party who was present as A.Z. and B.Z. each signed the form and orally considered its import.

The six cryopreservation consent forms signed over the course of the next three years were completed in a different fashion. A.Z. signed the form while it was still blank and B.Z. subsequently filled in the dispositional language and signed the form in his absence.[102] Often the form was witnessed much later by a third party who was not present when either A.Z. or B.Z. signed the form.[103] No one from the IVF Clinic explained the cryopreservation consent forms to A.Z.[104] A.Z. never reviewed with anyone the available choices of disposition, storage, destruction, or donation in the event of separation or divorce. Neither A.Z. nor B.Z. consulted with counsel before signing any of the forms.[105]

Following the dicta in *Davis*, the Suffolk County Probate and Family Court reiterated the Tennessee court's mandate that prior agreements regarding the disposition of embryos should be enforced. The courts stated that enforcing the progenitors' advance directives regarding the future treatment of frozen embryos serves several functions. First, it "allows all parties involved . . . to rely on the agreement as a fundamental means for

97. *Id.* at 8.
98. *Id.* at 8-11.
99. *Id.* at 8-9.
100. *Id.* at 9.
101. *Id.*
102. *Id.* at 9-11.
103. *Id.*
104. *Id.*at 11.
105. *Id.*

resolving disputes which may arrive."[106] Second, it provides incentives for parties to think carefully about the decisions facing them.[107] If parties know they will be bound to such agreements, they will, reasoned the court, approach them seriously and attentively. Such thoughtful and careful deliberation will "minimize the cost and frequency of suits surrounding disagreement over the disposition of the preembryos which are sure to occur as IVF procedures become more common."[108] Lastly, the court stated that binding a couple to a prior agreement recognizes their procreational liberty.[109] For all of these reasons, the court concluded that, "[w]here the parties have knowingly contemplated the disposition of the preembryos based upon a contingency which later occurs, the agreement should be enforced."[110]

Applying this general rule to A.Z. and B.Z.'s particular set of agreements, the court indicated that the couple's dispositional agreement contained in the clinic's standardized forms ought to be enforced.[111] Later in its opinion, the court held that changed circumstances not contemplated by the parties at the time of contracting invalidated the agreements.[112] Still, it is worth noting that the court found nothing amiss in the nature of the agreements and the process by which they were reached.

This oversight was rectified, in dicta, by the Massachusetts Supreme Court, though the court affirmed on different grounds. The Massachusetts court is the first judicial body to find the location of a dispositional agreement in fertility consent forms problematic. The court stated that "the consent form's purpose is to explain to the donors the benefits and risks of freezing [and] to provide the clinic with guidance if the donors (as a unit) no

106. *Id.* at 23.

107. The court stated, "parties who know in advance that they will be bound by the agreement will be thoughtful of the decisions they make." *Id.*

108. *Id.*

109. *Id.*

110. *Id.*

111. *Id.* at 22.

112. The couple signed a series of forms containing dispositional agreements between 1988 and 1991. *Id.* at 3. The couple conceived twins in 1992. *Id.* at 2. Several years later, the couple's relationship deteriorated. *Id.* at 3. The wife sought a restraining order against the husband, they separated and the husband filed for divorce. *Id.* at 24. The court held that this combination of circumstances was unforeseeable, stating:

> What this court finds was never contemplated by the couple is that these events would be compounded, that the couple would have twins as a result of the IVF procedure, the wife would file a restraining order against the husband, the husband would file for a divorce and then the wife would seek to thaw the preembryos for implantation in the hopes of having additional children.

Id. at 24-25.

longer wish to use the frozen preembryos."[113] The court expressed doubt that either husband or wife intended the dispositional agreement contained in the form to be enforceable against each other.[114] The form, the court implied, was never intended to serve as a contract between husband and wife.[115] "Rather, it appears that it [the consent form] was intended only to define the donors' relationship as a unit with the clinic."[116]

The court also was troubled by the piecemeal and haphazard method by which the consent forms were signed and witnessed.[117] The court noted that the consent form at issue "was signed in blank by the husband, before the wife filled in the language indicating that she would use the preembryos for implantation on separation."[118] Consequently, the court was unconvinced that the consent form reflected the husband's true intentions regarding embryo disposition.[119]

These procedural critiques, however, were not central to the court's holding.[120] Rather, the court stated that it would not enforce an unambiguous, free-standing dispositional agreement between husband and wife if the agreement were to "compel one donor to become a parent against his or her will."[121] The Massachusetts court's dicta suggests that the court will look skeptically at carelessly signed and witnessed dispositional agreements located in informed consent documents.[122] However, the holding demonstrates that the court will ignore even the most flawlessly constructed contract if the contract requires implantation over one party's objection.[123] Far from encouraging fertility clinics and their clients to improve the process of crafting dispositional agreements, the *A.Z.* case may lead parties to dispense with contracting for fear that the courts will ignore their advance dispositional directives.[124]

The *A.Z.* court's approach has garnered one adherent.[125] But, it is not clear other courts will follow. This author believes that courts should enforce dispositional agreements that are properly conceived and

---

113. A.Z. v B.Z., 725 N.E.2d 1051, 1056 (Mass. 2000).

114. *Id.*

115. *Id.*

116. *Id.*

117. *Id.* at 1057.

118. *Id.*

119. *Id.*

120. *Id.* at 1057-58.

121. *Id.* ("As a matter of public policy, we conclude that forced procreation is not an area amenable to judicial enforcement.").

122. *Id.* at 1057.

123. *Id.* at 1057-58.

124. *See also* J.B v. M.B., 751 A.2d 613, 619 (N.J. Super. Ct. App. Div. 2000).

125. *Id.*

implemented. Dicta in the *Davis* and *Kass* opinions supports this view,[126] as does the majority of scholarly commentary.[127] Assuming other state courts follow *Davis* and *Kass*, one may hope they seriously consider the *A.Z.* court's criticisms in dicta and require dispositional agreements be taken out

126. *See supra* note 8 and accompanying text.

127. The New York State Task Force on Life and the Law, a prestigious body empaneled by executive order to recommend policy on bioethical issues, issued a 1998 report on Assisted Reproductive Technologies that specifically addresses the freezing, storage, and disposition of cryopreserved embryos. THE NEW YORK STATE TASK FORCE ON LIFE AND THE LAW, EXECUTIVE SUMMARY OF ASSISTED REPRODUCTIVE TECHNOLOGIES: ANALYSIS AND RECOMMENDATIONS FOR PUBLIC POLICY 318-19 (1998). The Task Force recommended that legislators enact regulations that would require individuals specify, in advance of the IVF cryopreservation procedure, what should be done with any cryopreserved embryos in the event of death, permanent loss of decision-making capacity, divorce, termination of the facility's storage period, or loss of contact with the storage facility. *Id.* at 319.

The American Society for Reproductive Medicine, an organization encompassing the Society of Reproductive Endocrinologists, the Society of Reproductive Surgeons, the Society for Assisted Reproductive Technology, and the Society for Male Reproduction and Urology, has also issued a report discussing the procurement of informed consent to artificial reproductive technology. The report strongly supports the creation of advance dispositional directives and appears to suggest that such directives should be folded into consent forms primarily devoted to the risks, success rates, and financial burdens of artificial reproduction. ASRM, PRACTICE COMMITTEE REPORT: ELEMENTS TO BE CONSIDERED IN OBTAINING INFORMED CONSENT FOR ART (June 1997).

The vast majority of legal commentary favors the creation and enforcement of pre-existing dispositional contracts as well. *See* Robertson, *Prior Agreements, supra* note 14; John A. Robertson, *In the Beginning: The Legal Status of Early Embryos*, 76 VA. L. REV. 437, 465-469 (1990) (arguing that agreements for disposition of extracorporeal embryos ought to be enforceable by one party against the other); *see also* ROBERTSON, CHILDREN OF CHOICE, *supra* note 39, at 113.

> The practice of freezing embryos will also raise questions about embryo disposition when the couple divorces, dies, is unavailable, is unable to agree, or is in arrears in paying storage charges . . . . [T]he best way to handle these questions is by dispositional agreements made at the time of creation or cryopreservation of embryos.

Id. A Greek Chorus of commentary follows Professor Robertson's lead. *See, e.g.*, Mario J. Trespalacios, *Frozen Embryos: Towards an Equitable Solution*, 46 U. MIAMI L. REV. 803, 826 (1992); Gregory A. Triber, *Growing Pains: Disputes Surrounding Human Reproductive Interests Stretch the Boundaries of Traditional Legal Concepts*, 23 SETON HALL LEGIS. J. 103, 137-40 (1998) (arguing that a contractual approach to dispositional disputes protects donors from misappropriation by storage facilities); Mark C. Haut, Note, *Divorce and the Disposition of Frozen Embryos*, 28 HOFSTRA L. REV. 493, 517-25 (1999) (arguing that dispositional agreements should be enforceable subject to traditional contract defenses); Donna Sheinbach, Comment, *Examining Disputes Over Ownership Rights to Frozen Embryos: Will Prior Consent Documents Survive if Challenged by State Law and/or Constitutional Principles*, 48 CATH. U.L. REV. 989, 1000-02, 1017-27 (1999) (generally supporting the enforcement of dispositional agreements, except where in conflict with state law or constitutional principles); Andrea Michelle Siegeal, Comment, *Legal Resolution to the Frozen Embryo Dilemma*, 4 J. PHARMACY & L. 43, 60 (1995). *But see* George J. Annas, *The Shadowlands—Secrets, Lies, and Assisted Reproduction* 339:13 NEW ENG. J. MED. 935, 936-37 (1998); Coleman, *supra* note 13, at 95, 97-104; Daar, *supra* note 13; Moskowitz, *supra* note 13; William A. Sieck, Comment, *In Vitro Fertilization and the Right to Procreate: The Right to No*, 147 U. PA. L. REV. 435, 464-75 (1998).

of fertility clinic consent documents and subjected to rigorous procedural scrutiny. The following Parts demonstrate why.

IV. The Problem With Reading Informed Consent Forms Signed by an Infertile Couple To Obtain Treatment as Valid Dispositional Contracts

As noted, courts and most scholarly authorities would transform documents designed to record the transmission of medical information from clinic to couple, and the couple's acceptance of medical treatment, into a binding agreement between the couple itself. This approach is problematic because, despite their aspirational title, informed consent forms often reflect accessions to recommended treatment that are neither deliberate, thoughtful, nor informed.[128] Numerous commentators have suggested that reading informed consent forms as contracts between patient and provider is speculative because it requires reading the patient's signature as a manifestation of informed, deliberate choice.[129] This interpretation, they contend, is fanciful, because informed consent remains a fairytale: a pretty story largely accepted by the courts but belied by the clinical reality.[130] If it is tenuous to read informed consent forms as a valid contract between patient and provider, it is infinitely more implausible to read such forms as constituting a contract between patients jointly seeking medical care.

A. *Limitations Inherent in Informed Consent Forms*

Informed consent forms are a by-product of the effort to enhance patient autonomy in the doctor-patient relationship.[131] In the last forty years,

128. CARL E. SCHNEIDER, THE PRACTICE OF AUTONOMY 9 (1998).

129. *See infra* notes 137-49 and accompanying text.

130. Jay Katz, *Informed Consent—Must It Remain a Fairy Tale?*, 10 J. CONTEMP. L. & POL'Y 69, 91 (1993).

131. Judith F. Daar, *Informed Consent: Defining Limits Through Therapeutic Parameters*, 16 WHITTIER L. REV. 187, 188 (1995).

> The evolution of the physician's duty to disclose over this past century reflects the characterization of the physician-patient relationship as one that has evolved from being perceived as rightly paternalistic to one in which pleas for patient autonomy have helped shape disclosure requirements which, at least theoretically, promote informed decision-making.

Id.; *see also* Stephen H. Behnke & Elyn Saks, *Therapeutic Jurisprudence: Informed Consent as a Clinical Indication for the Chronically Suicidal Patient with Borderline Personality Disorder*, 31 medical ethicists, lawyers, philosophers, and some physicians have joined forces to shift the balance of power between doctors and their patients.[132] To this end, they have successfully lobbied for laws and ethical guidelines that constrain physician paternalism and encourage patient self-determination.[133] The jurisprudence of informed consent stands at the center of this movement.

The goal of informed consent is to enable patients to determine the course of their own care.[134] This can only occur when patients are provided sufficient information to evaluate knowledgeably available medical choices.[135] Physicians who fail to disclose material risks associated with recommended treatment may be found negligent if the undisclosed risk occurs and the patient suffers injury.[136]

Legal requirements, however, do not always translate into clinical successes.[137] Many physicians avoid having the conversations about medical risk and uncertainty that informed consent doctrine contemplates.[138] Some

---

LOY. L.A. L. REV. 945, 958 (1998) ("From an ethical perspective, informed consent underscores the value of individual autonomy, a value that both flows out of and protects human dignity.").

132. *See generally* TOM L. BEAUCHAMP & JAMES F. CHILDRESS, PRINCIPLES OF BIOMEDICAL ETHICS 142 (4th ed. 1994); DAVID J. ROTHMAN, STRANGERS AT THE BEDSIDE: A HISTORY OF HOW LAW AND BIOETHICS TRANSFORMED MEDICAL DECISION MAKING (1991); Susan M. Wolf, *Toward a Systemic Theory of Informed Consent in Managed Care*, 35 HOUS. L. REV. 1631, 1640 (1999) ("Informed consent aspiration and doctrine are the product of both bioethics and law.").

133. One example of this effort is the Patient Self Determination Act, passed in 1991. 42 U.S.C. 1395cc (1994). This statute requires health care providers to inform patients of their rights, under state law, to complete advance directives and include them as a part of their medical record.

134. Schloendorff v. Soc'y of New York Hosp., 105 N.E. 92, 93 (N.Y. 1914) ("Every human being of adult years and sound mind has a right to determine what shall be done with his own body . . . ."); *see also* Fosmire v. Nicoleau, 75 N.Y.2d 218, 226 (1990).

135. Scott v. Bradford, 606 P.2d 554, 557 (Okla. 1979) ("True consent to what happens to one's self is the informed exercise of a choice. This entails an opportunity to evaluate knowledgeably the options available and the risks attendant upon each.").

136. Canterbury v. Spence, 464 F.2d 772, 790 (D.C. Cir.1972); ARNOLD J. ROSOFF, INFORMED CONSENT: A GUIDE FOR HEALTH CARE PROVIDERS 33-63 (1981).

137. Elizabeth B. Cooper, *Testing for Genetic Traits: The Need for New Legal Doctrine of Informed Consent*, 58 MD. L. REV. 346, 381 (1999) ("Current informed consent doctrine has been criticized as inadequate to protect the needs, and the rights, of most patients."); *see also* Clarence H. Braddock III et al., *Informed Decision Making in Outpatient Practice*, 282 JAMA 2313, 2317 (1999) (analyzing 1,057 audiotaped informed consent discussions, few of which meet the criteria for completeness envisioned by legal or ethical theory); Joan H. Krause, *Reconceptualizing Informed Consent in an Era of Health Care Cost Containment*, 85 IOWA L. REV. 261, 275-78, 305-07 (1999) (summarizing critiques of informed consent practice and concluding that "there is a significant gap between theoretical pronouncements regarding informed consent and the way the doctrine functions in practice").

138. Edmund L. Erde, *Informed Consent to Septoplasty: An Anecdote from the Field*, 24 J. MED. & PHIL. 11, 12-13 (1999) (relating patient's experience of surgical correction for a deviated septum in which consent was procured solely through the "shadow of an anemic consent form," with no offer of further explanation).

physicians avoid these conversations because they find them awkward and personally uncomfortable.[139] Others avoid them because they do not believe that any amount of dialogue can enable patients to make truly informed medical decisions.[140] Others avoid in-depth discussion of medical options because they intrude on appointments and procedures that can be billed out at a higher rate.[141] In order to satisfy the legal requirement to obtain "informed" consent, most hospitals and clinicians rely on pre-printed forms that contain a description of the treatment being offered and the associated risks.[142] The patient's signature on the forms serves as an acknowledgment that the patient has read the information detailing the medical disasters that might occur, and agrees to proceed with treatment. What was intended as a process of dialogue and discussion has devolved into an event in which papers are signed and minimal legal requirements are satisfied.[143]

---

139. Katz, *supra* note 130, at 81-82 (arguing that physician discomfort with medical uncertainty remains a barrier to the effective implementation of informed consent principles); *see also* Arthur Caplan, *Can We Talk? A Review of Jay Katz, The Silent World of Doctor and Patient*, 9 W. NEW ENG. L. REV. 43, 48 (1987) (suggesting that students who select medicine as a career may have less aptitude and interest in the communication skills necessary for effective physician-patient dialogue).

140. Cathy J. Jones, *Autonomy and Informed Consent in Medical Decisionmaking: Toward a New Self-Fulfilling Prophecy*, 47 WASH. & LEE L. REV. 379, 406-07 (1990) (reporting that physicians are skeptical about the benefits of informed consent because they believe "patients neither understand nor remember what they are told, in large part because the information to be conveyed is too technical for patients to grasp and is knowable and understandable only by physicians after years of schooling and training"); Jay Katz, *Physician-Patient Encounters "On a Darkling Plain,"* 9 W. NEW ENG. L. REV. 207, 211 (1987); *see generally* Jon F. Merz & Baruch Fischhoff, *Informed Consent Does Not Mean Rational Consent: Cognitive Limitations on Decision-Making*, 11 J. Legal Med. 321 (1990).

141. Jones, *supra* note 140, at 407 (reporting physician objections to testing patients' understanding of what they have been told because to do so is "too time consuming and too expensive in terms of the physician's additional duties to this patient and others").

142. Alan Meisel & Mark Kuczewski, *Legal and Ethical Myths About Informed Consent*, 156 ARCHIVES OF INTERNAL MEDICINE 2521, 2522 (1996) ("Consent forms are used as a matter of routine in both treatment and research settings because many hospital administrators, physicians, and their attorneys see these forms as providing protection against liability, despite the fact that they actually provide little protection."); *see also* IRENE S. SWITANKOWSKY, A NEW PARADIGM FOR INFORMED CONSENT 2 (1998) Switankowsky argues that:

> [M]inimalist disclosure that is implicit in the framework of the harm avoidance paradigm of informed consent is insufficient for preserving a patient's autonomy and cannot ensure the patient's decision is autonomous. Consent to treatment is considered to be a mere legal formality of signing a consent form. This formality does not honor and respect a patient's individual and personal autonomy, which is the ultimate purpose of obtaining an informed consent.

Id.

143. *See* Rebecca D. Pentz, *The Vagaries of Informed Consent: Experiences in Oncologic Care*, 9 CLINICAL ETHICS REP. 1, 5 (1995) ("[I]nformed consent's birth in the legal realm has damaged its image among some physicians. They see it as a burden imposed by the courts that is to

Physician use of consent forms to accomplish the information flow required by informed consent doctrine creates a documentary record of patient intention that overstates the patient's exercise of conscious will.[144] The problem resides both in the content of the forms and the way they are presented to patients. Consent forms tend to be long and dense, despite the fact that patient understanding is inversely related to form prolixity.[145] Written in complex language dappled with technical description, form vocabulary and structure often confound patient comprehension.[146] The manner in which forms are presented similarly affects the quality of the consent achieved. Because many physicians perceive consent forms to be a "medical Miranda" requirement,[147] they present informed consent topics to patients as if procuring patient signatures, rather than provoking thoughtful deliberation and dialogue, is the true purpose of the exercise. Patients, like doctors, come to see the forms as simply a bureaucratic hurdle to be jumped

---

be met in letter and not in spirit."); *see also* Stephen Wear, *Enhancing Clinician Provision of Informed Consent and Counseling: Some Pedagogical Strategies*, 24 J. MED. & PHIL. 34, 37 (1999) (attributing physician deficiencies in discussing medical risks and benefits to "the common clinician perspective of informed consent as a legal entity").

144. Peter H. Schuck, *Rethinking Informed Consent*, 103 YALE L.J. 899, 933 (1994). In discussing informed consent, Schuck states:

> Regardless of the formal doctrinal requirements, the usefulness of informed consent depends on a meaningful dialogue between physician and patient. Yet the minimally necessary ingredients of such a dialogue—questions by the patient, full and discursive responses by the physician that invite the patient to ask follow-up questions—are usually absent in most clinical situations.

Id.; *see also* Charles S. White et al., *Informed Consent for Percutaneous Lung Biopsy: Comparison of Two Consent Protocols Based on Patient Recall After the Procedure*, 165 AM. J. RADIOLOGY 1139, 1140-41 (1995) (reporting that when a standard informed consent protocol is used, patient recall of procedure risks and complications is poor).

145. PAUL S. APPELBAUM ET AL., INFORMED CONSENT: LEGAL THEORY AND CLINICAL PRACTICE 182 (1987) (footnote omitted); *see also* Jones, *supra* note 140, at 410 n.106.

146. APPELBAUM, *supra* note 145, at 183-85; *see also* Kenneth D. Hopper et al., *The Readability of Currently Used Surgical/Procedure Consent Forms in the United States*, 123 SURGERY 496, 498-99 (1998) (presenting data that only 3 to 20% of adults can understand most informed consent forms).

147. Meisel & Kuczewski, *supra* note 142, at 2522. Meisel & Kuczewski compare consent forms to warnings:

> As practiced, and certainly as symbolized by consent forms, informed consent is often no more than a medical Miranda warning. Just as police are required to tell criminal suspects that "you have a right to remain silent, you have a right to a lawyer, and if you choose to speak, anything you say can be used against you," some physicians believe that informed consent has been obtained if they warn patients of the risks of treatment.

Id.; Larry R. Churchill et al., *Genetic Research as Therapy: Implications of "Gene Therapy" for Informed Consent*, 26 J.L. MED. & ETHICS 38, 42 (1998) (discussing routinization of informed consent, in which "consent for routine patient care is seen as a legal encumbrance, introduced with words such as, '[w]e have to consent you now'").

before the real work of medicine can begin.[148] This is especially true when the patient is handed the form right before the surgery or other proposed treatment is about to begin.[149] In these situations, the consent form serves merely to protect the doctor from exposure to a medical malpractice suit; it does not facilitate informed, deliberate, and voluntary patient choice.

B. Limitations on Informed Consent in the Fertility Treatment Context

Securing meaningful informed consent is particularly challenging when patient emotions run high. When individuals experience strong feelings, their tendency to engage in selective perception increases.[150] Selective perception is a cognitive response to "information overload," in which individuals selectively construct evidence that confirms their existing beliefs and desires.[151] Selective perception leads individuals to emphasize information that supports preconceived hypotheses while filtering out or selectively reinterpreting dissonant data.[152] Patients beset by strong hopes and anxieties have difficulty absorbing medical information and rationally

148. APPELBAUM, *supra* note 145, at 185-86; Jones, *supra* note 140, at 400-02. Jones describes the presentation of consent forms in ways that discourage informed decision-making.

> Although the information set forth on the consent forms may in fact have disclosed the alternatives available to the patients and the material risks inherent in those alternatives, the nature of the presentations—in one case a written form presented immediately prior to the procedure and in the other a written form accompanied by a nonspecific, rather off the cuff discussion with a physician—were not designed to enhance or test the patients' understanding of the material presented.

Id.

149. Jones, *supra* note 140, at 400-01; *see also* Cooper, *supra* note 137, at 385.

> [I]t is not unusual for health care providers, or their assistants, to seek a patient's written consent immediately prior to the performance of a procedure, when a patient is not in the physical or emotional condition to consider rationally whether consenting to the proposed procedure is advisable. Although the patient is likely to sign the form, one must question the nature and quality of her consent.

Id. (footnotes omitted).

150. JEFFREY Z. RUBIN ET AL., SOCIAL CONFLICT: ESCALATION, STALEMATE AND SETTLEMENT 103-04 (2d ed. 1994).

151. *Id.* at 102-05.

152. For example, people interpret an actor's behavior very differently depending upon their pre-existing assessment of the actor's motivation and character. *See* Stuart Oskamp, *Attitudes Toward U.S. and Russian Actions: A Double Standard,* 16 PSYCHOL. REP. 43, 43-46 (1965) (discussing how American college students interpreted Russian military maneuvers as belligerent, while interpreting the same behavior by the United States as conciliatory); *see also* MUZAFER SHERIF & CAROLYN W. SHERIF, GROUPS IN HARMONY AND TENSION 289 (1953) (noting that stereotypes persist in the face of contrary evidence—cases that challenge the prevailing stereotype are disregarded as aberrational).

evaluating the risks and benefits of various treatment options. This poses particular difficulties in the realm of assisted reproduction, where infertility generates strong emotional currents.[153]

Infertile couples describe the experience of infertility and its treatment as a profoundly disorienting and wrenching one.[154] As many as 49% of women interviewed in one study characterized infertility as "the most upsetting experience in their lives."[155] Couples struggling with infertility report high rates of depression, loss of self-esteem, stress, and anger.[156] Common complaints include feelings of loss of control, feelings of defectiveness, stress on marital and sexual relations, feelings of alienation from the "fertile world," and social stigma.[157] As Professor Judith Daar has noted, infertility patients present "a unique, dichotomous psychological profile . . . ."[158] Hungry for information, these patients are well-educated regarding the mechanics of reproduction, their condition, and the newest technological innovations designed to supplement and support natural conception. Possession of a high level of technical information, however, does not necessarily yield an appreciation of the low likelihood of success promised by these innovations. The power of wishful thinking obscures rational deliberation. Infertile women will often opt for any treatment option presented, regardless of the physical, psychological, or financial price.[159]

---

153. *See* Linda D. Applegarth, *Emotional Implications*, *in* 2 REPRODUCTIVE ENDOCRINOLOGY, SURGERY AND TECHNOLOGY 1954, 1954-62 (Eli Y. Adashi et al. eds., 1996) (describing the extreme emotional response engendered by infertility).

154. Melvin L. Taymor & Ellen Bresnick, *Infertility Counseling*, *in* INFERTILITY: A CLINICIAN'S GUIDE TO DIAGNOSIS AND TREATMENT 105, 105-08 (1990).

155. Ellen W. Freeman et al., *Psychological Evaluation and Support in a Program of In Vitro Fertilization and Embryo Transfer*, 43 FERTILITY & STERILITY 48, 50 (1985); *see also* BETH COOPER-HILBERT, INFERTILITY AND INVOLUNTARY CHILDLESSNESS 32 (1998) (Infertile couples "feel at odds with society, betrayed by nature, their bodies, and each other"); *see, e.g.*, Applegarth, *supra* note 153, at 1954-55 (describing infertility as a life crisis notable in its depth, chronicity and pervasiveness).

156. Patricia P. Mahlstedt, *The Psychological Component of Infertility*, 43 FERTILITY & STERILITY 335, 335-41 (1985); *see also* COOPER-HILBERT, *supra* note 155, at 39-46 (listing shock and disbelief, denial, anxiety, anger, loss of control, isolation and alienation, guilt, depression and grief as the emotional stages of the infertility cycle).

157. Arthur L. Greil, *Infertility and Psychological Distress: A Critical Review of the Literature*, 45 SOC. SCI. & MED. 1679, 1682 (1997); *see also* COOPER-HILBERT, *supra* note 155, at 47 (describing negative effects of infertility on couples' sexual relations, as well as individual feelings of inadequacy); *see also* DEBBY PEOPLES & HARRIETTE ROVNER FERGUSON, WHAT TO EXPECT WHEN YOU'RE EXPERIENCING INFERTILITY 106-07 (1998) (listing typical reactions to loss).

158. Judith F. Daar, *Regulating Reproductive Technologies: Panacea or Paper Tiger?*, 34 HOUS. L. REV. 609, 629 (1997) [hereinafter Daar, *Regulating Reproductive Technologies*].

159. Judith Daniluk, *Helping Patients Cope with Infertility*, 40 CLINICAL OBSTETRICS & GYNECOLOGY 663, 665 (1997) ("If a viable treatment option is available, the infertile woman often

This is true even where the chances for success are distinctly remote.[160] As Professor Daar observes with great understatement, "[t]he world of fertility medicine . . . presents unique challenges to the smooth operation of the doctrine of informed consent . . . ."[161] Put more strongly, one might argue that the effort to promote informed and considered medical decision-making is seriously hindered by the emotional vortex in which reproductive medicine occurs.

To the degree that consent forms document the risks associated with proposed treatment, they are certain to contain anxiety-producing information a patient might be inclined to resist or ignore. Consent forms for in vitro fertilization discuss potential maternal injuries.[162] Hazards discussed include hyperstimulation syndrome, fertility medication side effects, bleeding, infection or injury to abdominal organs from ultrasound needle aspiration, and multiple births.[163] Consent forms also discuss the paucity of data regarding risks to offspring.[164] Consent forms for cryopreservation raise the possibility that some or all embryos may not survive freezing and thawing. The forms explain that the risks of freezing, thawing and transfer are not well established, and that the failure of storage containers can result in the loss of liquid nitrogen and the destruction of the embryos inside.[165] Patients often resist thoughtfully considering these possibilities and must be pressed to seriously evaluate the medical risks that artificial reproductive technology entails.[166]

Adding informed consent provisions to the same form which asks couples to determine what should be done with the embryos if they die, become disabled, or choose to divorce, adds yet another layer of information that is

is very willing to submit to any type of medical intervention in the hopes of producing a child, irrespective of how invasive the treatment or how remote the possibility of success."); *see also* Brenda S. Houmard & David B. Seifer, *Infertility Treatment and Informed Consent: Current Practices of Reproductive Endocrinologists*, 93 CLINICAL OBSTETRICS & GYNECOLOGY 252, 256 (1999) (noting that women receiving fertility treatment "are willing to accept a two- to ten-fold increase in their lifetime risk of ovarian cancer," while failing to appreciate ovarian cancer's dismal morbidity rates).

160. Houmard & Seifer, *supra* note 159, at 256.

161. Daar, *Regulating Reproductive Technologies*, *supra* note 158, at 628.

162. Mark Perloe, M.D., Assisted Reproduction Health Center, *In Vitro Fertilization Permit (IVF-ET)*, *at* http://www.ivf.com/ivfpr.html (last visited Nov. 27, 1999).

163. *Id.*

164. *Id.*

165. Mark Perloe, M.D., Assisted Reproduction Health Center, *Informed Consent* (Cryopreservation of Embryos), http://www.ivf.com/cryoperm.html (last visited Oct. 11, 1999).

166. Interview with Dr. Seth E. Katz, Assistant Professor of Reproductive Endocrinology and Infertility, University of California, San Diego School of Medicine (Jan. 14, 2000) (stating that fertility patients' desire to become pregnant leads them to disregard or devalue the risks attendant to ART procedures).

difficult to process and thoughtfully evaluate. In the best of circumstances, individuals do not like to consider their own mortality.[167] It is similarly unsurprising that couples, on what they fervently hope will be the cusp of parenthood, would be disinclined to contemplate seriously what should be done in the event they lose capacity or divorce before having a child.[168] Inserting dispositional agreements into documents already brimming with emotionally forbidding information will likely lead to psychological overload, and a glossing over the import of the information being conveyed.

If dispositional agreements are to represent truly the will of each gamete provider, it would seem important to devise contracting procedures that enhance, rather than defeat, the couple's ability to focus and deliberate upon the available options. The emotional stresses under which fertility patients labor require that the couple's consideration of the risks of in vitro fertilization and cryopreservation be separate from the process of choosing what should be done with the embryos if the couple dies, becomes disabled, or divorces. The signing of consent documents and the creation of dispositional agreements treat different subjects, implicate different concerns, and deserve separate contracting procedures. Further, couples should be provided counseling as they make dispositional choices.[169] These procedural reforms not only make sense from a psychological standpoint; they also rescue the dispositional agreements from charges of unconscionability.

---

167. If the underwhelming lay response to the promotion of living wills has proven anything, it is that people avoid conducting thought experiments regarding their own death and disability. Greg A. Sachs et al., *Empowerment of the Older Patient? A Randomized, Controlled Trial to Increase Discussion and Use of Advance Directives*, 40 J. AM. GERIATRICS SOC'Y, 269, 269-73 (1992); *see also* Linda L. Emanuel & Ezekiel J. Emanuel, *Decisions at the End of Life: Guided by Communities of Patients*, HASTINGS CENTER REP., Sept.-Oct. 1993 at 6-14; Nicole Lurie et al., *Attitudes Toward Discussing Life-Sustaining Treatments in Extended Care Facility Patients*, 40 J. AM. GERIATRICS SOC'Y, 1205, 1205-08 (1992).

168. Sieck, *supra* note 127, at 466 n.179 and accompanying text (discussing data that suggests couples on the eve of marriage greatly underestimate the likelihood of divorce and suggesting IVF participants suffer from similar cognitive distortions); *see also Consistently Inconsistent*, THE ECONOMIST, Aug. 7, 1999, at 66 (noting that many individuals irrationally discount future harms in quest of immediate gratification); *Rethinking Thinking*, THE ECONOMIST, Dec. 18, 1999, at 63, 64 (explaining that, according to prospect theory, people regularly miscalculate probabilities. One common miscalculation discounts the probability of outcomes that are, in fact, quite likely to occur.).

169. *See* Andrea Mechanick Braverman et al., *Characteristics and Attitudes of Parents of Children Born with the Use of Assisted Reproductive Technology*, 70 FERTILITY & STERILITY 860, 863 (1998) (surveying parents who successfully bore children through ART techniques and reporting that 16.2% of those surveyed stated that if they were to procure fertility treatment again in the future they would like to see counselors provide greater emotional support).

V. LINKING CONSENT FORMS AND DISPOSITIONAL AGREEMENTS—AN UNCONSCIONABLE CONTRACT

Dispositional agreements that are encrypted in informed consent documents smack of unconscionability. Unconscionability, a defense that allows for the voiding of contractual duties, is said to have two components: procedural and substantive.[170] The hallmark of procedural unconscionability, "bargaining naughtiness,"[171] is a defect in the bargaining process that suggests that one party to the contract did not exercise meaningful choice.[172] Indices of procedural unconscionability include the use of standardized forms, presentation of the form as a take it or leave it proposition, and form language that is incomprehensible to a layperson with key contractual provisions hidden in fine print.[173] Substantive unconscionability looks to the actual terms of the contract and whether the obligations are unreasonably favorable to one of the parties, such that it manifests an outrageous degree of

---

170. Arthur Allen Leff, *Unconscionability and the Code—The Emperor's New Clause*, 115 U. PA. L. REV. 485, 487 (1967).

171. *Id.*

172. *See, e.g.*, Denise E. Lascarides, *A Plea for the Enforceability of Gestational Surrogacy Contracts*, 25 HOFSTRA L. REV. 1221, 1256 (1997) ("Procedural unconscionability focuses on the procedure of the agreement and whether there existed an absence of meaningful choice.") (footnote omitted); *see also* Kinney v. United Healthcare Servs., 70 Cal. App. 4th 1322, 1329 (Ct. App. 1999).

> "Procedural unconscionability" concerns the manner in which the contract was negotiated and the circumstances of the parties at that time. It focuses on factors of oppression and surprise. The oppression component arises from an inequality of bargaining power of the parties to the contract and an absence of real negotiation or a meaningful choice on the part of the weaker party.

Id.; Gillman v. Chase Manhattan Bank, 534 N.E.2d 824, 828 (N.Y. 1988).

173. Resource Mgmt. Co. v. Weston Ranch, 706 P.2d 1028, 1042 (Utah 1985) (citations omitted). This case lists the hallmarks of procedural unconscionability as

> [t]he use of printed form or boilerplate contracts drawn skillfully by the party in the strongest economic position," generally offered on a take-it-or-leave-it basis, phrasing contractual terms "in language that is incomprehensible to a layman or that divert[s] his attention from the problems raised by them or the rights given up through them," hiding key contractual provisions in a maze of fine print or in an inconspicuous part of the document . . . .

Id. (citations omitted); *see also* Lagatree v. Luce, Forward, Hamilton & Scripps, 88 Cal. Rptr. 2d 664, 679 (Ct. App. 1999) ("The procedural element focuses on the unequal bargaining positions and hidden terms common in the context of adhesion contracts . . . ."); *Gillman*, 534 N.E.2d at 828.

> The focus [of a procedural unconscionability inquiry] is on such matters as the size and commercial setting of the transaction . . . whether deceptive or high-pressured tactics were employed, the use of fine print in the contract, the experience and education of the party claiming unconscionability, and whether there was disparity in bargaining power.

Id. (citations omitted).

unfairness.[174] In the Victorian prose of one recent court, a substantively unconscionable contract contains terms that "shock the conscience."[175]

Courts are split as to whether substantive or procedural unconscionability alone can void a contract. While some jurisdictions will void a contract based solely on substantive unfairness,[176] many others require a showing of both substantive and procedural unconscionability.[177] Commentators and courts have suggested that, in practice, the two elements of unconscionability are measured according to a sliding scale.[178] A grotesquely one-sided contract might be voided with only a slight showing of procedural defectiveness. Conversely, clear defects in the bargaining process might be sufficient to nullify a contract whose terms, though problematic, cannot be said to "shock the conscience."

The dispositional agreements at issue in disputed embryo cases might best be described as substantively problematic and procedurally defective. While their terms are not so one-sided or oppressive as to "shock the

174. "Substantive unconscionability requires proving that the terms of the contract are unreasonable and unfair." Garrett v. Janiewski, 480 So. 2d 1324, 1326 (Fla. Dist. Ct. App. 1985) (citations omitted); *see also* Maxwell v. Fidelity Fin. Servs., Inc., 907 P.2d 51, 58 (Ariz. 1995) ("Indicative of substantive unconsionability are contract terms so one-sided as to oppress or unfairly surprise an innocent party, an overall imbalance in the obligations and rights imposed by the bargain . . . ."); Martin Rispens & Son v. Hall Farms, Inc., 621 N.E.2d 1078, 1087 (Ind. 1993) ("A substantively unconscionable contract is one that no sensible man would make and such as no honest and fair man would accept.") (citation omitted).

175. *Lagatree*, 88 Cal. Rptr. 2d at 679 (quoting 24 Hour Fitness, Inc. v. Superior Court, 78 Cal. Rptr. 2d 533 (Ct. App. 1998)).

176. *See Maxwell*, 907 P.2d at 58 (concluding that a claim of unconscionability can be established with a showing of substantive unconscionability alone); *see also* Sosa v. Paulos, 924 P.2d 357, 361 (Utah 1996) ("Gross disparity in terms, absent evidence of procedural unconscionability, can support a finding of unconscionability.") (citations omitted).

177. Edward A. Dauer, *AAA Waives the Rules and Consumer Arbitration May Never Be the Same*, 9 WORLD ARB. & MEDIATION REP. 222, 223 (1998) (arguing that "a contract may be avoided only if there has been *both* a procedural defect . . . *and* substantive unfairness in the contract's terms"); *see also Maxwell*, 907 P.2d at 58 ("Many courts, perhaps a majority, have held that there must be some quantum of both procedural and substantive unconscionability to establish a claim, and take a balancing approach in applying them.") (citation omitted); *Gillman*, 534 N.E.2d at 828 ("A determination of unconscionability generally requires a showing that the contract was both procedurally and substantively unconscionable when made . . . ."); Harry G. Prince, *Unconscionability in California; A Need for Restraint and Consistency*, 46 HASTINGS L.J. 459, 472 (1995) ("Most successful claims involve a combination of procedural and substantive unconscionability, but it is debatable whether both elements must be present.") (footnotes omitted).

178. Prince, *supra* note 177, at 472-73 ("Some courts have also indicated that a sliding scale applies: for example, a contract with extraordinarily oppressive substantive terms will require less in the way of procedural unconscionability.") (footnote omitted); *see also Lagatree*, 88 Cal. Rptr. 2d at 679 n.16 (stating that "there is a 'sliding scale relationship between the two concepts: the greater the degree of substantive unconscionability, the less the degree of procedural unconscionability that is required to annul the contract or clause . . . .'") (citations omitted); *Sosa*, 924 P.2d at 361 n.1.

conscience,"[179] they are significantly more constraining for the women who enter into them than for the men. The agreements' asymmetry lies in their prohibition of post-divorce implantation of the embryos. An agreement to discard or donate frozen embryos upon divorce will not significantly affect the parenting opportunities of individuals, generally men, able to produce gametes and parent children in other relationships. The same agreement, however, will be an irrevocable bar to genetic parenthood for individuals, generally women, no longer able to produce additional gametes.

In most instances, the disadvantaged individual is a woman who, having entered into fertility treatment in her reproductive prime, finds herself divorced in the twilight of her reproductive years. While men are capable of producing sperm, and thus able to contribute to additional embryos well into their seventies, a woman's ability to produce viable eggs diminishes precipitously after age thirty-five and virtually vanishes after age forty-five.[180] If, as in the *Kass* case, the divorce occurs several years following the cryopreservation procedure, the divorcing wife may no longer be able to generate viable eggs for fertilization. Thus, the cryopreserved embryos represent her last opportunity to parent a genetically related child.

In these instances, dispositional agreements that preclude the unilateral use of embryos in the event of divorce are substantively skewed against the woman. Such a contract should survive review under unconscionability principles only if generated pursuant to an open and fair process.

---

179. In my view, a dispositional agreement that precludes a spouse from parenting post-divorce (by dictating that frozen embryos, upon divorce, be either discarded or donated to other couples) is not, in and of itself, so oppressive that it should be voided on substantive unconscionability grounds alone. To void these agreements on the basis of their terms alone would preclude women from entering into these types of bargains under any circumstances, a position that is too restrictive of women's contracting rights. Other commentators, however, have reached different conclusions. *See* Annas, *supra* note 127; Moskowitz, *supra* note 13. Although these analysts do not explicitly maintain that dispositional agreements are unconscionable, their arguments are grounded in the same concerns that animate unconscionability doctrine. *See* Coleman, *supra* note 13, at 95, 97-104 (arguing that dispositional agreements should not be enforced because: 1) they waive important rights in situations where such waivers cannot be "knowing" or "intelligent;" 2) their inclusion in take-it-or-leave-it adhesion contracts makes them inherently coercive).

180. "A woman's age is the most important factor affecting the chances of a live birth when her own eggs are used." 1997 ART SUCCESS RATES, *supra* note 16, at 20.

> As women get older, cycles that have progressed to pregnancy are less likely to result in a live birth. Cumulatively, live births occurred in 31% of cycles started in 1997 among women younger than 35, 26% among women aged 35-37, 17% among women aged 38-40, and 8% among women older than 40.

Id. at 21; *see also* American Society for Reproductive Medicine, *Patient's Fact Sheet: Prediction of Fertility Potential in Older Female Patients* (August, 1996) ("Approximately one-third of couples in which the female partner is age 35 or older will have problems with fertility. It is estimated that two-thirds of women will not be able to get pregnant spontaneously by the age of 40."), *at* http://www.asrm.org/Patients/FactSheets/Older-Female-Fact.pdf.

The process currently used to generate dispositional agreements does not pass muster under this standard. Dispositional agreements, like the consent forms in which they lie buried, are primarily contracts between the fertility clinic and the husband and wife as a marital unit. Viewed as an enforceable contract between husband and wife, the agreements are procedurally deficient in at least three ways: 1) they are drafted by the fertility clinic which frequently offers a constricted set of dispositional options and presents those options to the couple on a take-it-leave-it; 2) they are embedded in forms that treat entirely different subject matter; and 3) their language is both intellectually and emotionally hard to assimilate.

Taking each objection in turn, the first procedural problem is connected to the substantive problems discussed above. As noted, when fertility clinics draft these agreements they frequently do not offer options that would allow either husband or wife to unilaterally claim the embryos for post-divorce use.[181] A woman's choice to erect a barrier to her own use of the embryos post-divorce is untroubling if it indeed represents a choice. However, if the only options presented are donation or destruction of the embryos upon divorce, her selection of one of these options does not necessarily reflect her true preferences. This is especially true where the terms of the agreement are presented on a take it or leave it basis. Unfortunately, in at least two of the disputed embryo cases that have reached the courts, *Wendel v. Wendel*[182] and *Kass v. Kass*,[183] destruction or donation of the embryos were the only post-divorce possibilities offered in the agreements, with no possibility provided for negotiation or modification of terms.[184]

A second procedural deficiency arises from enfolding the dispositional agreements in medical consent forms that treat entirely different subject matter. Parties are bound to terms in a standardized form only if they could reasonably expect such terms to be part of the form.[185] Two factors

181. Robertson, *Prior Agreements*, *supra* note 14, at 412 n.19 (citing Cleveland Clinic Foundation, "Embryo Freezing Agreement" (Jan. 25, 1988)); Attorney John V. Heutsche who represented Mrs. Wendel, stated that his client was not afforded the opportunity to modify or amend the dispositional agreement presented to her. Interview with John V. Heutsche, *supra* note 47; *see* J.B. v. M.B., 751 A.2d 613 (N.J. Super. Ct. App. Div. 2000); *see Kass* Informed Consent Form No. 2, *supra* note 72.

182. 696 N.E.2d 174 (N.Y. 1998)

183. No. D 191962 (Ohio C.P. Dom. Rel. Ct. filed July 21, 1989).

184. Robertson, *Prior Agreements*, *supra* note 14, at 412 n.19; *Kass*, Informed Consent Form No. 2, *supra* note 72.

185. *See, e.g.*, RESTATEMENT (SECOND) OF CONTRACTS § 211 (1981):

> 1) Except as stated in Subsection (3), where a party to an agreement signs or otherwise manifests assent to a writing and has reason to believe that like writings are regularly used to embody terms of agreements of the same type ,

important in determining whether a reasonable person would expect the inclusion of a particular term are: 1) the relationship of the term to the subject matter of the transaction, and 2) whether the term eliminates the dominant purpose of the transaction.[186]

It is clear that medical consent forms and dispositional agreements treat different subject matter. An informed consent form to IVF and cryopreservation details the risks associated with the medical treatment the patient is about to undergo. It is focused entirely on the here and now. A dispositional agreement treats matters hypothetical. It asks couples to consider hypothetical scenarios that, at first blush, must appear unlikely to the point of absurdity. The disparity between the temporal focus of medical consent forms and dispositional agreements is dizzying. Their subject matter is entirely distinct.

A dispositional agreement that precludes post-divorce parenting can also be said to thwart the dominant purpose of the medical consent form. The primary purpose of the consent form, from the patient's perspective, is to facilitate the creation of a baby. A dispositional agreement that mandates discard or destruction of the embryos upon divorce eliminates this possibility for both members of the couple.[187] While it has been argued that patients' primary purpose in seeking fertility treatment is to create a child solely

---

> he adopts the writing as an integrated agreement with respect to the terms included in the writing.
>
> (2) Such a writing is interpreted wherever reasonable as treating alike all those similarly situated, without regard to their knowledge or understanding of the standard terms of the writing.
>
> (3) Where the other party has reason to believe that the party manifesting such assent would not do so if he knew that the writing contained a particular term, the term is not part of the agreement.

Id.

186. A reasonable person would not expect a term to be included in a standardized form if the term is bizarre, oppressive, or eliminates the dominant purpose of the transaction. RESTATEMENT (SECOND) OF CONTRACTS § 211 cmt. f; *see also* E. ALLAN FARNSWORTH, 1 FARNSWORTH ON CONTRACTS § 4.26 (2d ed. 1998) ("[I]n hard cases [involving standard forms], courts have strained to avoid applying [the] principle [that a person is presumed to know and understand the contents of a document that he executes] and, in doing so, they have developed several techniques. One . . . is to refuse to hold a party to a writing on the ground that it was not of a type that would reasonably appear to the recipient to contain the terms of a proposed contract . . . . A second judicial technique in dealing with standard forms is to refuse to hold a party to a term on the ground that, although the writing may plainly have been an offer, the term was not one that an uninitiated reader ought reasonably to have understood to be a part of that offer.").

187. The dispositional provisions in the *Wendel* case, as well as in *Kass*, provided only for the donation or destruction of excess frozen embryos in the event of divorce. No other options were presented. *See supra* note 182-83 and accompanying text.

within the bonds of marriage,[188] there is simply nothing in the agreements themselves that supports such a limited construction. Indeed, the fact that the appellants in *Davis*, *A.Z.* and *Kass* took the extraordinary step of invoking the power of the courts in order to obtain access to embryos that might permit post-divorce parenthood suggests otherwise.

The last procedural difficulty stems from the complex and emotional nature of both informed consent forms and dispositional agreements. Courts have looked askance at contracts in which the key contractual provisions are camouflaged "in a maze of fine print."[189] As discussed, dispositional agreements are nestled amidst complex medical information that requires a high level of sophistication to read and understand. The consent form signed by the Kasses, for example, was twelve pages, single-spaced and required a college-level education to understand.[190] Moreover, the information

188. *See* Heidi Forster et al., *Comment on ABA's Proposed Frozen Embryo Disposition Policy*, 71 FERTILITY & STERILITY 994, 995 (1999) ("Generally, when a person donates for the IVF process, the gametes are intended for use only within the couple's relationship. The unilateral use of frozen embryos is therefore distinguished."). In *Bohn v. Ann Arbor Reprod. Med. Assocs.*, No. 97-16310-CK (Mich. Cir. Ct. Jun. 24, 1998), the court held that the four page informed consent document signed by Ms. Bohn, in combination with Mr. Mobley's oral agreements to supply sperm to fertilize the eggs retrieved from Ms. Bohn's ovary, created a part oral/part written contract that requires mutual consent to the future utilization of the embryos. *Id.* at 10-11. Neither the document nor the discussions, however, explicitly or implicitly suggested that the parties' wish to become parents was contingent on their remaining married. Similarly, the appellate and final New York courts in *Kass* held that Mr. and Mrs. Kass only sought parenthood within the bonds of matrimony. Kass v. Kass, 696 N.E.2d 174, 182 (N.Y. 1998); Kass v. Kass, 663 N.Y.S.2d 581, 587 (N.Y. App. Div. 1997) (The parties' very participation in the IVF program is premised on their status as a married couple committed to a single joint decision to use IVF in an attempt to achieve parenthood."). The courts made much of the fact that Mr. and Mrs. Kass seemed to speak as a single unit in the fertility clinic informed consent forms. Decisions appear to emanate from a joint entity; plural pronouns—"we", "us", "our"—abound. Of course, the use of such language signifies nothing other than that the hospital attorney who drafted the form found it more convenient to use those terms than to have Mr. and Mrs. Kass agree separately, in separate forms, speaking in the first person singular. *Kass*, 663 N.Y.S.2d at 587.

189. Resource Mgmt. Co. v. Weston Ranch and Livestock Co., 706 P.2d 1028, 1042 (1985) (quoting Williams v. Walker Thomas Furniture Co., 350 F.3d 445, 449 (D.C. Cir. 1965)).

190. *See* Daar, *Regulating Reproductive Technologies*, *supra* note 158, at 622-23 (describing forms as well-intentioned but ambiguous); *see also* Annas, *supra* note 127, at 936 (characterizing the *Kass* forms as "technical, boilerplate . . . [and] difficult to understand"). Readability indices are used to calculate the "grade level" at which technical material is written. A simplified version of a readability index developed by Robert Gunning (Gunning Fog Index, "GFI"), involves selecting a 100-word segment of text, adding the calculated average sentence length in the segment to the number of three or more syllable words in the segment, multiplying the sum by 0.4, and rounding the result to the nearest whole number. Donald F. Doell, *Gunning Fog Index*, *at* http://pimacc.pima.edu/ ~ddoell/tw/gfiex.html (last visited Sept. 18, 2000). "The GFI is fairly effective in estimating the reading difficulty of a document for readers who are not familiar with the technical material." *Id.* GFI of 13 corresponds to a college freshman reading level; 16 to a college

presented in the form is emotionally charged, demanding patients contemplate the occurrence of serious risks and devastating disappointments. Enfolding dispositional agreements into the informed consent form's recitation of worst case scenarios virtually ensures their neglect. While the fertility clinics likely do not intend to "pull a fast one" over would-be parents seeking their services,[191] the merging of the two separate agreements—the one to treatment itself, the other to embryo disposition—defeats careful consideration of the dispositional provisions. The current placement of dispositional agreements within consent forms is, thus, both substantively and procedurally problematic and vulnerable to attack on unconscionability grounds.

VI. JUDICIAL AND LEGISLATIVE RESPONSES TO REPRODUCTIVE WAIVERS IN THE ADOPTION AND SURROGACY CONTEXTS SUGGEST GREATER SCRUTINY OF DISPOSITIONAL WAIVERS

Doctrinal consistency should prompt courts to scrutinize the process by which dispositional agreements are formed. In the adoption and surrogate contract context, a formidable matrix of legal constraints guards against flippant and ill-considered surrender of reproductive opportunities. Adoption proceedings, in which the "natural" parent divests herself of all parental rights and responsibilities, are stringently regulated to protect the parent-child bond and ensure that such divestiture is voluntary, informed, and deliberate.[192] Most state statutes refuse to recognize prenatal agreements to

graduate, and a GFI of 20 to the equivalent of a PhD reading level. *Id.* Applying this to the *Kass* Informed Consent Form No. 2 results in a GFI of 15. *See supra* note 72.

191. Most unconscionable contracts are entered into by two parties, one of whom enjoys considerably greater bargaining power than the other, and is able, by virtue of that greater bargaining power, to extract extremely favorable terms from the other. As a result, the contract is one-sided in the stronger party's favor. In the case of dispositional agreements, the party wielding the bargaining power—the fertility clinic—is not necessarily benefitting from the terms imposed. Rather, in most cases, it is the husband who benefits from a dispositional agreement that doesn't allow for post-divorce parenting. However, the fact that the party enjoying greater bargaining power is not the party benefitting from the oppressive quality of the terms does not weaken the unconscionability argument. In determining whether a contract is unconscionable, it is necessary to determine whether a party with lesser degrees of bargaining power is drawn into a contract that is substantively disadvantageous to her. Ms. Kass and Ms. Wendel both suffered from a lack of bargaining power vis-a-vis the fertility clinics and signed dispositional agreements that were unfavorable to them.

192. *See infra* notes 193-98.

surrender a child to adoption.[193] Post-birth relinquishment of parental rights is generally effective only after a statutory grace period has elapsed.[194]

Relinquishments that are immediately self-executing are generally subject to a series of safeguards protecting the parent from hasty or ill-informed decisions.[195] In New York, for example, where a judicial consent to a private placement adoption is irrevocable upon execution, the courts have established a set of inquiries designed to test the capacity of the consenting parent. Judicial questioning is oriented toward ascertaining whether the mother has received counseling about options for keeping the baby, whether she needs more time to consider alternate plans, whether her emotional state is sound, and whether she is operating under duress or fraud.[196] In California, where relinquishment of a child to a licensed adoption agency is final and can only be rescinded with the consent of the adoption agency, the process of termination is, similarly, closely regulated.[197] The agency must provide counseling, ensure that the parent knows she has the right to legal counsel, provide information regarding alternative plans for the child, and make referrals where appropriate.[198]

---

193. *Cf.* CARMEL SHALEV, BIRTH POWER: THE CASE FOR SURROGACY 52 (1989); NAT'L COMM'N ON ADOPTION, ADOPTION FACTBOOK 102 (1985).

194. *See, e.g.*, MISS. CODE ANN. § 93-17-5(1) (1994) (declaring that valid and enforceable consent to adoption may be given by the natural parent only after 72 hours have elapsed following the birth of the child); N.Y. DOM. REL. LAW ANN. § 115-b(3) (McKinney 1999) (stating that consent to a private placement adoption shall become irrevocable forty-five days after the adoption proceeding in which consent is provided); UNIF. ADOPTION ACT § 2-404(a) (amended 1994), 9 U.L.A. 30 (Supp. 1994) (stating that a parent may revoke consent within 192 hours after the birth of the child).

195. *See* Tyler v. Children's Home Soc. of Cal., 29 Cal. App. 4th 511, 540 (1994) ("[T]he manifest overall purpose of the regulations is to assure that relinquishments are given voluntarily and knowingly.").

196. *See In re* Anonymous, 393 N.Y.S.2d 900, 902 (N.Y. Sup. Ct. 1977). While apparently not the norm throughout all of New York State, these inquiries have become routine practice for the Surrogate and Family Courts of New York County. *See* Nancy Mendelker Frieden, Note, *The Constitutional Rights of Natural Parents Under New York's Adoption Statutes*, 12 N.Y.U. REV. L. & SOC. CHANGE 617, 629 (1983-84).

197. CAL. FAM. CODE § 8700 (West 1994 & Supp. 2000); *see also* CAL. CODE REGS. tit. 22, § 35128 (1999) (freeing a child for adoption).

198. CAL. CODE REGS. tit. 22 §§ 35128-35239 (1999).

> Before accepting the relinquishment of a child for adoption . . . the agency shall:
>
> . . . (2) Provide counseling that, at a minimum, is intended to assist the parent to:
>
> (A) Understand his or her feelings regarding relinquishing the child for adoption and the long range implications of relinquishing the child for adoption, and
>
> (B) Freely make his or her choice regarding relinquishing the child to the agency for adoption

In the surrogacy context, many state legislatures have enacted laws declaring surrogate contracts void and unenforceable.[199] In other states, common law decisions render them a nullity.[200] States that do recognize surrogate contracts often require numerous conditions be met before the contract becomes enforceable. For example, New Hampshire deems legally binding only those surrogate contracts that have received judicial pre-authorization.[201] Pre-authorization is granted only if the judge finds all parties to the contract have provided informed consent, the contract contains no unconscionable terms, and the surrogate has received counseling regarding her ability to "adjust to and assume the inherent risks of the contract. . . ."[202] Additionally, New Hampshire's statute allows the birth mother to rescind the contract any time up until seventy-two hours after birth.[203] Virginia is similarly skittish about recognizing the surrogate's consent to adoption in surrogacy agreements. That state's statute sets forth a list of criteria to be met before surrogacy contracts can obtain judicial authorization.[204] Such contracts must include a home study of the surrogate, her husband and the intended parents, as well as physical and psychological examinations and counseling.[205] Additionally, the judge is directed to ensure that "[a]ll parties have voluntarily entered into the surrogacy contract and understand its terms and the nature, meaning, and effect of the proceeding . . . ."[206] Where the contract is not judicially pre-approved, the courts will only enforce it to the degree its terms can be reformed to meet the statutory standards required for judicial preapproval.[207] Additionally, the surrogate's

---

Id. § 35129(a).

199. *See, e.g.*, ARIZ. REV. STAT. ANN. § 25-218 (West 1999); LA. REV. STAT. ANN. § 9:2713 (West 1999); N.D. CENT. CODE § 14-18-05 (1997); N.Y. DOM. REL. LAW ANN. § 122 (McKinney 1999); UTAH CODE ANN. § 76-7-204 (1999).

200. Moschetta v. Moschetta, 25 Cal. App. 4th 1218, 1231 (Ct. App. 1994). With respect to the enforcement of the surrogacy contract, the court stated:

> We thus decline to enforce the traditional surrogacy contract in this case because to do so would mean we would have to ignore both the analysis used by our Supreme Court in *Johnson v. Calvert* and the adoption statute that requires a formal consent to a child's adoption by his or her birth mother.

Id.; *see also In re* Baby M, 537 A.2d 1227, 1240, 1246-48 (N.J. 1988) (finding the surrogate contract in conflict with existing state statutes and public policies).

201. N.H. REV. STAT. ANN. § 168-B:23(III) (1994).

202. *Id.* § 168-B:16(I)(B).

203. *Id.* § 168-B:25(IV); *see also* FLA. STAT. ANN. § 742.15 (West 1999) (consent to adoption agreed to in surrogate contract rescindable by birth mother up until seven days following birth).

204. VA. CODE ANN. § 20-160(B) (Michie 1999).

205. *Id.* § 20-160(B)(2), (7), (11).

206. *Id.* § 20-160(B)(4).

207. *Id.* § 20-162(A).

consent to adoption in a non-judicially pre-authorized contract is not valid until twenty-five days following birth.[208]

The judicial and statutory restrictions placed upon enforcement of reproductive waivers in the adoption and surrogate contexts recognize the uniqueness of reproduction. These restrictions respect the biological tie between mother and child and acknowledge that intention regarding child rearing can change dramatically over time.

The more progressive state laws treating waiver of parental rights take great care to ensure that the waiver occurs with complete information and with as great an appreciation of the consequences as is possible. State refusal to enforce prenatal adoption consents and reluctance to recognize surrogate contracts simply assumes a mother's inability to foresee the effect of gestation and childbirth on her decision to claim or relinquish parental rights. As one commentator explains, "[c]hildbirth is such a major change in circumstances that one should not reasonably be held to foresee how one arguably would feel about child rearing until after birth has occurred."[209] Consequently, contractual bonds assumed prior to gestation and parturition are easily shrugged off.

A spouse seeking to repudiate a pre-existing agreement regarding embryo disposition has not experienced the gestation or parturition of that embryo. So, arguably, no change of circumstance has occurred that would render the earlier signed agreement unenforceable. But the fact that embryo disposition does relate to the advancement or relinquishment of reproductive opportunities should lead courts and legislatures to concern themselves with the quality of the agreement reached.

Judicial and legislative concern is warranted because the determination to relinquish reproductive opportunities may be affected and shaken by life events apart from pregnancy and birth. Time, relatively unimportant to men, but of crucial importance to women, may work rather dramatic changes in a woman's interest in using a particular embryo for reproduction. Disinterest at age thirty in using frozen embryos to procreate outside of marriage may, a decade later, become an overriding desire. Conditions such as single parenthood that may have looked unattractive initially, may become more palatable if they constitute the only remaining options for parenthood. Aging, a potent circumstance-changer in the reproductive context, is not unforeseeable; however, its effect on the desire to reproduce in less than optimal circumstances may be. And though this change in circumstance may not, unlike gestation and birth, be the type of intervening event that should

208. *Id.* § 20-162(A)(3).

209. Robertson, *Prior Agreements*, *supra* note 14, at 421.

lead courts to strike down previously signed dispositional agreements,[210] it is of sufficient concern to lead courts to restrict the form and manner by which such agreements are reached. Where substantively skewed agreements are located in informed consent documents, presented as nonnegotiable, squeezed into fine print, phrased ambiguously, and unaccompanied by counseling or legal advice, the agreements should not be judicially enforced. Only freestanding dispositional agreements, arrived at after thorough consideration and counseling, warrant judicial enforcement.

VII. STATUTORY EFFORTS TO REGULATE THE FORM OF DISPOSITIONAL AGREEMENTS

Legislatures have recently begun to provide guidance regarding the disposition of frozen embryos. To date, only one state, Florida, has explicitly endorsed a contractual approach to dispositional disputes[211] by requiring couples pursuing fertility treatment to sign a written agreement providing for the disposition of the couple's eggs, sperm, and embryos in the event of death or divorce.[212] Unfortunately, Florida's statute says nothing about the process or form such agreement should take.[213]

Recently, however, legislatures in New York and New Jersey have considered bills that not only mandate the creation of advance written directives for the disposition of frozen embryos, but specify what such

---

210. Arguing to the contrary, Carl Coleman contends that an individual's response to infertility over time is sufficiently difficult to predict that prior agreements to dispose of embryos in a particular fashion should not be enforced. Coleman, *supra* note 13, at 101-02. Coleman states:

> The difficulty of predicting one's future feelings about cryopreserved embryos is compounded by the fact that disposition decisions may not be implemented for decades after the embryos are created. There is simply not enough societal experience with the practice of embryo cryopreservation to presume that most people's decisions about the disposition of their frozen embryos will remain stable over such long periods of time. In the absence of such experience, the law should err on the side of greater flexibility, given the profoundly emotional nature of the issues.

Id.

211. Other states have implicitly limited the contractual options of a couple contemplating cryopreservation of excess embryos by prohibiting destruction of a fertilized egg under certain circumstances. *See, e.g.*, LA. REV. STAT. ANN. § 9:123 (West 1999) (declaring an in vitro fertilized human ovum to be a juridical person and thus prohibiting its destruction under any circumstances). It is not clear that these statutes comport with *Roe v. Wade*. *See* Daar, *Regulating Reproductive Technologies*, *supra* note 158, at 646-51.

212. FLA. STAT. ANN. § 742.17 (West 1999).

213. *Id.*

directives should contain.[214] The bills currently being considered in the New York Senate and Assembly and New Jersey Assembly are substantially similar. They each require medical facilities providing in vitro fertilization and embryo cryopreservation to secure informed consent for those services. In addition, they require that facilities obtain from couples a written advance directive that addresses what shall be done with the cryopreserved embryos in the event of death, divorce, abandonment of the embryos by request, or failure to pay storage fees.[215] The bills further require that the written directive forms offer a number of dispositional choices in the event the stated contingencies occur. These choices must include: transfer of the embryo to the other partner (if alive), donation for research purposes, donation to another individual or couple, and thawing of the embryo with no further action taken.[216] If the donor individual or couple is not satisfied with the options provided, another disposition can be chosen so long as the disposition is clearly stated.[217]

These bills, if passed, will improve the manner by which dispositional agreements are crafted because they require that couples and individuals seeking to cryopreserve embryos be given a panoply of dispositional choices. As noted earlier,[218] many fertility clinics require patients to sign dispositional agreements, but the forms provided offer a constricted set of options. Specifically, individuals are not given the option to use the embryos for implantation if their partner were to die or leave the marriage. The New York and New Jersey bills rectify this problem by mandating that all forms allow individual members of a couple to claim unilateral use of the embryos post-divorce or in widowhood.[219] Additionally, the bills require all forms

214. Assemb. 1116, 209th Leg., 2000 Sess. (N.J. 2000) (supplementing Title 26 of the Revised Statutes) [hereinafter N.J. Bill]. The text of the proposed New York State Senate and Assembly Bills are identical, proposing identical modifications to the New York Public Health Law, adding a new section 2507. S. 1120, 1999 S., Reg. Sess. (N.Y. 1999) [hereinafter N.Y. Bill]; Assemb. 1932, 1999 Assemb., Reg. Sess. (N.Y. 1999) [hereinafter N.Y. Bill]. References to the "N.Y. Bill" refer to both the New York State Senate and New York State Assembly Bills.

215. N.J. Bill, *supra* note 214, § 2(a)-(c); N.Y. Bill, *supra* note 214, § 3(A)-(G).

216. *Id.*

217. *Id.*

218. *See supra* notes 181 and accompanying text.

219. N.J. Bill, *supra* note 214, § 2(c) states:

> The form . . . shall provide, at a minimum, the following choices for disposition in the circumstances indicated: (1) In the event of the death of the male partner: (a) made available to the female partner . . . (2) In the event of the death of the female partner: (a) made available to the male partner . . . (4) In the event of the separation or divorce of the partners: (a) made available to the female partner; (b) made available to the male partner . . . .

Id. N.Y. Bill, *supra* note 214, § 3 states:

allow individuals to write in preferred options that are not listed in the forms.[220] The bills' insistence that individuals and couples seeking to cryopreserve their embryos be given maximum flexibility in exercising their reproductive choice represents a vast improvement over the ad hoc arrangements devised by fertility clinics to date.

The bills, however, could do more to perfect the contracting process. Each bill, as currently proposed, would permit dispositional agreements to remain a part of the clinic's informed consent form. The New Jersey Bill explicitly contemplates one form that would include both provisions for obtaining consent to medical procedures as well as a dispositional agreement determining what should be done with excess frozen embryos.[221] The New York bill is drafted such that the consent and dispositional agreement may, though need not, be located on the same form and signed pursuant to the same contracting process.[222] To ensure that dispositional agreements are

---

> The form . . . shall provide at a minimum the following direction and choices for disposition in the following circumstances: (A) In the case of death of the male partner . . . (I) Transfer to the female partner . . . (B) In the case of death of the female partner . . . (I) Transfer at the discretion of the male partner . . . (D) In the event of the couple's separation or divorce . . . (I) Made available to female partner; (II) Made available to male partner. . . .

Id.

220. N.J. Bill, *supra* note 214, § 2(c)(1)-(7) (allowing individuals to choose "[another] disposition which shall be clearly stated."); N.Y. Bill, *supra* note 214, at § 3(A)-(G) (allowing individuals to choose "other disposition, provided that such other disposition shall be clearly stated").

221. N.J. Bill, *supra* note 214, § 2(a)-(b). The bill requires entities doing business in New Jersey and providing assisted reproductive services obtain:

> [A]dvance written consent for these services and advance written directives as to the disposition of the cryopreserved eggs or embryos. The consent and directive shall be provided by the couple or individual prior to receiving an in vitro or other assisted reproduction service on a form prescribed by the Commissioner of Health and Senior Services . . . . The form containing the advance written consent and directive shall include the name of the patient, the type and number, if applicable, of sperm, ova or embryos donated, the name of the clinic or storage facility, or the name of another donee for a specified purpose which shall be clearly stated.

Id.

222. N.Y. Bill, *supra* note 214, §§ (1)-(3). The bill requires entities located in New York providing assisted reproduction services to require:

> [Commissioning] couples or individuals to provide advance written consent for such services and directives in writing as to the disposition of such cryopreserved eggs or embryos . . . . The form requiring advance written consent for such services shall at a minimum state the name of the patient, the type and number, if applicable, of sperm, ova or embryos donated . . . which shall be clearly stated . . . . The form prescribing directives as to the disposition of cryopreserved eggs or embryos shall provide at a minimum the

thoughtfully considered in their own right, not as adjuncts to the more immediate and emotionally engaging concerns raised by the consent requirement, the bills should explicitly require that the consent and dispositional agreements be disaggregated. These agreements should be contained in different forms, generated by different contracting procedures. Ideally, when individuals are asked to sign dispositional agreements, they would, at the same time, receive counseling regarding how they might feel if the contingencies discussed in the forms occurred. If courts and legislatures truly believe that dispositional agreements enhance reproductive autonomy, then the legal mechanisms designed to encourage their formation should include provisions ensuring that such agreements are made in a deliberate and considered manner.

VIII. CONCLUSION

With assisted reproductive technologies developing at their current pace, disputes over the disposition of frozen embryos are certain to continue. Judicial and legislative approaches to existing disputes suggest a contract model is ascendant.[223] While generally supportive of this trend, this article has cautioned that more attention must be paid to the process by which these contracts are reached.

---

following direction and choices for disposition in the following circumstances

. . . .

Id.

223. The recent decisions of *A.Z. v. B.Z.* and *J.B. v. M.B.* have dimmed this ascent somewhat. It remains unclear whether courts will follow *Davis* and *Kass* and enforce dispositional agreements or adopt the reasoning of the courts in *A.Z. v. B.Z* and *J.B. v. M.B.*, and void such agreements on public policy grounds. In this author's view, the courts should allow couples to plan their reproductive future, whether that entails the use, donation, or destruction of stored embryos. To refuse to do so is paternalistic and intrudes unnecessarily in the private decisions of fertility patients. *See generally* note 6 and accompanying text.

Moreover, adapting a baseline view that implantation should not occur over the contemporaneous objection of one party unfairly restricts the reproductive options of the spouse who contracts to use the embryos if her spouse leaves the relationship. The right to procreate is every bit as compelling and worthy of respect as the right to avoid procreation. Where parties have agreed to vest custody with one parent in the event of divorce, that parent should be able to rely on the agreement. Her ability to plan her reproductive future should not be held hostage to her partner's capriciousness.

Contracts are useful precisely because they enable individuals to plan and order their lives. Contracts in the frozen embryo setting are particularly useful, because reproductive options are neither constant nor eternal. Because the ability to plan and preserve one's reproductive future is so important, dispositional agreements deserve more, not less judicial respect than agreements forged in business or other settings.

Currently, embryo disposition agreements are located in fertility clinic informed consent documents. Thus, at the same time that fertility patients are considering the risks and dangers associated with in vitro fertilization and cryopreservation procedures, they are asked to consider what they want done with excess cryopreserved embryos in the event of death, disability, and divorce. As argued above, placement of dispositional agreements in consent forms is unwise for several reasons. First, the forms used to secure informed consent rarely inspire the rich deliberative process that informed consent jurisprudence envisions. Patients are generally loathe to fully consider the risks involved in medical treatment. When the medical service sought is infertility treatment, careful attention to the content of the informed consent forms is even more unlikely. Text imported into these forms will likely be glossed over as patients erect cognitive barriers to the thoughtful consideration of undesirable outcomes.

Second, even if patients were inclined to treat informed consent documents with more attention than they frequently do, dispositional agreements should not be imported into them because the agreements treat different subject matter. The considerations associated with determining what should be done with excess embryos are separate and unrelated to those associated with determining if a desired medical treatment is worth the danger it creates. The disjunction between the thrust of informed consent documents and dispositional agreements, when combined with the one-sided nature of these agreements, raise unconscionability concerns. These concerns can only be remedied through the types of procedural safeguards that are already in place in the adoption and surrogate contexts. In these contexts, courts and legislatures have sought to regulate the manner in which reproductive rights waivers take place to ensure that they are careful and deliberate.

Recently proposed legislation would mandate couples seeking fertility treatment sign contracts determining embryo disposition. Unfortunately, this legislation does not address how these contracts should be constructed and whether they should be free standing or folded into informed consent documents. This article has argued that the legislation must make clear that dispositional agreements should be free-standing contracts, located in separate forms and reached through a separate contracting process in which counseling is available to the signatories. Such attention to process is necessary if advances in reproductive technology are to achieve the goal of enhancing procreational liberty.

Posthumous Reproduction

[6]

POSTHUMOUS REPRODUCTION AND THE MEANINGS OF AUTONOMY

BELINDA BENNETT*

[In recent years there has been considerable debate over the legal and ethical issues associated with posthumous reproduction. This article analyses recent cases and legal regulation of reproductive technologies in Australia. The issues associated with posthumous reproduction are explored through a consideration of the nature of an individual's interest in their reproductive material. The suitability of a property-based model as a means of conceptualising interests in reproductive material is explored. The article concludes that the issues in this area need to be analysed in terms of autonomy interests that are understood relationally.]

In July 1998 Australian newspapers reported that a widow had won the right to have sperm removed from her late husband's body after he died suddenly as a result of a road accident.[1] The decision by Gillard J in the Victorian Supreme Court[2] sparked debate in Australia over the legal and ethical aspects of posthumous reproduction.[3] In many respects, this debate has much in common with public debate over other aspects of reproductive technology, such as the use of in-vitro fertilisation ('IVF') for older women or for single women, that have pushed out the boundaries of traditional understandings of parenthood. In all of these areas there is debate over whether assisted conception techniques, such as IVF or artificial insemination, should be used to create non-traditional families. However posthumous reproduction adds an additional layer of complexity to the debate for it raises concerns over the ethics of using gametes from a dead person. In addition, the debate in these areas highlights the inadequacies of existing legal concepts in dealing with reproductive issues.

The Victorian case resonates with the much publicised case of Diane Blood in Britain in which Mrs Blood fought for the right to access her dead husband's sperm.[4] Both of these cases reveal the tensions created between scientific and

* BEc, LLB (Hons) (Macquarie), LLM, SJD (Wisconsin); Senior Lecturer, Faculty of Law, University of Sydney. I am grateful to Hilary Astor, Isabel Karpin, Roger Magnusson and Loane Skene for their valuable comments on a draft of this article.

1 Peter Gregory, 'Court Lets Widow Save Husband's Sperm', *The Sydney Morning Herald* (Sydney), 22 July 1998, 3. See also Rachel Hawes and Kimina Lyall, 'Widow's Wishes Come First for IVF Doctor', *The Australian* (Sydney), 23 July 1998, 4; Rachel Hawes, Kimina Lyall and Tania Branigan, 'Father-in-Law Backs Sperm Row Widow', *The Australian* (Sydney), 24 July 1998, 4.

2 *A B v A-G (Vic)* (Unreported, Supreme Court of Victoria, Gillard J, 21 July 1998).

3 Editorial, 'Agonising Choices of Death and Life', *The Australian* (Sydney), 23 July 1998, 12; Deborah Smith, 'Sperm Counts', *The Sydney Morning Herald* (Sydney), 23 July 1998, 11; Kimina Lyall, 'Dead Men Walking', *The Weekend Australian* (Sydney), 25–6 July 1998, 19; Helga Kuhse, 'The Moral Right to Reproductive Freedom', *The Australian* (Sydney), 23 July 1998, 13. See also Anne Winckel, 'The Dead Man's Sperm Case' (1998) 23 *Alternative Law Journal* 288.

4 *R v Human Fertilisation and Embryology Authority; Ex parte Blood* [1997] 2 All ER 687 (CA) ('*Blood*').

reproductive possibilities on the one hand and legal regulation on the other. In a very real sense, posthumous reproduction simultaneously leads us to question the limits of life and the meaning of death,[5] and to consider the challenges posed to law by the scientific possibilities of both.[6] This article seeks to explore the issues raised by posthumous reproduction through an analysis of the posthumous use of sperm. The possibilities of posthumous reproduction pose fundamental questions about the significance of reproductive material, the meaning(s) of autonomy in the context of reproductive decision-making, and the balancing of interests between the living and the dead.

I The *Blood* Case

Debate over posthumous reproduction is not new. In 1984 a French court decided that Corrine Parpalaix could retrieve her dead husband's frozen sperm from the centre at which it was kept so that she could try to conceive a child.[7] While the best known case is probably that of Diane Blood in the UK, there have also been cases in the United States.[8]

Diane Blood had married her husband Stephen in the Anglican Church in 1991. In 1994 Mr and Mrs Blood decided to try to have a child. Tragically, Mr Blood contracted meningitis on 26 February 1995, before Mrs Blood could conceive a child. Two days later, and with Mr Blood in a coma, Mrs Blood asked doctors if a sample of her husband's sperm could be taken. Two samples were taken by electro-ejaculation: the first on 1 March 1995 and the second the following day 'shortly before her husband was certified clinically dead'.[9] Mrs Blood wanted to use the samples so she could have her husband's child. However, the Human Fertilisation and Embryology Authority was of the view that Mrs Blood could not be treated in Britain using her husband's sperm as to do so would contravene the provisions of the *Human Fertilisation and Embryology Act 1990* (UK).[10] Mrs Blood was prepared to go abroad for treatment and the Authority had the power to authorise export of the sperm, however it declined to grant the necessary permission. Mrs Blood applied unsuccessfully for judicial review of the Authority's decision,[11] and subsequently appealed to the Court of Appeal.[12]

5 Derek Morgan and Robert Lee, '"In the Name of the Father?" *Ex parte Blood*: Dealing with Novelty and Anomaly' (1997) 60 *Modern Law Review* 840, 856.

6 One is reminded of Windeyer J's comment, 'Law, marching with medicine but in the rear and limping a little': *Mount Isa Mines Ltd v Pusey* (1970) 125 CLR 383, 395.

7 For discussion of the Parpalaix case see Derek Jones, 'Artificial Procreation, Societal Reconceptions: Legal Insight from France' (1988) 36 *American Journal of Comparative Law* 525. See also 'The Parpalaix Case and Post-Mortem Insemination' (1984) 58 *Australian Law Journal* 627.

8 See Lyall, above n 3.

9 *Blood* [1997] 2 All ER 687, 690 (CA).

10 For an excellent analysis of the background to the Act and the Act's provisions see Derek Morgan and Robert Lee, *Blackstone's Guide to the* Human Fertilisation and Embryology Act 1990: *Abortion and Embryo Research — The New Law* (1991).

11 *R v Human Fertilisation and Embryology Authority; Ex parte Blood* [1996] 3 WLR 1176 (QBD).

12 *Blood* [1997] 2 All ER 687 (CA). For further discussion of *Blood* see Morgan and Lee, 'In the Name of the Father?', above n 5.

The *Human Fertilisation and Embryology Act 1990* (UK) establishes a licensing system for assisted conception techniques and prohibits gametes or embryos being used or stored otherwise than in accordance with a licence. The Act also contains conditions of licences under the Act, including provisions requiring written consent for storage and use of gametes. The Authority is also empowered under the Act to give directions on certain matters, including the export of gametes and embryos.

On the issue of storage of Mr Blood's sperm, the Court of Appeal concluded that under the Act there should be no preservation of sperm without written consent.[13] The storage of Mr Blood's sperm without written consent meant that '[t]echnically therefore, an offence was committed by the licence holder as a result of the storage under s 41(2)(b) of the 1990 Act by the licensee.'[14] However, on this point Lord Woolf MR said that there was 'no question of any prosecution being brought in the circumstances of this case and no possible criticism can be made of the fact that storage has taken place'.[15] Lord Woolf described the case as 'an unexplored legal situation where humanity dictated that the sperm was taken and preserved first, and the legal argument followed'.[16] However, Lord Woolf noted that the situation was unlikely to be the same in the future:

> Because this judgment makes it clear that the sperm of Mr Blood has been preserved and stored when it should not have been, this case raises issues as to the lawfulness of the use and export of sperm which should never arise again.[17]

One issue that the case raises is that of consent by Mr Blood to the actual taking of the sperm.[18] However, the issue of consent, which was governed by the common law, had not been argued before the court and consequently it was not necessary for the Court of Appeal to analyse the issue.[19] What was clear though was that 'treatment was being provided to Mr Blood even though he was unconscious when the sperm was obtained'.[20] The issue then arose as to whether Mr and Mrs Blood were being treated 'for the woman and man together' as required under s 4(1)(b) of the Act.[21] On this point Lord Woolf concluded that

[13] *Blood* [1997] 2 All ER 687, 695.

[14] Ibid.

[15] Ibid.

[16] Ibid.

[17] Ibid.

[18] As Lord Woolf noted: 'The question of the lawfulness of the storage is quite separate from the lawfulness of the taking of the sperm from Mr Blood as he lay unconscious' (ibid).

[19] Ibid.

[20] Ibid.

[21] Section 4(1) of the Act provides:

> No person shall—
>
> (a) store any gametes, or
>
> (b) in the course of providing treatment services for any woman, use the sperm of any man unless the services are being provided for the woman and the man together or use the eggs of any other woman …
>
> except in pursuance of a licence.

> it is really not possible to regard treatment as being together for the purposes of section 4(1)(b), once the man who has provided the sperm has died. And, in any event, the exception to the need for written consent in the case of gametes for 'treatment together' only applies where the sperm is used at once and so does not need to be preserved. The keeping of sperm requires written consent under section 4(1)(a) and the terms of the licence ... The absence of the necessary written consent means that both the treatment of Mrs Blood and the storage of Mr Blood's sperm would be prohibited by the 1990 Act. The authority has no discretion to authorise treatment in the United Kingdom.[22]

As treatment of Mrs Blood would be unlawful in the United Kingdom, the final issue to be resolved in *Blood* concerned the Authority's decision to refuse to permit the export of the sperm so as to allow Mrs Blood to be treated abroad. The Court of Appeal was of the view that the Authority did not adequately take into account the effect of European Community law,[23] nor the fact that there should be no future cases involving sperm being stored without consent.[24] In allowing Mrs Blood's appeal, the Court concluded that 'Mrs Blood has the right to receive treatment in Belgium with her husband's sperm unless there are good public policy reasons for not allowing this to happen.'[25] Diane Blood was ultimately successful in her battle against the authorities and late in 1998 the media reported that she had given birth to a healthy child.[26]

II Australian Regulation of Reproductive Technology

These recent cases show that the issues related to posthumous reproduction are very real. In Australia the issue is complicated by the federal structure of Australian laws which leaves legislation on matters such as reproductive technology in the hands of the states. Only three Australian states, Victoria, South Australia and Western Australia, currently have legislation that specifically regulates assisted conception techniques,[27] although some other states do have legislation regulating surrogacy arrangements[28] and all states have legislation addressing the status of children born as a result of assisted conception.[29]

This section is quoted in *R v Human Fertilisation and Embryology Authority; Ex parte Blood* [1996] 3 WLR 1176, 1178 (QBD).

22 *Blood* [1997] 2 All ER 687, 697.

23 For analysis of European Community law and *Blood* see Tamara Hervey, 'Buy Baby: The European Union and Regulation of Human Reproduction' (1998) 18 *Oxford Journal of Legal Studies* 207.

24 *Blood* [1997] 2 All ER 687, 702.

25 Ibid 703–4.

26 'Life Comes from Death', *The Sun-Herald* (Sydney), 13 December 1998, 51.

27 *Infertility Treatment Act 1995* (Vic); *Reproductive Technology Act 1988* (SA); *Human Reproductive Technology Act 1991* (WA). In 1997 the NSW Department of Health released a discussion paper on whether NSW should also introduce laws regulating reproductive technology: New South Wales Health, *Discussion Paper: Review of the* Human Tissue Act 1983 — *Assisted Reproductive Technologies* (October 1997).

28 *Infertility Treatment Act 1995* (Vic) pt 6; *Surrogacy Contracts Act 1993* (Tas); *Family Relationships Act 1975* (SA) pt IIB; *Surrogate Parenthood Act 1988* (Qld); *Substitute Parent Agreements Act 1994* (ACT).

29 *Family Law Act 1975* (Cth) s 60H; *Status of Children Act 1996* (NSW); *Status of Children Act 1974* (Vic); *Status of Children Act 1978* (Qld); *Family Relationships Act 1975* (SA); *Artificial*

In Victoria, the *Infertility Treatment Act 1995* provides that a woman who has an infertility treatment procedure must be married (or in a de facto relationship), and that prior to the treatment procedure both she and her husband must consent to the type of procedure to be performed.[30] In addition, for a woman to be eligible for treatment either (a) a doctor must be satisfied on reasonable grounds either from examining or treating the woman, that she is unlikely to become pregnant with her eggs and her husband's sperm without an infertility treatment procedure, or (b) a doctor, with specialist qualifications in human genetics, must be satisfied that if the woman conceived a child naturally by her husband that any child born to them could inherit a genetic abnormality or disease.[31] The consent must be written, it must 'specify that the woman and her husband have consented to undergo the kind of treatment procedure specified in the consent' and when the procedure is performed the consent must not have been withdrawn or lapsed.[32] The Act requires that before a woman gives her consent to a treatment procedure, she and her husband must be given a list of approved counsellors and 'enough information about the procedure and the alternatives to the procedure to enable the woman and her husband to make an informed decision about whether or not to undergo the procedure'.[33] The woman and her husband must have received counselling (including counselling on prescribed matters) from an approved counsellor before the woman consents to have a treatment procedure.[34]

Even if a husband and wife decide to have an infertility treatment procedure and give their consent in accordance with the Act while the husband is still alive, it is still not possible to use a dead husband's sperm for treatment of his widow in Victoria. The *Infertility Treatment Act 1995* bans procedures that use gametes from persons known to be dead. Section 43 provides:

> A person must not—
>
> (a) inseminate a woman with sperm from a man known to be dead; or
>
> (b) transfer to a woman a gamete from a person known to be dead; or
>
> (c) transfer to a woman a zygote or an embryo formed from a gamete from a person known to be dead; or
>
> (d) form a zygote with sperm from a man known to be dead; or
>
> (e) form a zygote, if the woman who produced the oocyte used to form the zygote is known to be dead.
>
> Penalty: 240 penalty units or 2 years imprisonment or both.

Although this means that a widow could not be inseminated with her dead husband's sperm in Victoria, the Infertility Treatment Authority does have power

Conception Act 1985 (WA); *Status of Children Act 1974* (Tas); *Status of Children Act 1978* (NT); *Artificial Conception Act 1985* (ACT).

30 *Infertility Treatment Act 1995* (Vic) s 8(1), (2).

31 *Infertility Treatment Act 1995* (Vic) s 8(3).

32 *Infertility Treatment Act 1995* (Vic) s 9.

33 *Infertility Treatment Act 1995* (Vic) s 10(1).

34 *Infertility Treatment Act 1995* (Vic) s 11(1).

under the Act to authorise gametes being taken out of the State.[35] The Act also provides that a zygote or embryo can only be removed from storage for certain designated reasons which include the death of one or both of the gamete providers.[36]

The only other Australian states with legislation regulating reproductive technologies are South Australia and Western Australia. In South Australia, access to treatment under the *Reproductive Technology Act 1988* is limited to married couples where either (a) one or both partners appears to be infertile; or (b) there is a risk that any child born to the couple as a result of natural conception could have a genetic defect.[37] The definition of 'married couple' includes long-term de facto couples.[38] Regulations under the *Reproductive Technology Act 1988* require that infertility treatment must not be given to a person unless that person and their spouse have consented to the treatment in accordance with the Regulations.[39] Furthermore, semen or ova must not be stored unless consent has been given to storage.[40] Although the Regulations provide that a licensee must dispose of an embryo that is stored for future use by an infertile couple if the licensee becomes aware that either spouse has died, that their marriage has been dissolved or that consent to the storage of the embryo has been revoked by one or both spouse(s),[41] the provision in relation to the storage of gametes only provides that a licensee must dispose of stored semen or ova if the consent to their use or storage is revoked.[42]

In Western Australia the *Human Reproductive Technology Act 1991* also establishes a licensing system for assisted conception procedures. The Act provides that an IVF procedure can be carried out where 'it would be likely to benefit' either individuals who are infertile 'as a couple', or a couple whose child is likely to have a genetic abnormality or disease.[43] In addition, each of the

35 *Infertility Treatment Act 1995* (Vic) s 56.

36 *Infertility Treatment Act 1995* (Vic) s 53(1)(c).

37 *Reproductive Technology Act 1988* (SA) s 13(3)(b).

38 Section 13(4) of the *Reproductive Technology Act 1988* (SA) provides that

> 'married couple' includes two people who are not married but who are cohabiting as husband and wife and who—
>
> (a) have cohabited continuously as husband and wife for the immediately preceding five years; or
>
> (b) have, during the immediately preceding six years, cohabited as husband and wife, for periods aggregating at least five years.

In *Pearce v South Australian Health Commission* (1996) 66 SASR 486 the plaintiff was granted a declaration that s 13(3)(b) of the *Reproductive Technology Act* was inconsistent with s 22 of the *Sex Discrimination Act 1984* (Cth) and was therefore invalid to the extent of the inconsistency due to s 109 of the *Australian Constitution*.

39 *Reproductive Technology (Code of Ethical Clinical Practice) Regulations 1995* (SA) cl 15(1).

40 *Reproductive Technology (Code of Ethical Clinical Practice) Regulations 1995* (SA) cl 17.

41 *Reproductive Technology (Code of Ethical Clinical Practice) Regulations 1995* (SA) cl 26(1). This provision does not apply if the gamete providers have specified conditions for dealing with or disposing of an embryo in the event of one of these situations arising: cl 26(2).

42 *Reproductive Technology (Code of Ethical Clinical Practice) Regulations 1995* (SA) cl 25.

43 *Human Reproductive Technology Act 1991* (WA) s 23(a).

participants must have given an effective consent.[44] The individuals seeking treatment as a couple must be either married to each other or be in a long-term de facto relationship.[45] Furthermore, the reason for the infertility must not be age or another prescribed cause,[46] and consideration must have been given to the welfare and interests of the participants and any child likely to be born.[47]

The Act provides that gametes, an ovum in the process of fertilisation or an embryo may not be used or stored without the consent of the gamete provider(s).[48] Furthermore, a consent to storage of gametes, an ovum in the process of fertilisation or an embryo must specify a maximum storage period if that is to be less than the statutory maximum, and must provide instructions indicating what is to be done with stored material if the person consenting to the storage is unable to vary or withdraw the consent due to incapacity or for some other reason.[49] The Act requires that consent to the keeping or use of reproductive material must be in writing.[50] The Act envisages the development of a Code of Practice and s 18(1) provides that the Code may make provisions relating to, inter alia:

> (f) the donation, use, supply, export from the State, posthumous use, or other dealing in or disposal of, gametes, eggs in the process of fertilisation or embryos by licensees.

Directions issued under the Act also contain relevant provisions.[51] In relation to the giving of consent to the keeping of gametes or embryos, '[t]he person responsible must ensure that no consent is given for a use not permitted under the Act, including the use of gametes of a person known to be dead'.[52] The Directions also provide: 'Any person to whom the licence applies must not knowingly use or authorise the use of gametes in an artificial fertilisation procedure after the death of the gamete provider.'[53]

No other states have legislation regulating reproductive technologies in this way. However, in 1996 the National Health and Medical Research Council ('NHMRC') issued guidelines in this area entitled *Ethical Guidelines on Assisted Reproductive Technology* ('*Guidelines*'). The *Guidelines* include '[t]he use in ART [Assisted Reproductive Technology] treatment programs of gametes or embryos harvested from cadavers' in a list of practices that 'are ethically unac-

44 *Human Reproductive Technology Act 1991* (WA) s 23(b).

45 *Human Reproductive Technology Act 1991* (WA) s 23(c). The couple must be 'co-habiting in a heterosexual relationship as husband and wife and have done so for periods aggregating at least 5 years, during the immediately preceding 6 years': s 23(c)(ii).

46 *Human Reproductive Technology Act 1991* (WA) s 23(d).

47 *Human Reproductive Technology Act 1991* (WA) s 23(e).

48 *Human Reproductive Technology Act 1991* (WA) s 22(1).

49 *Human Reproductive Technology Act 1991* (WA) s 22(6).

50 *Human Reproductive Technology Act 1991* (WA) s 22(8).

51 'Directions Given by the Commissioner of Health to Set the Standards of Practice under the *Human Reproductive Technology Act 1991* on the Advice of the WA Reproductive Technology Council', *Western Australian Government Gazette*, No 171, 3 October 1997.

52 Ibid [3.3].

53 Ibid [8.5].

ceptable and should be prohibited'.[54] However, apart from this provision, the *Guidelines* do not specifically prohibit the use of gametes from a person who is known to be dead. In relation to the consent to storage and use of gametes, the *Guidelines* do address the issue of use of gametes and embryos after death. The *Guidelines* provide that consent for the storage and use of gametes should, inter alia,

> give an advance directive as to what should be done with the gametes if the gamete provider dies, becomes incapable of varying or revoking the consent, or fail to give further instructions at the expiry of the maximum period of storage.[55]

There is an equivalent provision in relation to consent by couples for the storage and use of their embryos.[56] In addition, the *Guidelines* contain the following provision:

> Should one member of a couple with the responsibility to make decisions about an embryo die, the surviving member has the responsibility to make the relevant decisions about the keeping or use of the embryo, taking into consideration any advance directive from the deceased partner.
>
> Should both members of the couple die, where possible any advance directive from the couple should be complied with or, if there is no such directive or it cannot be complied with, the embryo should be allowed to succumb.[57]

As ethical guidelines issued by the NHMRC, these guidelines do carry some weight. However, the issue of posthumous use of gametes remains a live issue in those jurisdictions without legislation in this area.

The legal regulation of posthumous reproduction obviously varies around Australia. These variations have highlighted the need for consistency and have led to calls for national uniform laws to regulate assisted conception techniques.[58] Whether we opt for a uniform approach, or whether we prefer instead to pursue 'harmonisation' of state laws[59] in this area, we must be able to conceptualise a framework for decision-making about the body, both on the individual level and at the social level, that can inform the processes of law reform and law-making.

[54] NHMRC, *Ethical Guidelines on Assisted Reproductive Technology* (1996) [11.11].

[55] Ibid [3.2.6].

[56] Ibid [3.2.7].

[57] Ibid [3.2.9].

[58] Bryan Gurry, Marcus Hoyne and Nicki Mollard, 'The *Blood* Case — A Need for National Uniformity' (1997) 5 *Australian Health Law Bulletin* 76. The need for uniform legislation has also been recognised in the introduction to the NHMRC *Guidelines*:

> In particular, AHEC [Australian Health Ethics Committee] considers that without uniform legislation, regulation of national data collection and maintenance of a centralised data base and monitoring of research in this area cannot be achieved.

NHMRC, above n 54, v.

[59] For an analysis of harmonisation of health law in Australia see Brian Opeskin, 'The Architecture of Public Health Law Reform: Harmonisation of Law in a Federal System' (1998) 22 *Melbourne University Law Review* 337.

III Decision-Making and the Body

In the search for an adequate decision-making framework for posthumous reproduction, it is necessary to conceptualise the nature of the interest that individuals have in their reproductive material. In terms of posthumous reproduction, there are two separate issues to be considered. The first is the nature of the interest in the sperm once it has been removed from the body of the provider. The second issue is that of the nature of the interest that an individual has in whether or not his sperm is used after his death.

In relation to the first of these issues the concept of property has been applied to the issue of decision-making over the body. As a general rule, there is no property in the human body or in tissue taken from the body. This is not to say that the body has never been property. It is quite clear that people have, in the past, been regarded as property — most notably in the case of slavery.[60] The 'no property' proposition is drawn from a line of English cases holding that a corpse could not be the subject of property.[61] In Australia, the High Court considered the issue in the 1908 case of *Doodeward v Spence*.[62] The case arose following prosecution of the plaintiff for publicly exhibiting a bottle containing the corpse of a still-born two-headed child. The bottle and its contents were seized by the police. Although the plaintiff demanded its return, the corpse was retained at a University museum. The plaintiff then brought a suit for conversion.[63]

In determining whether a corpse could be the subject of property, Griffith CJ said:

> I entertain no doubt that, when a person has by the lawful exercise of work or skill so dealt with a human body or part of a human body in his lawful possession that it has acquired some attributes differentiating it from a mere corpse awaiting burial, he acquires a right to retain possession of it, at least as against any person not entitled to have it delivered to him for the purpose of burial, but subject, of course, to any positive law which forbids its retention under the particular circumstances.[64]

Barton J indicated that he 'entirely agree[d]'[65] with the judgment of Griffith CJ, adding however 'that I do not wish it to be supposed that I cast the slightest doubt upon the general rule that an unburied corpse is not the subject of property, or upon the legal authorities which require the proper and decent disposal of the dead'.[66] Higgins J gave a dissenting judgment, stating that there could be no property in a corpse:

60 See Patricia Williams, *The Alchemy of Race and Rights* (1991).

61 For discussion of these cases and the principles of property in the body generally see Roger Magnusson, 'Proprietary Rights in Human Tissue' in Norman Palmer and Ewan McKendrick (eds), *Interests in Goods* (2nd ed, 1998) 25, 27–37.

62 (1908) 6 CLR 406 ('*Doodeward*').

63 Ibid 417.

64 Ibid 414.

65 Ibid 417.

66 Ibid.

> From first to last, I can find no instance of any Court asserting any property in a corpse except in favour of persons who wanted it for purposes of burial, and who by virtue of their close relationship with the deceased might be regarded as under a duty to give the corpse a decent interment. I confess that I am unable to see how we can ignore such definite decisions and pronouncements as to the law.[67]

The decision in *Doodeward* would appear to stand for the proposition that although there is generally no property in a corpse, if the application of human work or skill changes the corpse into something other than simply a corpse awaiting burial, it may be able to be the subject of property.

The issue was considered more recently by the English Court of Appeal in *Dobson v North Tyneside Health Authority*,[68] in which the plaintiff sued the first defendant alleging a failure to diagnose the deceased's brain tumor, and the second defendant for failing to keep and preserve the deceased's brain or sections of the brain tumor. Peter Gibson LJ, with whom Thorpe and Butler-Sloss LJJ agreed, said that 'in the present state of the English authorities there is no property in a corpse',[69] although this is qualified by a recognition that the deceased's administrators or executors or others who have a duty to inter the body have a right to custody and possession of the body until its burial.[70]

The second qualification to the general 'no property' rule considered by the Court of Appeal was that where skill had been applied, or where the corpse had undergone a process, it could be the subject of property.[71] Considering the facts of the case, Peter Gibson LJ said that preserving a brain after a post-mortem was not

> on a par with stuffing or embalming a corpse or preserving an anatomical or pathological specimen for a scientific collection or with preserving a human freak such as a double-headed foetus that had some value for exhibition purposes.[72]

Peter Gibson LJ held that a brain fixed in paraffin for a post-mortem was not 'an item to possession of which the plaintiffs ever became entitled for the purpose of interment or any other purpose, still less that the plaintiffs ever acquired the property in it.'[73]

From *Doodeward* and *Dobson* it would appear that there is generally no property in a corpse, although there may be a right to possession of it for the purposes of interment. However, it seems possible that a corpse that has been altered through a process such as embalming or some other form of preservation may be able to be the subject of property.

67 Ibid 421–2.
68 [1997] 1 WLR 596 ('*Dobson*').
69 Ibid 600.
70 Ibid.
71 Ibid.
72 Ibid 601.
73 Ibid 601–2.

Even in relation to excised human tissue, there are few instances of the courts applying a model of proprietary rights.[74] In the case of *Moore v Regents of the University of California*[75] the Californian Supreme Court held that Moore had not stated a case for conversion in relation to the use of cells from his spleen in research and commercial development.[76] Developments in genetic technology are likely to highlight the interests of individuals in control over the uses of tissue samples for genetic testing and control over the uses to which information derived from testing will be put.[77]

IV CONCEPTUALISING THE INTEREST

Even though there is no property in the body or in tissue once separated from the body, it is clear that individuals can have an interest in any use made of their tissue. Yet if there are interests in tissue generally, the interests of individuals in their gametes (sperm and ova) are even more significant. There is one vital factor that makes sperm and ova so totally unlike any other human tissue and that one factor is *reproductive potential.*[78] There is a very clear and definite interest in controlling any uses made of reproductive material, for as Robert Jansen has commented, it is the very fact that gametes have this potential that makes them so unique:[79]

> [E]ach ejaculate or each ovulation hardly constitutes a major drain on an individual's resources. One simply does not care if ejaculates or ova are lost — provided that they are *actually* lost and that their information content, their genetic potential, is not going to be realised in a way one's not happy with.[80]

The reproductive potential inherent in gametes is then at the heart of an individual's interest in control over gametes and their use. These interests are recognised in the legislative framework that exists in Victoria, South Australia and Western Australia, as well as in the NHMRC *Guidelines*, in the provisions containing requirements as to consent,[81] storage of gametes[82] and limits on their use,[83] as

[74] See Magnusson, above n 61, 44–5 for a discussion of cases in which tissue has been regarded as property.

[75] 793 P 2d 479 (1990) ('*Moore*').

[76] For discussion of *Moore* see Magnusson, above n 61, 52–3.

[77] For discussion of privacy concerns with genetic testing see Privacy Commissioner, Human Rights and Equal Opportunity Commission, *The Privacy Implications of Genetic Testing* (Information Paper No 5, 1996).

[78] Robert Jansen, 'Sperm and Ova as Property (1985) 11 *Journal of Medical Ethics* 123, 125.

[79] Ibid. A similar point has also been made in *Hecht v Superior Court (Kane)*, 20 Cal Rptr 2d 275, 283 (Cal App 2 Dist, 1993):

> Sperm which is stored by its provider with the intent that it be used for artificial insemination is thus unlike other human tissue because it is 'gametic material' (*Davis v Davis, supra*, 842 SW 2d 588, 597) that can be used for reproduction. Although it has not yet been joined with an egg to form a preembryo, as in *Davis*, the value of sperm lies in its potential to create a child after fertilization, growth, and birth.

[80] Jansen, above n 78, 125.

[81] *Infertility Treatment Act 1995* (Vic) ss 9, 10(1), 11(1); *Reproductive Technology (Code of Ethical Clinical Practice) Regulations 1995* (SA) cll 23–6; *Human Reproductive Technology Act 1991* (WA) ss 22(1), 22(8), 23(b).

well as the more general provisions relating to the licensing of providers of treatment services.

If reproductive material is different from other human tissue because of its reproductive potential, how then are we to conceptualise an individual's interest in their gametes or embryos? As we have seen, the property model does not sit easily with discussion of interests in dead bodies or excised tissue. It sits even less easily with considerations of interests in gametes and embryos. Furthermore, in considering the nature of the interest that individuals have in their gametes and embryos, we are not looking at whether that reproductive material can be regarded as property in the sense of whether it could be stolen. It is clear that stored reproductive material could be regarded as property if we are considering its theft. However, this does not mean that we should be limited to the property paradigm when endeavouring to conceptualise the nature of the interest that individuals have in their gametes and embryos.

The legal status of frozen embryos is a topic that has occupied the attention of official committees of inquiry and commentators on reproductive technology. In the mid-1980s, the Waller Committee in Victoria rejected a property-based approach to stored embryos, stating:

> The Committee does not regard the couple whose embryo is stored as owning or having dominion over that embryo. It considers that those concepts should not be imported into and have no place in a consideration of issues which focus on an individual and genetically unique human entity. ... The Committee nevertheless does consider that the couple whose gametes are used to form the embryo in the context of an IVF programme should be recognized as having rights which are in some ways analogous to those recognized in parents of a child after its birth. The Committee does not consider that those rights are absolute, just as the rights of parents are limited by the rights and interests of the child, and by the larger concerns of the community in which they all live.[84]

This approach was met with approval by the majority report of the Senate Select Committee on the Human Embryo Experimentation Bill 1985 (Cth) when it adopted its guardianship approach to human embryos:

> Thus, the preferred model is to regard the embryo not as 'property belonging to', but as an entity enjoying the protection of a guardian. Under this model the property rights of gamete donors are exhausted on fertilisation when a genetically new human life organised as a distinct entity oriented towards further development comes into being. At that point guardianship arises and would be ordinarily and properly exercised by the intending social parents (whether or not these are the same persons as the gamete donors).[85]

82 *Reproductive Technology (Code of Ethical Clinical Practice) Regulations 1995* (SA) cl 17; *Human Reproductive Technology Act 1991* (WA) s 22(6).

83 *Infertility Treatment Act 1995* (Vic) s 43; *Reproductive Technology (Code of Ethical Clinical Practice) Regulations 1995* (SA) cll 25, 26.

84 The Committee to Consider the Social, Ethical and Legal Issues Arising from In Vitro Fertilization (Prof Louis Waller, Chair), *Report on the Disposition of Embryos Produced by In Vitro Fertilization* (Victoria, 1984) [2.8] ('Waller Committee').

85 Senate Select Committee on the Human Embryo Experimentation Bill 1985, *Human Embryo Experimentation in Australia* (1986) [3.41]. For discussion of the report see Pascal Kasimba and

This 'not property' approach to embryos has been reflected in case law. In the United States case of *Davis v Davis*, which concerned a dispute over control of frozen embryos, the Supreme Court of Tennessee concluded

> that preembryos are not, strictly speaking, either 'persons' or 'property', but occupy an interim category that entitles them to special respect because of their potential for human life.[86]

While the Court concluded that the couple did not have a 'true property interest' in the embryos, it did recognise that they

> have an interest in the nature of ownership, to the extent that they have decision-making authority concerning disposition of the preembryos, within the scope of policy set by law.[87]

The difficulties that clearly exist in relation to the application of property concepts to gametes and, to an even greater degree to embryos, highlight the inadequacy of existing legal concepts when applied to reproduction, reproductive material, and the female body.[88] In relation to gametes and embryos the shortcomings of the property model are evident. Gametes and embryos are not just forms of property like TV sets, cars or houses.[89] Even though we may not be prepared to grant personhood, and in particular *legal* personhood to embryos,[90] the view taken by the Waller Committee back in 1984 that gamete providers' interests 'are in some ways analogous to those recognized in parents of a child after its birth'[91] takes us some way towards an understanding and a conceptualisation of our interest in gametes and embryos and demands that we look beyond a simple property paradigm.

V The Importance of Connection

A property model does not reflect the value of gametes and embryos to the individual concerned. Property does not speak to the significance of genetic links, genetic continuity and potential personhood inherent in our relationship

Stephen Buckle, 'Embryos and Children: Problems Raised by the Majority Report of the Senate Select Committee on Human Embryo Experimentation' (1988) 2 *Australian Journal of Family Law* 228; Pascal Kasimba and Stephen Buckle, 'Guardianship and the IVF Human Embryo' (1989) 17 *Melbourne University Law Review* 139; Rebecca Albury, 'Inquiring into Ethics: The Australian Senate and Human Embryo Experimentation' (1989) 24 *Australian Journal of Social Issues* 269.

86 *Davis v Davis*, 842 SW 2d 588, 597 (Tenn, 1992).

87 Ibid.

88 Isabel Karpin, 'Legislating the Female Body: Reproductive Technology and the Reconstructed Woman' (1992) 3 *Columbia Journal of Gender and Law* 325; Roxanne Mykitiuk, 'Fragmenting the Body' (1994) 2 *Australian Feminist Law Journal* 63.

89 In Victoria there is a penalty for receiving or holding oneself out as willing to receive compensation for gamete donation: *Infertility Treatment Act 1995* (Vic) s 57.

90 Embryos are not persons, although they undoubtedly have the potential to develop into them. Furthermore, to regard embryos as persons and to attach legal significance to this will have implications for other aspects of reproductive decision-making, such as in the abortion context. In any event, the concept of 'persons' has little relevance to gametes and so is of little practical use in finding an appropriate framework in this context.

91 Waller Committee, above n 84, [2.8].

with our gametes and embryos. As Jennifer Nedelsky has argued, property does not speak of attachment:

> In the case of property as the legal category for potential life, I think a relational analysis reveals that the promises of hope are illusory, at least in the long run, and that the concept of property will not help, but will distort our understanding of what matters in disputes over potential life. The values at stake in the cases turn out to be about honouring and protecting the kind of attachment to potential life that is appropriate for fostering relations of respect and appreciation of children. I think the issues in the cases also touch the most general concern of fostering people's capacities to form relationships of intimacy, trust and responsibility. These issues involve allocation of control and decision-making authority, but they are not about ownership.[92]

The terminology we choose is important, for as Nedelsky points out, the 'choice of legal category is a strategic one'.[93] When thinking about conceptualising structures for decision-making in the reproductive context we need to inquire 'into the values we want to promote by permitting and protecting certain kinds of control'.[94] As we seek to formulate a framework for decision-making over gametes and embryos of both the living and the dead, we need to look beyond debates based in 'rights', 'ownership' and 'property' and look towards articulating the interest(s) we have in the potential inherent in reproductive material.

Within the context of the new reproductive technologies, with the possibility of gametes and embryos frozen in storage for later use, the issue of control over reproductive material takes on a new importance. It is precisely because we recognise the special nature of the interest of an infertile individual or couple in having a child of their own, that the use of their gametes or embryo for some other purpose or some other person, is unthinkable.[95] What we are concerned with, in the reproductive context, is not whether we *own* our gametes or embryos, for even as parents we do not *own* our children.[96] As Nedelsky argues, rather than *ownership* we are instead concerned with *authority* to make decisions.[97]

What is at stake here is the meaning of reproductive autonomy. Within bioethics, the principle of autonomy looms large as a basis for structuring health care decision-making and weighing conflicting priorities.[98] Yet while as a society we clearly value autonomy in the sense that we believe that, in general, a competent adult patient has a right to make decisions about his/her own health care, we should not take the meaning of autonomy for granted. Even the basic liberal concept of the autonomous, self-owning individual fails to speak to the realities of women's lives in which women's 'self-ownership' has traditionally

92 Jennifer Nedelsky, 'Property in Potential Life? A Relational Approach to Choosing Legal Categories' (1993) 6 *Canadian Journal of Law and Jurisprudence* 343, 363.

93 Ibid 354.

94 Ibid 362.

95 Jansen, above n 78, 124.

96 Nedelsky, 'Property in Potential Life?', above n 92, 358.

97 Ibid 361–2.

98 For a thorough analysis of autonomy and other bioethical principles see Tom Beauchamp and James Childress, *Principles of Biomedical Ethics* (3rd ed, 1989).

been undermined by men's interest in control over women's reproductive capacity.[99] Liberalism's autonomy has always been one of an individual separated from others by 'a wall (of rights).'[100] Nedelsky argues that property is the 'central symbol' for this individualised form of autonomy.[101] In the search for an ethical framework that can be used to sift the sands of posthumous reproduction, it is difficult to see what individualised autonomy provides us with other than a basis for formulating competing rights which must then be mediated with reference to some other principle.

Feminist theory provides an alternative theoretical framework for bioethical decision-making by providing an analysis that is based on interpersonal relations and connections rather than individualised rights. Feminists have argued the need for greater acknowledgment and valuing of the role of caring and nurturing relationships in our lives and our decision-making.[102] Yet what is the meaning of autonomy when conceptualised in terms of an ethic of care? Leslie Bender argues that the value of autonomy is not diminished by an ethic of care: the differences are seen not in the value placed on autonomy, but rather 'in the sources and meanings of autonomy'.[103] As Bender argues:

> In a care-based ethic, individual autonomy is a *process* nurtured in webs of relationships and responsibilities instead of a static condition pre-existing them. … The autonomy of an ethic of care can be melded with the autonomy concerns in a rights-based medical ethic, if it is understood to mean self-governing moral agency, rather than independent or self-contained decision-making. Self-governing in an ethic of care does not mean governing alone by abstract reasoning and distant observations, but means choosing options with respect to responsibilities, relationships, conversations, and dialogues with others.[104]

Jennifer Nedelsky has also argued for autonomy to be reconceived in terms of caring. She argues that autonomy should be seen as grounded not in isolation from others, but rather in connections and relationships with others.[105]

99 As Ngaire Naffine points out:

> The structure of self-ownership therefore, of necessity, applied only to the male body which was thought to be free from the encumbrances of sex and reproduction and yet which still depended on ready and exclusive access to the fertile body of a woman for its reproductive needs (both physical and economic).

Ngaire Naffine, 'The Legal Structure of Self-Ownership: Or the Self-Possessed Man and the Woman Possessed' (1998) 25 *Journal of Law and Society* 193, 204.

100 Jennifer Nedelsky, 'Reconceiving Autonomy: Sources, Thoughts and Possibilities' (1989) 1 *Yale Journal of Law and Feminism* 7, 12.

101 Ibid.

102 See, eg, Nedelsky, 'Property in Potential Life?', above n 92; Carol Gilligan, *In a Different Voice: Psychological Theory and Women's Development* (1982); Claudia Card (ed), *Feminist Ethics* (1991); Susan Sherwin, 'Feminist and Medical Ethics: Two Different Approaches to Contextual Ethics' in Helen Holmes and Laura Purdy (eds), *Feminist Perspectives in Medical Ethics* (1992) 17; Virginia Warren, 'Feminist Directions in Medical Ethics' in Helen Holmes and Laura Purdy (eds), *Feminist Perspectives in Medical Ethics* (1992) 32; Leslie Bender, 'A Feminist Analysis of Physician-Assisted Dying and Voluntary Active Euthanasia' (1992) 59 *Tennessee Law Review* 519; Sara Ruddick, *Maternal Thinking: Toward a Politics of Peace* (1989); Nel Noddings, *Caring: A Feminine Approach to Ethics and Moral Education* (1984).

103 Bender, above n 102, 536.

104 Ibid 536–7 (emphasis in original).

105 Nedelsky, 'Reconceiving Autonomy', above n 100, 12.

> To be autonomous a person must feel a sense of her own power (which does not mean power over others), and that feeling is only possible within a structure of relationships conducive to autonomy. But it is also the case that if we lose our feeling of being autonomous, we lose our capacity to be so. Autonomy is a capacity that exists only in the context of social relations that support it and only in conjunction with the internal sense of being autonomous.[106]

Instead of a property model as a symbol for individualised autonomy, Nedelsky proposes childrearing as the symbol for a related and interdependent understanding of autonomy.[107]

What is clear is that, to the extent that it stands in sharp contrast to liberal conceptions of autonomy, caring autonomy is also an embodied autonomy. While liberalism has rested on the Cartesian split between body and mind (as well as other dualisms such as public–private and reason–emotion), it is the male body and traditionally masculine attributes that have been privileged and the female body problematised.[108] The generic, yet defined nature of the male body within liberalism's legal and social analyses is challenged by alternative theories of the body articulated within feminist theory.[109] Embodiment has been a central concern of feminist theory. The claims of liberalism and liberal legalism to an abstract, disembodied and universal knowledge have been questioned by feminist scholars who have countered universal stories with stories of specificity, and of individuals whose lived realities are mediated through the embodied intersections of race, class, gender, sexuality, disability, and fertility.[110] Autonomy is not found in an extra-corporeal individual carrying a bag full of rights as a safeguard against the world. Instead, autonomy is articulated by an embodied self, through relationships with others. Reconceptualising reproductive autonomy in terms of embodiment can provide a new framework for thinking about contested or controversial reproductive issues.[111] Within the context of the new reproductive

106 Ibid 24–5.

107 Ibid 12.

108 For discussion see Nicola Lacey, *Unspeakable Subjects: Feminist Essays in Legal and Social Theory* (1998) 107–8.

109 See, eg, Mykitiuk, above n 88; Karpin, above n 88; Ngaire Naffine, 'The Body Bag' in Ngaire Naffine and Rosemary Owens (eds), *Sexing the Subject of Law* (1997); Carl Stychin, 'Body Talk: Rethinking Autonomy, Commodification and the Embodied Legal Self' in Sally Sheldon and Michael Thomson (eds), *Feminist Perspectives on Health Care Law* (1998).

110 The need to move beyond an essentialist view of the body and towards an appreciation of the multiple selves that constitute each of us has been the subject of feminist debate. See Elizabeth Spelman, *Inessential Woman: Problems of Exclusion in Feminist Thought* (1988); Diana Fuss, *Essentially Speaking: Feminism, Nature and Difference* (1989); Angela Harris, 'Race and Essentialism in Feminist Legal Theory' (1990) 42 *Stanford Law Review* 581; Marlee Kline, 'Race, Racism, and Feminist Legal Theory' (1989) 12 *Harvard Women's Law Journal* 115; Kimberle Crenshaw, 'Demarginalizing the Intersection of Race and Sex: A Black Feminist Critique of Antidiscrimination Doctrine, Feminist Theory and Antiracist Politics' [1989] *University of Chicago Legal Forum* 139; Martha Minow, 'Beyond Universality' [1989] *University of Chicago Legal Forum* 115. In the context of the new reproductive technologies it is important that feminist theories of embodiment are not premised on reproductive capacity as to do so risks excluding infertile or childless women. For discussion of infertility and feminist theory see Margarete Sandelowski, 'Fault Lines: Infertility and Imperiled Sisterhood' (1990) 16 *Feminist Studies* 33; Linda J Lacey, '"O Wind, Remind Him That I Have No Child": Infertility and Feminist Jurisprudence' (1998) 5 *Michigan Journal of Gender and Law* 163.

111 Stychin, above n 109.

technologies, an autonomy premised on connectedness and embodiment provides an alternative ethical framework within which the interests of the parties in debates over posthumous reproduction can be weighed and balanced.

VI Posthumous Reproduction: Weighing the Interests

What is it about posthumous reproduction that causes concern? Is it the sense that we have somehow failed to adequately respect the dead? Is it annoyance at the legal obstacles placed in the way of a deserving widow? Or is it concern for the welfare of a child born to a dead father? The interests of all these parties — the deceased, the widow, the child — as well as the broader social interest, must be weighed if we are to decide on the ethics of posthumous reproduction.

It may seem strange to consider whether a dead person has reproductive interests. After all, they are dead. Yet if we consider that sperm and embryos can be stored and used at a much later date, or that sperm can be retrieved from the body of a newly deceased man, it is clear that there are reproductive interests that can extend after death. Considering the interests of the deceased also makes sense when we look at the issues through a filter of caring-based autonomy.

The question of whether the deceased's interests have been upheld or violated cannot be determined by application of a blanket rule Each case must be considered individually. There is, after all, a fundamental difference between posthumous use of sperm stored by a man with a terminal disease in the knowledge that he may not survive the disease,[112] and the posthumous use of the sperm of a man who has died suddenly and has given no consent and expressed no wishes about the retrieval and use of his sperm in the event of his death. In the former case, the posthumous use of sperm may be furthering the interests and reproductive autonomy of the deceased, although there would, of course, be no obligation on his widow to actually put those wishes into effect unless she so desired.

A man who expresses wishes and views contrary to posthumous reproduction has a clear interest in having those wishes respected after his death.[113] The intervention of death does not necessarily abolish interests that flow from decision-making during life. Furthermore, as Schiff points out,

> it would be ironic indeed if the law were to protect pre-mortem wishes regarding the disposition of property, but ignore pre-mortem wishes concerning a

[112] Jansen has noted the importance of a sense of continuity for some terminally ill men:

> [M]en often store semen when they learn they have a life-threatening disease. On the face of it the motive may seem to be that they are to receive cancer-killing drugs which are likely, as a side effect, to destroy the sperm-forming tissues in the testes. But from my contact with these men I am aware they often have another motive: to preserve their genetic potential in the event that they die as a result of their disease. Many dying patients take comfort in the fact that they have children, that it is not the end of the road genetically. On the other hand among the causes of anguish adolescents have in facing death is unfulfilment of their procreative instincts.

Jansen, above n 78, 125.

[113] Anne Reichman Schiff, 'Arising from the Dead: Challenges of Posthumous Procreation' (1997) 75 *North Carolina Law Review* 901, 943.

matter as central to a person's identity as the desire not to create another human being.[114]

Where the deceased has clearly indicated that he objects to his sperm being used posthumously, there is no countervailing interest of the widow that overrules this. Although it is possible to argue that the widow's interest is in having her husband's child, the fact that while alive he objected to posthumous reproduction must be respected as an expression of his reproductive autonomy. To act contrary to an individual's wishes about posthumous reproduction where a person had expressed their opposition to it during their lifetime would be a gross violation of that person's interests and reproductive autonomy.

Even if posthumous reproduction were to be permitted, and this is undoubtedly a contentious issue, we should be very careful to ensure that appropriate legal safeguards are in place so that posthumous reproduction is only possible in cases in which clear consent had been given by the deceased during his lifetime. Although requiring consent will exclude those individuals who would not have objected to posthumous reproduction but who did not explicitly consent to the procedure,[115] as Schiff points out, 'it is difficult to see why it is any more fair to presume consent on the part of those who have contemplated posthumous conception but who decided against it while omitting to record their objections for posterity.'[116]

Permitting posthumous reproduction may of course present the need for some statutory reform. It would, for example, be necessary to amend relevant reproductive technology legislation that limits access to assisted conception procedures to married or de facto couples,[117] for without such amendments a widow would not qualify for treatment in those states with such requirements. One might also wish to impose limitations such as time limits (both a maximum period of time after the death for the use of the gametes to prevent a child being born 10 or 20 years after the death of his or her father, and perhaps also a time period stipulating that gametes must not be used before a certain period of time had elapsed so as to allow the widow a period of mourning and reflection). It would also be necessary to clarify whether the posthumous child would be regarded as a child of the marriage,[118] and to resolve any inheritance issues that may arise.[119] It

[114] Ibid. Schiff also argues:

> Posthumous conception likewise affects the deceased's interests, because it recasts the content and contours of the deceased's life. When it occurs without the person's consent, it deprives an individual of the opportunity to be the conclusive author of a highly significant chapter in his or her life.

Anne Reichman Schiff, 'Posthumous Conception and the Need for Consent' (1999) 170 *Medical Journal of Australia* 53, 53–4.

[115] Schiff, 'Arising from the Dead', above n 113, 951.

[116] Ibid.

[117] *Infertility Treatment Act 1995* (Vic) s 8; *Reproductive Technology Act 1988* (SA) s 13(3); *Human Reproductive Technology Act 1991* (WA) s 23(a).

[118] Under current laws, a child must be born within a specified period of time to be presumed to be a child of the marriage. For example, under the *Status of Children Act 1996* (NSW), a child is presumed to be a child of a marriage if 'born to a woman within 44 weeks after her husband dies': s 9(2).

is important to realise, however, that posthumous reproduction with consent is likely to be limited to a very small number of cases in which the man had knowledge of his impending death, such as in the case of a terminal disease, and was able to discuss the issues related to posthumous reproduction with both his family and his medical advisers.

For the man who has not given consent, or has not expressed any wishes, the issues are much more complex for we must ask ourselves, to what extent does it make sense to speak of reproductive autonomy after death? John Robertson has argued that posthumous reproduction has little in common with what we value in reproduction:

> With posthumous reproduction, the most important question is whether it is a meaningful reproductive experience to know in advance that one's genes might (or might not) be used to produce offspring after one's death. Ordinarily, reproduction is valued because of the genetic, gestational, and rearing experiences involved. Reproduction connects individuals with future generations and provides personal experiences of great moment in large part because persons reproducing see and have contact with offspring, or are at least aware that they exist.[120]

Robertson is undoubtedly correct in his argument here. There is obviously no way in which posthumous reproduction can share the nurturing and caring aspects we generally associate with and value in reproduction.

It is where the deceased has not made his views on posthumous reproduction known during his lifetime that the balancing of interests is most complex. And indeed this is the situation that is most likely to arise since there are likely to be very few men who will have discussed with their families and/or medical advisers whether they wish their sperm to be used after their death. In part this is because the whole concept of posthumous reproduction is still so new that it has yet to enter the popular consciousness, although media coverage of the Diane Blood case will obviously go some way towards changing this. It is also true that in general people do not like to contemplate their own mortality or the uses to which their body parts might be put in the event of their sudden death.

If the deceased's wishes are not known, there are strong arguments against the posthumous retrieval and use of his sperm. The decision to reproduce is so deeply personal and important that it is difficult to see how a person's interests are extinguished on death. In the absence of some indication of the person's

119 In *Re Estate of the Late K; Ex parte The Public Trustee* (Unreported, Supreme Court of Tasmania, Slicer J, 22 April 1996) it was held that a child born from a frozen embryo could have a right of inheritance. For discussion see Derek Morgan, 'Rights and Legal Status of Embryos' (1996) 4 *Australian Health Law Bulletin* 61. In the mid-1980s there was discussion of whether frozen embryos could, if implanted and born alive, inherit from their parents' estate after the parents were killed in a plane crash. See George P Smith II, 'Australia's Frozen "Orphan" Embryos: A Medical, Legal and Ethical Dilemma' (1985) 24 *Journal of Family Law* 27. For discussion of inheritance issues in this context see Rosalind Atherton, '*En Ventre sa Frigidaire*: Posthumous Children in the Succession Context' (1999) 19 *Legal Studies* 139. See also James Bailey, 'An Analytical Framework for Resolving the Issues Raised by the Interaction Between Reproductive Technology and the Law of Inheritance' (1998) 47 *De Paul Law Review* 743. I am grateful to Les McCrimmon for bringing this article to my attention.

120 John Robertson, 'Posthumous Reproduction' (1994) 69 *Indiana Law Journal* 1027, 1031.

wishes or views on these matters, consent cannot simply be assumed, even in the context of marriage. Even where a man and his partner have been planning or actively trying to conceive a child, it is difficult to assume consent to posthumous reproduction. A man who was happy to plan and have a child with his partner may nonetheless have reservations about *posthumous* reproduction.[121] The use of a person's reproductive material after their death, in the absence of their consent or knowledge of their wishes, violates not only the reproductive autonomy of the deceased but devalues its currency for the living.[122] We must ensure that the dead are treated with the respect with which we would like ourselves to be treated after death.

It is important to recognise the differences between reproductive tissue and other forms of human tissue. The posthumous use of sperm is not the same as posthumous use of non-reproductive tissue such as a kidney. As Anne Reichman Schiff points out, gamete donation 'is life-creating rather than life-sustaining or life-enhancing'.[123] It is precisely because of this difference that posthumous reproduction must be seen as distinct from organ donation.

Furthermore, we need to recognise that the widow has no special claim to access infertility treatment services. Her infertility appears to be only in relation to her dead husband[124] and, apart from the fact that she wishes to use the sperm of a particular man (her husband), her position is similar to single or lesbian women who wish to use infertility treatment services. Yet the widow is often portrayed as a deserving recipient of these services,[125] in contrast to single or lesbian women who are often seen as less deserving.[126]

While a grieving widow may wish to have her partner's child, the fact of death cannot be ignored. It is not simply a question of whether the widow has a right to possession of the sperm vis-à-vis a clinic holding the sperm, although the law may characterise the claim in terms of rights. Nor is it simply an issue of whether the rights of the widow outweigh the rights of the deceased.

As argued above, the language of property is inadequate as a framework for decision-making over gametes and embryos. We are concerned instead with

121 Schiff, 'Arising from the Dead', above n 113, 950.

122 Schiff argues:

> [I]f the state allowed family members to utilize the gametes of the dead for procreation without the deceased's consent, the lack of assurance that individuals would have about the fate of their own body parts could be a source of apprehension to the living.

Ibid 946.

123 Ibid 932.

124 Hazel Biggs, 'Madonna Minus Child. Or — Wanted: Dead or Alive! The Right to Have a Dead Partner's Child' (1997) 5 *Feminist Legal Studies* 225, 231–2.

125 Ibid 231–2.

126 Davina Cooper and Didi Herman, 'Getting "The Family Right": Legislating Heterosexuality in Britain, 1986–1991' (1991) 10 *Canadian Journal of Family Law* 41. As Michael Thomson has argued:

> The desire for a male presence appears so extreme as to privilege those who may provide a clinician with a macabre, disembodied and spectral presence over those who may seek treatment services with an embodied, corporeal and supportive partner who happens to be the same sex.

Michael Thomson, *Reproducing Narrative: Gender, Reproduction and Law* (1998) 188.

decision-making authority. This can only be exercised in a meaningful way within a matrix that conceives reproductive autonomy not as rights but as connection. It is for this reason that we need to evaluate the widow's claim in *relational* rather than rights-based terms.

How then do we conceptualise the widow's claim relationally? Consideration of these relational issues involves a consideration of the impact of posthumous reproduction on relationships. Posthumous reproduction changes the shape of the deceased individual's life and the relationships of that individual with others. In this respect, the potential impact of posthumous reproduction should not be underestimated:

> The use of an individual's reproductive material for posthumous procreation significantly affects the way that individual's life is remembered and regarded by the decedent's community and family — not least by the resultant child. Posthumous reproduction can alter in ways emotional, psychological, and financial the relationship between the deceased and any offspring already in existence.[127]

In addition, a relational analysis of posthumous reproduction requires consideration of the relationship between the widow and the deceased. When death intervenes, the corporeal bond between husband and wife is broken. While for the widow the emotional tie may live on, perhaps indefinitely, the husband's physical presence is no more. The process of grieving is the process of coming to terms with the absence of the person and their companionship. Part of that grieving process may be to grieve for the loss of future children that the couple could have had Once death has intervened, the relationship within which reproductive potential and autonomy could have been realised is at an end. Death does sever corporeal and relational bonds. Perhaps this sounds harsh. The temptation to have a living legacy of a dead loved one is enormous. Yet there is a time to let go There is a time at which nature's realities must be faced. There is a time at which it *is* too late.

VII Conclusion

Posthumous reproduction using assisted conception techniques is not simply about whether a widow has a right to have her dead husband's child. Central to this debate are questions about the significance of reproductive potential and the implications of this potential for decision-making over the body. This issue of decision-making cannot be separated from the issue of autonomy, and in this context, reproductive autonomy. The need to move away from a rights and property based conceptualisation of autonomy and towards an understanding of autonomy based on caring and relationships gains clarity in the reproductive context. It is this alternative understanding of autonomy that.provides a basis for determining that there are very few cases in which posthumous reproduction using assisted conception techniques can be justified. While the temptation to allow science to help is strong, at a policy level some limits must be imposed.

127 Schiff, 'Arising from the Dead', above n 113, 944–5.

Before translating scientific possibilities into actualities we must give careful consideration to past, present and future relationships between the individuals concerned for it is only by thinking relationally, rather than through rights, that we can determine the ethics of the new possibilities offered by science.

Research Subjects' Rights

[7]

The Suppressed Legacy of Nuremberg

by Robert A. Burt

The story of patient self-determination cannot be told without the Nuremberg trials. Patient autonomy was the first criterion enunciated by the Nuremberg judges and has served as a touchstone for human subject research and patient care ever since. Yet this ideal was in an important sense irrelevant at the moment it was originally proclaimed.

Nuremberg has a special resonance in the annals of law and biomedical ethics. Though it was not the first jurisprudential appearance for the principle of patient autonomy, the Nuremberg judgment gave central importance to this principle as an ideal that should govern physician-patient relations. When we retell the history of this relationship today—its evolution from "doctor knows best" to "patient self-determination"—honorific citation to Nuremberg is a conventional starting point in the narrative.

Depending on the narrator, there are two typical variations of the story. Most frequently, the plotline is a progression onward and upward for the application of the Nuremberg autonomy ideal: from research subjects to all patients, from the right to "informed choice" about extraordinary therapies to the right to refuse "ordinary" life-prolonging interventions such as tube feeding or antibiotics, from the right to refuse treatment to the right to obtain physician assistance in suicide.[1] In other, less common, recountings, the plotline puts Nuremberg at a pinnacle followed by decline; in this version, the vision of patient autonomy held aloft by the Nuremberg judges has subsequently been given lip-service but never fully honored in practice.[2] In either variation, the story has a triumphalist implication—a moral victory was won at Nuremberg and that victory serves as a beacon (or as a righteous rebuke) for us today.

Like many oft-told family stories, however, this narrative has a darker side that the constant retelling obscures and yet, at the same time, paradoxically keeps alive by the simple fact of its repetition. The self-determination ideal is, of course, much celebrated in our political tradition; it was the guiding ideal in this country for our War of Independence from Great Britain. Since that foundational moment, the ambit of this ideal has been a continuously contested proposition. The terms of this contest have had the same recurrent theme: that some social relationships are outside the self-determination ideal and are more properly (or even more "naturally") depicted as based on dependency and correlative inequality between caretaker and ward. This was the argument advanced in the nineteenth century by men of property regarding landless laboring men, by white slaveholders regarding black slaves, by men regarding women, by physicians regarding patients. The case for dependency and inherent inequality has, however, been a losing battle: the dominant narrative in our intellectual history has been the progressive spread of the self-determination ideal as the sole legitimate depiction of all these social relationships (however haltingly or imperfectly that ideal has been implemented in practice).

The application of the ideal to physician-patient relations is the most recent in this progression but it hardly seems surprising; and its invocation in the 1947 doctors' trial at Nuremberg is even less surprising in light of the fact that all of the judges in this proceeding were Americans, whereas the judges in the immediately preceding Nuremberg trials of high Nazi officials and German military officers were drawn from all of the Allied nations. There is, nonetheless, one surprising aspect to the conjuring of the self-determination ideal in the Nuremberg doctors' trial that seems, on close inspection, to raise some disconcerting questions about the legitimacy of its application there.

Consider the foundational example of the self-determination ideal in the American Revolution. In that context, the proponents of the ideal understood that if they had consented to the measures imposed by Great Britain regarding taxation or other matters, their consent in itself would have validated the British actions. At Nuremberg, however, it was clear that the consent of the experimental subjects would not have justified the experiments. The ideal of patient self-determination whose lineage is so proudly traced to Nuremberg was in an important sense irrelevant at the very moment that it was originally proclaimed. This is an odd beginning for a family history.

Patient self-determination was the first criterion that the Nuremberg judges enunciated—that "the voluntary consent of the human subject is absolutely essential"[3]—and this self-consciously awarded pride of place established the central role of the Nuremberg judgment in subsequent recitations of this ideal. But the

Robert A. Burt, "The Suppressed Legacy of Nuremberg," *Hastings Center Report* 26, no. 5 (1996): 30-33.

Hastings Center Report, September-October 1996

judges also invoked eight other criteria which, they said, "all [medical ethicists] agree . . . must be observed" in human experimentation. Only two of these standards dealt with self-determination: the first, as quoted, and the ninth, which specified that the subject must remain free to discontinue the experiment at any time. The other eight criteria all depended, more or less explicitly, on the application of "reasonable professional judgment." The second, for example, provided that "the experiment should be such as to yield fruitful results for the good of society, unprocurable by other methods . . . "; the sixth stated that "the degree of risk to be taken should never exceed that determined by the humanitarian importance of the problem to be solved. . . ."

The application of these standards faced a very different direction from the tribunal's initial insistence on patient consent. We have become so accustomed today to the norm of patient consent that we easily miss the disturbing implications of the differing perspectives between this norm and the other criteria in the Nuremberg pantheon. At the moment that the Nuremberg tribunal promulgated these standards, however, the disturbance—an undercurrent of loss and disillusion—was almost impossible to ignore.

We might recapture this sense by imagining that we ourselves had been judges at Nuremberg and that, before writing the ten standards in our formal judgment, we had presided over the 133 days of testimony about the concentration camp experiments. During those 133 days, we would have heard about camp inmates placed in pressure chambers where the simulated altitude was increased until their lungs and other body organs exploded; we would have heard about inmates plunged into ice water clothed in heavy military uniforms, or stripped naked and thrown outdoors in winter temperatures, where they remained (clothed or naked) until they had frozen to death; we would have heard about inmates purposefully burnt or cut by ground glass and left untreated until they died from the infection of their wounds; we would have heard about inmates whose healthy arms or legs were severed simply to test various surgical techniques for amputations.

After hearing all of this, during more than four months of testimony, imagine now that we adjourned to our conference room and talked among ourselves to arrive at a verdict. How plausible is it, in these discussions, that any of us would say: "The basic problem with these experiments is that the subjects did not agree to participate"? How truly important, or even relevant, was the question whether any subject had consented before his lungs were exploded in a high altitude chamber, before he was tossed into ice water until he froze to death, before he was burnt and left to die of infection, before his healthy arm was amputated to provide training experience for the surgeon? To insist on the importance, or even the relevance, of consent in these matters is surely peculiar. But the Nuremberg tribunal judges did indulge in this almost fantastic imagining. How could they have come to this? After hearing about these barbaric experiments for 133 days, how could they begin their judgment by proclaiming that their primary standard of moral evaluation was: "The voluntary consent of the human subject is absolutely essential"?

There is a plausible answer to this question, but it is a disturbing answer. This answer is that other imaginable criteria offered no comfort for the future. The fact was, as the 133 days of testimony clearly demonstrated, that these experiments had been approved and carried out by recognized leaders of the German medical profession, by holders of university chairs, by respected teachers and researchers of worldwide reputation. In the face of this social reality, other more apparently plausible condemnatory criteria—in particular, the criteria subsequently set out in the tribunal's judgment that good physicians never purposefully inflict death or disabling injury on anyone—lacked convincing effective force.

Considerable effort was expended after the war, both inside and outside Germany, to claim that the physicians in the Nuremberg dock were not well-respected scientists and that the Nuremberg experiments were not "good science" or "real science." This effort cannot withstand critical scrutiny.[4] But the Nuremberg judges did not in any event pursue this chimera; they followed a different strategy. They did not put their trust in the existence of "civilized standards" among future professionals—neither in doctors who might consider whether to perform experiments nor in government officials who might prospectively or retrospectively judge the propriety of those experiments. The Nuremberg judges established, as their first line of defense against recurrence of these barbarities, the individual subject-patient armed with the principle of self-determination.

The implicit lesson that the Nuremberg judges drew from the trial testimony was that they could not place principal reliance on the self-restraining decency of traditional embodiments of social authority. This was the lesson taught not only by the doctors' trial but by the preceding war crimes trials of high government officials. The Nuremberg judges were led to their reliance on the protection of individual self-determination by the same route that had conveyed Thomas Hobbes to this conclusion three centuries earlier. Sitting in Nuremberg in 1947—surrounded by the physical wreckage of war and confronted by a human spiritual degradation beyond any previous experience—the judges could readily have imagined themselves plunged into Hobbes's state of nature where no one could trust another for protection or comfort; a time without social bonds, a "war of all against all" where everyone was at the mercy of others' unconstrained avarice and aggression. As Hobbes had seen in the aftermath of the seventeenth-century English civil war, the only predictable source for human protection in such a world was each individual's solitary instinct for self-preservation.

Hobbes also saw that perpetual warfare, where each individual could rely only on himself, was an intolerable state for human affairs since life would necessarily be without valued meaning, would be "nasty, brutish and short." We need not endorse Hobbes's proposed solution, that each of us should enter a social contract surrendering personal authority to one absolute sovereign, to understand the powerful truth in his diag-

Hastings Center Report, September-October 1996

nosis that this endless sense of personal vulnerability and consequent perpetual wariness in all human relations is unbearable. But this unendurable world is precisely what the judges at Nuremberg glimpsed—and then tried strenuously to avoid.

If we look closely at contemporary American invocations of the self-determination ideal in doctor-patient relations, we can see the same underlying sense of betrayal and helpless vulnerability that framed the Nuremberg judgment.

If we look closely at contemporary American invocations of the self-determination ideal in doctor-patient relations, we can see the same underlying sense of betrayal and helpless vulnerability that framed the Nuremberg judgment—and even implicit parallels with the German concentration camp experiments in the expressed fears that medical technology imprisons and inflicts torture on many people. This nightmare vision was epitomized in the first state court case to apply the self-determination ideal specifically regarding the regulation of death in doctor-patient relations. In 1976, the New Jersey Supreme Court invoked this principle to free Karen Ann Quinlan, a young woman in a persistent vegetative state, from the mechanical respirator that apparently was keeping her indefinitely but insensibly alive.[5] The U.S. Supreme Court effectively endorsed this precedent in 1990, in a case like *Quinlan* involving an unconscious young woman.[6] In separate opinions, two justices testified to this same bad dream: "a seriously ill or dying patient whose wishes are not honored may feel a captive of the machinery required for life-sustaining measures" (Justice O'Connor) (p. 288); "the thought of an ignoble end, steeped in decay, is abhorrent" (Justice Brennan) (p. 310). The shadow of the Nazi experiments hovers in the background of these cases in the image of predatory doctors subjecting vulnerable people to inhumane scientific procedures in order to benefit some dogmatic social policy unrelated to the individual welfare of their patient-subjects.

In these cases, as in the Nuremberg judgment itself, the triumphalist recitation of the self-determination ideal masks several nagging background questions: How did these once-trusted caretakers become transformed into heartless predators? If they no longer can be trusted to protect vulnerable people, who can be trusted? Can I trust no one but myself when I am helplessly vulnerable? And, even more poignantly, is it enough to trust myself when I am helplessly vulnerable? To understand the self-determination ideal not as a transhistorical postulate but as the answer offered to these questions, questions that erupted urgently in a specific cultural and historical context, is to see the fragility and pathos that underlies our contemporary invocation of the ideal of self-determination.

This is our full connection with Nuremberg, a genealogy that is suppressed but nonetheless implicitly conveyed beneath the surface of our constant repetition of the triumphalist version of this family history. There is, however, a substantial cost to this mode of recollection, this unmentioned but nonetheless atmospherically conveyed dark suspicion of weakness that underlies our protestations of confident strength. The most compelling contemporary expression of this suppressed recollection is in the arguments for a right to physician-assisted suicide. The proponents of this right base their claim on the principle of patient self-determination. But the invocation of this principle in this context carries the darker aspects of Nuremberg along with the text of the tribunal's judgment. Just as the Nuremberg citation to self-determination did not resolve the issue before the tribunal, since the subjects' consent to the experiments would not have justified them, so too the self-determination principle is radically incomplete as a justification for physician-assisted suicide. In both contexts, the confident assertion of the self-determination right leaves unacknowledged and unanswered a crucial background question: who can be trusted to care for me when I am too vulnerable and fearful to care for myself?

The self-determination principle cannot answer this question since the question itself rests on the premise that the subject is too weak for effective self-protection. In the context of physician-assisted suicide, this unasked question arises in the gap between the professed principle of self-determination and the demand for the assistance of another person, a professional caretaker, to carry out the subject's wishes. If self-determination truly were the core value at issue in this demand, then the practicably available and legally recognized opportunities for self-administered suicide would have an obvious relevance. For terminally ill, mentally competent people in particular—the group for whom the right is exclusively claimed in the current cases[7]—existing law already provides the option not only of refusing high-technology life-prolonging treatment but also food and water. And when a terminally ill, mentally competent person makes this choice, existing law does not bar physicians from providing palliative care which, well within current technological capacity but without purposefully hastening death, can effectively address any physical discomforts that might accompany this path toward death.

The exercise of this option, which is fully justified by the internal logic of the self-determination principle, is not, however, enough for the current claimants. They want more than self-

Hastings Center Report, September-October 1996

determination. They want active assistance from physicians. They want active support from state officials in order to assure that physicians will care for them. They want a reassuring answer to the question that hovered behind the Nuremberg doctors' trial: whether physicians and/or state officials can be trusted to protect rather than abuse vulnerable people. The principle of self-determination was invoked by the Nuremberg judges in effect to mask the fact that they could not provide any reassuring answer. The same principle is also invoked today, most notably though not exclusively in the claims for physician-assisted suicide, more as an expression of mistrust toward physicians and the state than as a convincing refutation of that mistrust.

The staggering fact about our contemporary comprehension of the Nazi era in Germany is that we still cannot understand how and why it happened—whether it reflects some deep fault line in German character, in modern technological societies, in human nature; whether it was a unique historical event produced by a combination of forces unlikely to come together again, or whether its preconditions are readily replicable; whether any possible repetition can be averted by self-consciously devised preventive measures and, if so, precisely what those administrations might be. These large, terrible, unanswered questions are the full legacy of the Nuremberg trials. We are walking through these questions today in the specific context of claims for physician-assisted suicide. No wonder that a hasty conclusion, even a quick death, might appear preferable to an answer that we do not want to hear.

References

1. For example, Justice O'Connor's concurring opinion in Washington v. Harper, 494 U.S. 210, 238 (1990); Justice Brennan's separate opinion in United States v. Stanley, 483 U.S. 669, 687 (1987).

2. See Jay Katz, "The Consent Principle of the Nuremberg Code: Its Significance Then and Now," in *The Nazi Doctors and the Nuremberg Code*, ed. George J. Annas and Michael A. Grodin (New York: Oxford University Press, 1992), pp. 227-38.

3. "Judgment and Aftermath," *The Nazi Doctors*, pp. 94-107.

4. See Robert N. Proctor, "Nazi Doctors, Racial Medicine, and Human Experimentation," *The Nazi Doctors*, pp. 18-31; Christian Pross, "Nazi Doctors, German Medicine, and Historical Truth," *The Nazi Doctors*, pp. 32-52; Mario Biagioli, "Science, Modernity, and the 'Final Solution'," in *Probing the Limits of Representation: Nazism and the 'Final Solution,'* ed. S. Friedlander (Cambridge: Harvard University Press, 1992), pp. 185-205, at 185.

5. In re Quinlan, 70 N.J. 10, 355 A.2d 647 (1976).

6. Cruzan v. Director, Missouri Department of Health, 497 U.S. 261 (1990).

7. See Compassion in Dying v. Washington, 79 F.3d 790 (9th Cir. 1996); Quill v. Vacco, 80 F.3d 716 (2d Cir. 1996).

[8]

Research in Developing Countries: Taking "Benefit" Seriously

by LEONARD H. GLANTZ, GEORGE J. ANNAS, MICHAEL A. GRODIN and WENDY K. MARINER

An April 1998 *New York Times Magazine* article described Ronald Munger's efforts to obtain blood samples from a group of extremely impoverished people in the Philippine island of Cebu.[1] Munger sought the blood to study whether there was a genetic cause for this group's unusually high incidence of cleft lip and palate. One of many obstacles to the research project was the need to obtain the cooperation of the local health officer. It was not clear to Munger, or the reader, whether the health officer had a bona fide interest in protecting the populace or was looking for a bribe. The health officer asked Munger a few perfunctory questions about informed consent and the study's ethical review in the United States, which Munger answered. Munger also explained the benefits that mothers and children would derive from participating in the research. The mothers would learn their blood types (which they apparently desired) and whether they were anemic. If they were anemic, they would be given iron pills. Lunch would be served, and raffles arranged

Leonard H. Glantz, George J. Annas, Michael A. Grodin, and Wendy K. Mariner, "Research in Developing Countries: Taking 'Benefit' Seriously," *Hastings Center Report* 28, no. 6 (1998): 38-42.

so that families could win simple toys and other small items.

Munger told the health officer that if his hypotheses were correct, the research would benefit the population of Cebu: if the research shows that increased folate and vitamin B6 reduces the risk of cleft lip and palate, families could reduce the risk of facial deformities in their future offspring. The reporter noted that the health officer "laughs aloud at the suggestion that much of what is being discovered in American laboratories will make it back to Cebu any time soon." Reflecting on his experience with another simple intervention, iodized salt, the health officer said that when salt was iodized, the price rose threefold "so those who need it couldn't afford it and those who didn't need it are the only ones who could afford it."

The simple blood collecting mission to Cebu illustrates almost all the issues presented by research in developing countries. First is the threshold question of the goal of the research and its importance to the population represented by the research subjects. Next is the quality of informed consent, including whether the potential subjects thought that participation in the research was related to free surgical care that was offered in the same facility (although it clearly was not) and whether one could adequately explain genetic hypotheses to an uneducated populace. Finally, there is the question whether the population from which subjects were drawn could benefit from the research. This research intervention is very low risk—the collection of 10 drops of blood from affected people and their family members. The risk of job or insurance discrimination that genetic research poses in this country did not exist for the Cebu population; ironically, they were protected from the risk of economic discrimination by the profound poverty in which they lived.

Even this simple study raises the most fundamental question: "Why is it acceptable for researchers in developed countries to use citizens of developing countries as research subjects?" A cautionary approach to permitting research with human subjects in underdeveloped countries has been recommended because of the risk of their inadvertent or deliberate exploitation by researchers from developed countries. This cautionary approach generally is invoked when researchers propose to use what are considered "vulnerable populations," such as prisoners and children, as research subjects.[2] Vulnerable populations are those that are less able to protect themselves, either because they are not capable of making their own decisions or because they are particularly susceptible to mistreatment.[3] For example, children may be incapable of giving informed consent or of standing up to adult authority, while prisoners are especially vulnerable to being coerced into becoming subjects. Citizens of developing countries are often in vulnerable situations because of their lack of political power, lack of education, unfamiliarity with medical interventions, extreme poverty, or dire need for health care and nutrition. It is the dire need of these populations that may make them both appropriate subjects of research and especially vulnerable to exploitation. This combination of need and vulnerability has led to the development of guidelines for the use of citizens of developing countries as research subjects.

CIOMS Guidelines

In 1992, the Council for International Organizations of Medical Sciences (CIOMS), in collaboration with the World Health Organization, published guidelines for the appropriate use of research subjects from "underdeveloped communities."[4]

Like other human research codes, the CIOMS guidelines combine the protection of subjects' rights with protection of their welfare; as subjects become less able to protect their own rights (and therefore become more vulnerable), researchers and reviewers must increase their efforts to protect the welfare of subjects.[5] Perhaps the most important statement in these guidelines is what appears to be the injunction against using subjects in developing countries if the research could be carried out reasonably well in developed countries. Commentary to guideline 8 notes, for example, that there are diseases that rarely or never occur in economically developed countries, and that prevention and treatment research therefore needs to be conducted in the countries at risk for those diseases. The conclusion to be drawn from the substance of these guidelines is that in order for research to be ethically conducted, it must offer the potential of actual benefit to the inhabitants of that developing country.

In order for underdeveloped communities to derive potential benefit from research, they must have access to the fruits of such research. The CIOMS commentary to guideline 8 states that, "as a general rule, the sponsoring agency should ensure that, at the completion of successful testing, any product developed *will* be made reasonably available to inhabitants of the underdeveloped community in which the research was carried out: exceptions to this general requirement should be justified, and agreed to by all concerned parties before the research is begun."[6] This statement is directed at minimizing exploitation of the underdeveloped community that provides the research subjects. If developed countries use inhabitants of underdeveloped countries to create new products that would be beneficial to both the developed and the underdeveloped country, but the underdeveloped country cannot gain access to the product because of expense, then the subjects in the underdeveloped countries have been grossly exploited. As written, however, this CIOMS guideline is not strong or specific enough to prevent exploitation. Exemplifying this problem are recent short course zidovudine (AZT) studies in Africa that were approved and conducted despite the existence of the CIOMS guidelines.[7]

The African Maternal-Fetal HIV Transmission Studies

The goal of the short course AZT studies was to see if lower doses of the drug AZT than those used in the United States could reduce the rate of maternal-child transmission of HIV. It was well established that doses of AZT that cost $800 (not taking into account screening and other related costs) reduced maternal-fetal transmission of HIV by as much as two-thirds in the United States.[8,9] If the developed countries had been willing to subsidize the cost of this regimen in Africa, no additional research would have been needed. But because many African countries could not afford this expense, the decision was made to attempt to see if lower (and therefore cheaper) doses would prevent maternal-fetal HIV transmission. Several impoverished countries were chosen as research sites. The justification for conducting research in those countries was not that they suffered from a disease that did not afflict people in developed countries, and not because no treatment existed, but because their impoverishment made an existing therapy unavailable to them (as long as developed countries refused to subsidize the costs).[10]

The issue, as always, is to determine the ethical acceptability of the proposed research *before* it is conducted. In a case like this, where the researchable problem exists *solely* because of economic reasons, the research hypothesis must contain an economic component. The research question should be formulated as follows:

1) We know that a given regimen of AZT will reduce the rate of maternal-child transmission of HIV.

2) Maternal-child transmission of HIV in many African countries is a serious problem but the effective AZT regimen is not available because it is too expensive.

3) If an effective AZT regimen costs $X, then it will be made available in the country in which it is to be studied.

4) Therefore, we will conduct trials in certain African countries to see if $X worth of AZT will effectively reduce maternal-child transmission of HIV in those countries.

The most important part of the development of this research question is number 3. Without knowing what dollar amount X actually represents, it is impossible to formulate a research question that can lead to any benefit to the citizens of the country in which the research is to be conducted. There is no way to determine what $X represents in the absence of committed funding. Therefore, an essential prerequisite to designing ethical research in underdeveloped countries is identifying the source and amount of funding for providing the fruits of the research to the people of the developing country in which it is to be studied as a condition of the research being approved.

If a study found, for example, that $50 worth of AZT has the same effect as $800 worth of AZT, it would greatly benefit the developed world. Developed countries, which currently spend $800 per case on drugs alone, could pay substantially less for this preventive measure, and, because the research was conducted elsewhere, none of their citizens would have been put at any risk. At the same time, if the underdeveloped country could not afford to spend $50 any more than it could spend $800, then it could not possibly derive information that would be of any benefit to its population. This is the definition of exploitation.[11]

It is only now that an effort is being made to determine how to raise the money to actually provide AZT to prevent maternal-child HIV transmission (as well as the other costly services that go with the appropriate administration of the drug) to the impoverished African countries that provided the human subjects.[12] These efforts began after parallel studies conducted in Thailand reported that lower doses of AZT reduced maternal-fetal transmission of HIV.[13] The Thai government had committed to providing the AZT before its trials began. In the African trials, however, no one "ensured" that at the completion of successful testing the product would be made reasonably available, thereby violating the CIOMS guidelines.[14] The guidelines say that there can be exceptions to this general requirement, but that exceptions must be "justified" and "agreed to by all concerned parties." It is not clear to whom the exception must be "justified" or on what grounds. Moreover, if the "concerned parties" are the sponsor and/or the investigator and the host country, they may not adequately represent the interests of the research subjects. The fact that representatives of the research community and officials of the host countries agree to exploit the population does not make the research any less exploitive.[15]

Rules for Ethical Research in Developing Countries

We believe the standards for research in developing countries should include the following.

There should be a rebuttable presumption that researchers from developed countries will not conduct research in developing countries unless it can be shown that a direct benefit *will* be bestowed upon the residents of that country if the research proves to be successful. The person or entities proposing to conduct the study must demonstrate that there is a realistic plan, which includes identified funding, to provide the newly proven intervention to the population from which the potential pool of research subjects is to be recruited. In the absence of a realistic plan and identified funding, the population from which the research subjects will be drawn cannot derive benefit from the research. Therefore, the benefits cannot outweigh the risks, because there are, and will be, no benefits. Only by having committed funding and a plan to make a successful intervention available can it be determined that there will be sufficient benefit to justify conducting research on the target population. The distribution plan must be realistic. Where the health care infrastucture is so undeveloped that it would be impossible to deliver the intervention even if it were free, research would be unjustified in the absence of a plan to improve that country's health care delivery capabilities.

Some might argue that this standard is too strict and that it would reduce the amount of research that could be conducted in certain countries. The answer, of course, is that if the benefits of the research are not made available to the inhabitants of that country, they have lost nothing by the lack of such research. Others might argue that research in underdeveloped countries is justified if it might benefit the individual research subjects, even if it will not benefit anyone else in the population. However, research is, by definition, designed to create generalizable knowledge, and is legitimate in a developing country only if its purpose is to create generalizable knowledge that will benefit the citizens of that country. If the research only has the potential to benefit the limited number of individuals who participate in the study, it cannot offer the benefit to the underdeveloped country that legitimizes the use of its citizens as research subjects. It should be emphasized that research whose goal is to prevent or treat large populations is fundamentally public health research, and public health research makes no sense (and thus should not be done) if its benefits are limited to the small population of research subjects.

It might be argued that there is no requirement that such a plan be devised prior to conducting research in the United States, and, therefore, that by adopting such a requirement we would be imposing a higher standard for research conducted in developing countries than we do for research conducted in the United States.

This argument only further demonstrates the differences between wealthy and poor countries. The reality in the United States is that regardless of the very significant gaps in insurance and Medicaid coverage and the health care discrepancies between the rich and poor, medical interventions are relatively widely available, especially when compared to developing countries. Upon the successful completion of the research that demonstrated the effectiveness of the 076 regimen in reducing maternal-child transmission, the primary beneficiaries of this new preventive intervention in the United States were poor women and their newborns. Unlike the United States, absent a plan to pay for a new intervention and lacking the infrastructure to deliver an intervention, it is virtually guaranteed that the intervention will not be generally available in a developing country.

The more accurate analogy to the African AIDS trials would be if investigators proposed the 076 protocol in the United States knowing that only poor women would be recruited as research subjects and that, if successful, the intervention would not be made generally available to poor women. Such research would be clearly unethical. Not only would this be a gross violation of the ethical principle of distributive justice, it would be a violation of the regulatory obligation of the equitable selection of subjects.[16]

A further objection is that one cannot always trust what a government or another potential funder promises. What is to prevent the promisor from reneging? The answer is, nothing. One can try to expose the funder to embarrassment and other pressures that might cause it to live up to the promise upon which researchers and subjects relied. However, the potential unethical behavior in the future by the funder is no excuse for not having a realistic plan at the outset. Furthermore, if we take this obligation seriously, this should only occur once per funder. After reneging once, they cannot be relied upon again to justify research in the future.

An additional objection to our position is that it will restrict access to new interventions because once a new intervention is developed, the price will come down and therefore the intervention will become available to the people of the impoverished country. The answer is to ask those who control the pricing of interventions if this will be the case in any particular instance. One could have asked Glaxo if it would reduce its price once it was shown that lower doses of AZT were effective. If the answer is yes, one can proceed. If the answer is no, or "we have not decided," there seems to be no justification to proceed if the current price would significantly restrict availability. There is nothing magical about pricing. Pricing is in the absolute control of manufacturers and there is no need to guess or speculate about what will happen to price. Indeed, this objection to our argument would justify conducting the full 076 trial itself in developing countries. The price *might* come down enough so that determining the efficacy of short course AZT regimens might not be needed at all. Such speculation should not be sufficient to put subjects at risk.

Finally, it might be argued that there are diseases that only affect people in developing countries for which there are no effective treatments, but that the treatments that might be discovered could be expensive. The argument continues that it is not right to fail to develop treatments that could benefit some affected people because it will not be available to most affected people. This objection raises quite a different issue from the one addressed in this article. The impetus for such research is the absence of effective treatment and not the absence of economic resources. We have discussed research intended to determine whether effective but unaffordable interventions would work if used in lower, less expensive dosages. The researchable issue arises from an economic circumstance. The only way such research could offer any benefit is by "curing" the economic problem by establishing that the less expensive form of the intervention will be affordable and available. Absent knowledge of financial resources, one might well be creating a new unaffordable, and therefore useless, intervention. In contrast, in the case in which one is developing a new intervention, not because of poverty, but because no known effective intervention exists, and the disease is prevalent in a particular geographic area, the issue is quite different. In such a case one is not conducting research to try to "cure" the effects of poverty but rather because of the need to create new knowledge to treat a currently untreatable disease. However, even this case may raise problems similar to the ones addressed here. If one were to try to develop an intervention for such a condition and chose research subjects from impoverished segments of a society, knowing that only the richest segment of that society could benefit from that intervention, such subject selection would be unethical for many of the reasons we have discussed.

Our proposal to require researchers and their funders to develop realistic plans to make their interventions available to the relevant population of the developing country in which the research is proposed should not be controversial. It is well accepted in principle not only by groups like CIOMS, but by the funders of many of the African HIV trials, including the Centers for Disease Control and Prevention and the National Institutes of Health.[17] The principle is often honored in the breach, however. Research funders who hope that their studies will yield beneficial knowledge may neglect the steps necessary to ensure that the benefits will be made available. Ethical codes have not been sufficiently specific or enforceable to protect research subjects from exploitation. It is essential to replace vague promises with realistic plans that must be reviewed and approved before the research commences.

In at least one other instance it has been suggested that economic issues be addressed in the review of proposed research projects. The U.S. National Research Council's Committee on Human Genome Diversity recommended that "Arrangements regarding financial interests in the products or outcomes of the research should be negotiated as *part of the original project review* and informed-consent process."[18]

It is essential that the wealthier countries of the world use their resources, both financial and technological, to help resolve the health problems that afflict the poor of the world. Doing so will undoubtedly require research. But research is a means to solving health problems, not an end in itself. The goal must be to create interventions that will benefit the people of the countries in which the research is conducted. They will benefit only if the knowledge gained produces interventions that are affordable and accessible. This needs to be determined as a condition of approval before research is conducted so that limited research funds are not wasted, and research subjects are not drawn from populations that will not be able to benefit from the research.

References

1. Lisa Belkin, "The Clues Are in the Blood," *New York Times Magazine*, 26 April 1998.

2. Michael Grodin and Leonard Glantz, eds., *Children as Research Subjects: Science, Ethics, and Law* (New York: Oxford University Press, 1994).

3. Wendy K. Mariner, "Distinguishing 'Exploitable' from 'Vulnerable' Populations: When Consent Is Not the Issue," in *Ethics and Research on Human Subjects: Proceedings*, ed. Zbigniew Bankowski and Robert J. Levine (Geneva: CIOMS, 1993), pp. 44-55.

4. Zbigniew Bankowski and Robert J. Levine, eds., *Ethics and Research on Human Subjects: International Guidelines* (Geneva: CIOMS, 1993), pp. 25-32, 43-46.

5. Sharon Perley, Sev S. Fluss, Zbigniew Bankowski, and Francoise Simon, "The Nuremberg Code: An International Overview," in *The Nazi Doctors and the Nuremberg Code*, ed. George J. Annas and Michael A. Grodin (New York: Oxford University Press, 1992), pp. 149-73.

6. Bankowski and Levine, *Ethics and Research*, p. 26. Emphasis added.

7. George Annas and Michael Grodin, "Human Rights and Maternal-Fetal HIV Transmission Prevention Trials in Africa," *American Journal of Public Health* 88, no. 4 (1998): 560-63.

8. Edward Connor, Rhoda Sperling, Richard Gelber et al., "Reduction of Maternal-Infant Transmission of Human Immunodeficiency Virus Type 1 with Zidovudine Treatment," *NEJM* 331 (1994): 1173-80.

9. "Recommendation of the U.S. Public Health Service Task Force on the Use of Zidovudine to Reduce Prenatal Transmission of Human Immunodeficiency Virus," *MMWR Morbidity and Mortality Weekly Reports* 43 (1994): 1-20.

10. Harold Varmus and David Satcher, "Ethical Complexities of Conducting Research in Developing Countries," *NEJM* 337 (1997): 1003-1005.

11. The per capita health care expenditures of most of the African countries involved in mother-to-child HIV transmission prevention trials range from $5 to $22 U.S. *World Bank Sector Strategy Health Nutrition and Population*, 1997.

12. M. Bunce, "Chirac Seeks Worldwide Relief for AIDS in Africa," *Boston Globe*, 8 December 1997.

13. "Administration of Zidovudine During Late Pregnancy and Delivery to Prevent Perinatal HIV Transmission—Thailand 1996-1998," *MMWR Morbidity and Mortality Weekly Reports* 47, no. 8 (1998): 151-54. The editorial note states that "to implement these findings, ministries of health, donor agencies, and other interested agents *should* develop policies and practices to strengthen access to prenatal care, testing and counseling for HIV infections, and provision of ZDV for HIV-infected pregnant woman."

14. Bankowski and Levine, *Ethics and Research*, p. 45.

15. As the National Research Council's Committee on Human Genome Diversity properly put it, in the context of research on human subjects, "[s]ensitivity to the special practices and beliefs of a community cannot be used as a justification for violating universal human rights." Committee on Human Genetic Diversity, *Evaluating Human Genetic Diversity* (Washington, D.C.: National Academy Press, 1997), p. 65.

16. 45 CFR 46.111(a)(3).

17. Varmus and Satcher, "Ethical Complexities of Conducting Research in Developing Countries."

18. *Evaluating Human Genetic Diversity*, at pp. 55-68. Emphasis added.

[9]

Experimental Treatment
Oxymoron or Aspiration?

by Nancy M. P. King

Giving up the increasingly troubled distinction between "experiment" and "treatment" would make it easier to focus on informed consent and harder to beg questions about uncertainty and shared decisionmaking in medicine.

A lead article in the *New England Journal of Medicine* describes a retrospective cohort study comparing clinical outcomes in patients with patent ductus arteriosus (a common cardiopulmonary complication of prematurity) who had undergone standard surgical closure of the ductus with patients who had undergone transcatheter placement of a new device designed to occlude the ductus nonsurgically.[1] The authors state: "Placement of the occluder is currently considered investigational by the Food and Drug Administration." Nonetheless, in their methods section they describe the population of patients receiving occluders in the following way: "Although the choice of treatment reflected the physician's judgment, policies at the six occluder centers generally favored use of the device in eligible patients." And in the discussion section they observe: "New procedures are infrequently evaluated in randomized trials. . . . No randomized trial comparing the two strategies for closure of patent ductus arteriosus has been performed. . . . The rapid, almost universal adoption of the occluder device in some centers coincided with the continued exclusive use of surgery in comparable institutions." They conclude: "Despite the inherent promise of the new procedure, our results do not provide support for its widespread dissemination."

Later in the same issue, an editorial challenges those results.[2] The author first observes that the device is commercially available outside the United States, despite its investigational status here. Next he identifies some flaws in the study, concluding:

> Finally, and most important, the study compared the results of the first 4 ¼ years of experience with catheter occlusion with the results of 50 years of experience with surgery. . . . With the cumulative effects of time, competition, and new technology, catheter occlusion of the ductus should become cheaper and more effective. Premature acceptance of the results of the comparison . . . of an established method with one in its infancy could stifle innovation and be disadvantageous to patients.

Together these articles constitute a classic example of the venerable debate about the status of new treatments: Are they experiment, or are they therapy? It is striking that neither article calls for the randomized trial that has never been done to compare these procedures, each considering such a trial unnecessary in light of the available data, even though the conclusions they draw from those data are in diametric opposition. It is even more striking that neither appears to wonder about the patients who are offered a treatment that reflects "the physician's judgment," even though the device has investigational status only, surgical ligation is effective, and catheter occlusion is "in its infancy." Reading these articles I wondered what these patients (or, rather, their parents, because virtually all such patients are infants and young children) had been told about the investigational status of the occluder, the relative lack of information about its efficacy and safety, and the availability of a proven standard therapy. Their physicians, I am certain, were acting for the benefit of their patients in recommending the occluder instead of surgery. But should they have seen themselves as engaged in research instead?

Experiment: A Meaning in Context

Historically, medical treatments have long been distinguished from "experiments." Experimentation bears connotations of heroism—the risk-taking researcher who struggles altruistically, ultimately making the intuitive leap that saves patients' lives. But it also bears connotations of inhumanity, even monstrosity—of amoral or evil researchers and maimed and betrayed subjects.

In particular, the term *experiment* embodies societal ambivalence about what is new in medicine. We embrace innovation and recoil from it at once. New AIDS drugs, new cancer treatments, prenatal surgery, gene therapy, and a host of other examples from the nightly news have forcefully and repeatedly raised questions about when and how new technologies should be made available, who should have access to them, and who should pay for them. Very often, those questions are cast in terms of whether what is new is experimental

---

Nancy M. P. King is an associate professor in the Department of Social Medicine, School of Medicine, University of North Carolina, Chapel Hill.

Nancy M. P. King, "Experimental Treatment: Oxymoron or Aspiration?" *Hastings Center Report* 25, no. 4 (1995): 6-15.

Hastings Center Report, July-August 1995

or therapeutic. Why should this distinction hold so much interest, and have so much power?

Many medical technologies are labeled "experimental" at some point during their careers.[3] Although every medical treatment has been called an experiment with an *n* of 1, experiments are nonetheless generally thought to be exceptive cases in the practice of medicine as a whole. Examining how the term *experimental* has been and is defined and used in health law and policy should, then, provide some insights about how physicians, patients, and the public think—or ought to think—about what is worth doing in medicine.

What marks a medical technology as "experimental" rather than standard? What are—and what should be—the consequences of that label? The term is rarely, if ever, simply descriptive; instead, its application springs from particular concerns and often has significant consequences. The three principal contexts in which the designation "experimental" is currently applied to medical technology are medical malpractice, reimbursement, and research regulation. In medical malpractice, distinguishing between experimentation and therapy determines whether injured patients have been treated appropriately and provided with sufficient information about their treatment. In the context of insurance reimbursement, the choice of label determines whether a procedure will be paid for. And the federal regulations governing research with human subjects contain a definition that determines whether federal oversight is necessary. Research—experimentation—is the principal modern source of evidence about what works and doesn't work in medicine. Drawing the distinction between experiment and treatment addresses fundamental and long-standing questions about technology assessment and diffusion—that is, about how we determine what "works" in medicine, and about the nature of medical progress.

"Experiment" in Medical Malpractice

The experimentation label found its first application in medical malpractice law. What has been called the first malpractice case as well as the first consent to treatment case, decided in England in 1767,[4] concerned an apparently experimental device used in place of conventional treatment for a broken leg.

In early malpractice law, physicians experimented at their peril. Experiment was a pejorative term used by courts to justify holding physicians strictly liable for the adverse results of treatments deviating from the standard of care. Later, the term also began to be employed to imply use of the scientific method; thus, physicians defending themselves from malpractice or quackery charges would argue that they had experimentally devised a superior treatment method.[5]

Before the twentieth century, the practice of medicine was not organized into the powerful, self-regulating "scientific" profession recognized today. Instead, physicians struggled, on the one hand, against competition from nonmedical practitioners, and on the other, against the indisputable fact of medicine's own inefficaciousness, even dangerousness. The medical profession could use the experiment label to judge treatment acceptable or unacceptable, thus both claiming control over its members and drawing lines between its members and those outside mainstream medicine. Courts embraced both of these professional interests while claiming as their primary concern the limitation of innovation in the name of consumer safety. It was not until medicine became well recognized as a science, and the profession's power and reputation had grown considerably, that the chilling of medical progress came to be a concern of the courts.[6]

Cases raising the question of experimentation in the modern era generally apply the standards of medical malpractice and, increasingly, of informed consent. An experimentation case based in malpractice would condemn as experimental new or unproven treatments that deviate unreasonably far from the standard of care, especially when standard treatment is available. One based in informed consent might impose a requirement that patients be specifically informed of the experimental nature of the proffered treatment.

In addition, some plaintiffs have alleged that the physician deceptively claimed to offer treatment but in reality sought only to gather experimental data. This claim brings to mind the societal concerns about the integrity of medical research that have been raised by cases like the Tuskegee experiment[7] and the mid-century radiation experiments sponsored by the Departments of Energy and Defense and other federal agencies.[8] The courts are generally sympathetic to plaintiffs who claim to have been experimented upon against their will, particularly when there was an accepted treatment available, but such cases are uncommon.

Malpractice cases about experimentation thus set forth a variety of propositions about what patients need to know, about how much deviation from standard medical treatment is acceptable. Unfortunately it is difficult to learn much from them. Case law is not a subtle or precise definitional tool. Most of the cases contain little in the way of definition or analysis and focus simply on whether the treatment given was considered acceptable practice by the medical profession, generally making no distinction between medical treatments that are not yet accepted, treatments that fall below accepted standards, and treatments that are altogether outside medicine. However, some cases seem to embrace an intent-based distinction between experimentation and therapy, emphasizing that patients thought they were getting therapy (that is, treatment prescribed with their best interests in mind) when in fact they were the subjects of experimentation (that is, treatment offered primarily for its learning value to the experimenter). Others are willing to call treatments "experimental" where the physician's therapeutic intent is clear but his skill, his judgment, the quality of his disclosure, or the success or safety of the experimental alternative is in question. In at least some of these cases it is possible, albeit neither easy nor, indeed, necessary to the success of plaintiffs' claims, to read between the lines to discern a judicial concern about the potentially mixed inten-

Hastings Center Report, July-August 1995

tions of physicians who offer treatment innovations. Finally, though, the only thing that is clear from these cases about the employment of the term *experimental* in this context is that it is linked to avoidable injury to patients.

Desperate patients argue that technology assessment takes too long—it isn't fair to patients or physician-scientists to have to wait in the face of life-threatening illness.

Controlling "Experimentation" through Reimbursement

Insurers and other third-party payers have attempted to define "experimental" in the reimbursement context with a different object in mind: the limitation of their payment obligations. Although their agenda is clear, their success has been limited, for patient-centered reasons.

Treatment ordered for a patient by a physician is almost always paid for by someone other than the patient: by one of the many commercial health insurers, a Blue Cross/Blue Shield plan, a health maintenance organization, or federal and state plans like Medicare, Medicaid, and CHAMPUS. Virtually all such third-party payers have developed coverage and reimbursement criteria that are quite deferential to medical judgment, although in recent times additional oversight has been added through managed care (for example, precertification and second opinion requirements). The primary coverage criterion is often whether the treatment ordered is "reasonable and necessary," and disagreement about coverage lies in the standards by which reasonableness and necessity are to be judged. Should the criteria be patient-centered, evidence-based, or something else? How much risk is too much? How much cost is too high? What likelihood of success is too low? Whereas patients and physicians prefer the physician's individual therapeutic intuition to govern insurer reimbursement decisions, insurers are increasingly attempting to curb their responsibility to pay for treatments that are often both extremely costly and unlikely to succeed by seeking to apply more "scientific" definitions and standards of acceptability.[9] High dose chemotherapy with autologous bone marrow transplantation as a cancer treatment is the foremost current example of this kind of dispute. Third-party payers want most of all to get a return for their money. "Experimental" captures insurers' desire to know that what they pay for has a reasonable chance of working.

In a sense, these reimbursement disputes pit an intent-based definition of experimentation against an evidence-based definition. Patients and their physicians argue that the treating physician's desire to benefit the patient makes a proffered intervention reasonable and necessary; insurers answer that the likelihood of benefit, measured by scientific consensus, must be definitive. In response, desperate patients argue that technology assessment takes too long, and that, in any event, experimental treatments can't be treated like other technologies being assessed—it isn't fair to patients or physician-scientists to have to wait in the face of life-threatening illness. Litigation over the reimbursement status of technologies happens because patients who have run out of standard treatment options are offered treatments by their physicians that their insurers won't pay for. These reimbursement disputes are very affected by media publicity; they involve identified lives and are usually heart-rending, and they often result in liberalizing changes in insurers' practices in the first instance, and the rewriting of exclusionary language to limit payment in the second.

Although the outcomes of particular disputes depend upon specific contractual or regulatory language, the general effort to engage in coverage decisionmaking that is both less deferential to the judgment of individual physicians and less costly to insurers and other payers highlights some of the most significant issues for the future of technology assessment and the meaning of medical progress in the face of shrinking resources: Who is to have the responsibility for controlling the development and delivery of new medical care, scientists, physicians, patients, or payers? Should that control be centralized or decentralized? And upon what bases can we justify the controls we believe necessary, without curtailing medical progress or curbing patients' access to care?[10]

Concern about the lack of definitive technology assessment has often been expressed by those who purchase new medical technology and those who pay for its use. A variety of public and private assessment bodies have come and gone over the years, the most recent being the Agency for Health Care Policy and Research. Advocates of a centralized, authoritative assessment scheme might well look to the Food and Drug Administration's control of the development and introduction of new drugs and medical devices, and to the federal "common rule" regulating all government-sponsored research using human subjects, as guides. But does the current federal regulatory process serve us well?

Regulating "Experimentation"

The history of research regulation springs in significant part from the concern that physician-researchers may deliberately or inadvertently misrepresent their intent, with the result that patients may become research subjects without their knowledge or consent. The Nuremberg trials and Henry Beecher's 1960 exposé of modern institutional research formed the basis for public concern that external oversight was necessary in order to protect human subjects and

Hastings Center Report, July-August 1995

ensure the integrity of the research process.[11] In this context, the definition of *experiment* determines what conduct will be federally regulated. The conduct of research activities involving human subjects is governed by standards designed to prevent situations in which patients are experimented upon rather than treated, to ensure that the human subjects of experimentation are treated fairly and not exposed to excessive risks and harms, and to promote research that has both scientific validity and societal value. If the activities in question are not considered research but treatment, their conduct is not governed by this regulatory scheme, with its protective standards of oversight and relatively detailed informed consent requirements.

The key to distinguishing between research and treatment in this context has been held to be the physician's intent regarding the activities in question. The National Commission's *Belmont Report*, charged with defining research for purposes of protecting human subjects, defined medical "practice" as "interventions . . . designed solely to enhance the well-being of an individual patient . . . and that have a reasonable expectation of success." *Research* was then defined as "an activity designed to test a hypothesis, permit conclusions to be drawn, and thereby to develop or contribute to generalizable knowledge."[12] Current federal regulations continue to perpetuate this intent-based dichotomy between research and treatment, defining research strictly in intent terms, as "systematic investigation designed to develop or contribute to generalizable knowledge."

"Experimental Treatment": A Third Thing?

This intent-based dichotomy between research and treatment presents clearly a special problem of categorization that is only hinted at in the malpractice and reimbursement settings. What is to be done with those categories of activities in which the physician's intent is (or should be) *both* to benefit the patient *and* to gain generalizable knowledge about an insufficiently understood new technology? Or, to put the problem another way, what about treatments that are intended to benefit the patient, when there are questions about the reasonableness of the expectation of success?

According to the *Belmont Report*, "innovation does not, in and of itself, constitute research," but major innovations should "be made the object of formal research at an early stage to determine whether they are safe and effective."[13] Robert Levine, in preliminary papers prepared for the National Commission, urged that "innovative therapy" be conducted and reviewed as if it were research, reasoning that "if for purposes of review, innovative therapy (practice) is classified as research and reviewed by IRBs . . . the likelihood of introduction of 'bad' innovative practices should be minimized." He recommended that

> any innovative practice in which the deviation from customary practice is substantive should be conducted so that it most closely approximates the standards of good research . . . without obstructing the intent to bring direct health benefit to the patient-subject. . . . [This] means that the proposed innovative activity should be reviewed by an IRB, that the consent negotiation indicate that the activity is being performed with—at least in part—research intent, and so on.[14]

Levine would permit use of innovative therapies in "pure practice" contexts only if the physician-researchers involved are held accountable after the fact by the hospital board or the IRB.

In contrast, in another paper prepared for the National Commission, John Robertson took the position that not all innovative therapies need to be treated as research. He reasoned that to do so would greatly increase the workload of IRBs without necessarily protecting patients' interests any better than tort remedies. He focused on the physician's ability and inclination to calculate accurately and convey honestly the risks and benefits of innovative treatments. He saw no great difference in these respects between standard and innovative treatment, and no reason to presume that before-the-fact review would police these matters better than after-the-fact lawsuits.[15]

Although Robertson's analysis is persuasive, it does not consider that choosing to treat innovative therapy like standard therapy has wider implications for how progress in medicine is appropriately evaluated, as well as for the practices of physician-researchers (like those at centers using the ductus occluder of our first example). As Jay Katz explains:

> First, the establishment of regulations for the conduct of human research has led investigators both wittingly and unwittingly to label their interventions "therapy" rather than "research" in order to avoid the requirement of protocol review. For example, at a national meeting I listened to an interesting paper on the treatment of leukemia in young children. . . . During the discussion period I expressed surprise that [the investigator] had been able to receive IRB committee approval for a project that exposed infants to considerable discomfort. He responded that committee review had been unnecessary because his was not a research project, but a therapeutic intervention. I pressed him for an explanation and he told me that he had employed these procedures only in order to be more helpful to his infant-*patients* in the therapeutic management of their disease.
>
> Second, a related problem emerges in the all-too-quick decision to designate procedures . . . therapeutic ones . . . before careful experimental studies on efficacy have been conducted. . . .
>
> Third, investigators . . . have employed informed consent as a justification for their research studies without first posing and answering the following crucial question: Are the innovative or experimental procedures at a stage of development to justify approaching patients and asking for their consent?[16]

But the problem of how to regard "experimental treatment" is not only

Hastings Center Report, July-August 1995

one of determining whether to include *more* interventions under the umbrella of regulation and oversight. The confusion surrounding the intent-based definition also works to undermine our current understanding of the regulation of research on interventions aimed at treating seriously debilitating and life-threatening conditions and conditions for which effective standard therapy does not exist. The confusion between research and treatment has had an important effect on the development of drug treatments for AIDS[17] and on the conduct of clinical trials for many advanced cancers and other conditions.[18] Even that most futuristic of research avenues, experimental gene therapy, has not escaped this confusion, as access to experimental modalities is considered a last chance for cure.[19] Gene therapy protocols are conducted according to the federal regulations for research with human subjects.[20] But even when, as here, it should be clear that the purpose of the research is to determine *whether* an intervention can ameliorate a disease, the researchers themselves, and the committees set up to consider the research protocols, get confused by the ultimate goal of benefiting patients. Consider the following example.

The minutes of the Recombinant DNA Advisory Committee and its Human Gene Therapy Subcommittee (HGTS), published in the *Recombinant DNA Technical Bulletin*, contain many discussions of informed consent in experimental gene therapy. The committee's and subcommittee's consideration of a protocol for gene therapy of familial hypercholesterolemia (FH)[21] provide an excellent illustration of the conceptual confusion between research and treatment that follows from an intent-based distinction and the resulting problem of so-called therapeutic research.

Conventional medical, pharmacological, and dietary treatments for patients with FH have only a small effect in ameliorating its damage to the heart and liver. Liver transplant, which would replace the patient's liver with one capable of producing the low-density-lipoprotein (LDL) receptor that is needed, carries the not inconsiderable risk of rejection. The experimental protocol involves isolating hepatocytes from the patient's liver, combining them with a retroviral vector carrying genes that express the LDL receptor, and reinfusing the genetically altered hepatocytes into the liver through the portal vein. The hope is that these altered hepatocytes will "seed" the liver and lower the patient's blood cholesterol level. An increase of 5 percent in the expression of LDL receptors and thus a modest decrease in serum cholesterol—for example, from 900 to 700 mg/dl—would be considered a success. Successful gene therapy is therefore not a cure, but researchers hope that it would permanently diminish the patient's baseline serum cholesterol enough to make conventional therapies more successful.

At its meeting of 29 July 1991, the HGTS discussed the inclusion of children in the FH protocol. Children too young to consent for themselves are generally included in human subjects research only if the research carries few or no risks or promises significant benefit to subjects. This research carries risks, some of which are unknown, and there is no promise of benefit to individual research subjects. Thus, lawyer-ethicist Alexander Capron argued that because there are many adults with FH, who can consent for themselves, the involvement of children should be postponed until the experimental treatment is proven efficacious and reasonably safe:

> Mr. Capron said that because this disease affects children as well as adults, the safety and efficacy of the treatment first should be determined in adults. Dr. Parkman said that treating adults before children is discriminatory against children. . . . The only other option for these children might be a liver transplant. However, they might not receive the transplant because of the cost issue, whereas they could participate in this clinical protocol free of charge. . . . Mr. Capron said if markedly beneficial results are achieved in adults, the treatment of children should be initiated. . . . Mr. Capron moved to limit treatment to subjects who are capable of giving their own consent. . . . Dr. Parkman said this is an important issue. However, it is important that children have equal access to innovative therapy.[22]

Here Dr. Parkman's suggestion that restricting enrollment to adults in the first stage of the FH protocol is discrimination against sick children appears to illustrate a conviction that participation in the protocol will benefit subjects—a conviction that is not warranted in research. His conviction was buttressed, however, by his concerns about the efficacy and availability of "standard" treatments, like liver transplantation, and by his use of the term *innovative therapy*—an attempt to sidestep the research-treatment distinction. Note that even the person taking the minutes could not avoid conceptual confusion, stating: "Mr. Capron moved to limit *treatment*," when Capron's point in putting his motion forward was that the FH protocol is research, *not* treatment.

Professor Capron's motion to restrict enrollment to patients who can give their own consent failed. On 8 October the full RAC considered the issue again, and Professor Capron reiterated his argument:

> He expressed concern, as he had at the subcommittee meeting, that this research, which is still at a very early stage of gene therapy, should not be performed with children. This is a disease which does not express itself only in children but also expresses itself in adults. The committee has to recognize the fact that this remains experimental, and the researchers say there is only a small possibility that there will be any benefits. This is a learning process. Learn first with people who can consent to participate in that context. . . . Mr. Barton moved that the treatment be restricted to adults. Dr. Leventhal refused to accept the amendment, because she said that the treatment should be available to patients on the basis of symptoms, not age. . . . It is a deprivation, not a protection, to disallow a patient that needs treatment. . . Ms. Buc said recog-

Hastings Center Report, July-August 1995

nizing that there are risks, the question is not really who is most likely to benefit but from whom it is appropriate to elicit consent. . . . Dr. B. Murray added that because of the risk of other experimental therapies, such as liver transplantation or heart-lung transplantation, she would be opposed to the age limit restriction.[23]

This motion to restrict patient selection to persons eighteen or older also failed.

Here the full committee had a discussion very similar to that held in the HGTS. Dr. Leventhal's concern that restricting participation in the protocol to adults would deprive children of needed treatment correlates with the minutes' description of the protocol as treatment. The recorder's attempts to capture the discussion resulted in many inappropriate uses of the term *treatment*, but also in a paraphrase of Professor Capron's argument that employed the tortuous notion of "research at a very early stage of gene therapy." In discussion before both groups, disagreement over whether to view the protocol as essentially experimental or essentially therapeutic was influenced by the severity of the condition, by the nature of alternative therapies, both standard and experimental, and by the intent of researchers.

Maybe the right question to ask is whether experimental treatment is more like standard therapy or more like research. Considering it like one or the other essentially has to do with the way medical progress is conceptualized. To view it as therapy is to place one's faith in the individual physician's desire to help patients, and to view it as research is to claim that only the scientific method holds out the hope of benefit, even to the individual patient currently in need.[24] But as the FH example illustrates, the uses of this third term, *experimental treatment*, are complex enough to defy the dichotomy.

Is a Larger Discussion Needed?

The three settings in which the attempt is made to distinguish "experiment" from "treatment" are different enough to make comparisons among them difficult. Medical malpractice law is primarily concerned about assigning responsibility for injuries suffered by patients. Insurance companies and other payers draft policy exclusion language to limit reimbursement for treatments that are costly and arguably ineffective. Federal research regulations serve to determine when their elaborate oversight mechanism should be applied (and it is certainly true that IRBs already have plenty of work to do, and that many substantial issues remain for them to address if they are to do it well).

Given the same example, then, decisionmakers in the three settings might well draw different conclusions about where the line between experiment and treatment should be drawn. However, the elements informing their considerations about the distinction have much in common. All include, in some way, a recognition of intent; a consideration of reasonableness, like the degree of deviation from accepted treatment, or the likelihood of success, or the need for systematic and generalizable knowledge; and some role for the patient's or subject's informed choice. All three seek to avoid harm to current patients, on the one hand, and to avoid chilling scientific progress, on the other.

The question, then, is whether examining the experiment/treatment dichotomy in these contexts can help determine how to draw the proper line between them, or how to define, describe, and deal with experimental treatment as a third thing. The examination appears to have resulted in a recipe that consists of nothing but ingredients—no proportions, no directions for their combination.

Experimental treatment has been controversial at least since the Declaration of Helsinki first permitted the use of the therapeutic privilege to bypass the need for physician researchers to obtain consent to "clinical research."[25] "Experimental treatment," as it jumps from one side of the intent-based dichotomy to the other, potentially both expands and contracts the meaning of "experiment." Should "experiment" be contracted to mean only organized research using the federal regulatory model of IRB-approved randomized control trials? Or should it be expanded? Already, the FDA's changes in its new drug and device approval process include fast tracking, parallel tracking, treatment applications, investigational new drug and compassionate use exemptions. But an expanded definition of what is experimental could go much further and include all therapeutic experimentation in medicine and surgery. Like the ductus occluder and countless other examples, this kind of treatment innovation is usually undertaken after internal peer review, uses research methods other than RCTs, such as case collection, and anticipates publication in professional journals—but it is not currently subject to standardized external oversight like that promised by federal regulators, and it is usually paid for by third-party payers, who would often prefer not to.[26]

Intent would be a clean and logical point on which to hang the distinction between experiment and treatment, from which all else could follow—except that experimental treatment has an intent problem. The *Belmont Report* envisioned that therapeutic intent would work in concert with

Maybe the right question to ask is whether experimental treatment is more like standard therapy or more like research.

Hastings Center Report, July-August 1995

evidence-based technology assessment criteria to determine how innovative therapy should be regarded and regulated. But the examples discussed herein, and many others, demonstrate that therapeutic intent tends to overwhelm other considerations in that determination. Moreover, both patient-subjects and physician-researchers suffer from the confusion of therapeutic and research intentions. Researchers may offer patient-subjects participation in research, wrongly characterizing it as for their benefit; and when they participate in research, patient-subjects may also wrongly feel betrayed when they are treated as subjects rather than as patients.

For these reasons, it is necessary to examine critically the desirability of perpetuating the intent-based distinction between research and treatment, and of continuing to try to describe experimental treatment as embodying two intentions. But it is not easy to wipe intent out of the equation either. Therapeutic intent is a powerful thing; springing as it does from the motivations at the heart of the physician-patient relationship, it cannot easily be discounted.[27] Perhaps the desire for the patient's benefit ought instead to be classed with hope: necessary and inevitable, but having meaning only when success is reasonably possible. Since intent to benefit the patient is not enough, we must go on to examine the consequences of concluding that more than intent is necessary to protect patients. We must define and measure the reasonableness of the possibility of success in the context of experimental treatment.

And surprisingly, these questions turn out to be almost indistinguishable from those being raised by the futility debate.

Doing this requires us to ask some hard, fundamental questions about medicine. As we have seen, underlying the question of what constitutes research are questions about how much and what kind of evidence about the safety and efficacy of new treatments is needed; how such things are to be measured; and whether, when, and how new treatments should be made available to patients. And surprisingly, these questions turn out to be almost indistinguishable from those being raised by the futility debate: If we ought not to do what doesn't work to benefit patients, what "works"? How well does it have to work? What amount and kind of evidence of efficacy is sufficient? How does safety fit in? Is greater promise of efficacy required if the safety risks are greater? Is a lesser promise of efficacy required if there is no other treatment that works?[28]

These questions call up a longstanding and far-reaching debate about the need for and nature of a fair and universal standard of safety and efficacy, and about whether the RCT constitutes that "gold standard." This debate, which ranges far beyond the confines of the current inquiry, explores the validity and practicality of the randomized clinical trial in research, the differences between clinical and scientific skills and values, and the physician's intent-based "double agent" problem of tempering patient advocacy with scientific judgment in the decision to offer experimental treatment, either as treatment or as research. "Experimental treatment" is often viewed by respectable physicians as promising enough to recommend. This has happened with many medical and surgical innovations. Some of these have proven effective, others have been shown to be ineffective, and the efficacy of others is still in question—like the ductus occluder, about which the proof is disputed, and where the disputes themselves raise the question of what constitutes sufficient proof.[29]

Not only is the "gold standard" of the RCT disputed; it may even be outmoded. The promise of genetic medicine is turning us toward individually tailored treatments that are ill-suited to conventional evaluation through research. The stakes are high and getting higher in experimental treatment; "hard facts" about safety and efficacy are harder to come by as the standards for the introduction of new therapies change, changing researchers' ability to collect data. Perhaps, then, it is time to address more systematically the role of the scientific method in medicine—to ask how the standard of care is developed in malpractice, how technology assessment should proceed in medicine, and how the two and reimbursement policy should fit together.[30]

Giving up the Distinction

The attempt to distinguish "experiment" from "treatment" and "researcher" from "physician" seems especially doomed precisely when these terms appear most troublesome and in need of sorting out. They are most troublesome when patients are desperately ill and standard therapies are risky and of low efficacy; when treating physicians are also engaged in or associated with clinical research on their patients' conditions; and where there is disagreement about how the available evidence should be interpreted, so that the status of the intervention as experimental or standard is in doubt but individual physician-researchers have strong views. The richness and complexity of the toughest examples of the problem make any neat distinction appear not only implausible but counterproductive, tending, as Katz noted, to beg important questions about the interventions at issue. If physicians and researchers find that applying the distinction confuses or oversimplifies their own understanding of an intervention, surely it will similarly affect their ability to explain and describe the intervention to patients and subjects.

Hastings Center Report, July-August 1995

Robertson argued that the physician's ability and willingness to engage in an honest and meaningful informed consent process is of critical importance regardless of whether research or treatment is at issue. I propose that giving up "experiment" versus "treatment" makes it easier to focus on the informed consent process and harder to beg questions about uncertainty, authority, and the elusive ideal of shared decisionmaking in medicine.

Once we give up the labels, what remains, I propose, is the requirement that physicians offer meaningful justification for their recommendations to patients. In a genuine decisionmaking partnership, meaning is negotiated; therefore, this is an informed consent requirement. I intend it to apply equally well to the informed consent ingredients for both "treatment" and "research," as defined in common law and federal regulations, and to informed consent in cases that might or might not fall in between, like our two examples: the ductus closure device and FH gene therapy. Every rich and complex example of "experimental treatment" that has been debated in the literature and in the press has a distinctive social and historical context, as regards the disease and its treatments, patients and physicians, institutions and financing. Knowing and understanding this context for each "experimental treatment" is essential to understanding and explaining them for the purpose of shared decisionmaking.

The ductus closure example might be taken as a paradigm case for Benjamin Freedman's notion of clinical equipoise:[31] Physicians at two groups of institutions have come to opposite, strongly held, conclusions about which of two therapies is superior, but the question is not settled in the profession as a whole. Reputable physicians therefore make different recommendations to patients.

This alone is indisputable evidence of the existence of uncertainty and the subjective nature of medical judgment. But uncertainty must be acknowledged and managed. What makes a recommendation meaningful in this context? Certainly the existence of an alternative treatment, viewed by other reputable physicians as the better choice, is an extremely significant factor. The labels "standard" and "experimental" provide less information to parents here than would explanations of the nature of each choice, the amount of experience with it, and the evidence of its risks and likelihood of success that has been amassed from that experience.

The physician's reasons for preferring one choice must have more content for parents than the circular "this is standard" and "this is promising." After all, in the institutions that have made policy choices about which therapy to use, proponents of the new occluder device had to make a case for it (for example, "this is less invasive"), and those sticking to the status quo presumably had reasons as well (for example, "surgery works fine and there is insufficient experience with the device to date"). If there are other reasons at issue (for example, "this brings in more revenue for less labor" versus "nobody here has learned the new technique yet"), some of those reasons may have meaning for parents, though their meaning may not be the same as for physicians; other reasons may not survive scrutiny when offered for examination.

The context for this example includes some other significant features, though. The condition is one common complication of prematurity, itself a complex and sometimes serious, but by no means always life-threatening condition. Parents are often at a serious information disadvantage in the decisionmaking partnership for their ill premature newborns, because they lack experience with the illnesses, they often lack experience as parents, and the technological complexities of the treatments leave many of them highly inclined to rely on their physician's judgment. Treatment of a patent ductus arteriosus often appears as one component of a multifaceted treatment plan of interdependent parts, and the ductus treatment plan itself may have several stages, beginning with minimally invasive components like fluid management and medication. Thus, an informed consent process that focused on meaningful justification for a part of such a treatment plan might have little apparent effect on parents' choices in most instances, though there could be some instances in which parents had strong preferences (for example, against surgery).

The gene therapy example might play out somewhat differently. Because FH is an inherited disorder, patients or their parents are more likely to bring knowledge and experience to the decisionmaking process, and also to have ongoing long-term relationships with physician-researchers. FH patients can be of any age, and are affected with varying degrees of severity; thus, the weighing of risks and benefits for each possible treatment will differ for each patient. The context for decisionmaking encompasses a lifetime goal of reducing the impact of a chronic condition that ranges from serious to very dangerous. And the treatment choices—drugs, liver transplantation, and experimental gene therapy—are extremely disparate. Meaningful justification for a recommendation regarding experimental gene therapy might include comparison with the degree of effect drug therapy can have; consideration of the risk, expense, and life-course of transplantation; and the significant unknowns of gene therapy, including whether there will be any effect, how great and how permanent any effect might be, and the possibility of other unanticipated effects. Possible reasons for choosing among these alternatives seem especially likely to reflect underlying values, as well as the health and circumstances of particular patients: risk aversion; financial considerations; the attractiveness of a "complete cure" as offered by transplantation; altruism; contributing to medical progress, or being on the cutting edge; avoidance of harm; and confidence, or lack thereof, about the unknown. Patients, parents, and physicians might all hold strong views about which choice is best. In addition, the systematic collection of data so as to produce generalizable knowledge may, in this case, have an effect on the experience of one choice, and so must be considered in the decision.

But wait: If we are getting rid of the labels, shouldn't we be systematically gathering knowledge, one way or another, from every treatment?

Hastings Center Report, July-August 1995

Certainly we need more data on liver transplantation, because there isn't all that much yet, but also from both choices in the ductus example, because that was the problem in the first place. And while we're at it, why take one treatment choice—one component of a treatment plan—and subject it to the meaningful justification standard unless we subject all components to it? Just as in both our examples the "experimental" option can only be made sense of in the context of the treatment plan as a whole, so each component of treatment informs the others, both from the standpoint of the production and ordering of the physician's knowledge and understanding and for the purpose of shared decisionmaking between physician and patient. Which is precisely the idea.

To begin applying a meaningful justification standard, it is necessary to encourage physicians and patients to talk more about some things that aren't often talked about well: medicine's limits, patients' expectations, and physicians' recommendations. Once again, similarities to the futility problem are striking. Tom Tomlinson and Howard Brody argued some time ago that patients' autonomy is not served by allowing them to choose ineffective therapies, but that it might be increased through discussion with their physicians of both patient's and physician's reasoning about treatment choices.[32] Such discussions are challenging, to say the least. They are especially difficult because physicians and patients have been using medical progress and its attendant labels to avoid them for many years. But it is exactly this kind of discussion that Alexander Capron wrote about twenty years ago as helping to promote autonomy, to protect the patient-subject's status as a human being deserving of respect, to prevent fraud and duress, to encourage self-scrutiny by the physician-researcher, to promote rational decisionmaking, and to involve the public in discourse about significant questions of policy in health care and research.[33]

Within the decisionmaking partnership between physician and patient, discussion of evidence and reasoning about medical choices, about mixed and complicated roles and intentions, and about hope and limits does more than begin the process of rethinking "experimental treatment." Discussion of these issues really amounts to negotiating and renegotiating the meaning of treatment and of treatment choices. Moving away from labels to work with a meaningful justification standard thus holds out the possibility of directly engaging physicians and patients along with institutions and policymakers in a deep and ongoing critical inquiry about the nature of medical power and medical progress.

Acknowledgments

I am indebted to my former research assistant, William L. Christopher; to my colleagues, especially Larry R. Churchill, Gail E. Henderson, and Keith A. Wailoo; and to the Triangle Bioethics Group for their creative and critical contributions to the ideas in this paper. An earlier version of this paper was presented at the Annual Meeting of the Society for Health and Human Values, Washington, D.C., 6 November 1993.

References

1. Darryl T. Gray et al., "Clinical Outcomes and Costs of Transcatheter as Compared with Surgical Closure of Patent Ductus Arteriosus," *NEJM* 329 (1993): 1517-23.

2. Michael Tynan, "The Ductus Arteriosus and Its Closure," *NEJM* 329 (1993): 1570-72.

3. Stanley J. Reiser, "Criteria for Standard versus Experimental Therapy," *Health Affairs* 13, no. 3 (1994): 127-36.

4. Slater v. Baker and Stapleton, 95 Eng. Rep. 860, 2 Wils. K.B. 359 (1767).

5. Carpenter v. Blake, 60 Barb. 488 (N.Y. Sup. Ct. 1871), *aff'd*, 75 N.Y. 12 (1878).

6. Brown v. Hughes, 94 Colo. 295, 30 P.2d 259 (1934); Fortner v. Koch, 272 Mich. 273, 261 N.W. 762 (1935).

7. James H. Jones, *Bad Blood: The Tuskegee Syphilis Experiment* (New York: Free Press, 1981).

8. Advisory Committee on Human Radiation Experiments, *Interim Report* (21 October 1994).

9. The many legal disputes are comprehensively discussed in Mark A. Hall and Gerard F. Anderson, "Health Insurers' Assessment of Medical Necessity," *University of Pennsylvania Law Review* 140 (1992): 1637-1712. See also the article, editorial, and Sounding Board piece on this issue in the *New England Journal of Medicine* of February 1994. If the current system pays for much that does not work, then the problem of distinguishing between experiment and treatment is only a subset of the problem of uniform, efficient, accurate, and meaningful technology assessment. See, for example, Wendy K. Mariner, "Medical Technology Assessment—Intended for Whom?" *American Journal of Public Health* 83 (1993): 1525-26; Maxwell J. Mehlman, "Health Care Cost Containment and Medical Technology: A Critique of Waste Theory," *Case Western Reserve Law Review* 36 (1986): 778-877.

10. George J. Annas, "Faith (Healing), Hope and Charity at the FDA: The Politics of AIDS Drug Trials," *Villanova Law Review* 34 (1989): 771; Nancy M. P. King and Gail E. Henderson, "Treatments of Last Resort: Informed Consent and the Diffusion of New Technology," *Mercer Law Review* 42 (1991): 1007-50.

11. Ruth R. Faden and Tom L. Beauchamp with Nancy M. P. King, *A History and Theory of Informed Consent* (New York: Oxford University Press, 1986); Jay Katz, "'Ethics and Clinical Research' Revisited: A Tribute to Henry K. Beecher," *Hastings Center Report* 23, no. 5 (1993): 31-39.

12. National Commission for the Protection of Human Subjects of Biomedical and Behavioral Research, *The Belmont Report: Ethical Principles and Guidelines for the Protection of Human Subjects of Research*, DHEW Pub. No. (OS) 78-0012 (Washington, D.C.: U.S. Government Printing Office, 1978), pp. 2-3.

13. Federal Policy for the Protection of Human Subjects, appearing in DHHS regulations at 45 CFR §46.102(d).

14. Robert J. Levine, "The Boundaries between Biomedical or Behavioral Research and the Accepted and Routine Practice of Medicine," *Belmont Report*, Appendix vol. 1, pp. 1-37-43.

15. John A. Robertson, "Legal Implications of the Boundaries between Biomedical Research Involving Human Subjects and the Accepted or Routine Practice of Medicine," *Belmont Report*, Appendix vol. 2, pp. 16-1-53.

16. Jay Katz, "The Regulation of Human Experimentation in the United States—A Personal Odyssey," *IRB: A Review of Human Subjects Research* 9, no. 1 (1987): 1, 5-6.

17. See Annas, "Faith (Healing), Hope and Charity at the FDA"; Benjamin Freedman, "Nonvalidated Therapies and HIV Disease," *Hastings Center Report* 19, no. 3 (1989): 14-20; Wendy K. Mariner, "Equitable Access to Biomedical Advances: Getting beyond the Rights Impasse," *Connecticut Law Review* 21 (1989): 571-603.

18. Don Marquis et al., "Case Study: The Doctor's Unproven Beliefs and the Subject's Informed Choice," *IRB: A Review*

of *Human Subjects Research* 10, no. 3 (1988): 3-5 and 11, no. 3 (1989): 8-11; Lawrence K. Altman, "Insurer to Pay Costs to Study Experiment in Treating Cancer," *New York Times*, 12 November 1990; Gina Kolata, "When the Dying Enroll in Studies: A Debate over False Hopes," *New York Times*, 29 January 1994.

19. Charles Marwick, "'Desperate Use' Gene Therapy Guidelines Ready," *JAMA* 269 (1993): 843; Bette-Jane Crigger, "The Quality of Mercy," *Hastings Center Report* 23, no. 3 (1993): 3.

20. David A. Kessler et al., "Regulation of Somatic-Cell Therapy and Gene Therapy by the Food and Drug Administration," *NEJM* 329 (1993): 1169-73.

21. James M. Wilson et al., "Ex Vivo Gene Therapy of Familial Hypercholesterolemia," *Human Gene Therapy* 3 (1992): 179-222.

22. Human Gene Therapy Subcommittee, "Minutes of the July 29, 1991 Meeting," *Recombinant DNA Technical Bulletin* 15 (1992): 174-82.

23. Recombinant DNA Advisory Committee, "Minutes of the October 7-8, 1991 Meeting," *Recombinant DNA Technical Bulletin* 15 (1992): 29-37.

24. Robert J. Levine, "The Impact of HIV Infection on Society's Perception of Clinical Trials," *Kennedy Institute of Ethics Journal* 4 (1994): 93-98.

25. See, for example, Renée C. Fox and Judith P. Swazey, *The Courage to Fail* (Chicago: University of Chicago Press, 1974), Chapter 3: "The Experiment-Therapy Dilemma"; Jay Katz and Alexander M. Capron, *Experimentation with Human Beings* (New York: Russell Sage Foundation, 1972); Ruth Macklin, "Ethical Implications of Surgical Experiments," *ACS Bulletin* 70, no. 6 (1985): 2-5; Faden et al., *A History and Theory of Informed Consent*, pp. 156-57; "Declaration of Helsinki: Recommendations Guiding Medical Doctors in Biomedical Research Involving Human Subjects," adopted by the 18th World Medical Assembly, Helsinki, Finland, 1964, published in *NEJM* 271 (1964): 473.

26. Expansion of oversight for these technologies has been proposed. See Linda Oberman, "Group Backs FDA-Like Review of Tests and Treatments," *American Medical News*, 24/31 October 1994, pp. 6-7.

27. See Jay Katz, "Human Experimentation and Human Rights," *St. Louis University Law Journal* 38 (1993): 7-54; Edmund D. Pellegrino, "Autonomy, Beneficence, and the Experimental Subject's Consent: A Reply to Jay Katz," *St. Louis University Law Journal* 38 (1993): 55-62.

28. See, for example, Robert Truog, Allan Brett, and Joel Frader, "The Problem with Futility," *NEJM* 326 (1992): 1560-64; E. Haavi Morreim, "Profoundly Diminished Life: The Casualties of Coercion," *Hastings Center Report* 24, no. 1 (1994): 33-42.

29. This wide-ranging, complex, and fascinating debate is addressed in the writings of Benjamin Freedman, Thomas Chalmers, Dale Cowan, David Eddy, Robert Levine, Robert Veatch, and many others. For thoughtful discussion of some of these issues in the context of a particular "experimental treatment," see Valerie Miké, Alfred N. Krause, and Gail S. Ross, "Neonatal Extracorporeal Membrane Oxygenation (ECMO): Clinical Trials and the Ethics of Evidence," *Journal of Medical Ethics* 19 (1993): 212-18; John Lantos and Joel Frader, "Extracorporeal Membrane Oxygenation and the Ethics of Clinical Research in Pediatrics," *NEJM* 323 (1990): 409-13.

30. See, for example, Harris Meyer, "Reform Debate Skirts Issue of Costly New Technology," *American Medical News*, 25 April 1994; Angela R. Holder, "Medical Insurance Payments and Patients Involved in Research," *IRB: A Review of Human Subjects Research* 16, nos. 1-2 (1994): 19-22.

31. Benjamin Freedman, "Equipoise and the Ethics of Clinical Research," *NEJM* 317 (1987): 141-45.

32. Tom Tomlinson and Howard Brody, "Futility and the Ethics of Resuscitation," *JAMA* 264 (1990): 1276, 1279. See also George J. Annas, "Informed Consent, Cancer, and Truth in Prognosis," *NEJM* 330 (1994): 223-25.

33. Alexander M. Capron, "Informed Consent in Catastrophic Disease Research and Treatment," *University of Pennsylvania Law Review* 123 (1974): 340, 364-76.

Genetics

[10]

THE CONTROL OF GENETIC RESEARCH: INVOLVING THE "GROUPS BETWEEN"

*Henry T. Greely**

Table of Contents

---

* Professor of Law, Stanford University; A.B., Stanford University, 1974; J.D., Yale Law School, 1977. The author is also a member of the North American Regional Committee of the proposed Human Genome Diversity Project (HGDP) and the chair of that Committee's ethics subcommittee. He would like to thank the many people involved in the HGDP, as members and as critics, for their roles in the development of this Article's analysis, particularly the past and present members of its North American Regional Committee. He also would like to thank the diligent assistance of Joshua Wagner, Stanford Law School class of 1998. This research was supported in part by a bequest from the Claire and Michael Brown Estate.

I. INTRODUCTION

For twenty years, one paradigm for the control of biomedical research has ruled the United States.[1] The federal government has controlled that research in two ways, to one end. It has used both its power of the purse, as the main source of funding of research,[2] and its regulatory power, as the approver of new drugs and devices,[3] to require that almost all biomedical research be governed by federal regulations, enforced through Institutional Review Boards (IRB).[4] In addition, those federal regulations, supported both by international declarations[5] and the domestic growth of patient autonomy,[6] insisted almost always on the consent, properly informed, of the individual subjects of the research.[7] This American paradigm rules not only the United States, but, through the spread of ideas, the international flow of federal money, and the universal interest of commercial firms in selling products to the American market, it has come to dominate the entire research world.[8]

Yet, in many cases, this paradigm is strikingly incomplete. It ignores almost entirely the groups *between* national governments and individuals. In at least one important area of biomedical research, human genetics, that incompleteness has important consequences. Research in human genetics is rarely about either national governments or individuals; rather, the

1. *See* RUTH R. FADEN ET AL., A HISTORY AND THEORY OF INFORMED CONSENT 87-113, 151-67, 200-32 (1986) (detailing the history and development of informed consent in the United States and describing the mechanisms of federal control).

2. *See* Anthony Szczygiel, *Beyond Informed Consent*, 21 OHIO N.U. L. REV. 171, 195 (1994).

3. *See* FADEN ET AL., *supra* note 1, at 203 (describing the development of the informed consent doctrine within the Food & Drug Administration, which initially provided "that researchers inform subjects of a drug's experimental nature and receive their consent before starting an investigation").

4. *See* 45 C.F.R. § 46.111 (1995) (establishing IRB approval requirements for studies involving human subjects); *see also* Szczygiel, *supra* note 2, at 195 (providing that before initiating a project, a researcher must ensure an IRB that risks have been minimized and that benefits of the experiment exceed the risks).

5. *See* Robert J. Levine, *Informed Consent: Some Challenges to the Universal Validity of the Western Model*, 19 L. MED & HEALTH CARE 207, 207-08 (1991) (containing an account of the ethical grounding of informed consent in the Western world, pointing out that the "term first appeared in American common law in the late 1950s and subsequently has been reflected in international codes").

6. *See* FADEN ET AL., *supra* note 1, at 87 (describing the rise of patient autonomy and the promulgation in 1972 of the Patient's Bill of Rights by the American Hospital Association).

7. *See id.* (noting that the patient autonomy movement sought recognition for the need to have practitioners and researchers honor refusals of treatment).

8. Refer to Part II *infra*.

research is almost always about *groups* of people,[9] defined not by their citizenship but by a common tie of heredity or disease. These groups—ethnic groups, disease organizations, and families—are, in a real sense, the usual *subjects* of genetic research, but they are subjects to whom the dominant paradigm gives no formal role in the control of research about them.[10] This Article argues that both researchers and national governments should give these groups some measure of control over such research.

Part II of this Article sketches briefly the prevailing paradigm for control of research. Part III then demonstrates how much biomedical research, particularly genetic research, can most directly affect neither national governments nor individuals, but these groups between—in reputation, commercialization, and autonomy. Part IV proposes some ways to increase the control these groups have over research that affects them. In doing so, this Article builds on the experiences to date of the proposed Human Genome Diversity Project (HGDP),[11] which has begun to directly confront these issues.

II. THE DOMINANT PARADIGM

Existing regulation of biomedical research in the United States works at two levels. At one level, federal law in effect requires researchers to submit proposals for studies of human subjects to expert panels, which must judge those proposals based on their adherence to federal regulations for the protection of human subjects.[12] Those regulations, bolstered by both international declarations[13] and trends in United States domestic

---

9. *See* L. LUCA CAVALLI-SFORZA ET AL., THE HISTORY AND GEOGRAPHY OF HUMAN GENES 20 (1994) (recognizing that while, in principle, individuals can be the subject of genetic studies, "the amount of information soon becomes prohibitive," thus, experiments are more suited to populations).

10. *See* Larry Gostin, *Ethical Principles for the Conduct of Human Subject Research: Population-Based Research and Ethics*, 19 L. MED. & HEALTH CARE 191, 191, 193 (1991) (noting that ethical considerations for genetics testing, including the importance of ensuring subjects' rights through consent provisions and the ability to withdraw from a study, are principally focused on an *individual* patient's autonomy regarding the subject's involvement in the study).

11. For a discussion of the efforts of the HGDP, refer to Part IV *infra*.

12. *See* 45 C.F.R. § 46.111 (1995) (detailing requirements for IRB approval of research, including that risks are minimized and reasonable, subject selection is equitable, and informed consent is obtained); *see also* PAUL M. MCNEILL, THE ETHICS AND POLITICS OF HUMAN EXPERIMENTATION 85-86 (1993) (explaining that IRBs are responsible for reviewing and monitoring human subject experimentation in the United States to protect subjects and improve the quality of scientific research); Szczygiel, *supra* note 2, at 195 (noting that IRBs must approve experimental research to ensure that risks are minimized).

13. *See* Leonard H. Glantz, *The Influence of the Nuremberg Code on U.S. Statutes and Regulations*, *in* THE NAZI DOCTORS AND THE NUREMBERG CODE: HUMAN

law,[14] also enshrine the second level of control: the requirement that individual research subjects be fully informed about the nature, scope, and risks of the research and agree formally to participate in it.[15]

Substantial federal regulation of biomedical research began in the aftermath of the disclosure of research that abused human subjects,[16] notably the notorious Tuskegee syphilis study.[17] This regulation is indirect but overpowering.[18] First, any research funded by the federal government—and any research institution that receives federal funds—is required by regulation to take

---

RIGHTS IN HUMAN EXPERIMENTATION 183, 185-99 (George J. Annas & Michael A. Grodin eds., 1992) (tracing the influence of the Nuremberg Code on United States statutes and regulations); Sharon Perly et al., *The Nuremberg Code: An International Overview*, *in* THE NAZI DOCTORS AND THE NUREMBERG CODE: HUMAN RIGHTS IN HUMAN EXPERIMENTATION 149, 158 (George J. Annas & Michael A. Grodin eds., 1992) (explaining that "the 1964 Declaration of Helsinki requires that research be based on laboratory and animal experiments"); *id.* at 159 (describing Helsinki II as providing "fundamental guiding principles for the conduct of biomedical research involving human subjects").

14. *See* Glantz, *supra* note 13, at 185-91 (reviewing notions of consent from the 1950s to the revised rules of the 1980s that focus on detailed informed consent provisions); Levine, *supra* note 5, at 207-08 (noting that the term "informed consent" first appeared in American common law in the 1950s).

15. *See* 42 U.S.C. § 3515b (1994) (disallowing government funding for research on human subjects without the written informed consent of each participant); Grethe v. Trustmark Ins. Co., 881 F. Supp. 1160, 1162 (N.D. Ill. 1995) (detailing the procedure required before a patient may receive treatment under an IRB proposal). Under IRB protocols, the informed consent procedure demands that the consent document explain "(1) the risks of the proposed therapy, (2) any alternatives to the proposed therapy, and (3) that the therapy is part of a research study." *Id.* The government may dispense with the consent requirement in certain circumstances. *See, e.g.*, MCNEILL, *supra* note 12, at 35 (disapproving of the policy of the FDA and Department of Defense that allows experimentation without consent during times of war, such as the nonconsensual use of experimental drugs and vaccines on American troops during the Gulf War).

16. *See* Henry K. Beecher, *Ethics and Clinical Research*, 274 NEW ENG. J. MED. 1354, 1354-60 (1966); Henry K. Beecher, *Consent in Clinical Experimentation: Myth and Reality*, 195 JAMA 34, 34-35 (1966). *See generally* MCNEILL, *supra* note 12, at 59-60 (discussing the work of Henry Beecher, a professor of anesthesiology at Harvard).

17. For a detailed chronology of the United States Public Health Service's (PHS) notorious study on the effects of untreated syphilis on nonconsenting black males, see JAMES H. JONES, BAD BLOOD: THE TUSKEGEE SYPHILIS EXPERIMENT (1993). For a general discussion of the development of ethical oversight of research, see Susan M. Wolf, *Quality Assessment of Ethics in Health Care: The Accountability Revolution*, 20 AM. J.L. & MED. 105, 115-25 (1994) (arguing that ethics should be used to help consumers evaluate health care professionals' performance and that quality assessment techniques are needed to determine ethical behavior within health care organizations).

18. *See* HUMAN SUBJECTS RESEARCH: A HANDBOOK FOR INSTITUTIONAL REVIEW BOARDS xi (Robert A. Greenwald et al. eds., 1982) [hereinafter IRB HANDBOOK] (estimating that 20% of the health care dollar is spent on compliance with regulations).

certain steps to protect human research subjects.[19] These regulations may be promulgated separately by federal agencies that fund research, but they are largely identical.[20] Substantively, the rules demand that the research risks to subjects be justified by the potential benefits of the research,[21] that broad informed consent be provided,[22] and that special protections be applied to particularly vulnerable populations.[23] Procedurally, the regulations force all such research to be approved by IRBs, which determine whether the research meets federal standards.[24]

Second, any research to be used in supporting applications to the Food and Drug Administration (FDA) must also satisfy regulations for protecting subjects.[25] The regulations are largely similar to those of the funding agencies, but they expand the reach of those provisions to research performed by institutions that do not receive federal grants: notably pharmaceutical and biotechnology companies.[26] Importantly, these regulations apply not only to companies from the United States and those doing research in the United States, but to companies from any country doing biomedical research anywhere that plan to use the research in support of an application to the FDA.[27] Those firms must also have their relevant research approved by IRBs.[28]

---

19. *See* 42 U.S.C. § 3515b (1994) (forbidding government funding for projects that fail to ensure that informed consent is obtained); 45 C.F.R. § 46.111 (1995) (detailing the mandates that must be followed in order to obtain research approval from an IRB).

20. The regulations of the Department of Health and Human Services, which provides the greatest amount of funding for medical research, are found in 45 C.F.R. pt. 46. These regulations were largely adopted by 16 federal departments or agencies, not including the FDA, as the "Common Rule." *See Federal Policy for the Protection of Human Subjects*, 56 Fed. Reg. 28,002 (1991).

21. *See* 45 C.F.R. § 46.111(a)(2) (1995) (explaining that the IRB should consider only those risks and benefits that may result from the research and exclude the possible long-term benefits of applying knowledge gained in the research).

22. *See id.* § 46.111(a)(4).

23. *See id.* § 46.111.

24. *See* IRB HANDBOOK, *supra* note 18, at xii (explaining that IRBs were established to guarantee the protection of human subjects and to ensure full compliance with federal regulations).

25. *See* 21 C.F.R. § 50.1 (1995) (providing that the scope of subsequent regulations govern applications seeking approval for "drugs for human use, medical devices for human use, [and] biological products for human use").

26. *See id.* (noting that "all clinical investigations" under FDA authority, including "applications for research or marketing permits" for FDA regulated products, are governed by the regulations).

27. *See id.* FDA regulations do not allow an official to apply equivalent foreign rules to research done overseas—the full FDA rules must apply. *See id.* § 50.23 (delineating the exceptions to the provisions of the regulations and not including an exception for applications made by foreign companies); *id.* § 50.1 (requiring Protection of Human Subjects rules to be followed for all investigations for applications to the FDA); *id.* § 56.103 (mandating the use of IRBs).

28. *See id.* § 56.103 (requiring that all clinical investigations obtain IRB ap-

Thus, the federal government effectively regulates biomedical research, not by asserting its direct governmental power to require that research follow certain rules, but by withholding federal benefits—research funding or regulatory approval—from institutions that have not met federal rules. This federal mandate is largely enforced by nonfederal, in fact nongovernmental, bodies,[29] but it remains a federal mandate.[30]

This federal initiative effectively preempts any less stringent state regulation of research. The states may regulate as they wish, but they cannot force the federal government to provide funds or to approve medical drugs or devices.[31] The federal scheme does not, however, preempt more stringent state or local regulation of research.[32] Some states have passed legislation on various aspects of research,[33] particularly those connected to the politically charged issue of abortion,[34] and state

---

proval, and noting that research results not submitted may be refused consideration if no previous application has been filed).

29. *See id.* §§ 56.102, 56.107 (delineating the makeup of IRBs and mandating that membership be composed from scientific and nonscientific communities and not government officials).

30. *See id.* § 50.1 (noting that the regulations apply to *all* clinical investigations in support of an application to the FDA).

31. *See* U.S. CONST. art. VI, § 2, cl. 2 (establishing the laws of the federal government to be "the supreme Law of the Land").

32. The important issue when deciding whether state regulation is preempted by federal law is the intent of Congress. *See* Cipollone v. Liggett Group, Inc., 505 U.S. 504, 516, 518-20 (1992) (deciding that federal laws on cigarette warning labels preempted any state warning label laws). The assumption is that Congress is not preempting state law unless there is evidence of intent to the contrary. *See id.* Congress may express its intent either explicitly in the statute, or implicitly in its structure and purpose. *See id.* at 516. Implied preemption may occur when Congress intends to occupy an entire field, where compliance with federal and state law is impossible, or where the state law frustrates federal law. *See* Mazur v. Merck & Co., 742 F. Supp. 239, 245 (E.D. Pa. 1990) (finding that a federal regulation of vaccines was comprehensive and, thus, superseded state packaging, labeling, and handling laws); *see also* Brown v. Medtronic, Inc., 852 F. Supp. 717, 718, 721 (S.D. Ind. 1994) (finding that the FDA intended to preempt state law on the regulation of some components of a medical device, but that there was a question of material fact on its intention towards regulation of other parts).

33. *See, e.g.*, ARIZ. REV. STAT. ANN. § 31-321 (West 1996) (requiring written consent from a prisoner prior to participation in a medical research study); ARK. CODE ANN. § 20-9-304 (Michie 1991) (requiring records of patients in medical research to be held confidential); CAL. GOV'T CODE § 27491.45 (West 1988) (describing rules for tissue use by hospitals and medical research institutions); COLO. REV. STAT. § 25-4-1402.5 (Supp. 1996) (exempting medical researchers from reporting requirements regarding HIV).

34. *See, e.g.*, Lifchez v. Hartigan, 735 F. Supp. 1361, 1376-77 (N.D. Ill. 1990) (striking down a criminal statute as unconstitutionally vague and as violating a woman's right to an abortion); Margaret S. v. Edwards, 488 F. Supp. 181, 219-21 (E.D. La. 1980) (rejecting constitutional attacks on state limits for experimentation on embryos or fetuses); Wynn v. Scott, 449 F. Supp. 1302, 1322 (N.D. Ill. 1978)

and local governments have regulated various health and safety aspects of biomedical research.[35] For the most part, however, the federal government has been the sole significant regulator of the treatment of human research subjects.[36]

National government control over some aspects of genetic research is encouraged by at least one international treaty, the Convention on Biological Diversity (Convention).[37] The Convention concludes that "[r]ecognizing the sovereign rights of States over their natural resources, the authority to determine access to genetic resources rests with the national governments and is subject to national legislation."[38] The "Contracting Parties,"[39] national governments and "regional economic integration organizations," agree to "endeavour to create conditions to facilitate access to genetic resources for environmentally sound uses by other Contracting Parties."[40] Access to those resources is to be "on mutually agreed terms"[41] and "subject to prior informed consent of the Contracting Party providing such resources."[42] The parties are to "endeavour to develop and carry out scientific research based on genetic resources provided by other Contracting Parties with the full participation of, and where possible

---

(upholding an Illinois statute restricting use of fetal tissue for biomedical research).

35. *See, e.g.*, IOWA CODE ANN. § 455B.501 (West 1990) (controlling disposal of infectious waste generated by medical research facilities); ME. REV. STAT. ANN. tit. 38, § 1546 (West 1995) (detailing legislative findings regarding the health and safety risks of low-level radioactive waste generated by research).

36. Refer to notes 49-65 *supra* and accompanying text (examining federal regulation of experimental human subject use and the informed consent doctrine). *See* CAL. HEALTH & SAFETY CODE § 439.901 (West Supp. 1996) (detailing California legislative findings that the National Institutes of Health is the major source for funding medical research in the United States); Gary S. Becker, *The Painful Political Truth About Medical Research*, BUS. WK., July 29, 1996, at 18, 18 (finding that the $12 billion budget of the National Institutes of Health is by far the majority of money spent on medical research by the United States government).

37. Convention on Biological Diversity, *opened for signature* June 5, 1992, S. TREATY DOC. NO. 103-20 (1993) [hereinafter Convention on Biodiversity]. As of August 1996, the Convention had been ratified by 149 countries. *See* United Nations Environment Programme, *List of Ratifications for the Convention on Biological Diversity* (visited Jan. 27, 1997) <http://www.unep.ch/bio/ratifica.html#g>. The United States is the most prominent country that has not ratified the Convention. *See id.*

38. Convention on Biodiversity, *supra* note 37, art. 15, § 1, S. TREATY DOC. NO. 103-20, at 10.

39. *See id.* art. 2 (defining "regional economic integration organization" as an organization of sovereign states in a region having competence to sign, ratify, approve, accept, or accede to the Convention in accordance with its own internal procedures).

40. *Id.* art. 15, § 2, S. TREATY DOC. NO. 103-20, at 11.

41. *Id.* § 4, S. TREATY DOC. NO. 103-20, at 11.

42. *Id.* § 5, S. TREATY DOC. NO. 103-20, at 11.

in, such Contracting Parties."[43]

The most interesting provision concerns the financial consequences of the use of genetic resources:

> Each Contracting Party shall take legislative, administrative or policy measures, as appropriate, and in accordance with Articles 16 and 19 and, where necessary, through the financial mechanism established by Articles 20 and 21 with the aim of sharing in a fair and equitable way the results of research and development and the benefits arising from the commercial and other utilization of genetic resources with the Contracting Party providing such resources. Such sharing shall be upon mutually agreed terms.[44]

Article 19 of the Convention contains a further obligation that Contracting Parties "take all practicable measures to promote and advance priority access on a fair and equitable basis by Contracting Parties, especially developing countries, to the results and benefits arising from biotechnologies based upon genetic resources provided by those Contracting Parties."[45]

The Convention, although it probably should not be read to apply to human genetic resources,[46] does squarely vest control

43. *Id.* § 6, S. TREATY DOC. NO. 103-20, at 11.

44. *Id.* § 7, S. TREATY DOC. NO. 103-20, at 11. Articles 20 and 21, referred to in the quoted passage, describe and create a financial mechanism for developed countries to provide funds to developing countries for purposes of protecting biodiversity. *See id.* arts. 20-21, S. TREATY DOC. NO. 103-20, at 14-16. Article 39 provides that the Global Environment Facility shall be the financial mechanism referred to in article 21 on an interim basis, if it has been restructured in accordance with article 21. *See id.* art. 39, S. TREATY DOC. NO. 103-20, at 24.

45. *Id.* art. 19, § 2, S. TREATY DOC. NO. 103-20, at 13.

46. Although the language of the Convention does not expressly exclude human genetic material, there are good reasons to think that the Convention does not apply to human genetic resources. The Convention defines "biological resources" as "genetic resources, organisms or parts thereof, populations, or any other biotic component of ecosystems with actual or potential use or value for humanity," *id.* art. 2, S. TREATY DOC. NO. 103-20, at 4, and "genetic material" as "any material of plant, animal, microbial or other origin containing functional units of heredity." *Id.* The Convention then defines "genetic resources" as "genetic material of actual or potential value." *Id.* art. 2. The Convention also states that "[d]omesticated or cultivated species means species in which the evolutionary process has been influenced *by* humans to meet *their* needs." *Id.* (emphasis added).

Humans would seem to be "organisms . . . [or] populations . . . with actual or potential use or value for humanity" and human DNA certainly is "material of . . animal . . origin containing functional units of heredity." *See id.* It even seems likely that humans are a species "in which the evolutionary process has been influenced by humans to meet their needs" and therefore are "domesticated." *See id.* (defining "domesticated or cultivated species"). The Convention, however, gives no indication that its drafters considered human DNA as within its scope. *See id.* arts. 1 & 3, S. TREATY DOC. NO. 103-20, at 4-5 (setting forth Convention objectives, but making no reference to human DNA, and stating the Convention's principles in terms of protecting the environment).

over nonhuman genetic resources within a nation's territory in the national government[47]—not in the "owners" of the lifeforms or the lands in which they are found, nor in any human populations that have used, preserved, or improved them.[48] This result is perhaps not surprising in an international agreement negotiated by, and intended for signature by, national governments.

Individual informed consent is the other prong of the current paradigm for control of research of human subjects. It is enshrined in the federal "Common Rule," which generally requires informed, written consent from individual research subjects,[49] and contains a fairly detailed description of the disclosures required.[50]

Stressing individual informed consent in research is undoubtedly related to the movement to increased patient autonomy in medical decision making. Although the doctrine of consent to medical treatment has deep roots in Anglo-American jurispru-

---

The casual concession of national government control over "their own biological resources," *see id.* pmbl., S. TREATY DOC. NO. 103-20, at 2, seems unlikely to have been written with humans or their genetic material in mind. Such a reading certainly squares poorly with international conventions on human rights as against their governments. Similarly, the Convention's mandate that Contracting Parties "[d]evelop national strategies, plans or programmes for the conservation and sustainable use of biological diversity," *see id.* art. 6(a), S. TREATY DOC. NO. 103-20, at 6, seems unlikely to have been intended to include human biological diversity. Nor does it seem likely that humans were considered within the Convention's article 8, which requires states both to take steps to preserve biological diversity and to "prevent the introduction of, control or eradicate those alien species which threaten ecosystems, habitats or species," *id.* art. 8(a), (h), S. TREATY DOC. NO. 103-20, at 7, among which humans, at least those outside of Africa, might certainly be numbered.

47. *See id.* art. 3, S. TREATY DOC. NO. 103-20, at 5 (recognizing nations' sovereign rights under the United Nations Charter and principles of international law "to exploit their own resources pursuant to their own environmental policies").

48. The Convention's Preamble focuses almost entirely on states and their rights and responsibilities, although it does make one brief reference to indigenous and local communities. *See id.* pmbl., S. TREATY DOC. NO. 103-20, at 2-3 ("Recognizing the close and traditional dependence of many indigenous and local communities embodying traditional lifestyles on biological resources . . . .").

49. *See* 45 C.F.R. § 46.117 (1995) (requiring written documentation of informed consent, except in cases where an IRB finds the principal risk to the subject to be potential harm from a breach of confidentiality, the research presents only a minimal risk, and does not invoke a procedure that usually requires written consent).

50. *See id.* § 46.116(a) (listing eight basic elements of informed consent, including an explanation of the research purpose, risks, discomforts, benefits, and the extent to which the subject's identity will remain confidential). When four strict requirements are met, the Common Rule does allow an IRB to alter or waive elements of informed consent or waive entirely the informed consent requirement. *See id.* § 46.116(d) (permitting alteration or waiver when the research involves only minimal risk, the alteration or waiver does not jeopardize a subject's rights or welfare, the waiver or alteration is necessary to make the research practical, and, when appropriate, the subjects receive pertinent post-participation information).

dence,[51] the modern era of informed consent litigation in medicine began in 1972, with nearly simultaneous decisions in the California Supreme Court[52] and the United States Court of Appeals for the District of Columbia Circuit.[53] These cases require that a patient be fully informed of the risks of medical interventions and knowingly consent to the procedure.[54] They did not, themselves, deal with research settings,[55] nor were there any notable opinions dealing with informed consent in research at that time. But those cases, and their progeny, formed a large part of the background when, after Tuskegee, the research subject protection regulations were written.[56] If a patient faced with a decision about a standard medical procedure was in a poor position to evaluate the physician's advice, how much worse was the position of the subject in medical research?

This requirement of individual informed consent has also been adopted widely across the world.[57] Although many nations do not agree with all aspects of the American informed consent regulations, particularly their stress on written, legalistic documents, the concept is widespread, although not entirely uncontroversial.[58]

---

51. *See* Schloendorff v. Society of New York Hosp., 105 N.E. 92, 93 (N.Y. 1914) (stating that every adult of sound mind has the right to determine what is to be done with his body and that a doctor that performs an operation without consent commits assault). *See generally* FADEN ET AL., *supra* note 1, at 116-25 (addressing the development of the informed consent doctrine from eighteenth-century England through *Schloendorff*).

52. *See* Cobbs v. Grant, 502 P.2d 1 (Cal. 1972).

53. *See* Canterbury v. Spence, 464 F.2d 772 (D.C. Cir. 1972).

54. *See id.* at 786-87 (recognizing "the patient's right of self-decision" and the patient's need to know "all risks potentially affecting the decision" before the patient can effectively exercise the right); *Cobbs*, 502 P.2d at 9, 11 (postulating that adults of sound mind have a right to decide whether to submit to medical treatment and citing *Canterbury* for the physician's duty to inform the patient of all perils material to that decision).

55. *See Canterbury*, 464 F.2d at 776-77 (involving a medical malpractice claim related to back surgery); *Cobbs*, 502 P.2d at 4-5 (dealing with medical malpractice in the context of abdominal surgery).

56. Refer to notes 16-28 *supra* and accompanying text (discussing post-Tuskegee federal regulations).

57. *See* Marcia Angell, *Ethical Imperialism? Ethics in International Collaborative Clinical Research*, 319 NEW ENG. J. MED. 1081, 1082 (1988) (noting the related concept of voluntary consent and recognizing the incorporation of these restrictions in international agreements, such as the Nuremberg Code and the World Medical Association Declaration of Helsinki, revised in 1975). For a discussion of the Nuremberg Code and the Declaration of Helsinki, refer to notes 59-65 *infra*. *See generally* Dorothy C. Wertz, *International Perspectives on Ethics and Human Genetics*, 27 SUFFOLK U. L. REV. 1411, 1447-48 (1993) (recognizing that the World Health Organization has incorporated principles governing international ethics, which include informed consent provisions, in published guidelines involving medical genetics).

58. *See, e.g.*, Levine, *supra* note 5, at 210 (asserting the impossibility of providing a widely applicable definition of informed consent). Different cultural per-

Individual informed consent also drew force from the international background. After World War II and the Nuremberg trials, the United States proceeded to put various German doctors and scientists on trial for their atrocious abuse of human subjects in biomedical experiments.[59] From these trials came the ten principles of the "Nuremberg Code" for medical research.[60] The Nuremberg Code stressed the central importance of informed consent,[61] the opposite of what occurred in the Nazi experiments.[62] Its first principle begins:

> The voluntary consent of the human subject is absolutely essential.
>
> This means that the person involved should have legal capacity to give consent; should be so situated as to be able to exercise free power of choice, without the intervention of any element of force, fraud, deceit, duress, overreaching, or other ulterior form of constraint or coercion; and should have sufficient knowledge and comprehension of the elements of the subject matter involved as to enable him to make an understanding and enlightened decision.[63]

Although these principles were promulgated only by the American court in trying Nazi researchers, they have been quite influential. Their lofty position was reinforced when the principles were largely adopted in the Declaration of Helsinki in 1964.[64] This statement, as adopted and several times amended

---

spectives of personhood make a uniform definition of informed consent very difficult. *See id.* The American perspective, for example, relies heavily upon rational legalistic principles expressed in documents like the Declaration of Independence and the Constitution. *See id.* at 209. *But see* Angell, *supra* note 57, at 1083 (noting that some commentators believe researchers should adhere to Western ethical standards regardless of their research subjects).

59. *See* FADEN ET AL., *supra* note 1, at 153; Robert D. Mulford, *Experimentation on Human Beings*, 20 STAN. L. REV. 99, 102 (1967).

60. *See* FADEN ET AL., *supra* note 1, at 155.

61. *See The Nuremberg Code, reprinted in* 19 L. MED. & HEALTH CARE 266, 266 (1991) (declaring voluntary consent absolutely essential and mandating disclosure of the general nature of the experiment and all dangers possibly linked to participation); Mulford, *supra* note 59, at 102 (noting that informed consent was a significant part of the Nuremberg code).

62. *See* FADEN ET AL., *supra* note 1, at 154-55 (observing that Nazi victims could not "qualify as volunteers, much less *informed* volunteers").

63. *The Nuremberg Code, supra* note 61, at 266.

64. *See* World Medical Association, *Declaration of Helsinki, reprinted in* 19 L. MED. & HEALTH CARE 264 (1991). *See generally* FADEN ET AL., *supra* note 1, at 156 (noting the Declaration's 1964 adoption and the centrality of consent to both the Declaration and the Nuremberg Code).

by the World Medical Assembly, continues to stress the importance of informed consent.

> In any research on human beings, each potential subject must be adequately informed of the aims, methods, anticipated benefits and potential hazards of the study and the discomfort it may entail. He or she should be informed that he or she is at liberty to abstain from participation in the study and that he or she is free to withdraw his or her consent to participation at any time. The physician should then obtain the subject's freely-given informed consent, preferably in writing.[65]

Thus, in the United States and many other parts of the world, national governments have taken control over research at one level, and individual research subjects have been given control at the other.[66] But no one talks about other kinds of groups that could be given some power to control research. In many situations, that makes sense because there are no obvious groups between the government and the individual. Research in human genetics, however, almost always involves those kinds of groups and often produces problems, and opportunities, for them as groups.

III. HUMAN GENETICS RESEARCH AND THE PROBLEM OF THE GROUPS BETWEEN

For purposes of this Article, the "groups between" in human genetics research are groups of people who share some genetic characteristics of interest. Often, they are families in whom a particular genetic characteristic or disease is common. Frequently, they are groups of families that suffer from high levels of genetic disease, organized into a formal or informal "disease organization." Such organizations exist for many genetic conditions of medical significance, such as the CF Foundation, the Fanconi Anemia Research Fund, Inc., or National Tay-Sachs and Allied Diseases Association. Finally, sometimes entire ethnic groups are the subjects of genetic research.[67] This is necessarily

65. *Declaration of Helsinki*, *supra* note 64, at 265. The Helsinki Declaration goes on to demand special care for patients in a "dependent relationship" with the researching physician and patients who are legally incompetent. *See id.*

66. Refer to notes 12-36 *supra* and accompanying text (discussing national government control over research).

67. *See* C. Thomas Caskey, *Molecular Medicine: A Spin-Off from the Helix*, 269 JAMA 1986, 1989 (1993) (noting that screening for Tay-Sachs disease in Ashkenazi Jews and sickle cell anemia in African-Americans is conventional medical practice); Gina Kolata, *Scientist Closes in on Rare Gene*, HOUS. CHRON., July 22, 1996, at 8E (describing research on Dysautonomia, a disease that affects Ashkenazi Jews almost

the case in the proposed HGDP, which, among other things, is seeking genetic evidence about the origins, relatives, and migrations of different human populations.[68] It is also the case with some medical research, where a particular ethnic group provides a useful population for studying a disease. The Old Order Amish provide one example of an ethnic or cultural group useful for genetic studies:

> The Old Order Amish community has large, extended families, and information on their ancestry is well known and available—genealogical records can trace their ancestry back to only 30 or so European progenitors. In addition to information on ancestry, medical and hospital records with demographic details are also available. The group is located within a small geographic location, and even individuals who leave the community tend to remain in the immediate area, making them accessible for genetic studies. The group is both genetically and culturally homogenous, thereby reducing the variables that can complicate genetic studies. In addition, cultural taboos essentially eliminate alcohol or drug abuse, which is important for the study of affective disorders since the symptoms of these disorders can be masked by alcohol or drug use. Furthermore, individuals within this community have very well-defined roles, and close interactions between its members mean that behavior that differs from the norm is readily detectable. Finally, this community, as a whole, is very concerned about health issues and particularly about mental illness. They have therefore been extremely cooperative with researchers interested in understanding the basis for such disorders.[69]

Whether family, disease organization, or ethnic group, these groupings, intermediate between the individual and the national government, are crucial to, and crucially affected by, research in human genetics. Research in human genetics is by its nature collective research.[70] One person's genome is only revealing in

---

exclusively); *see also* Marty Racine, *She Defied the Predictions*, HOUS. CHRON., Sept. 18, 1996, at 1D (discussing a woman with sickle cell anemia, a blood disorder that affects mostly African-Americans and a smaller percentage of those descended from some Mediterranean and Middle Eastern countries).

68. For information on the HGDP, visit the Project's web site at Human Genome Diversity Project, http://www-leland.stanford.edu/group/morrinst/HGDP.html.

69. Neil Risch & David Botstein, *A Manic Depressive History*, 12 NATURE GENETICS 351, 352 fig.1 (1996).

70. *See* ANNE J. KRUSH & KATHLEEN A. EVANS, FAMILY STUDIES IN GENETIC DISORDERS ix (1984).

the context of the genomes of others.[71] Typically, disease-related research starts by locating families with a high incidence of a condition thought to have a genetic link.[72] The researchers categorize the family members as affected or unaffected by the condition and create pedigrees, demonstrating how the family is related.[73] At that point, the research can move from clinical medicine and genealogy into molecular biology, as the researchers will try to determine what portions of genetic material those with the disease share with each other, but not with their unaffected relatives.[74] This may result in learning the location of one or more genes that, in those families, contribute to the disease. The same process can be employed when working with unrelated families that share the same disease or with ethnic groups in which the disease is common.[75]

One genome is usually of very little value, as knowledge is gained only by comparing the genomes of many individuals, some with the condition and some without.[76] Both the positive cases and the negative cases are essential to finding out what genetic location is important.[77] One individual with one genome is almost meaningless without a background for comparison,[78] and, as the Amish example reveals, the closer the background—genetically and environmentally—the better.[79]

This may not always be the case. At some point, we may know enough about both the common human genome and the nature and extent of variation within that genome to use that background knowledge for comparison. At the extreme, this is already true. We know that humans usually have their nuclear genetic material in the form of forty-six chromosomes.[80] If a person has an unusual condition and forty-five or forty-seven chromosomes,

---

71. *See id.* at ix, 132-34 (discussing the comparisons for risks between the person studied and his relatives, and between relatives and the general population).

72. *See id.* at 13 (relating that family studies begin with a patient discussing a disease that several relatives have, which leads the physician to contact other family members).

73. *See id.* at 45-65 (describing how and when to use a pedigree chart).

74. *See id.* at 131, 134 (discussing how clues from disease transmission can be derived from pedigrees and environmental factors).

75. *See id.* at 4 (noting that certain techniques for genetic study can be employed for a series of families).

76. *See id.* at 132-34 (discussing various subgroups for analysis and reviewing proportion of each affected in relation to the general population).

77. *See id.* (reviewing the importance of complete information on all relatives regardless of the absence or presence of the target characteristic).

78. *See id.* (highlighting the importance of comparing results among family members).

79. *See id.* (breaking comparison of subgroups down by closeness of relationship to the target individual).

80. *See* LYNN B. JORDE ET AL., MEDICAL GENETICS 7 (1995).

a strong initial inference might be drawn that the deviation from forty-six is important. As knowledge of the human genome, and of the extent of normal (or, at least, nondisease-associated) variation in the human genome grows, individual cases may take on more significance, but we are nowhere near that degree of knowledge. For now, group research remains essential.[81]

But as genetic researchers use groups of people to learn about normal and disease-producing genetic variants, their findings provide information about those groups. Research into a family or a group of families with a high incidence of a disease may reveal that those families are more likely than average to carry a "flawed" allele of a gene. That information necessarily has implications for every family member, whether she took part in the research or not. She knows that she, her parents, her children, and her other relatives are at a higher risk for this genetic disorder. She will often learn that she can be tested for the disease allele—and so will everyone else, including her potential employers and insurers. The same dynamic is at work in ethnic groups. The fact that sickle cell anemia, for example, is much more common among African-Americans than among European-Americans[82] necessarily provides some probabilistic information about African-Americans who did not take part in the genetic tests. Information about groups has implications for all the members of those groups. Three implications are particularly important: autonomy, reputation, and commercialization.

Genetic research on groups can limit autonomy at two levels.

---

81. Ironically, the single important judicial opinion concerning the rights of research subjects in the age of molecular biology involved one of the rare exceptions to the importance of collective research. In *Moore v. Regents of Univ. of Cal.*, 793 P.2d 479 (Cal. 1990), the California Supreme Court considered the claims of a research subject against a researcher who had created what seemed to be a commercially valuable cell line from a sample of his spleen. *See id.* at 480-81. The cell line appeared valuable because it created large quantities of certain chemicals called cytokines that are important to the immune system and normally produced only in tiny amounts. *See id.* at 481 n.2, 482. The cells involved, however, were apparently cancerous blood cells, symptomatic of a disease known as hairy cell leukemia. *See id.* at 481. Furthermore, they were unusual in being infected with a human retrovirus known as HTLV-II. *See id.* at 490-91 n.30. Whether the excess production of cytokines was caused by the hairy cell leukemia, the HTLV-II infection, Moore's healthy genetic code, or a combination of factors remains unclear. It is clear that the vast overproduction of these cytokines made the cell line from Moore stand out, without careful comparative work, and allowed researchers to work backwards from at least one of the chemicals being produced to the gene that coded for it. *See id.* at 490 n.29 (stating that a copy, or clone, of the original gene can be derived from an adequate source of MRNA).

82. *See* Mark A. Rothstein, *Employee Selection Based on Susceptibility to Occupational Illness*, 81 MICH. L. REV. 1379, 1385-86, 1421 tbl.viii (1983) (detailing the nature of sickle cell anemia and the occurrence of the disease predominantly among blacks).

At one level, it can limit the autonomy of an individual group member who does not choose to participate in the research. She may have refused to participate or may never have been asked, but the research results will tell her, her fellow group members, and perhaps the outside world, something about her. At the least, they may say that her risk of carrying a particular disease-linked allele is higher, or lower, than average. It might tell her, if her children are found to be affected with a recessive disease, that she carries the allele.[83] Her decision whether or not to participate may have little meaning if enough other members of her group do participate.

Looking at this as an issue of *individual* autonomy, however, seems somewhat artificial. The research inevitably provides information about a group, as well as the individuals who constitute it. The group—whether one family, a set of families in a genetic disease organization, or an ethnic group—is really the research subject. It is the group's collective autonomy that is challenged if researchers, with the informed consent of only a few individuals in the group, can probe for information about the whole group.

The implications of group genetic research for "reputation" seem straightforward. Research on a group provides information about all members of the group. Group members may have their reputations, defined broadly, harmed. They may find it harder to marry, harder to get insurance, or harder to find work, whether or not they had consented to the research. If strong genetic links are ever established to important behavioral characteristics, which remains in doubt, people might find themselves "scientifically proven" to be genetically violent, emotionally unstable, or stupid.

The reputational implications are not entirely one-sided, however. Genetic research might determine that a disease thought to be genetic often was not, thus limiting the negative implications described above. Even a finding that the condition is genetic might have beneficial "reputational" implications. For example, if mental illnesses that were widely thought to be the result of early childhood environment were shown to be largely genetic, parents might avoid an implication of bad parenting, and their own consequent sense of guilt.

Commercial interests may also come into play. Genetics

83. To be affected with a recessive disorder, a person must normally inherit one "bad" allele from each parent. *See* JORDE ET AL., *supra* note 80, at 56-82. Male children, who have only one X chromosome, may develop a genetic disease that is recessive in women by having only one "bad" allele, because they do not have another X chromosome with another, possibly safe, allele. *See id.* at 83-101.

research has already led to commercial testing for some genetic diseases. It may lead to successful therapies. If so, questions arise at two levels. Does anyone connected with the source of the research have any claim to some of the commercial value of the discovery? And, if so, who should have that claim—the affected group? the group members who participated in the research? the individual from whose cells the gene was cloned? Any one individual has a relatively minor claim. Nothing could have been discovered from research on her alone as the group context was essential. The group, whose existence and at least partial participation in the research was necessary, could have a stronger moral claim. That claim, however, could be undercut practically by the decisions of a few members of the group to participate in the research. And, once the discovery is made, material of commercial value might be obtained from any affected member of the group.

Thus, genetic research into a group with shared genetic characteristics may bring the group costs, particularly to its reputation. Or it may bring benefits, particularly through improved diagnosis and treatment of disease. But a group is not a government, so it has not been asked for its permission to conduct the research. It is not the individual research subject, either, so it has not been subject to rules requiring informed consent. It is a "group between," and although it is the effective subject of the research, no one has asked *it* how it balances the costs and benefits of going forward.

IV. PROTECTING THE INTERESTS OF THE GROUPS BETWEEN

It is one thing to say that genetics research has strong implications for groups that exist at a level below governments and above individuals. It is quite another to try to think through what interests should be protected and how to do so. That effort has been undertaken, at least as to ethnic groups, by the North American Regional Committee (NAmC) of the Human Genome Diversity Project (HGDP).[84] This section of the Article first describes the conclusions reached by the NAmC with respect to group autonomy, commercial rights, and reputation, as well as

84. *See generally Proposed Model Ethical Protocol for Collecting DNA Samples*, 33 HOUS. L. REV. 1431, 1433 (1997) [hereinafter *Model Protocol*]. For further information on the Human Genome Project, see VICTOR MCKUSICK, THE HUMAN GENOME PROJECT: PLANS, STATUS, AND APPLICATIONS IN BIOLOGY AND MEDICINE IN GENE MAPPING 18, 18-42 (George J. Annas & Sherman Elius eds., 1992). For an update on the HGDP, see *Human Genome Diversity Project*, <http://www-leland.stanford.edu/ group/morrinst/HGDP.html>.

the difficulties raised by those conclusions. It then extends that analysis to other intermediate groups, namely disease organizations and affected families.

A. *The Human Genome Diversity Project and "Populations"*

The Human Genome Project plans to map and sequence the three billion nucleotide pairs of the DNA forming "the" human genome.[85] But humans vary genetically, and there exist approximately six billion human genomes, not just one.[86] This vast diversity forms the subject of human population genetics and the *raison d'être* of the HGDP.[87]

The HGDP intends to collect a representative sample of human genetic variation.[88] It would like to collect DNA from members of about five hundred of the roughly five to ten thousand human populations in the world.[89] This DNA would be stored in repositories and made available to researchers.[90] The samples would all be subjected to analysis under a standard set of markers, and the results would be placed in a database, also generally available to researchers.[91] The result would be a reference library of human genetic diversity,[92] which the HGDP estimates could be completed in about five to seven years, for a cost of about twenty-five to thirty-five million dollars.[93]

Improved information about human genetic diversity can be important for at least four different reasons. First, thus far the vast majority of detailed research into human genetics has been done with Europeans or North Americans of European descent, and thus omits the eighty percent of the world's population that is not of European ancestry.[94] It is fundamentally unfair to the majority of humanity to describe the human genome without including a representative sample of all humans. Second, studying human genetic diversity will help us understand better the workings of evolution in humans, including the ways in which culture influences evolution. Third, greater knowledge of human

85. *See* MCKUSICK, *supra* note 84, at 18-42.

86. *See* THE HUMAN GENOME PROJECT: DECIPHERING THE BLUEPRINT OF HEREDITY 170 (Necia G. Cooper ed., 1994).

87. *See Human Genome Diversity Project*, <http://www-leland.stanford.edu.group/morrinst/HGDP.html>.

88. *See id.*

89. *See id.*

90. *See id.*

91. *See id.*

92. *See id.*

93. *See id.*

94. *See id.*

genetic diversity will improve medicine, both because it will advance the study of those genetic diseases found largely in non-European populations, and because genetic variation is basic to better understanding a host of diseases found in all peoples. Finally, studying human diversity will help us uncover our shared human history. Genetic results, when interpreted along with evidence from anthropology, archaeology, history, linguistics, and other fields, will help map human migrations and expansions in prehistoric times.[95]

The HGDP, first suggested in print in 1991,[96] was formally organized at an international meeting at Porto Conte, Sardinia, Italy in September 1993.[97] Currently, it consists entirely of an international executive committee and regional committees for Europe, China, and North America with other committees being formed.[98] Both the regional and the international committees are, at this point, engaged largely in seeking funding and planning the implementation of the HGDP. Currently, DNA collection is not yet taking place as a formal part of the HGDP.[99]

The HGDP seeks to collect DNA samples from populations—ethnic groups ranging in size from the more than one billion ethnic Chinese (the Han) to some indigenous populations that number no more than a few hundred people. This focus on populations has led to concern about the consequences of the HGDP from some populations and their advocates.[100] This focus also led the NAmC of the HGDP to write a proposed Model Ethical Protocol for Collection of DNA Samples (Model Protocol), to be used to guide researchers, populations, and IRBs.[101] The issues of importance were concerns that revolved around the group nature of the expected participants in the HGDP: autonomy, reputation, and commercialization.[102]

The Model Protocol holds that informed consent must be at

95. *See, e.g.*, CAVALLI-SFORZA ET AL., *supra* note 9; L. Luca Cavalli-Sforza, *Genes, People, and Language*, 265 SCI. AM. 104 (1991).

96. *See* L. Luca Cavalli-Sforza et al., 11 GENOMICS 490, 490 (1991) (calling for geneticists and both public and private agencies to collaborate in collecting genetic material to record human ethnic and geographic diversity); Leslie L. Roberts, *A Genetic Survey of Vanishing Peoples*, 252 SCIENCE 1614, 1615 (1991).

97. *See Human Genome Diversity Project, Report of International Planning Workshop*, <http://www-leland. stanford.edu/group/morrinst/HGDP.html>.

98. *See Model Protocol, supra* note 84, at 1434.

99. Related projects have started in Europe, with European Union funding, and in China, that may eventually become associated with the HGDP.

100. For an example of concerns regarding the HGDP, see *Rural Advancement Foundation International*, http://www.charm.net/~rafi/rafihome.html.

101. The Model Protocol was released by the NAmC for comments in the Fall of 1995. It has not been adopted by the NAmC, but has been put forward as a basis for discussion. *See Model Protocol, supra* note 84, at 1433.

102. *See id.*

the group level as well as at the individual level.[103] It "requires that researchers participating in the HGDP show that they have obtained the informed consent of the population, through its culturally appropriate authorities where such authorities exist, before they begin sampling."[104] It thus resolves the issue of group autonomy by giving the group authority to decide whether to participate in the research.[105] For example, if a group such as the Navajo decides collectively not to participate, the HGDP would not accept a sample from an individual Navajo, no matter how willing.[106] In theory, the problem of group autonomy is thus solved in a single stroke. But this is a solution that holds many problems. The two biggest, and most relevant to other groups between, are defining the population and determining its "culturally appropriate authorities."

If a researcher collects samples from a town in the Navajo Nation, from what population is she collecting? It might be the members of the village. It could be the Navajo. It might be all North American speakers of languages in the same language group as Navajo. These Na Dene languages are found among a few tribes in the Southwest, many tribes in inland Alaska and Northwestern Canada, as well as a few populations scattered elsewhere.[107] Or the group might be all Native Americans. Each of those definitions is relevant for some purposes—which is relevant for seeking group consent?

The Model Protocol begins with the position that the researcher must always discuss the HGDP with the people in the community to be sampled.[108] The town, the parish, or the school district will always be one definition of the population. They must be informed, their views must be sought, and, if a consensus emerges, it must be honored.[109]

But the local community may not be enough. In many cases,

---

103. *See id.* at 1437 (requiring researchers to obtain government consent and the informed consent of the populations and individuals sampled).

104. *Id.* at 1443-44.

105. *See id.* at 1443 (reasoning that it would be unethical to sample members of a group when the group as a whole has not consented because it would attack politically or economically marginalized populations).

106. *See id.* (providing that "it cannot be ethically appropriate to sample some members of a group when the group itself has not agreed to participate in the HGDP").

107. *See* PETER IVERSON, THE NAVAJO NATION 3 (1981).

108. *See Model Protocol, supra* note 84, at 1436-38 (suggesting that researchers collaborate with anthropologists and others familiar with the population before sampling begins, and requiring researchers to explain, in the language appropriate to the culture, the sampling process and the HGDP to both individuals and the population).

109. *See id.* at 1443-47 (discussing group consent requirements).

the population will identify itself as part of a larger group. The researchers need to determine whether that is the case and, if so, what that larger group is. If they identify such a group, they must move to the second difficult question. Namely, what are the culturally appropriate authorities?[110] If such authorities exist for that larger group, their informed consent must be sought and obtained.[111]

In many cases, an absence of culturally appropriate authorities who could grant or deny consent will prevent this higher level group consent. A predominately Irish-American catholic parish may be a local community, among whom the HGDP can be discussed, but there is no culturally appropriate authority for Irish-Americans as a whole. There is no person or body that would be generally recognized by Irish-Americans as speaking for them or as having authority over them.

In other cases, particularly with Native Americans, such bodies do exist.[112] Almost all Indian cultures in the United States and Canada have tribal governments, with a defined geographical and tribal jurisdiction.[113] Federally recognized tribal governments in the United States have "semi-sovereign" status and, in many cases, broad governmental powers.[114] These tribal governments will necessarily be a culturally appropriate authority, whose informed consent should be sought. Individual populations may have other nonofficial authorities whose permission would also be required. Defining a population and its culturally relevant authorities will often be difficult tasks. It will require deep knowledge of the population's culture and extended discussions with its members. In some cases, the problem may be so severe that the population cannot even consider participating in

110. *See id.* at 1443-44.

111. *See id.* at 1445-47.

112. *See* SHARON O'BRIEN, AMERICAN INDIAN TRIBAL GOVERNMENTS 7, 18-20 (1989) (discussing formal governmental bodies of the Choctaws, Oneida, Onondaga, Cayuga, Seneca, and Tuscaroro).

113. *See id.* at 93 (observing that "[m]ost tribes today have a governing council of some sort, although these governing bodies vary widely in their titles, structures, and powers.").

114. *See* Talton v. Mayes, 163 U.S. 376, 382, 384 (1896) (noting that tribal sovereignty is not "created by and springing from the Constitution" but instead "exist[ed] prior to the Constitution"). The federal law governing the relationships between Indian tribes and the federal and state governments is complex, if not chaotic, *see* Philip P. Frickey, *Congressional Intent, Practical Reasoning, and the Dynamic nature of Federal Indian Law*, 78 CAL. L. REV. 1137, 1189 (1990); Philip P. Frickey, *Marshalling Past and Present: Colonialism, Constitutionalism, and Interpretation in Federal Indian Law*, 107 HARV. L. REV. 381, 410 (1993), but, whatever their boundaries, the existence of "special" powers in Indian tribes is clear, *see* O'BRIEN, *supra* note 112, at 292 (describing the quasi-sovereign status of Indian nations, including the ability of tribes to dispose of land freely, conduct foreign relations, and administer their own criminal decisions).

the HGDP. There might, for example, be such sharp division within the population about which authorities are appropriate that no group decision is possible. But where populations and the relevant authorities within those populations *can* be defined, the group's autonomy can and should be respected.

The Model Protocol also speaks to reputational concerns as embodied in the term "confidentiality."[115] It first suggests a modified form of confidentiality for participating populations.[116] More directly, the Model Protocol recognizes that researchers have an obligation to try to avoid any harm coming to their subjects as a result of the research.[117] In the context of reputation and the HGDP, this will most often mean dispelling racist or stereotypical conclusions about participating populations. That will almost certainly be easy scientifically; there is enormous genetic variation within all populations and very little variation between them.[118] Genetically, humans are a fairly homogenous species.[119]

But, whatever the scientific reading of HGDP data, it seems likely that racists or nationalists will try to misuse it for their own purposes. Bosnian Serbs might well try to use any relevant HGDP data to claim genetic superiority to Bosnian Muslims. To prevent harm to participating populations, the Model Protocol recognizes that the HGDP must react to, and counteract, that kind of abuse.[120]

Finally, the Model Protocol also tries to protect populations' interests in the commercial use or patenting of products derived from their samples.[121] It does this by incorporating a discussion of controls on such uses into the process of group informed consent.[122] As part of that process, the group will be asked to de-

115. *See Model Protocol, supra* note 84, at 1462-64 (indicating that researchers must ensure the confidentiality of individual donors and participating populations).

116. *See id.* at 1463 (providing that instead of identifying exactly the village or town of population, by name or by map coordinates, the HGDP can provide a description that names an area but not a specific research site).

117. *See id.* at 1456.

118. *See* L. LUCA & FRANSECO CAVALLI-SFORZA, THE GREAT HUMAN DIASPORAS 237 (1996) ("The idea of race in the human species serves no purpose."); *see also* DANIEL L. HARTL, PRINCIPLES OF POPULATION GENETICS 66-67 (1980) (explaining that natural populations have a high degree of genetic variation within them, which reflects the population's evolutionary history).

119. *See* HARTL, *supra* note 118, at 66-67.

120. *See Model Protocol, supra* note 84, at 1464-65 (suggesting that researchers use lectures, seminars, interviews, and popular articles to dispel notions of ethnic superiority).

121. *See id.* at 1466-68 (recognizing the controversy surrounding the use of samples for commercial uses and proposing parameters to safeguard populations' interests in uses of products derived from their samples).

122. *See id.* (discussing the implementation of rules governing commercial uses

cide whether it wants to allow commercial use or patenting and, if so, on what terms.[123] The group may want to permit any use or ban all uses. The group may choose to allow uses only with the subsequently negotiated express agreement of the group.[124] The HGDP would strive to enforce whatever decision the group made.[125]

But, again, this solution creates its own problems. Enforcing a term of the informed consent discussion may not prove simple. The Model Protocol does outline one way to protect those interests.[126] Anyone seeking to take samples or data from the HGDP's repositories or database would have to agree to a materials transfer agreement or database access agreement.[127] That agreement would bind that person contractually to abide by all the terms and conditions imposed on samples by the populations that provided them.[128]

This contractual approach avoids the knotty question of the property status of human DNA, which has only been decided in one jurisdiction.[129] On the other hand, the reliance on contract rather than property could make effective enforcement difficult if the initial researcher passed the samples on to someone else who was not contractually bound. Even in such a case, the risks of uncertain title, as well as bad publicity, could deter a pharmaceutical company from spending millions of dollars to develop a product without a clear agreement with the population that provided the DNA.

This solution also avoids the unsavory results under the dominant paradigm. The national government, as codified in the

---

and the requirement that such rules be disclosed in the process of obtaining the populations' informed consent).

123. *See id.* (arguing this part of the process as one of three plausible approaches).

124. *See id.* at 1466-67 (suggesting a scenario whereby commercial users of samples or data must negotiate financial payments with a trustee, with the proceeds to be spent for the group's common benefit).

125. *See id.* at 1467 (assuming the HGDP will adopt policies, but stating that the NAmC would require researchers to give populations a choice among three proposed approaches, if the HGDP fails to adopt a policy).

126. *See id.* at 1468 (identifying a contractual alternative as the most promising way to protect a population's interests).

127. *See id.* at 1468-69 (requiring agreement to a set of rules concerning the sampled population's rights).

128. *See id.*

129. *See* Moore v. Regents of Univ. of Cal., 793 P.2d 479, 488-93 (Cal. 1990) (finding no cases that support a patient's asserted interest in a patented cell line). The Court rejected the patient's theory of conversion, reasoning that policy considerations weigh against extending the tort to such cases. *See id.* at 493. The Court decided that this issue was better left to the legislature. *See id.*

Biodiversity Treaty with respect to nonhuman genetic materials,[130] seems an inappropriate recipient for financial benefits based on genetic research with some of its populations, particularly if the national government had oppressed the population in question. On the other hand, individual research subjects may not have the legal ability under *Moore v. Regents of University of California*,[131] or the practical ability under the conditions of research, to garner any financial return from their role in the research. Under the Model Protocol's proposed solution, the population, which by its participation in the research effectively provided the information, gets the benefits.[132]

The Model Protocol seeks to give both control and protection to populations that participate in the HGDP. It avoids the dual focus on the national government and individual research subject, and instead focuses on the entity that is the real subject of the study—the group.[133] Whether the Model Protocol will succeed, and indeed whether the proposed HGDP will ever be implemented, remains uncertain. But the Model Protocol may provide a useful way to begin thinking about the interests of other kinds of groups between. If successful, it could be the basis for a broader requirement that researchers genuinely consult with populations, through the methods and authorities appropriate to them, before embarking on genetic research with ethnic groups.

B. Disease Organizations

The long-noted American love of voluntary organizations has created numerous disease organizations, private nonprofit groups dedicated to supporting research into and treatments for different maladies. These groups range from the giant American Cancer Society, American Heart Association, and American Lung Association, to smaller, more specialized organizations, such as the Cystic Fibrosis Foundation, the Huntington's Disease Society of America, and the Fanconi Anemia Research Fund, Inc. These organizations typically draw support from patients, their fami-

---

130. Refer to notes 12-50 *supra* and accompanying text (discussing national governmental authority to determine access to genetic resources and the Convention's call for international cooperation regarding access to resources and distribution of benefits derived from genetic resources).

131. *See Moore*, 793 P.2d at 489, 493 (doubting that the subject retained any interest in the cell sample, and concluding that the use of excised cells in research is not conversion).

132. *See Model Protocol*, *supra* note 84, at 1452-56 (vowing to ensure that populations get a fair share of financial rewards).

133. Refer to notes 101-14 *supra* and accompanying text (discussing the Model Protocol's emphasis on obtaining populations' informed consent and allowing populations the use of their samples).

lies, and the public generally.[134]

Some disease organizations focus on disease with a very direct and well-understood genetic cause, such as cystic fibrosis.[135] Others are concerned with diseases where genetics plays a less powerful role. In some, such as breast cancer, genetic variants strongly cause the disease in only a small percentage of those with the disease.[136] In others, such as Alzheimer's disease, genetic variants may have some effect on the risks of disease in a large number of people.[137]

When genetic variations are known to, or suspected of, affecting a disease, a disease organization can greatly assist researchers. They can provide funding for research and contacts with individuals and family members who may be willing to participate in the research.[138] It is prudent for researchers to contact disease organizations when relevant ones exist. But more than prudence is involved. Such contact, when possible, should be ethically required. The underlying reason is the same as with research into the genetics of human populations—research into genetic characteristics found in a group necessarily affects that group. But the specific reasons for such contact, and the role of the contacted groups, are importantly different from those in research with human ethnic groups.

---

134. *See, e.g.*, CYSTIC FIBROSIS FOUNDATION, FOUNDATION FACTS 1 (1996) (describing the Foundation's reliance on public support to carry out its mission).

135. *See* CYSTIC FIBROSIS FOUNDATION, GENE THERAPY AND CF 1 (1996) (noting the 1989 discovery of the defective CF gene and the potential for finding a cure); *see generally* G. Santis, *Basic Molecular Genetics*, *in* CYSTIC FIBROSIS 15, 18-21 (Margaret E. Hodson & Duncan M. Geddes eds., 1995) (describing in detail the structure of the CF gene).

136. It is thought that about 10% of women with breast or ovarian cancer are born with mutated versions of the BRCA1 or BRCA2 (Breast Cancer 1 or 2) genes. *See* STANFORD WORKING GROUP, GENETIC TESTING FOR BREAST CANCER SUSCEPTIBILITY (forthcoming 1997) (on file with author).

137. *See* Joan Stephenson, *Questions on Genetic Testing Services*, 274 JAMA 1661, 1661 (1995) (reporting a test for a gene that directs the production of apolipoprotein E, whose presence in one particular form, E-4, indicates an elevated risk for Alzheimer's disease). The Alzheimer's story is actually still more interesting. The risks of developing Alzheimer's disease vary to some extent for almost everyone depending on the combination of alleles of a gene called apolipoprotein E. *See* Akira Veki et al., *Phenotypes and Genotypes of Apolipoprotein E in Japanese Patients with Late-Onset Sporadic Alzheimer's Disease, Vascular Dementia, Down's Syndrome or Parkinson's Disease*, *in* ALZHEIMER'S AND PARKINSON'S DISEASES: RECENT DEVELOPMENTS 189, 189, 193 (Israel Hanin et al. eds., 1995) (noting the existence of three human apoe alleles and concluding that phenotype E4 is a factor in accelerating the Alzheimer disease process). At the same time, a small number of people have genetic variants that very strongly influence, if not determine, their risk of developing the disease.

138. *See, e.g.*, Gina Kolata, *Parents Take Charge, Putting Gene Hunt onto the Fast Track*, N.Y. TIMES, July 16, 1996, at B5 (describing how the parent-led Dysautonomia Foundation successfully financed research that led to genetic discoveries concerning the disease).

When dealing with genetic research, disease organizations, like tribal governments or the other culturally appropriate authorities in ethnic groups, face the same three issues of autonomy, reputation, and commercialization. At first glance, autonomy would not seem to be a relevant concern. Unlike tribal governments, other culturally relevant authorities, or, at the other end, families, disease organizations are associations with fully voluntary membership—and nonmembership. Disease organizations have no mandate, legal or cultural, to make decisions about research for nonmembers who suffer from the disease, nor do those who have joined them normally expect that they have given the organization this power. Disease organizations should not be viewed as having authority over these decisions.

On the other hand, disease organizations can play an important role in promoting the autonomy of the individuals, families, or ethnic groups affected by the disease. They can assist these exercises of autonomy by providing information and, when appropriate, recommendations. Disease organizations should have a much greater capacity than most individuals or families to evaluate research proposals. They can suggest the possible advantages and disadvantages of participation. They may be able to negotiate with the researchers for general changes in the research that would benefit people with the disease. And, they can communicate their views about the research to their members and others. In these ways, disease organizations can be useful expert intermediaries for people with the disease—not by making decisions, but by helping those people make better informed decisions.

The reputations of those with a given disease may well be affected by the results of genetic research. The researchers themselves should feel ethically compelled to minimize the adverse social effects of their research. Disease organizations can play an important role in helping limit such problems.

Disease organizations are better placed than individuals to see those possible disadvantages and to work with the researchers to mitigate them. On the one hand, they may be able to lobby for regulatory or legislative changes. More directly, if given advance notice of the planned research, and of its results, they can prepare information for people with the disease about these implications and advise them on how to limit or avoid them.

For example, research results may be conveyed in the newspapers in an incomplete and misleading way, often implying a stronger genetic link than actually has been shown. An organization involved in breast cancer could provide accurate information to people with breast cancer regarding the limited role played by the BRCA1 and BRCA2 genes in the disease. The patients' sisters or daughters could use that information to combat a belief, by insurers, employers, or others, that their family history means they will necessarily develop breast cancer.

Commercialization issues are somewhat more complicated. Commercial products derived from research aimed at a particular disease are likely to be either predictive tests, diagnostic tests, or, eventually, treatments for the disease. Unlike the case of genetic research into ethnic groups, these kinds of products necessarily have a direct, and often beneficial, effect on the people involved in the research. The tests and treatments are "compensation" for participation in the research, with or without any financial benefits.

On the other hand, the disease organization may be an appropriate focus for some financial benefits. The organization may have provided valuable assistance to both researchers and research participants in evaluating and discussing the proposed research. Its activities in promoting research, treatment, and support for people with the disease may be quite valuable. And, in a sense, such an organization is the only group that would plow back any financial benefits from the research to all those who contributed to the research, without raising concerns about the sale of an individual's genetic material. This kind of charitable financial interest, targeted generally to the benefit of those who participated in the research, seems an attractive compromise between giving research subjects no financial return from products developed with their genetic material and allowing a free market in such materials and has been endorsed in ethical guidelines from the Human Genome Organisation.[139] It may thus be appropriate for a disease organization to receive a financial interest in any commercial products arising from the research, to be used by the organization for the benefit of those with the disease.

Such a commercial interest does raise some problems. Having financial interests in the results of different research projects could certainly affect the impartiality of a disease organization's

139. Ethical, Legal, and Social Issues Committee, Human Genome Organisation, *Statement on the Principled Conduct of Genetics Research* (March 1996). The Statement takes the position

> [t]hat undue inducement through *compensation* for individual participants, families, and populations should be prohibited. This prohibition does not include agreements with individuals, families, groups, communities or populations that foresee technology transfer, local training, joint ventures, provision of health care or of information infrastructures, or the possible use of a percentage of any royalties for humanitarian purposes.

Id. Use by a disease organization for the benefit of those with the disease would seem to be a relevant "humanitarian" purpose.

evaluation of such research. The organization, while in theory devoted to helping those with the disease, could, in fact, spend funds for the immediate benefit of its leadership or some particularly favored beneficiaries. Ultimately, the possibility of medical advances may be all the compensation that people with the disease, or their organizations, have any right to expect. Nonetheless, in some circumstances, disease organizations may be appropriate beneficiaries of some financial interest in the commercial consequences of research.

If such organizations can play useful roles in autonomy, reputation, and commercialization as intermediaries for people with the disease, how could such a role be implemented? Researchers could be encouraged, or even required, to consult with the relevant disease organizations as a condition of human subjects approval of their research. IRBs should ask whether such organizations exist with respect to the diseases being researched. Where they do, the reviewers should require researchers to consult with all such organizations, unless they could show, to the reviewers' satisfaction, good reasons not to do so. They should not, however, require negotiations over control of commercial uses of the research, as the case for such control is weaker than it is with ethnic groups.

A requirement that researchers consult with disease organizations would raise some difficulties in implementation. Just as determining the relevant authority can be difficult for ethnic groups, determining what organization best speaks for those with a particular disease may also be difficult. Clearly, specialized organizations should be consulted for research on the specific conditions they cover, but should the American Cancer Society be consulted with respect to all genetic research into cancer? There are now myriad organizations, with very different approaches, concerning some diseases, such as breast cancer or AIDS. Some provide emotional, logistical, and financial support to those with the disease;[140] some specialize in promoting research;[141] others, such as ACT-UP, have strong political components.[142] Similar diversity exists for genetic diseases. A

140. *See, e.g.*, Doug Podolsky, *Inside the Cancer Charities: Why They Draw More Queries than Other Health Groups*, U.S. NEWS & WORLD REP., Dec. 4, 1995, at 84, 85 (describing how several cancer organizations provide support to cancer patients, including the Cancer Fund of Knoxville, Tennessee and National Children's Cancer Society of St. Louis, Missouri).

141. *See, e.g.*, Katherine T. Beddingfield et al., *Sizing Up the Biggest Stories and Stats of 50 Favorite American Charities*, U.S. NEWS & WORLD REP., Dec. 4, 1995, at 88, 90-91 (identifying major disease organizations whose goals include research, such as the American Cancer Society, American Heart Association, March of Dimes Birth Defects Foundation, and the Muscular Dystrophy Association).

142. *See* Serge F. Kovaleski, *Protesters Hold Capitol Funeral with Corpse of*

Cystic Fibrosis web page lists six different cystic fibrosis organizations in the United States, and another five overseas.[143] Which organizations, or what kinds of organizations, need to be consulted? Finally, in some cases, an organization for a particular disease might splinter into antagonistic factions. Which group should be consulted?

These are not questions that can be answered in the abstract, but need to be considered on a case-by-case basis. Where the organizations' roles are to be advisory, there seems no reason to restrict consultation to only one group. But, on the other hand, researchers, like everyone else, have limited time, energy, and resources. Imposing substantial consultation burdens will likely cut into the substantive research being done. Researchers, in seeking human subjects approval for their research, should be required to discuss what relevant disease organizations exist and to describe why they have chosen to consult with particular groups and not with others. The IRB should then be asked only to ensure that their choice was reasonable.

C. Families

Genetics research is, above all else, a family affair. Biological families necessarily share genetic variations as each child receives half her genome from her mother and half from her father.[144] Families in which a particular disease is unusually common are the primary focus of research on genetic diseases.[145] Ethnic groups are genetically interesting, as groups, because of

---

AIDS Victim, WASH. POST, July 2, 1993, at C2 (describing an ACT-UP political funeral for a member who wanted his body thrown upon the White House lawn in protest of the government's AIDS policies); *Mounted Police Break Up AIDS Protest at White House*, WASH. POST, Oct. 14, 1996, at B3 (relating an ACT-UP demonstration where members tossed funeral urns onto the White House lawn to protest President Clinton's AIDS policies); Linda Wheeler, *Varied Events Expected to Draw a Million Visitors to D.C.*, WASH. POST, Oct. 11, 1996, at B4 (expecting an ACT-UP rally to draw 5000 members to encircle the White House).

143. *See* CF Web: Support Groups, <http://www.ai.mit.edu/people/mernst/cf/support.html>.

144. *See* ALICE WEXLER, MAPPING FATE 90 (1995) (explaining that each organism inherits one set of chromosomes from the mother and one from the father); *see also* WALTER BODMER & ROBIN MCKIE, THE BOOK OF MAN: THE HUMAN GENOME PROJECT AND THE QUEST TO DISCOVER THE GENETIC HERITAGE 47 (1995) (defining a genome as the cell's total complement of chromosomes).

145. See Nancy Wexler, *Clairvoyance and Caution: Repercussions from the Human Genome Project*, *in* THE CODE OF CODES: SCIENTIFIC AND SOCIAL ISSUES IN THE HUMAN GENOME PROJECT 211, 216-17 (Daniel J. Kevles & Leroy Hood eds., 1992) (explaining that genetic researchers look for people affected by a disease to have a certain DNA marker, and for the unaffected relatives to have another form of the same marker).

their relatedness; genetic disease organizations are made up of people who, it is expected, share the same genetic variations within their families and, to a large extent, between their families.[146]

Information about one family member's genes necessarily provides some information about other family members.[147] Often, that information will not be determinative, but may strongly affect the probabilities that other family members will have a genetic variation or develop a genetic disease. Thus, although the incidence of Huntington's disease is around seven to ten persons in ten thousand in the general population,[148] the child or sibling of a person with the genetic variation leading to the condition faces odds of one in two.[149] Sometimes, the information will be determinative. If a person shares an unusual genetic variant with his father's mother, his father almost certainly has the variant.[150]

Just as researchers will often seek assistance from disease organizations, they will seek to recruit families to participate in research and will make contact broadly through an extended family, seeking affected and unaffected relatives to participate in the research. Just as with disease organizations, however, such contact is more than efficient science—it is ethically important for the same reasons of autonomy, reputation, and commercialization.

In the context of families, the concept of group autonomy is more complicated than for ethnic groups or disease organizations. Some ethnic groups, notably federally recognized tribes, have substantial legal powers under American law,[151] while other groups, such as African-Americans or the Amish, are recognized by our culture. Disease organizations clearly cannot make convincing claims, legal or cultural, to have the power to

---

146. In many cases, of course, more than one genetic variation will be linked to the same disease, in which case families involved in the disease organization may have different causative variants. *See* P.A. Baird, *The Role of Genetics in Population Health*, *in* WHY ARE SOME PEOPLE HEALTHY AND OTHERS NOT?: THE DETERMINANTS OF HEALTH OF POPULATIONS 133, 139 (Robert G. Evans et al. eds., 1994).

147. *See* WEXLER, *supra* note 144, at 90 (explaining that chromosomes are inherited from parents).

148. *See id.* at xxiv.

149. *See* THOMAS F. LEE, THE HUMAN GENOME PROJECT: CRACKING THE GENETIC CODE OF LIFE 191 (1991) ("Since a dominant gene is responsible, each child of a parent with the disease has a 50-50 chance of inheriting it.").

150. Of course, one can never be absolutely certain. The same variant might have transmitted from the mother or it could conceivably be a new mutation in the son. Nonetheless, when the variant is rare, the probability that it came from the father can be enormous.

151. Refer to notes 112-14 *supra* and accompanying text.

speak for all people with the disease. The status of families is still less clear, if not legally, then culturally.

Certainly, parents have substantial legal control over the raising of their children, which has some basis in the United States Constitution.[152] This control includes the general power to determine whether their minor children will participate in medical research.[153] Close family, including spouses in some circumstances, may make decisions concerning medical treatments, presumably including experimental treatments, for adult family members who are not competent to make their own decisions.[154] For most purposes, however, family members have no special legal rights concerning the participation of other family members in research.[155]

But apart from legal rights, do families have culturally-based expectations that they will be able to control, or influence, the decisions of family members about participating in research with implications for the entire family? The only plausible answers seem to be yes, no, and maybe. In the United States, family structures differ enormously. Some people have regular and meaningful contact with their extended families; others have no

152. *See* Pierce v. Society of Sisters, 268 U.S. 510, 535 (1925) (emphasizing that parents have a right to determine how their children are instructed); *see also* Meyer v. Nebraska, 262 U.S. 390, 401 (1923) (striking down a law that materially interferes with the power of parents to control the education of their children).

153. *See* Gwen O'Sullivan, *Studies Involving Children*, *in* IRB HANDBOOK, *supra* note 18, at 139-40 (noting that IRB provisions require the involvement of a parent, guardian, or advocate in the conduct of research with very young or disabled children).

154. States have provided competent adults with the opportunity to give family members such rights through living wills or durable powers of attorney for health care. *See* Cruzan v. Missouri Dep't of Health, 497 U.S. 261, 291 n.4 (1990) (O'Connor, J., concurring) (recognizing that 13 states have living will statutes authorizing the appointment of health care proxies); *id.* at 291 n.2 (listing 13 states and the District of Columbia as having durable power of attorney statutes expressly authorizing the appointment of proxies for making health care decisions). In some states, when an incompetent adult has not left a formal indication of his own wishes, family members may be able to make decisions on their own, even when the consequence may be to hasten the patient's death. *See In re* Guardianship of Estelle M. Browning, 568 So. 2d 4, 13 (Fla. 1990) ("[W]e do not limit the ability to exercise this right only to a legally appointed guardian, but recognize that it may be exercised by proxies or surrogates such as close family members or friends."); In the Matter of Sue Ann Lawrance, 579 N.E.2d 32, 41-43 (Ind. 1991) (holding that a court proceeding is not necessary for family members to order the discontinuation of life support in appropriate cases). In other states, however, judicial intervention may be necessary to appoint a guardian or to approve a treatment decision. *See* Drabick v. Drabick, 245 Cal. Rptr. 840, 841-42, 854-55 (Cal. Ct. App. 1988) (holding that the conservator of an incompetent person in a permanent vegetative state is authorized to decide that medical treatment in the form of life support can be withdrawn, even if the natural consequence is death).

155. *See* 45 C.F.R. § 46.111(a)(4) (1995) (requiring informed consent from the research subject or the subject's legally authorized representative).

connection even with their nuclear families. This variation certainly exists within the majority European-derived culture; it is doubtlessly multiplied when considering all the other national cultures represented in the United States. When considering research outside the United States, the possible cultural roles for the family become almost endless. Some families, in some cultures, will have expectations that the family unit, in some circumstances, should have the autonomy to make decisions that concern the family; other families will not.

Reputational concerns will also affect families. In many cases in the United States, the direct effect may seem small compared with the reputational effects felt by ethnic groups or people with a particular disease, in two different ways. First, a person is more likely to be known as an Irish, Navajo, or Chinese or as a person with cystic fibrosis or sickle cell anemia than as a member of a particular family. Second, genetic information about ethnic groups or diseases is more likely to be widely known than is information about a particular family's genetic variations. Neither of these may be true in every context, in the United States or elsewhere. For example, Dr. Nancy Wexler and others used an extended family in Venezuela to locate the gene for Huntington's disease.[156] In that region, both membership in the family and its genetic links to the disease were widely known.[157]

But even in the more anonymous situations, family reputations for genetic disease may be important, particularly for health insurance. If health insurance is subject to medical underwriting, an applicant may well be asked about family histories of diseases. Even the applicant's knowledge that a particular genetic disease is widely found in her family could end up preventing her from getting insurance, if she discloses it, or voiding any insurance she obtains, if she conceals it.[158] Her knowledge, as a result of her family's participation in a genetic research project, could be held against her *whether or not* she had chosen to participate in the project.

The last, and perhaps most controversial issue, is commer-

---

156. *See* LEE, *supra* note 149, at 192.

157. *See* Wexler, *supra* note 145, at 217 (stating that researchers were able to trace the disease back to a single woman that lived in the early 1800s). Of 11,000 descendants, there are 371 persons with Huntington's disease, 1266 at 50% risk, and 2395 at 25% risk for the disease. *See id.*

158. The medical underwriting process may ask for family histories of disease whether or not they are known to be genetic. A family's participation in genetics research may lead to a conclusion that a genetic disease is found in that family, information that insurers could seek to use in medical underwriting. Even if no genetic link was found, the research might give a family member so much more information about her family's history of a disease that an honest answer to an insurer's question would now reveal a family history of which she had been ignorant.

cialization. Whether individuals should benefit from the use of their genetic variations is strongly contested with many arguing that such sequence information should not be marketable.[159] In addition, it can be argued that families with genetic diseases, like disease organizations, may already receive a direct benefit from research through tests or treatments for their diseases.

It may well be that laws or social norms will, or should, forbid paying anyone for participating in genetic research, either directly or through some share of the proceeds. If, however, such compensation were possible, the family is a more appropriate unit than those individuals who chose to participate in the research. As pointed out above, useful advances come not from any individual, but from all family members about whom the research project collects information. This includes not just those from whom genetic material is tested, but also family members, perhaps long dead, who are useful to the research because they either had, or did not have, the disease in question. In addition, the family as a whole will bear the reputational costs of the research. Finally, a family financial interest in the commercialization of genetic discoveries could more plausibly be restricted to charitable or humanitarian ends than a personal interest. One could imagine a family trust or foundation that provided educational or financial support to members in need.

The argument for considering families as social units, as well as genetic units, in research certainly raises problems. The two major questions that raise difficulties in working with ethnic groups exist with families, and usually to a greater extent. Defining the "family" will often be difficult—how far up and down does it extend? Ascertaining the culturally appropriate authority for the family may be impossible—is a family ruled by its consensus, a majority vote, a patriarch or matriarch? The family will not have a federally recognized government or, usually, an organization with a set of bylaws. While anthropologists, expert in particular populations, might be able to help answer these questions for ethnic groups, outside experts will rarely if ever be able to answer questions about particular extended families.

For these reasons, a requirement that researchers "consult families" seems too vague to be appropriate. Researchers, and IRBs that review their protocols, should be sensitive to issues of family structure, however. Researchers need to talk with participants about what family means to them and how their families function, and, when appropriate, they should talk with the

159. *See, e.g.*, Bartha M. Knoppers et al., *Ethical Issues in International Collaborative Research on the Human Genome: The HGP and the HGDP*, 34 GENOMICS 272-82 (1996).

broader family. Ethical standards for research, inside and outside the United States, should require this kind of inquiry into their participants' families.

V. CONCLUSION

Genetics research is almost always research about groups of people, smaller than nation-states and larger than individuals. When the research creates knowledge about a group, the whole group is affected. As a result, the group, whenever possible, should have some say in the research.

The existing rules governing medical research, national and international, do not fit that reality. Some kinds of researchers, as a matter of necessity, have long sought group consent for research. The anthropologist or the epidemiologist usually needs de facto group consent, whether regulations require it or not. Although there have been exceptions, clinical medical research has usually dealt with individuals or sets of individuals, not with groups defined in some way beyond their own health condition and their participation in the research.

One solution cannot fit every group. Ethnic groups are different from disease organizations and from families. And different ethnic groups, genetic disease organizations, and families will all differ. There can be no one form for ethical treatment in genetic research of all the groups between. But the ethical questions raised by the existence of such groups should be addressed by all researchers and all those charged with ensuring the ethical conduct of such research.

[11]

HOW WILL WE REGULATE GENETIC ENHANCEMENT?

*Maxwell J. Mehlman**

Genetic enhancement technologies present difficult and novel regulatory issues, including the problem of measuring and comparing risks and benefits and dealing with the impact of these technologies on social values. This Article describes and evaluates the potential approaches that may be taken to regulate these technologies. The author concludes that a variety of approaches will be necessary, involving self-regulation, government restrictions on access and use, licensing, and a national lottery.

INTRODUCTION

On September 11, 1997, the National Institutes of Health ("NIH") convened the first of its "Gene Therapy Policy Conferences." The subject was the regulation of genetic enhancement. This meeting marked a new attitude toward the subject; previously, genetic enhancement was regarded largely as science fiction, and serious discussion of its attendant ethical, legal, and social issues was conspicuously absent from serious genetics journals.[1] The meeting was prompted by a request to NIH to approve a protocol for conducting a

---

* B.A. Reed College; B.A. Oxford University; J.D. Yale Law School. The author is Arthur E. Petersilge Professor of Law and Director, The Law-Medicine Center, Case Western Reserve University, and Professor of Biomedical Ethics, Case Western Reserve University School of Medicine. This article was written under a grant from the Ethical, Legal, and Social Implications Research Program, Human Genome Research Institute, National Institutes of Health (No. 1 RO1 HG01446-01A1). The author thanks Tom Murray and Eric Juengst for their helpful comments on earlier drafts; John Stam, Michael Cosgrove, Jennifer Walker, and Catherine Hess for their research help; and the participants in the NIH Gene Therapy Policy Conference, September 11, 1997.

1. No doubt the legitimization of the topic of genetic enhancement was aided by the successful cloning of "Dolly" in Scotland, an accomplishment previously dismissed as science fiction. *See* Gina Kolata, *Little-Known Panel Challenged to Make Quick Cloning Study*, N.Y. TIMES, Mar. 18, 1997, at C1 ("Dr. Wilmut's feat shocked the world, for even most scientists had assumed that the cloning of adults was biologically impossible and was merely the stuff of science fiction.").

gene therapy experiment on healthy volunteers, rather than on patients.[2] Although the experiment was part of an effort to develop treatments for cystic fibrosis, the proposed use of healthy subjects raised, for the first time, the question of whether and in what circumstances it was appropriate to use gene insertion technology in "normal" individuals.[3] Officials at NIH realized that it was a short step from preliminary testing in healthy subjects of a genetic treatment for disease to experiments intended to genetically enhance a normal person's physical or mental characteristics.[4]

In a sense, genetic enhancement has been with us for some time if we include within that category genetically engineered drug products used to alter physical traits. Human growth hormone ("HGH"), which had been obtainable prior to 1985 only in limited quantities from cadaveric pituitary glands,[5] now can be produced in a virtually inexhaustible supply using recombinant DNA technology.[6] When its supply was more limited, HGH was prescribed for children with short stature caused by classical growth hormone deficiency.[7] With the advent of recombinant DNA manufacturing, however, some physicians have begun recommending use of HGH for non-hormone-deficient children who are below "normal" height.[8] A survey of pediatric endocrinologists, for example, found that as many as thirty-three percent of the respondents would recommend HGH for children who were not hormone-deficient, but who were in the lowest three percent of their age group in terms of height.[9] Endocrinologists also report being asked by parents of "normal" children to prescribe HGH in order to give their children an advantage in competi-

2. *See* Rick Weiss, *Gene Enhancements' Thorny Ethical Traits*, WASH. POST, Oct. 12, 1997, at A1 (describing a meeting between the NIH and the Food and Drug Administration ("FDA") that considered regulation of cosmetic gene therapy).

3. *See id.*

4. *See id.*

5. *See* Mark McDonald, *A Growth Industry: Some Athletes Are Turning to Hormone for Competitive Edge, but Safety Debated*, DALLAS MORNING NEWS, May 21, 1995, at 1A.

6. *See* American Academy of Pediatrics, *Considerations Related to the Use of Recombinant Human Growth Hormone in Children*, 99 PEDIATRICS 122 (1997).

7. *See id.*

8. *See id.*; *see also* Leona Cuttler et al., *Short Stature and Growth Hormone Therapy: A National Study of Physician Recommendation Patterns*, 276 JAMA 531, 531 (1996) (indicating many pediatric endocrinologists consider growth hormone treatment appropriate for non-growth hormone deficient children).

9. *See* Cuttler et al., *supra* note 8, at 533 fig.1. Children in the survey were two standard deviations from the mean height for their age. *See id.* Approximately 90,000 of the three million children born each year will fall into this category. *See* Barry Werth, *How Short Is Too Short?*, N.Y. TIMES, June 16, 1991, § 6, at 14.

tive sports.[10] Adult athletes are believed to use HGH to spur bone and muscle growth.[11]

Although the use of recombinant drugs such as HGH raises important regulatory issues, as we shall see, the NIH conference was inspired by the prospect of genetic enhancement achieved by more radical technologies—in particular, gene insertion. This involves the introduction of actual genetic material into a person's cells. When the goal is therapeutic, the genetic material may consist of a "normal" gene that compensates for a missing or defective gene.[12] When the goal is enhancement, the gene may supplement the functioning of normal genes or supersede them with "supergenes" that have been engineered to produce a desired enhancement effect.[13] Gene insertion may be intended to affect a single individual, or it may target a person's reproductive cells, in which case the resulting effect, if complemented by the cells of the person's reproductive partner, will be produced in their children and passed on to succeeding generations.[14]

Genetic enhancement raises a host of ethical, legal, and social questions. When should parents give drugs such as HGH to children of "normal" stature? For that matter, what is meant by "normal"—i.e., when is a genetic intervention "enhancing" or "therapeutic"? (This distinction is critical, for example, in determining whether the intervention will be covered by health insurance.) How should the benefit from a genetic enhancement be calculated in comparing its risks and benefits? Would people who have been genetically enhanced enjoy an unfair advantage in competing for scarce resources, from sports awards to the allocation of academic and professional opportunities? If so, how should these competitions be conducted to avoid or reduce the unfairness? Concerns like these

10. *See* McDonald, *supra* note 5, at 1A.

11. *See Chinese Takeaway: HGH*, IRISH TIMES, Jan. 10, 1998, at 57 (noting that while HGH burns fat and promotes bone, connective tissue, and muscle growth, the muscle is weak in relation to its size); *On the Track of the Drug Cheats: The Battle Between the Sports Authorities and Athletes Who Break the Rules Is Being Fought at Ever Higher Levels, Says Clive Cookson*, FIN. TIMES (London), July 20, 1996, Comment and Analysis, at 9 (noting that Atlanta Olympics officials worried about use of HGH by competing athletes).

12. *See* Theodore Friedman, *Overcoming the Obstacles to Gene Therapy*, SCI. AM., June 1997, at 96, 97-98.

13. For an overview of gene insertion techniques, see generally *Special Report: Making Gene Therapy Work*, SCI. AM., June 1997, at 95, 95-123 (offering five articles that outline current developments in genetic technology). The insertion of normal genes or "supergenes" to supplement the working of normal genes also can be intended to achieve therapeutic objectives, such as providing added immunity to disease. *See* Eric Juengst, *What Does "Enhancement" Mean?*, *in* ENHANCING HUMAN TRAITS: ETHICAL AND SOCIAL IMPLICATIONS (Erick Parens ed., 1998). This complicates both the definition of "genetic enhancement" and the regulatory response.

14. *See* Steve Mirsky & John Rennie, *What Cloning Means for Gene Therapy*, SCI. AM., June 1997, at 122, 123.

arguably would be exacerbated by germ cell genetic enhancement, in which these risks and benefits, advantages and harms, would be transferred to successive generations.

As genetic enhancement technology emerges, responses to these and similar concerns necessarily will be forthcoming. The nature of these responses, and how successfully they resolve the problems that they target, will depend in the first instance on identifying the responding individuals or institutions, and the principles and decision-making algorithms that they will employ.

I. DEFINING GENETIC ENHANCEMENT

Identifying what we mean by genetic enhancement presents two major difficulties. First, when is an enhancement "genetic?" Second, when is a genetic manipulation "enhancement?" People constantly try to improve themselves and their children by means of diet, exercise, education, marriage, job changes, cosmetic surgery, and the like. Some of these efforts are successful, at least in part, by virtue of the person's genetic endowment. For example, someone who has inherited good looks is likely to find it easier to marry someone attractive, which may enhance their social standing and lead, in turn, to the production of handsome children.[15] Getting into a prestigious college is influenced by the applicant's aptitude—to some degree a matter of genetic endowment. In addition, one's genetic make-up helps determine how much improvement is required to achieve a desired effect. Someone who inherits a fine facial bone structure, for example, may require less radical plastic surgery to continue to appear young than someone with coarser features.

For purposes of this Article, an enhancement will be deemed genetic when it is produced by biotechnological processes, such as by a pharmacological product made using recombinant DNA technology or by gene insertion. These processes raise significant, new challenges to our regulatory capabilities. There is little precedent for germ cell enhancement engineering modifications at the genetic level that biologically affect succeeding generations. Techniques such as education and exercise are apt to be far more gradual and less pronounced than genetic enhancement. Even the relatively rapid changes produced by cosmetic surgery and the use of performance enhancement drugs in sports lack the potential depth and breadth of genetic alteration.

Obviously, not all genetic interventions will be enhancements. Some, indeed almost all at the outset, will aim to treat or to prevent disease or disorders. A genetic *enhancement*, then, refers to an in-

15. While discussing herself and other top models, Linda Evangelista stated, "We were blessed with genetic good fortune, and we have long bodies and a lot of us have hardly any body fat. . . . I hate using this term, but we are genetic freaks." *Model Says Super Looks Just a Freak of Nature*, PLAIN DEALER, May 16, 1996, at 2A.

tervention that is not undertaken for purposes of treating or preventing diseases or disorders.[16] Instead, an enhancement is aimed at improving a characteristic that, but for the enhancement, would be within what is generally regarded as a "normal" range,[17] or at installing a characteristic that would not normally be present.[18]

II. REGULATORY CONCERNS

A. *Efficacy*

As genetic enhancement technologies are developed, serious questions will arise concerning the appropriateness of their use. Answers to these questions will depend, in the first instance, on the effectiveness of these technologies in achieving their intended effects. Consider a genetically engineered drug or gene insertion technique that purports to improve mental acuity. Does it work? If so, how well does it work? The answers to these questions are necessary to enable individuals or regulators to compare the positive and negative consequences of the technology in order to decide

16. There is burgeoning, insightful literature dealing with the distinction between enhancement and therapy. *See, e.g.*, LEROY WALTERS & JULIE G. PALMER, THE ETHICS OF HUMAN GENE THERAPY (1997); Norman Daniels, *Growth Hormone Therapy for Short Stature: Can We Support the Treatment/Enhancement Distinction?*, 8 GROWTH GENETICS & HORMONES 46, 46-48 (Supp. I 1992); Eric T. Juengst, *Can Enhancement Be Distinguished from Prevention in Genetic Medicine?*, 22 J. MED. & PHIL. 125, 125-42 (1997); Eric Parens, *The Goodness of Fragility: On the Prospect of Genetic Technologies Aimed at the Enhancement of Human Capabilities*, 5 KENNEDY INST. ETHICS J. 141, 141-51 (1995). As Eric Juengst observes, it is not satisfactory to classify an intervention as an enhancement merely because the intervention is aimed at improving the functioning of healthy systems and normal traits; like enhancements, preventive medicine, especially immunizations, "'fixes' bodily functions that aren't 'broken.'" Juengst, *supra* note 13, at 33.

17. The concept of "normalcy" is so value-laden, arbitrary, and subjective that the term must be placed in quotation marks. Typically, it refers to a certain distribution of the population around an average measure for a particular trait. Clinicians generally consider a person to be clinically "short" or "tall" if their height is more than two standard deviations from the mean of the population. *See* Werth, *supra* note 9, § 6, at 14. Since two standard deviations comprise, by definition, approximately 95% of the population, 5% of the population automatically becomes defined as above or below "normal" height. *See* GARY L. TEITJEN, A TOPICAL DICTIONARY OF STATISTICS 4-5 (1986). A more sophisticated attempt defines "normalcy" as a level of functionality that allows an individual to enjoy the opportunity range typical of their species, an approach championed by Norman Daniels. *See* Daniels, *supra* note 16, at 47. This approach falters when it attempts to delineate the boundary between therapy and enhancement. As Eric Juengst observes, Daniels' thesis assumes that we can define "species-typical function" and that an individual's "skills and talents" are fixed according to the "natural lottery" of human genetics, neither of which obtains once genetic enhancements become available. *See* Juengst, *supra* note 13, at 36.

18. These might be cosmetic alterations of appearance, such as creating human hair or eye colors that were not found in nature.

whether or not the benefits are worth the risks. Suppliers of the product need efficacy information in order to gauge how much they should charge for it. Potential purchasers, whether patient-consumers or third-party payers, need the information to know whether or not the charge is worth it.

Establishing the efficacy of genetic enhancements will present many of the same difficulties as establishing the efficacy of medical and biological interventions. The effect of the intervention will have to be detected and measured. For enhancements that achieve their effect in the next generation, this will necessitate waiting until the enhanced person has matured enough to display the effect, if any.

Measuring the effect will require appropriate instruments and standardized scales. In some cases, the degree of the effect that is achieved will be measurable in objective terms. The effect of an enhancement that improved visual acuity could be ascertained by conventional, standardized techniques such as reading an eye chart. Similar tests exist for height, strength, and even memory and intelligence.[19] But some traits that might be the subject of genetic enhancement, such as beauty or charisma, do not lend themselves to traditional measurement approaches.[20] Perhaps instruments and scales for these traits will be developed in the future in response to the emergence of enhancement technologies.

Once the effect of a genetic enhancement technology is measured, the effect must be valued. For a health effect, the first step usually is assessing the effect in terms of its clinical benefit and then expressing that benefit in standardized units. Drugs used to treat heart attacks, called "clot-busters," are a good example. They dissolve blood clots that interfere with circulation to the heart muscle, causing the infarct or heart attack. Determining their efficacy, however, requires more than simply ascertaining if they dissolve blood clots, for that is only a means to achieve their clinical benefits: reducing the severity of the heart attack, preventing a recurrence, easing discomfort, increasing recovery time, restoring functionality, and, ultimately, prolonging life. These effects must be measured over many years if the question is how well the drugs prolong life.[21]

19. *See, e.g.*, CLINICAL NEUROPSYCHOLOGICAL ASSESSMENT: A COGNITIVE APPROACH (Robert L. Mapou & Jack Spector eds., 1995) (discussing neuropsychological testing); ALAN S. KAUFMAN, ASSESSING ADOLESCENT AND ADULT INTELLIGENCE (1990) (discussing intelligence tests); MUSCLE STRENGTH TESTING: INSTRUMENTED AND NON-INSTRUMENTED SYSTEMS (Louis R. Amundson ed., 1990) (testing muscle strength in physical therapy settings). Even these tests are subjective in that they depend upon the cooperation of and the accurate performance by the subject.

20. *Cf.* John T. Molloy, *Acquiring Charisma Demands a Change in Attitude*, HOUS. CHRON., Nov. 16, 1995, at 7 (declaring that the only way to measure charisma is in terms of its effect); Simon Perry, *That's Beauty Baby: Why Good Looks Dazzle Even Those Only Three Months Old*, EVENING STANDARD (London), May 28, 1996, at 3 (testing for the effects that beauty has on infants).

21. *See* BARUCH A. BRODY, ETHICAL ISSUES IN DRUG TESTING, APPROVAL, AND

Finally, in order to compare the effectiveness of different interventions, clinical benefit must be expressed in standardized ways, such as in terms of providing additional years of life.

Up to this point, we have been largely objective. We measure effects such as functionality, recovery time and prolongation of life by observation, and we protect against observer bias by various techniques such as blinding the observers to whether the patients they are evaluating have or have not received the experimental modality. But we also employ subjective measures, such as relief from pain. Most importantly, the ultimate value that we place on the observed benefits is subjective: an additional year of life, for example, may be worth more to one person than to another.[22]

The same tasks would be necessary in assessing the efficacy of genetic enhancements. We would need to evaluate their effect not only in terms of the magnitude of their direct impact—extra inches of height or IQ points, for example—but in terms of the ultimate benefits that these effects produced: the increased probability of becoming a professional basketball player or of getting into Harvard. In addition, we would need to place a value on being a professional basketball player or a Harvard graduate. This value is likely to

---

PRICING 23 (1995) (discussing concept of clinical efficacy).

22. Researchers have struggled to develop ways to standardize these values. One approach attempts to convert benefits into a scale based on the person's willingness to pay for them. For example, if a person would be willing to pay $10,000 for an additional year of life and only $5000 for a year of restored function, then we can conclude that they value life above functionality. However, this system breaks down when we extend it to more than one individual, as we might if we were a regulatory agency determining whether the benefit from a genetic technology exceeded the risk. In this case, the willingness to pay approach falsely assumes that everyone has the same wealth and needs, so that a sum of money—say $10,000—is worth the same to all. *See generally* Elizabeth Hoffman & Matthew L. Spitzer, *Willingness to Pay vs. Willingness to Accept: Legal and Economic Implications*, 71 WASH. U. L.Q. 59, 61-97 (1993) (analyzing divergence between willingness to accept and willingness to pay models); Ted R. Miller, *Willingness to Pay Comes of Age: Will the System Survive?*, 83 NW. U. L. REV. 876, 886-91 (1989) (explaining willingness to pay approach and its use in regulatory analysis); Dennis C. Taylor, *Your Money or Your Life?: Thinking About the Use of Willingness-to-Pay Studies to Calculate Hedonic Damages*, 51 WASH. & LEE L. REV. 1519, 1552-55 (1994) (criticizing willingness to pay approach for majority of torts contexts). The subjectivity of valuing benefit confounds another standardization technique, called quality-adjusted life years ("QALYs"), which attempts to adjust the additional years of life produced by a medical intervention in order to take into account the patient's quality of life. Valuing different qualities of life is highly subjective; the state of being deaf may be much worse for a musician, for example, than for a computer programmer. In fact, advocates for persons with disabilities contend that disabilities are often valued as more serious detriments than they are perceived by those who have them. *See* Alexander M. Capron, *Oregon's Disability: Principles or Politics?*, HASTINGS CTR. RPT., Nov. 1992, at 18; Paul T. Menzel, *Oregon's Denial: Disabilities and Quality of Life*, HASTINGS CTR. RPT., Nov. 1992, at 21.

vary substantially from person to person.

An analogy might be cosmetic surgery. How would we establish that the surgery was efficacious? One way would be to construct a visual image of the desired outcome and compare it to the surgical result. But one could argue that we have still failed to measure the ultimate effect, such as whether the patient gains a better self-image or is more successful at business or at attracting a mate. These effects are highly subjective, as was recognized by a panel of outside experts advising the FDA on the efficacy of liposuction devices.[23] The panel decided that it could only characterize the benefits from these devices in terms of patient satisfaction.[24]

In one respect, moreover, evaluating the efficacy of genetic enhancements is likely to prove particularly difficult: valid and reliable efficacy data for genetic enhancement technologies are likely to be extremely scarce. This will be the case for two reasons. First, depending on how genetic enhancement is achieved, providers and suppliers may not be required to submit safety and efficacy data to the government and obtain government approval before marketing enhancement technologies. To the extent that genetic enhancement is deemed a surgical or medical procedure, as opposed to the administration of a drug, biological, or medical device,[25] it will not require prior approval by the FDA, which would be based on adequate and well-controlled clinical investigations.[26] Without being required to submit this data, it is unlikely that anyone would go to the enormous expense of creating it.[27] More importantly, even if regulators regard genetic enhancements as drugs, biologicals, or medical devices, these technologies are likely to emerge first as unapproved or "off-label" uses of therapeutic technologies—that is, uses for which the manufacturers are not labeling or promoting the technologies—and manufacturers are not required to conduct clinical investigations to support such uses.[28] The experience with HGH,

23. *See* Notice of Panel Recommendation, 61 Fed. Reg. 58,195-96 (1996) (giving notice that the FDA General Surgery and Plastic Surgery Devices Panel voted to reclassify liposuction devices from Class III to Class II).

24. *See id.* at 58,197.

25. For a description of these different modalities and a discussion of the differences in their regulation by the FDA, see *infra* Section III.E.

26. *See* 21 U.S.C.S. § 321(g)(1), (h) (Law. Co-op. 1997) (defining requirements for drugs and medical devices); 42 U.S.C.S. § 262 (Law. Co-op. 1994 & Supp. 1999) (outlining current regulation of biological products).

27. It is estimated that it costs an average of $359 million to research a new drug and send it through the FDA approval process. *See* Theresa Beeby Lewis, Comment, *Patent Protection for the Pharmaceutical Industry: A Survey of the Patent Laws of Various Countries*, 30 INT'L LAW. 835, 842 (1996).

28. However, manufacturers and providers are required by the FDA to submit reports of adverse events that occur in connection with the use of their products, whether through approved or unapproved uses. *See* 21 U.S.C.S. § 360i (Law. Co-op. 1997). Prior to mandatory reporting, some amount of safety data would be available, although it is not clear how complete this information

mentioned earlier, is a good example. The drug was approved by the FDA for use in individuals who were deficient in growth hormone. Nevertheless, pediatric endocrynologists began prescribing it for other individuals with short stature. There are reports that parents are seeking the drug—and no doubt obtaining it—for use in children who are of normal height and even for use in some who are tall, in the hopes that the drug will enable them to grow tall enough to become successful basketball players.[29] Efficacy data exists for the approved use of HGH, but there are likely to be only unconfirmed reports from uncontrolled case studies for the off-label uses.[30]

B. Adverse Effects

The same difficulties in determining the efficacy of genetic enhancements will interfere with assessing their risks. The likelihood that genetic enhancement will not trigger regulatory requirements applicable to drugs, biologics, or medical devices or that enhancement technologies will emerge as unapproved uses of approved drugs and devices will limit the availability of safety and efficacy information. Safety information may be especially deficient since the hazards of genetic enhancement may only manifest themselves in succeeding generations, and therefore may not be apparent for many years. Even if safety data were available, standardized measurement tools are lacking for effects such as pain. Furthermore, the valuation of harms, like that of benefits, is subjective; the shortening of life by a year, for example, may be viewed much more seriously by one person than another.

These limitations confound the central regulatory function of comparing risks and benefits. No intervention is completely safe; even the most innocuous treatment carries with it some element of risk however improbable or trivial. The question is whether the expected benefit is worth the potential risk. Given the problems in assessing the safety and efficacy of genetic enhancements, the most that may be possible may be to compare the risks involved in employing different means to achieve similar enhancement effects. For example, suppose that eye color can be changed using either genetic manipulation or colored contact lenses. Holding the desired benefit constant—producing a certain eye color—may allow us to compare the hazards without as much uncertainty and subjectivity as if we

---

would be since reporting of adverse events is not rigorously enforced. *See, e.g.*, Kathleen Kerr, *FDA Didn't Link Heart-valve Damage to Diet Drugs*, SEATTLE TIMES, Dec. 22, 1997, at A2 (criticizing FDA for limited follow-up of serious adverse event reports).

29. *See* Rita Rubin, *Giving Growth a Synthetic Hand: Use of Hormone Sparks Debate*, DALLAS MORNING NEWS, July 7, 1986, at 1A.

30. The FDA Modernization Act of 1997 changed the law to permit manufacturers to distribute literature on unapproved uses of drugs so long as the manufacturers are conducting studies intended to lead to eventual approval for the uses. 21 U.S.C.S. § 360aaa (Law. Co-op. 1997).

were comparing, say, changing eye color versus increasing height. Yet even this limited comparison of risks assumes that safety data are known.

Still, these problems also beset the regulation of technologies other than genetic enhancement. For example, the FDA is constantly struggling with the problem of regulating off-label uses of drugs and devices.[31] The gaps in the regulation of medical and surgical interventions, as opposed to new drugs and devices, is well-known and much-lamented.[32] The subjectivity of risk is a fundamental complication in all types of regulatory decision-making.[33] These problems may be exacerbated in the case of genetic enhance-

31. Off-label use within the medical community is accepted as part of a physician's discretion and considered essential to medical care. The FDA acknowledges the need for this discretion as do courts and Congress, which enacted legislation to prohibit FDA intrusion into medical practice by restricting off-label use. *See* 21 U.S.C.S. § 396 (Law. Co-op. 1997); James M. Beck & Elizabeth D. Azari, *FDA, Off-label Use, and Informed Consent: Debunking Myths and Misconceptions*, 53 FOOD & DRUG L.J. 71, 78 (1998). The FDA encounters problems regulating off-label use because it can be hard to draw the line between the legitimate flow of information (which is part of a doctor's practice and therefore not subject to FDA regulation) and a manufacturer's promotion of off-label use strictly for profit. *See* William L. Christopher, *Off-Label Drug Prescription: Filling the Regulatory Vacuum*, 48 FOOD & DRUG L.J. 247, 248-51 (1993). A federal district court ruled in July 1998 that the FDA's present rules regulating the dissemination of information regarding off-label use constituted a restriction of commercial free speech. *See* Washington Legal Found. v. Friedman, 13 F. Supp. 2d 51, 74 (D.D.C. 1998), *amended by*, 36 F. Supp. 2d 16 (D.D.C. 1999), *and amended by*, 36 F. Supp. 2d 418 (D.D.C. 1999). The court approved an injunction blocking enforcement of the existing rules. *See id.* at 74-75. This decision allows manufacturers to inform physician of uses of products even if those uses have not been approved by the FDA, subject to certain conditions. *See Federal Court Holds FDA May Not Restrict Information Involving Off-Label Use of Drugs*, 7 HEALTH LAW REP. (BNA) 1243 (Aug. 6, 1998).

32. New surgical procedures are typically subject only to approval from an institutional review board. *See* Jodi K. Fredrickson, *He's All Heart . . . And a Little Pig Too: A Look at the FDA Draft Xenotransplant Guideline*, 52 FOOD & DRUG L.J. 429, 438-43 (1997). However, the vast development of biotechnology products is pushing the limits of the FDA's definitions and approaches to regulation and challenging the traditional notion that the FDA doesn't regulate medical procedures. The dividing line as to the FDA's jurisdiction has become blurred by new cellular and related therapies that are often developed by processing cells and tissues. *See* Edward L. Korwek, *Human Biological Drug Regulation: Past, Present, and Beyond the Year 2000*, 50 FOOD & DRUG L.J. 123, 145-47 (1995); *see also* Jack M. Kress, *Xenotransplantation: Ethics and Economics*, 53 FOOD & DRUG L.J. 353, 381-84 (1998) (explaining that some transplant physicians argue xenotransplantation doesn't fall within FDA's jurisdiction because it is a surgical procedure and not a regulatory product).

33. Conclusive, direct evidence that a particular drug or device will threaten human health is rare. For example, science can establish the effects of high doses of formaldehyde in mice, "but quantification of the effects of low doses on humans currently lies beyond the reach of science." Wendy E. Wagner, *The Science Charade in Toxic Risk Regulation*, 95 COLUM. L. REV. 1613, 1619 (1995).

ment because of its novelty and the dearth of relevant data. But, by themselves, they do not indicate that the regulation of genetic enhancement would be fundamentally different than the regulation of other technologies, nor that regulating genetic enhancement would require the development of new regulatory approaches or entities.

Yet genetic enhancement does raise a host of truly unprecedented risks that are noteworthy not only for their novelty but for their subtlety. For, unlike the risks from traditional therapeutic interventions, which predominantly involve health hazards to the individual receiving the therapy, the principal risks from genetic enhancement are risks to third parties. They fall into three main categories: threats to social equality, "cheating," and the loss of personal autonomy. Let us turn to this last category first.

1. Personal Autonomy

Genetic enhancement threatens personal autonomy when it is imposed on persons without their consent. This could occur if enhancement were mandated by the government, say as part of a eugenics program, but a more likely scenario would be when a parent genetically enhanced a fetus or child, or when a person opted for germ cell enhancement for themselves or their offspring. These cases raise concerns because the effects of the enhancements, both positive and negative, are not chosen by those whom they will affect, and might not be chosen by them if they were given the choice.

We have had considerable experience with this problem in contexts other than genetic enhancement. Similar issues arise when medical treatment decisions are contemplated for persons who cannot make those decisions for themselves, such as when persons are unconscious;[34] when parents make treatment or lifestyle decisions for their children;[35] when researchers propose to experiment on em-

34. With respect to persons who are unconscious, the Supreme Court of New Jersey held that the only practical way to prevent destruction of an unconscious patient's right to privacy is to permit the guardian and family to make their best judgment as to how the patient would exercise her judgment. *See In re* Quinlan, 355 A.2d 647, 664 (N.J. 1976) (involving a father who sought to remove extraordinary treatment from daughter who was in persistent vegetative state). Furthermore, if the decision is to forgo treatment, then it should be a decision acceptable to a society in which the overwhelming majority would make the same choice in similar circumstances. *See id.*

35. Parental autonomy is constitutionally protected. The United States Supreme Court has extended the concept of a right to privacy to child rearing. *See* United States v. Orito, 413 U.S. 139, 142 (1973); Wisconsin v. Yoder, 406 U.S. 205, 213-14 (1972). "Parental autonomy, however, is not absolute." *In re* Philip B., 92 Cal. App. 3d 796, 802 (1979) (holding that the parents had a right to refuse surgery for their child with Down's syndrome even though it would significantly expand his life span and improve his physical functioning). Because the state has an interest in preserving life, if parents fail to provide their children with adequate care, the state is justified to intervene. However, since parental rights are sacred, they should only be invaded for the most compelling

bryos, fetuses, children, or persons who are mentally incompetent;[36] in connection with abortion;[37] and in treatment decisions by or for pregnant women that may affect their fetuses.[38] We respond to these situations in general by first trying to ascertain the wishes of the affected person or persons whenever possible and however imperfectly, such as by seeking statements by them of what they would prefer in related situations (the inaptly-named "substituted judgment" approach),[39] or by estimating what they would choose for themselves if they could do so, given what we know about them. If it is impossible to tell what the affected individual would have wanted, such as when the individual is *in utero*, the decision is made based on what "we" (society, family members, caregivers, legislators, judges, juries, ethics committee members—whoever is making or reviewing the decision) would want done if we were in the same cir-

---

reason. *See id.* In order to intervene, the state has the "burden of proving by clear and convincing evidence that intervening in the parent-child relationship is necessary to ensure the safety or health of the child, or to protect the public at large." Newmark v. Williams, 588 A.2d 1108, 1110 (Del. 1990) (allowing Christian Scientist parents to refuse chemotherapy to treat their child's cancer). Parents also have a right to decide their child's lifestyle to a degree. *See Yoder*, 406 U.S. at 211, 234-35 (holding that Amish parents have a right to teach their children the "specific skills needed to perform the adult role of an Amish farmer or housewife").

36. A mental illness does not necessarily mean that a person is incompetent. A mentally ill patient can still retain the ability to communicate and understand information. A patient diagnosed with schizophrenia still has the right to refuse treatment if her decision is made while she is competent. *See* United States v. Charters, 829 F.2d 479, 499 (4th Cir. 1987). Furthermore, life-sustaining treatment can be removed from an incompetent patient if it is clear that the patient would have wanted it removed. *See In re* Conroy, 486 A.2d 1209, 1229 (N.J. 1985). The decision "should be that which would be made by the incompetent person, if that person were competent, but taking into account the present and future incompetence of the individual as one of the factors which would necessarily enter into the decision-making process of the competent person." Superintendent of Belchertown State Sch. v. Saikewicz, 370 N.E.2d 417, 431 (Mass. 1977).

37. *See* Mary Mahowald & Virginia Abernethy, *When a Mentally Ill Woman Refuses Abortion*, HASTINGS CTR. REP., April 1985, at 22 (discussing a chronic paranoid schizophrenic woman's choice to continue her pregnancy against the advice of her mother who has legal custody).

38. *See* VAW v. Johnson Controls, Inc., 499 U.S. 187, 211 (1991) (holding that it was not appropriate for courts or employers to decide whether women should have children despite the fact that women, through their jobs, were exposed to lead which threatened the health of their fetuses); THOMAS H. MURRAY, THE WORTH OF A CHILD 96-115 (1996) (arguing that each individual should do her own balancing, considering all relevant factors as opposed to society treating pregnancy as a "moral trump card").

39. The substituted judgment approach, also known as the limited-objective test, states that "life-sustaining treatment may be withheld or withdrawn . . . when there is some trustworthy evidence that the patient would have refused the treatment, and the decision-maker is satisfied that it is clear that the burdens of the patient's continued life with the treatment outweigh the benefits . . . ." *Conroy*, 486 A.2d at 1232.

cumstances (the "best interests" approach).[40] Only in rare and controversial instances do we permit the interests of the affected individual to be overridden, such as in the case of abortion (where we sometimes content ourselves with the fiction that the affected entity has no real legal interests).[41]

Most importantly, we require decision-makers to act cautiously in these situations. Seldom can they act hastily or alone. Parents or family members seeking to make a treatment decision for a non-autonomous individual usually must consult at least a physician, and a physician usually must consult parents or next-of-kin. Review by a hospital ethics committee may be required. Researchers must obtain permission from an institutional review board and possibly from the FDA or NIH. In some jurisdictions, certain steps can only be taken pursuant to a court order.[42]

Similarly, we might expect that the regulation of genetic enhancement would include procedural protections for those who were proposed to be enhanced, but who could not choose for themselves. For example, parents might be required to get someone's permis-

40. The best interests approach, also known as the objective standard, incorporates what society considers to be reasonable medical choices. This standard is used when there is no evidence of an incompetent patient's former treatment preferences. *See* Rebecca Dresser, Bioethics and the Law (unpublished manuscript, on file with author). To justify removal of life-saving medical treatment, the burdens oo the patient's life with the treatment must clearly outweigh the benefits that the patient would derive from the treatment. In addition to this, there must be "recurring, unavoidable and severe pain . . . such that the effect of administering life-sustaining treatment would be inhumane." *Conroy*, 486 A.2d at 1232.

41. *See* John A. Robertson, *Genetic Selection of Offspring Characteristics*, 76 B.U. L. REV. 421, 444-46 (1996) (explaining how those who view the fetus as having no legal interests may not oppose abortion of fetuses with disabilities or abortion for gender selection).

42. The Supreme Court of Massachusetts outlined the required procedures for deciding whether to give or withhold life-prolonging treatment for an incompetent patient. *See Saikewicz*, 370 N.E.2d at 432-34. The court held that the first step was to petition for the appointment of a guardian or temporary guardian in Probate Court. Although the Probate Court was the proper court to determine the best interests of the incompetent patient, the appointed guardian ad litem was responsible for investigating the situation and representing the interests of the patient. If the judge, after listening to the guardian's report, was satisfied that the incompetent person would not have chosen treatment, then the judge would order treatment to be withheld. He would refuse to issue such an order if he was not satisfied that the patient would have so chosen or if he felt that the interests of the State required treatment. In developing this procedure, the Massachusetts Supreme Court expressly rejected the approach adopted by the New Jersey Supreme Court in *In re Quinlan*, which had held the decision should be entrusted to the patients, guardians, family, doctors, and hospital ethics committees. *See Saikewicz*, 370 N.E.2d at 434; *see also* John D. Hodson, Annotation, *Judicial Power to Order Discontinuance of Life- Sustaining Treatment*, 48 A.L.R.4TH 67 (1998) (analyzing federal and state cases in which courts have discussed under what conditions judicial authority exists to order discontinuance of life-sustaining treatment for incompetent patients).

sion, such as an ethics committee's or a court's, before they could enhance their children (whether before or after conception or birth). Such a regimen would require three components: (1) a set of decision-making rules; (2) a procedural mechanism, such as a court or a public or private administrative body; and (3) an enforcement method, including monitoring and sanctions.

Whatever "rules" or principles parents might justifiably use in deciding whether to pursue enhancements will depend in part on the particulars of the enhancement technologies in question. Some "enhancements" primarily will be for the child's benefit, while others may be directed more towards the parents' advantage or preference. Some enhancement technologies may carry very little risk to the children on whom they are used, while others may be quite risky. The guiding principles will rely on our conceptions of good parent-child relationships, on the values at the core of those relationships, and on the impact particular forms of enhancement technologies have on those values.

Procedural decision-making and enforcement mechanisms will be discussed below, but first, we need to address the two other major "safety" concerns: threats to social equality and "cheating." Both of these remaining social concerns stem from the fact that genetic enhancement will not readily be available to everyone. The primary roadblock will be cost.[43] Prenatal and germ cell enhancements most likely will involve expensive techniques such as *in vitro* fertilization ("IVF"), in addition to the cost of the enhancements themselves. IVF alone now costs an average of $38,000 per delivery.[44] Even somatic cell enhancement, which might be accomplished with drugs or drug-like techniques, is likely to be too expensive for most people to afford out-of-pocket. For a twenty kilogram child, growth hormone therapy costs approximately $14,000 per year.[45] Most people will need to rely on insurance to cover the costs of enhancement. If public and private health insurance coverage of analogous technologies today is

---

43. Other impediments will be infertility or post-reproduction age, in which cases germ cell enhancement will not be possible. Yet the age at which a woman can bear a child is advancing, and techniques such as cloning may enable reproduction to take place in cases where it is now impossible. The birth rate among women aged 30-34 rose from 61.9 per 1000 women in 1980 to 79.5 in 1991. *See* STEPHANIE J. VENTURA ET AL., U.S. DEPT. OF HEALTH AND HUMAN SERVICES, *Trends in Pregnancies and Pregnancy Rates: Estimates for the United States, 1980-92*, *in* MONTHLY VITAL STATISTICS REP. at 1, 7 (May 25, 1995). For an in-depth discussion of the reproductive possibilities of cloning technology, see LEE M. SILVER, REMAKING EDEN: CLONING AND BEYOND IN A BRAVE NEW WORLD (1997); Melinda Faier, *Cloning Breeds Contempt and Adulation: Now All Women May Have a Chance to Bring up Baby*, CHI. TRIB., Mar. 7, 1997, Commentary, at 23.

44. New York Taskforce Report 60.

45. Beth S. Finkelstein et al., *Insurance Coverage, Physician Recommendations, and Access to Emerging Treatments: Growth Hormone Therapy for Childhood Short Stature*, 279 JAMA 663, 663 (1998).

any indication, however, genetic enhancement will not be covered by most insurance policies.[46]

In case there is any doubt on this point, consider currently available products or services that might be thought of as "enhancements": cosmetics, cosmetic medicine and surgery, private education, fitness centers and trainers, and so on.[47] All of these must be purchased with personal funds rather than with funds furnished by third parties such as insurers or the government.[48]

Cosmetic surgery offers perhaps the best illustration. Medicare, for example, does not cover "items or services . . . which are not reasonable and necessary for the treatment of illness or injury, or to improve the functioning of a malformed body member," and there is an express statutory exclusion for "cosmetic surgery."[49] The same exclusions appear in private health insurance policies. An interesting consequence is that patients and their care-givers attempt to portray cosmetic interventions as necessary for the patient's mental and physical well-being in order to compel third-party payment. An illustration comes from an Idaho case, *Viveros v. Idaho Dept. of Health and Welfare*,[50] in which the state Medicaid program denied coverage of otoplastic surgery for an eight-year-old boy with unusually large ears.[51] The child's physicians attempted to portray the surgery as necessary for the child's self-esteem and not just to improve his appearance, but the state's rejection of their argument was upheld by the court.[52]

Although analogous services are not covered by current third-party payment systems, genetic enhancement is liable to be viewed as extremely desirable, especially if it is perceived to be relatively safe for the enhanced individual. Theoretically, genetic enhancement could improve any inherited trait, such as strength, stamina, height, weight, body type, beauty, intelligence, and even those that are multifactorial (that is, the product of the interaction of more than one gene) and those that are substantially affected by the individual's environment.[53] The demand for genetic enhancement, ac-

46. For a more extensive discussion of insurance limitations for genetic technologies, see MAXWELL J. MEHLMAN & JEFFREY R. BOTKIN, ACCESS TO THE GENOME: THE CHALLENGE TO EQUALITY 62-87 (1998).

47. The list focuses on products or services to exclude self-enhancement through, say, diet, exercise, or reading. Genetic enhancements will be provided, not self-generated.

48. The only exceptions might be training and fitness services provided by employers to boost productivity or by educational institutions or national sports associations to increase institutional or national prestige, and some degree of enhancement through social interactions such as "marrying up." Yet these enhancements also are available only to a few.

49. *See* 42 U.S.C.S. § 1395y(a)(1)(A), (a)(10) (Law. Co-op. 1993).

50. 889 P.2d 1104 (Idaho 1995).

51. *Id.* at 1105.

52. *See id.* at 1107.

53. There is a vigorous debate among scientists and social scientists over

cordingly, will be enormous. But this does not mean that third-party payers will add it to their list of covered services. The cost is likely to be enormous as well. Moreover, the very desirability of the services tends to disqualify them as candidates for true insurance coverage. There is no point in insuring a population for an expense that it is certain to incur, since the premium would be the same as the cost.[54] Public programs like Medicare and Medicaid might consider using government funds to cover genetic enhancement for those who could not otherwise afford them. The foregoing objection to regarding coverage of genetic enhancement as insurance could be eliminated if this coverage was viewed more as a redistribution of wealth via progressive taxation than as an insurance plan funded by enrollee premiums. Still, it is highly unlikely that the government would be able to afford the provision of genetic enhancement to everybody who might wish to obtain it. Even if it cost only $10,000,[55]

---

the degree to which genes or the environment control individual destiny—the so-called "nature versus nurture" controversy. Francis Galton, Charles Darwin's cousin, coined the phrase nature-nurture. His view was that "nature prevail[ed] enormously over nurture . . . ." ROBERT PLOMIN, GENETICS AND EXPERIENCE: THE INTERPLAY BETWEEN NATURE AND NURTURE 2-3 (1994) (quoting FRANCIS GALTON, INQUIRIES INTO HUMAN FACULTY AND ITS DEVELOPMENT 241 (1883)). Galton thought environment played a minor role in behavioral development. People in this school of thought became known as "hereditarians." The "environmentalists" argued that there was "no such thing as an inheritance of capacity, talent, temperament, mental constitution and characteristics" and that the environment determined our behavior. *Id.* at 3 (quoting J.B. WATSON, BEHAVIORISM 74 (1925)). Today, there is probably not a single scientist that would assert that behavior is ruled completely by the environment or completely by genetics. Research in the field of behavioral genetics has shown that "genetic influence is significant and substantial for most areas of behavioral development, even though it is not true that 'nature prevails enormously over nurture'." *Id.* Some argue that this conclusion leads to problems in and of itself. *See* Susan M. Wolf, *Beyond "Genetic Discrimination": Toward the Broader Harm of Geneticisim*, 23 J.L. MED. & ETHICS 345, 350 (1995) (pointing out that those who assert the importance of genetic factors are criticized by others for their "genetic discrimination" or "geneticism"). Nevertheless, it seems clear that even if genes are not the whole story, in that environmental conditions may moderate or modify genetic interventions, genetic manipulation will have a substantial impact on individual ability. *See* Natalie Angier, *Separated by Birth?*, N.Y. TIMES, Feb. 8, 1998, § 7, at 9 (mentioning the work of Thomas J. Bouchard, who conducted twin research at the University of Minnesota to study the effect of genes versus the environment, as well as his recent conclusion that the consensus figure for various studies is a heritability of 66% for IQ scores where heritability refers to the degree to which the difference between two people with regard to a trait is ascribed to genetic, rather than environmental factors).

54. Even life insurance, which arguably insures people against a certain event, depends for its profitability on betting on when the insured's death will occur.

55. The consensus seems to be that IVF costs at least $10,000 for each try. The national average for IVF programs is 20%, that is, there is a 20% chance that one egg in several will lead to a pregnancy, but not necessarily a baby. *See generally* Kristina Brenneman, *20 Years of In Vitro Test Tube Births Still Rais-*

and if only fifty million Americans sought coverage, the bill would be more than $500 billion. Furthermore, this would not be a one-time cost, since people might seek enhancement for each one of their children.[56]

The result, then, is that genetic enhancement will not be available to all, but only to the few who can afford to purchase it out of their personal finances. This, in turn, leads to the two major threats presented by genetic enhancement: the undermining of the principle of social equality that forms the foundation of Western democratic societies, and the related problem of "cheating"—the unfair advantage enjoyed by enhanced individuals in competitions for scarce societal resources.

2. *Social Inequality*

In the worst case scenario, unequal access to genetic enhancement will divide society into the enhanced and the un-enhanced. Germ cell enhancement will perpetuate enhancements from generation to generation, creating a hereditary aristocracy or "genobility." Added to their wealth, a prerequisite to being able to afford genetic enhancement, will be the advantages conferred by the enhancements themselves. The result will be a group of privileged individuals and families whose position in society will be virtually unassailable.[57]

This will pose grave threats to our political and social structure. The belief in social equality, reflected in the words of the Declaration of Independence that "all men are created equal," is the glue that holds our society together.[58] In the face of the evident disparities between us, we rely on the notion of equality of opportunity.

ing Questions, PATRIOT LEDGER (Quincy, Mass.), July 27, 1998, at 1 (explaining improvements in IVF technology).

56. One can imagine various efforts by the government to reduce this cost, such as limiting the number of children a person could have or the number of children who could be enhanced, but these all require government controls on private life that are unprecedented and extremely difficult to enforce.

57. The number of non-enhanced persons who become able to move upward into this social stratum is likely to be extremely limited, comprising only those who somehow accumulate enough wealth to purchase enhancements for themselves or their children, or who are able to marry into the genobility. *See* MEHLMAN & BOTKIN, *supra* note 46, at 99.

58. *See, e.g.*, FRANK PARKIN, CLASS INEQUALITY AND POLITICAL ORDER: SOCIAL STRATIFICATION IN CAPITALIST AND COMMUNIST SOCIETIES 48 (1971). Parkin writes:

> Inequality in the distribution of rewards is always a potential source of political and social instability. Because upper, relatively advantaged strata are generally fewer in number than disadvantaged lower strata, the former are faced with crucial problems of social control over the latter. One way of approaching this issue is to ask not why the unprivileged often rebel against the privileged but why they do not rebel more often than they do.

Id.

What matters is not that we are the same, or even that we are equal, so long as we believe that we have just as good an opportunity to succeed as the next person.[59]

Genetic enhancement of the few threatens the belief in equality of opportunity in three crucial ways. First, it increases actual inequalities between the enhanced and the "unadvantaged." Second, it gives the enhanced opportunities that others do not have, and that, in the case of germ cell enhancement, may be passed on to succeeding generations. Third, it freezes up the crucial safety valve of upward social mobility. The enhanced would tend to monopolize desirable occupations and fill high status social roles. The unadvantaged no longer would be able to count on traditional methods of social advancement, such as education and intermarriage, to improve their social standing.

The destruction of the belief in equality of opportunity threatens the foundations of our democratic order. Societies characterized by inherited, largely fixed social status are no stranger to the human condition, as evinced by feudalism, caste systems, and slavery. None of these states are compatible with Western democratic institutions.

3. *"Cheating"*

The preceding section dealt with the concern that the fact that only some people will be able to afford enhancement will create a societal division along genetic lines that threatens the fabric of democratic society. On a more specific level, it presents fairness problems in competitions for scarce societal benefits. These benefits include jobs, education, "good" marriages, and social status, as well as the routine, arms-length business and social transactions of daily life. Imagine evaluating the results of a law school admissions test administered to a group of applicants some of whom had genetically-enhanced cognitive functioning. Imagine a business or legal negotiation in which one party was represented by such an enhanced individual and the other was not.

We have some experience with this problem in the context of the use of performance-enhancing drugs in sports. Tom Murray, who serves on the United States Olympic Committee's advisory group, has written extensively on the difficulties of enforcing a no-drug policy in Olympic competition.[60] In part, the problem of perform-

59. *See, e.g.*, David B. Grusky & Azumi A. Takata, *Social Stratification*, *in* 4 ENCYCLOPEDIA OF SOCIOLOGY 1955, 1965 (Edgar F. Borgatta & Marie L. Borgatta eds., 1992) ("Whereas most Americans are willing to tolerate sizeable inequalities in the distribution of resources, they typically insist that individuals from all backgrounds should have an equal opportunity to secure these resources.").

60. *See, e.g.*, Thomas H. Murray, *Drugs, Sports and Ethics*, *in* FEELING GOOD AND DOING BETTER: ETHICS AND NON-THERAPEUTIC DRUG USE 107 (Thomas H. Murray et al. eds., 1984).

ance-enhancing drugs in sports is a problem of definition. The Olympics, for example, might be said to define its competition as being between non-drug-takers, with the gold medal going to the best drug-free athlete. A different competition that did not prohibit drug use might define its winner simply as, say, the fastest or strongest person. In fact, a division along these lines already has occurred in professional weight lifting, where there are drug-free and "open" events.[61]

Similarly, we could attempt to redefine competition for scarce societal benefits to accommodate the possibility that some contestants would be genetically enhanced and others would not. We could establish an admissions quota for enhanced college applicants, for example. Or, we could decide that being genetically enhanced was irrelevant in that it was not substantially different than other advantages that we ignore, such as being born into a wealthy family. What is the difference, for example, between being able to afford the best trainer in the world, which is allowed in the Olympics, and taking anabolic steroids, which is prohibited? In either case, some athletes possess a significant advantage over others.

In seeking to regulate genetic enhancement, in any event, society must attend not only to the traditional regulatory concerns of safety and efficacy, but to the problems of social inequality and cheating posed by the lack of universal access to enhancement technologies. Indeed, the problems of social inequality and cheating may well pose the greater threats.

III. POTENTIAL REGULATORY MECHANISMS

When we think of regulating an activity associated with medical interventions, we probably think first of traditional options such as the FDA or state medical licensing boards. These entities no doubt will play an important role. But we must not overlook other types of regulatory activity. As we will see, traditional regulatory actors may be ill-suited to respond to the special concerns raised by genetic enhancement.

A. *Self-Regulation*

Persons considering genetic enhancement for themselves or

61. *See generally* Ira Berkow, *This Lifter Is Fueled by Natural Power; Operating in a Drug-Free Environment, Ted Sobel Is Soaring Above the Field*, N.Y. TIMES, Feb. 6, 1994, § 8, at 2 (describing how drug-free or natural competitions such as the World Natural Power Lifting Championships are a relatively recent phenomenon); Olga Connolly, *Steroid Debate: 'Enhanced' vs. Natural Athletes*, WASH. POST, Sept. 13, 1988, at Z15 (explaining that two separate categories of champions have been established in power lifting, "open" and "natural"); Roger Mills, *562-pound Lift Makes Ferrantelli a Champ*, ST. PETERSBURG TIMES, Jan. 5, 1997, at 4. (describing how Mike Ferrantelli placed first in both the open and drug-free portions of a power lifting competition).

their offspring (and being able to afford it) may decline to go forward for a host of reasons. For example, a parent may feel that the enhancement choice ought to be left up to the child rather than be made by the parent. Although this would preclude germ cell and other pre-natal enhancements, parents might choose this option if effective somatic cell enhancement—the kind that can be done for adults—were available. This in turn suggests that, if we are worried about the hazards of germ cell enhancement, including the societal worries described in the preceding section, we should make sure that somatic enhancements are safe and effective, such as by devoting public research funds to their development. Parents also might resist germ cell enhancements for ethical or religious reasons, or because they feel an obligation to help prevent the social dislocations that might result from the creation of a "genobility" with inherited enhancement advantages. The same concerns might motivate individuals contemplating somatic enhancements for themselves. In all these cases, individual decision-making acts as a decisive regulatory mechanism.

Self-regulation becomes critical when we recall the earlier discussion concerning the uncertainties and subjective valuation of the risks and benefits of genetic enhancement. These factors call for leaving the choice of whether or not to proceed up to the affected individual. In medical decision making, this is known as the principle of informed consent. The patient is deemed to be the best gauge of her own values, preferences, and aversion to risk; armed with accurate, comprehensible information provided by health professionals, the patient should be allowed to decide, at least in broad terms, what will or will not be done for her.[62]

---

62. In *Natanson v. Kline*, 350 P.2d 1093, 1104 (Kan. 1960), the Kansas Supreme Court stated:

> Anglo-American law starts with the premise of thorough-going self determination. It follows that each man is considered to be master of his own body, and he may, if he be of sound mind, expressly prohibit the performance of life-saving surgery, or other medical treatment. A doctor might well believe that an operation or form of treatment is desirable or necessary but the law does not permit him to substitute his own judgment for that of the patient by any form of artifice or deception.

The court continued by adopting the standard applied in *Salgo v. Leland Stanford Jr. University Board of Trustees*:

> A physician violates his duty to his patient and subjects himself to liability if he withholds any facts which are necessary to form the basis of an intelligent consent by the patient to the proposed treatment. Likewise the physician may not minimize the known dangers of a procedure or operation in order to induce his patient's consent. At the same time, the physician must place the welfare of his patient above all else and this very fact places him in a position in which he sometimes must choose between two alternative courses of action. One is to explain to the patient every risk attendant upon any surgical procedure or operation, no matter how remote; this may well result in

Traditionally, we have abridged the individual's freedom of choice only in three situations: (1) when the individual is incompetent to choose, (2) when the choice will have a significant impact on the welfare of others, and (3) when leaving the choice up to the individual would be so inefficient that we delegate the decision to a better decision-maker. All three of these factors may affect our willingness to allow individuals to decide whether or not to obtain genetic enhancement. For example, in the same way that many question the appropriateness of permitting minors to obtain an abortion without parental consent, we may question minors' right to choose to enhance themselves. As suggested earlier, we might want to circumscribe the right of parents to enhance their children, on the ground that the children ought to be allowed to make this decision for themselves. This is particularly likely if enhancement carries with it significant risks to the enhanced individual. Moreover, society may try to deny persons the right to enhance themselves or their children because of fears of inequality or cheating described in the previous section. Finally, we have limited an individual's ability to purchase certain medical products and services when we have felt that the individual could not adequately inform herself of the risks and benefits, at least not without an unrealistic amount of effort. Thus, we have delegated to the FDA the responsibility for reviewing the safety and efficacy of drugs and medical devices and denied individuals the right to purchase unapproved products because the FDA, rather than the consumer, is deemed to possess the expertise, the access to data, and insulation from manufacturers' inducements and pressures needed to make this evaluation correctly.[63]

The FDA example, however, suggests a slightly different way of thinking about the role of self-regulation in deciding whether or not to obtain genetic enhancement. What FDA regulation accomplishes, it might be said, is to carve out a realm—that of approved products and services—within which individuals are free to make their own choices. This realm is one in which competent individuals are deemed capable of being given sufficient information to enable them to make meaningful choices, and in which the effects of their choices

---

> alarming a patient who is already unduly apprehensive and who may as a result refuse to undertake surgery in which there is in fact minimal risk; it may also result in actually increasing the risks by reason of the physiological results of the apprehension itself. The other is to recognize that each patient presents a separate problem, that the patient's mental and emotional condition is important and in certain cases may be crucial, and that in discussing the element of risk a certain amount of discretion must be employed consistent with the full disclosure of facts necessary to an informed consent . . . . "The instruction given should be modified to inform the jury that the physician has such discretion consistent, of course, with the full disclosure of facts necessary to an informed consent."

Natanson, 350 P.2d at 407 (quoting *Salgo*, 317 P.2d at 181).

63. *See* BRODY, *supra* note 21, at 192-97.

on the welfare of third parties is deemed sufficiently small or acceptable. Within this realm, regulatory mechanisms, such as the FDA and health professionals, see their function primarily as one of providing data and advice to assist individuals in making their decisions.[64] Particularly in view of the difficulty of objectively assessing the risks and benefits of genetic enhancement, we should strive to preserve as much individual decision-making as is compatible with our concerns about competence, efficiency, and effects on others. This suggests, among other things, that we should attend to the need to make readily available to the public comprehensible information about the risks and benefits of enhancement technologies.

One other point needs to be made regarding self-regulation. Individual choice can be influenced by social concerns. People act or refrain from acting on the basis of principle, and have been known to do so even at significant personal cost. Conceivably, individuals might eschew genetic enhancement for themselves or their offspring because of their belief in the principle of equality or because of the ethical problem raised by cheating. They might be encouraged to do so by political and religious leaders. If society felt that the threats from genetic enhancement outweighed the benefits, it would be likely to employ social pressures to affect individual decision-making, a sort of "Just Say No" approach to genetic enhancement. Society might use this approach if other regulatory options were costly or not fully effective. As with the "War on Drugs," self-regulation may end up being one of the most important regulatory techniques.

B. *Professional Self-Regulation*

Genetic enhancement is unlikely to be available on a do-it-yourself basis. Instead, it is likely to require the services of one or more health professionals. These include primary care physicians who are approached by their patients for information about, or referrals or prescriptions for, genetic enhancement; genetic counselors who explain options, risks, and benefits; infertility treatment specialists who provide the IVF services associated with germ cell enhancement; obstetricians and gynecologists who manage pregnancies involving enhanced fetuses; and a new medical specialty likely to emerge with the advent of genetic enhancement: the genetic enhancement specialist.[65] The involvement of these professionals opens up another regulatory avenue: relying on them to regulate themselves in providing access to enhancement services.

Professional self-regulation may be based on individual ethical, religious, social, or scientific beliefs, or it may be based on the views of professional organizations such as the American Medical Associa-

64. *See* 21 U.S.C.S. § 393(b) (Law. Co-op. 1997) (describing FDA mission).

65. Other health professionals may be involved as well, such as psychiatrists, psychologists, social workers, and nurses.

tion ("AMA") and the American College of Physicians; specialty groups like the American College of Obstetrics and Gynecology and the boards that govern specialty certification; prestigious organizations like the Institute of Medicine of the National Academy of Sciences; and views expressed in influential journals such as the *New England Journal of Medicine* or *Science*. In some cases, failure to adhere to the guidelines of professional associations can subject the health care professional to sanctions such as censure or loss of membership in the association.[66] In other cases, the professional merely suffers the pangs of conscience.

Professional self-regulation has played an important role in the regulation of genetic technologies. In 1974, scientists adopted a voluntary moratorium on research involving recombinant DNA technology until the potential risks were more clearly understood.[67]

It is especially noteworthy that one professional association, the AMA, has already issued a policy statement to provide ethical guidance to its members in dealing with genetic enhancement. This statement, put forward in 1994 by the AMA's Council on Ethical and Judicial Affairs, observes that efforts to enhance "desirable" characteristics through the insertion of a modified or additional gene, or efforts to "improve" complex human traits—the eugenic development of offspring—are contrary not only to the ethical tradition of medicine but also to the egalitarian values of our society.[68] The statement goes on to assert that "genetic interventions to enhance traits should be considered permissible only in severely restricted

66. *See* CODE OF MEDICAL ETHICS Rules XII-XIII (AMA Council on Ethical and Judicial Affairs 1996-1997 ed.) (providing that the Council may expel a person from membership in the association on grounds of ethical misconduct). Professional sanctions differ from adverse actions taken by state medical boards for failure to adhere to state licensing laws and regulations, in that professional sanctions are imposed for breaches of rules adopted by the professionals themselves rather than by the government. For a discussion of government regulation of genetic enhancement, see *infra* Section III.E-F. Note that the distinction between professional self-regulation and government regulation is not always clear, since government agencies in some cases delegate some of their regulatory oversight responsibilities to professional or industry self-regulatory bodies. A prime example is the Health Care Financing Administration's reliance on the Joint Commission for the Accreditation of Healthcare Organizations to certify hospitals to be eligible to receive Medicare reimbursement. *See* 42 U.S.C.S. §§ 1395x(e)(9), 1395bb (Law. Co-op. 1999) (noting accredited hospitals deemed to meet Medicare certification requirements).

67. *See* Paul Berg et al., *Potential Biohazards of Recombinant DNA Molecules*, SCIENCE, July 26, 1974, at 303 (1974). Apparently, the moratorium was universally adhered to until it was replaced by a regulatory review process within NIH in 1975. *See generally* Judith P. Swazey et al., *Risks and Benefits, Rights and Responsibilities: A History of the Recombinant DNA Research Controversy*, 51 S. CAL. L. REV. 1019 (1978) (outlining significant developments in the recombinant DNA debate from 1971-1977).

68. *Report on Ethical Issues Related to Prenatal Genetic Screening*, 3 ARCH FAM. MED. 633, 637-39 (1994).

situations."[69]

Without additional explanation, the Council lists three preconditions: (1) "clear and meaningful benefit to the fetus or child,"[70] (2) "no trade-off with other characteristics or traits,"[71] and (3) "equal access . . . irrespective of income or other socioeconomic characteristics."[72] A physician who failed to comply with these conditions would be violating the code of ethics of her profession.

The second of the Council's conditions is perplexing. What is meant by a "trade-off with other characteristics or traits"? Why should an individual not be permitted to accept, say, a slight reduction in dexterity for a significant increase in strength? Moreover, if health itself is regarded as a "characteristic," then the Council's statement, unwittingly perhaps, may call for a complete ban on genetic enhancement, since as mentioned earlier, no physical intervention in the human organism occurs without some chance of an adverse effect on health or well-being, however slight the probability or trivial the effect.

The Council's third condition responds to fairness concerns. It too is problematic. How is a physician or geneticist supposed to assure equal access to genetic enhancements regardless of a patient's income (which bears on the patient's ability to pay)? Only if the government provided universal coverage of genetic enhancements for all who desired them would the Council's statement seem to permit physicians and other health care professionals to provide enhancement to anyone.

Yet the fact that the AMA Council addresses the fairness question at all is highly significant. The services of health care professionals are likely to be indispensable to an individual seeking genetic enhancement, because enhancement will entail manipulating DNA *in vitro* or *in utero*, or prescribing a drug or biologic. A concerted refusal by professionals to supply genetic enhancement unless certain social conditions were met could block or at least substantially reduce access to genetic enhancement. The technology would be available only from non-cooperating professionals on the black market, or in foreign countries whose professionals did not recognize similar self-limitations.

It remains to be seen how successful professional self-regulation would be in solving the fairness and cheating problems. Genetic enhancement is certain to be lucrative. In an era of dwindling professional incomes, caused in part by the shift to managed care, physicians and other health care providers may be unable to resist the economic incentives to provide genetic enhancements to those will-

69. *Id.* at 640.

70. *Id.* The Council's statement focused on genetic interventions in children and fetuses, and did not address self-enhancement by adults.

71. *Id.*

72. *Id.* at 641.

ing to pay for them.[73] Not all professionals may agree with the egalitarian philosophy represented by the Council's statement. While the AMA, for example, has long endorsed the principle that physicians have a duty to provide health care services to the indigent,[74] the organization also supports the view that physicians should be permitted to charge Medicare patients any amount that the physician wishes, so long as the patient agrees not to seek Medicare reimbursement for any part of the fee,[75] which would lift existing restrictions on physician charges and, in the view of some, would undermine the egalitarian features of the Medicare program.[76] Regardless of the position taken by medical organizations, individual doctors and other health care professionals may follow their own consciences.

C. *Restrictions on Research Funding*

The federal government currently finances a substantial portion of the research associated with the Human Genome Project, and is likely to continue to do so for the foreseeable future.[77] A refusal by the government to fund research on genetic enhancement, or a refusal to do so unless certain conditions were met, could significantly affect the development of these technologies.

Historical precedent for this type of regulation is found in the activities of the NIH's Recombinant DNA Advisory Committee ("RAC").[78] The RAC was formed in 1975 to review applications for

73. *See Internal Medicine's Identity Crisis*, MED. ECON., May 12, 1997, at 110 (reporting the results of a survey by the American College of Physicians of 417 members' views on managed care, with half reporting a decrease in income).

74. *See* CODE OF MEDICAL ETHICS § 9.065 (AMA Council on Ethical and Judicial Affairs 1996-97 ed.).

75. *See* Sean Martin, *Private Contracting Heats Up: Right to Opt Out of Medicare at Issue in Lawsuit*, AM. MED. NEWS, Jan. 19, 1998, at 23.

76. *See Physician Contracting: Debate over KYL Amendment Grows*, HEALTH LINE, Nov. 26, 1997, *available in* LEXIS, Genmed Library, RXMEGA File (explaining the position of the American College of Physicians).

77. *See* Daniel S. Greenberg, *Bad Blood in U.S. Genome Research*, 351 LANCET 1939, 1939-40 (1998).

78. Other examples are the ban on funding of research using fetal tissue or embryos and the proposed ban on human cloning. *See infra* notes 126-128 and accompanying text for a discussion of the proposed ban on funding human cloning. The first ban related to research using fetuses accompanied the establishment of the National Commission for the Protection of Human Subjects of Biomedical and Behavioral Research. *See* National Research Service Award Act of 1974, Pub. L. No. 93-348, § 213, 88 Stat. 342, 392 (prohibiting research "on a living human fetus" that is not done "for the purpose of assuring the survival of such fetus"). The recommendations of the National Commission were codified in 45 C.F.R. § 46 (1998). 45 C.F.R. § 46.208 governs activities directed toward fetuses *in utero*, while 45 C.F.R. § 46.209 governs activities directed toward fetuses *ex utero*. Both are geared towards allowing only research posing a minimal risk to the fetus. Additionally, 45 C.F.R. § 46.204 provides for the establishment of Ethical Advisory Boards responsible for evaluating the merit of

NIH funding for experiments involving recombinant DNA technology. Following the creation of the RAC, scientists lifted their voluntary moratorium on recombinant DNA experiments mentioned earlier.[79] The RAC historically concerned itself chiefly with issues of safety and the protection of human research subjects, restricting the release of recombinant DNA-altered plants into the environment,[80] and limiting the conditions in which gene insertion could be attempted on patients.[81] The RAC also has addressed the conditions, if any, in which genetic enhancement experiments could be undertaken, and the committee has been mindful of the fairness and

individual research proposals that fall outside of 45 C.F.R. § 46. The creation of the President's Commission for the Study of Ethical Problems in Medicine and Biomedical and Behavioral Research drained resources from the Ethical Advisory Board, however, thus creating a de facto "moratorium on fetal research posing more than minimal risk, unless expected to enhance the health of the particular fetus." Robert Mullan Cook-Deegan, *Cloning Human Beings: Do Research Moratoria Work?*, *in* 2 CLONING HUMAN BEINGS: REPORT AND RECOMMENDATIONS OF THE NATIONAL BIOETHICS ADVISORY COMMISSION, at H8 (1997). In 1985, Congress amended the Public Health Service Act, banning funding for "any research or experimentation . . . on a nonviable living human fetus ex utero or a living human fetus ex utero for whom viability has not been ascertained" unless the research was geared towards increasing the survival prospects of the particular fetus or the research would not subject the fetus to increased risk of harm. Health Research Extension Act of 1985, Pub. L. 99-158, 99 Stat. 820, 877 (1985). The 1988 NIH authorization continued this moratorium. *See* Cook-Deegan, *supra*, at H9. Funding for experiments using fetal tissue became a concern soon thereafter. Assistant Secretary of Health Robert Windom responded to an NIH request for authorization to support research into using fetal tissue to treat Parkinson's disease by imposing a funding moratorium pending consideration by an *ad hoc* panel of his questions. *See* Letter from Robert Windom to Dr. Wyngaarden, *reprinted in* REPORT OF THE HUMAN FETAL TISSUE TRANSPLANTATION RESEARCH PANEL (1988). In 1993, the National Institutes of Health Revitalization Act of 1993 removed the legislative moratorium on fetal research that had been in place since 1985. Pub. L. No. 103-43, 107 Stat. 122, 129 (1993). This moratorium was restored in the NIH appropriations bills for fiscal years 1996 through 1998. *See* Departments of Labor, Health and Human Services, and Education Appropriations Act, Pub. L. No. 105-78, 111 Stat. 1467, 1517 (1998); Cook-Deegan, *supra*, at H10. For a discussion of these moratoria, see generally Cook-Deegan, *supra*.

79. See *supra* notes 66-75 and accompanying text.

80. The RAC provides guidelines specifying physical and biological containment conditions and practices suitable to the greenhouse conduct of experiments involving recombinant DNA-containing plants and plant-associated microorganisms. *See generally Guidelines for Research Involving Recombinant DNA*, app. P (1999) (visited June 6, 1999) <http://www.nih.gov/od/orda/apndxp.htm>.

81. NIH regulations required all proposals for federally funded research involving gene insertion into humans to be reviewed by the RAC. Germ line alterations were prohibited. Somatic cell alterations were to be considered if their aim was to protect the health and well being of human subjects being treated at the same time that generalized knowledge was being gathered. *See Guidelines for Research Involving Recombinant DNA*, *supra* note 80, at § III-c-1, app. M.

cheating concerns discussed above.[82] The RAC therefore might be an important regulatory mechanism. However, its mission recently has been redefined and its authority to rule on whether or not the NIH should fund specific research applications largely has been transferred to the FDA.[83] In order for the NIH to come to grips with the social policy issues raised by genetic enhancement, it either would have to restore the regulatory authority of the RAC or create a new entity with authority comparable to that which the RAC previously exercised.

NIH funding restrictions only affect government-sponsored research. Private companies are likely to sponsor genetic enhancement experiments that would avoid NIH controls, especially if the government restricted its own research funding. However, the government does impose a set of requirements on research conducted at hospitals and other institutions that receive reimbursement under government entitlement programs such as Medicare.[84] These institutions are required to establish "institutional review boards" ("IRBs") to review research proposals to ensure the protection of human subjects and compliance with the requirements of informed consent.[85] These controls apply not only to government-funded experiments, but to research funded by private manufacturers.[86] Moreover, the FDA imposes a similar set of requirements on privately-funded research which is submitted to FDA in support of an application to approve the marketing of a product within the agency's regulatory jurisdiction.[87]

Despite this web of regulation, loopholes exist that could allow a significant degree of non-complying research to be conducted. Historically, government research requirements have tended to avoid fairness issues, except those that would affect the willingness of individuals to participate as human subjects.[88] Even if the govern-

82. *See id.*

83. *See* FDC, *The Pink Sheet*, Dec. 16, 1997, TRADE & GOV'T, at 17. For a discussion of FDA regulation of genetic enhancement, see *infra* Section III.E.

84. *See* 45 C.F.R. §§ 46.102, 46.103 (1998); *see also* Jesse A. Goldner, *An Overview of Legal Controls on Human Experimentation and the Regulatory Implications of Taking Professor Katz Seriously*, 38 ST. LOUIS U. L.J. 63, 99 (1993) (explaining that federal regulations for research have been made applicable to all institutions doing research, including hospitals, universities, and medical schools, regardless of the source of funding).

85. *See* 45 C.F.R. § 103(h).

86. *See id.* at § 46.103(b).

87. *See* 21 C.F.R. § 56.103(a) (1998); *see also* Goldner, *supra* note 84, at 99 (explaining that FDA requirements "mandate IRB review of all investigational studies designed to support applications to the FDA for the marketing of drugs and medical devices").

88. For example, rules issued by the Department of Health and Human Services limit the incentives that researchers can offer members of certain populations, such as prisoners, to participate in biomedical experiments. *See* 45 C.F.R. § 46.305(a)(2) (1998).

ment sought to regulate research for fairness reasons, its efforts would be limited under current law to research funded by the government, and to privately-funded research only to the extent that it accompanied an application for FDA marketing approval. As the discussion in Section E below explains, genetic enhancement is likely to emerge as an unapproved use of an approved drug or biologic product, for which no marketing approval would be sought.[89] The government's current regulatory control over private research relating to such uses therefore is limited. Without substantial change in the law and the government's regulatory practices, restrictions on research in the name of social concerns such as fairness and cheating are likely to be incomplete and ineffective.

D. *Third-Party Payers*

As previously noted, access to specific medical technologies is controlled in substantial part by coverage policies established by government and private health insurers.[90] Few Americans can afford to purchase expensive health care services with personal funds. The fact that genetic enhancement would not be covered under third-party payment policies currently in effect is the major cause of the unfairness and cheating problems discussed earlier.

The coverage practice of private third-party payers in regard to genetic enhancements is unlikely to change in the future in response to these social problems. Private insurers view their businesses as competitive enterprises motivated by the need to make a profit.[91] They are unlikely to provide third-party payment for genetic enhancement if their competitors do not. Plans that covered genetic enhancement would have to charge higher premiums, a problem exacerbated by the likelihood of "adverse selection," the phenomenon in which individuals who know in advance that they will demand particular covered services will migrate to those plans that cover them, driving up premiums.[92] Similarly, third-party payers are not likely to be willing voluntarily to expend significant resources to police the behavior of providers and enrollees that does not affect the payers' costs; expecting payers on their own initiative to enforce genetic enhancement prohibitions or restrictions for purposes of achieving social goals is unrealistic unless the payers are forced to do so by law. Even if state or federal legislation attempted to impose such obligations on private third-party payers,[93] its reach would

89. *See infra* note 109 and accompanying text.

90. *See supra* note 46 and accompanying text.

91. Even not-for-profit insurers such as some Blue Cross/Blue Shield plans must operate in the black and, therefore, must compete effectively against for-profit plans.

92. *See* Steven P. Croley & Jon D. Hanson, *What Liability Crisis? An Alternative Explanation for Recent Events in Products Liability*, 8 YALE J. ON REG. 1, 28-29 (1991).

93. Under current law, state regulation of private health insurers is limited

not extend to persons who purchased genetic enhancement with their own funds.

In contrast to private insurers, government third-party payer programs such as Medicare and Medicaid might be expected to be more sensitive to social concerns. An example is the End Stage Renal Disease Program under Medicare, which covers kidney dialysis for all persons even though they are under age sixty-five or otherwise ineligible for Medicare.[94] Congress established this program in 1972 in response to concerns that poor people and others were dying because they could not afford kidney dialysis.

As noted earlier, however, the cost of providing universal access to genetic enhancement would be prohibitive.[95] Expecting a program like Medicare or Medicaid to cover enhancement is therefore unrealistic. Yet these programs might be employed as regulatory handles to control the behavior of health care providers. For example, the federal government imposes a number of requirements and restrictions on hospitals and health care professionals on pain of being disqualified from receiving Medicare reimbursement. Some of these regulations, such as the requirement that a hospital emergency room stabilize patients in emergency conditions or in active labor before transferring them, apply to all patients, not just to Medicare beneficiaries.[96] Similarly, the federal government might impose restrictions on access to genetic enhancement by threatening to disqualify non-compliant providers from participating in the Medicare program. This use of federal authority resembles the outright criminalization of genetic enhancement, which will be discussed later.

E. *FDA Regulation*

One of the more obvious sources of government regulation of genetic enhancement is regulation by the Food and Drug Administration. The FDA licenses the marketing of drugs, biological products and medical devices, all of which may be involved in the delivery of enhancement services. Moreover, the FDA regulates research on these products when the research is submitted in support of a licensing application or an approved product. As noted in Section C,

---

by the provisions of ERISA, which exempt employer self-insured health plans from state insurance regulation. *See* 29 U.S.C.A. § 1144(b)(2)(B) (Law. Co-op. 1999) (establishing the so-called "deemer clause"). Unless the ERISA preemption provisions were repealed, legislative control of payer policies toward genetic enhancement would have to be enacted by Congress. For a discussion of potential legislative controls on access to genetic enhancement, see *infra* text accompanying notes 126-28.

94. *See* Richard A. Rettig, *The Policy Debate on Patient Care Financing for Victims of End-Stage Renal Disease*, LAW & CONTEMP. PROBS., Autumn 1976, at 196, 198-201.

95. *See supra* note 43 and accompanying text.

96. *See* 42 U.S.C. § 1395dd (1997).

the FDA now asserts authority previously held by the RAC to regulate research on genetic technologies.[97]

To the extent that these genetic technologies are aimed at improving the appearance of the body, they might seem to be cosmetics, which the Federal Food, Drug, and Cosmetic Act defines as "articles intended to be . . . introduced into, or otherwise applied to the human body or any part thereof for . . . cleansing, beautifying, promoting attractiveness, or altering the appearance . . . ."[98] But the FDA exerts little regulatory effort on cosmetics. Unlike drugs or medical devices, they do not have to be approved prior to being marketed, and generally are subjected to FDA scrutiny only if they present a safety risk.[99] In order for the FDA to be able to control the introduction and use of genetic enhancement technologies, these techniques would have to be considered to be drugs, biologics, or medical devices.

The FDA possesses ample authority to regulate genetic enhancements within these categories, however. In regard to drugs used for enhancement purposes, the definition of a drug in the Federal Food, Drug, and Cosmetic Act includes not only "articles intended for use in the diagnosis, cure, mitigation, treatment, or prevention of disease in man" but "articles (other than food) intended to affect the structure or function of the body of man."[100] The FDA has relied on this definition to assert drug regulatory authority over products such as wrinkle creams and tanning agents that are intended to enhance the appearance of the body but that achieve their results by affecting the body's structural or functional components.[101] The Act similarly defines a medical device to include "an instrument, apparatus, implement, machine, contrivance, implant, in vitro reagent, or other similar or related article . . . which is . . . intended to affect the structure or any function of the body of man."[102]

---

97. *See supra* note 83 and accompanying text.

98. 21 U.S.C.S. § 321(i) (Law. Co-op. 1997).

99. *See* 21 U.S.C.S. § 361 (Law. Co-op. 1993).

100. 21 U.S.C.S. § 321(g)(1) (Law. Co-op. 1998).

101. *See* United States v. Line Away, 284 F. Supp. 107, 111 (D. Del. 1968) (holding that wrinkle creams are drugs); 43 Fed. Reg. 38,206 (1978) (codifying tanning agents as drugs).

102. 21 U.S.C.S. §321(h). The definition distinguishes a medical device from a drug in that a device "does not achieve its primary intended purposes through chemical action within or on the body of man . . . and which is not dependent on being metabolized for the achievement of its primary intended purposes." *Id.* Interestingly, the FDA presently regulates gene therapy products through its Center for Biologics Evaluation and Research ("CBER"), regarding them as "biologics." *See* FDA Notice, 58 Fed. Reg. 53,248, 53,249 (1993). The FDA has jurisdiction over biologics under the Virus, Serum, and Toxin Act of 1944, 42 U.S.C.S. § 262 (Law. Co-op. 1999). However, the definition of a "biologic" is a "virus, therapeutic serum, toxin, antitoxin, or analogous product *applicable to the prevention, treatment or cure of diseases or injuries of man.*" 21 C.F.R. § 600.3(h) (1998) (emphasis added). Therefore, the FDA would not have jurisdiction over an enhancement under this definition. Nevertheless, the FDA has

Nevertheless, FDA regulation of genetic enhancement is likely to be inadequate to address the efficacy and safety concerns described earlier. In the first place, the scope of FDA review is statutorily limited to safety and efficacy.[103] It currently does not have any statutory authority to consider the threat to personal autonomy posed by parental decisions to genetically enhance children, much less the social problems of fairness or cheating. To understand how limited the FDA's authority is, consider that the agency does not even have the authority to take into account the relative need for or cost of the products it regulates. For example, the agency could not decline to approve a product because there was another product already on the market that was equally safe and effective, even if the product already being marketed was less expensive.[104]

Even if the FDA were to assert the authority to consider the social implications of genetic enhancement, or to be given that authority by congressional amendment of its enabling legislation, the agency currently has no experience or expertise in this realm. It would be necessary to hire additional staff or to rely on panels of outside experts. There is precedent for the latter in the form of the agency's advisory committees,[105] but these committees provide expert advice to the agency on safety and efficacy matters within the agency's general expertise. The agency has no track record for employing outside experts to advise the agency on matters such as social fairness.

Moreover, even the FDA's ability to regulate genetic enhancements in the traditional areas of safety and efficacy would be compromised by the data deficiencies and subjectivity of judgments about risk and benefit described above. The example of liposuction devices for weight reduction mentioned earlier, where the benefit is purely cosmetic, illustrates the agency's difficulties: how can the government conclude that a risk of complications so clearly outweighs the subjective value to patients of an improvement in appearance that a liposuction device, assuming that it actually does remove fatty deposits, should not be approved because it is unsafe or ineffective?

---

taken the position that CBER can regulate drugs and devices as well as biologics in appropriate circumstances. *See* 21 C.F.R. § 5.33(a) (1998). Since an enhancement fits the definition of a drug or device even though it is not intended for therapeutic purposes, the allocation of regulatory authority to CBER is permissible.

103. *See* John Geweke & Burton A. Weisbrod, *Clinical Evaluation vs. Economic Evaluation: The Case of a New Drug*, 20 MED. CARE 821, 821 (1982).

104. *See* K. WARNER & B. LUCE, COST BENEFIT AND COST EFFECTIVENESS ANALYSIS IN HEALTH CARE PRINCIPLES AND POTENTIAL 198 (1982); Geweke & Weisbrod, *supra* note 103, at 821.

105. These are governed by the Federal Advisory Committee Act, 5 U.S.C.S. app. 2, § 1 (Law. Co-op. 1998), and by FDA regulations. *See* 21 C.F.R. §§ 14.1-14.174 (1998).

The FDA's problems with regulating enhancement-type technologies are also illustrated by its position in regard to cosmetic contact lenses and breast implants. In the latter case, the agency appears to have taken the view that the benefits from cosmetic use are outweighed by the risks, but not the benefits from therapeutic use. Thus, when the safety controversy over silicone gel-filled breast implants erupted in 1992, the agency limited their use to research for reconstructive purposes: i.e., in women who have had breast cancer surgery, severe injury to the breast, a birth defect affecting the breast, or a medical condition causing a severe breast abnormality.[106] The implants could not be used, much less studied, for cosmetic breast augmentation. At the same time, however, the FDA makes no distinction between cosmetic and reconstructive uses for saline breast implants: both are permitted.[107] This signifies either that the agency feels that the risks posed by saline implants are so small that they are outweighed by cosmetic as well as by therapeutic benefits, or that the agency simply has not come to grips with the enhancement/therapy distinction.

The possibility that the FDA lacks a clear appreciation of the enhancement/therapeutic distinction is reinforced by the agency's position on contact lenses. As with saline breast implants, the agency makes no regulatory distinction between contact lenses for corrective versus cosmetic use.[108] A manufacturer can market nonprescription lenses that change eye color under the same conditions as corrective lenses, despite the argument that, given the risks from contact lens use, the ratio of risks to benefits ought to be more favorable to justify the use of lenses for purely cosmetic purposes.

Finally, even if the FDA did establish a clear policy in regard to evaluating the relative safety of genetic enhancement, the agency would find itself virtually unable to enforce it. This stems primarily from the expectation that, as noted earlier, genetic enhancements may emerge as unapproved or off-label uses of approved products, uses over which the FDA lacks effective regulatory control. The agency might attempt to regulate off-label uses of genetic technologies by asserting jurisdiction over physician prescribing practices,[109] but the medical profession would be likely to view this as an unwarranted intrusion into their exercise of professional discretion. The other option would be for the FDA to prohibit or restrict the mar-

106. *See* FDC, *The Gray Sheet*, June 22, 1992, at 11.

107. *See* FDC, *The Gray Sheet*, May 9, 1994, at 17-19.

108. *See* Letter from Muriel Gelles to Maxwell Mehlman (July 13, 1998) (on file with author).

109. The agency would most likely need additional authority from Congress to do so. FDA regulations require prescriptions for controlled substances to be issued "for a legitimate medical purpose by an individual practitioner acting in the usual course of his professional practice." 21 C.F.R. § 1306.04(a) (1998). For the FDA to apply this regulatory requirement to genetic enhancements, however, they would first have to be classified as controlled substances.

keting of genetic technologies for therapeutic purposes because of fears about their enhancement uses. But it is completely unrealistic to expect society to forego therapeutic benefits in order to reduce enhancement risks. Imagine the reaction if the FDA sought to enjoin the marketing of a drug that alleviated the cognitive effects of mental retardation merely because it might be used by "normals" to "unfairly" boost their intelligence.

An additional set of constraints on the effectiveness of FDA regulation of genetic enhancements lies in the territorial limitations on the agency's jurisdiction. In the first place, under the Commerce Clause of the United States Constitution, the agency lacks jurisdiction over purely intra-state marketing.[110] But given the broad interpretation that the courts have given to interstate commerce, coupled with the likelihood that some elements of a genetic enhancement technology will cross state lines,[111] this is not likely to be a serious impediment. More significant by far will be the FDA's lack of jurisdiction over foreign providers.[112] A person seeking a genetic enhancement that the FDA restricted in the United States could simply travel to another country where the technology was freely available. The FDA might attempt to interdict the importation of an enhancement back into the United States,[113] but would be hard pressed to do so from a practical standpoint if the enhancement already had been introduced into the recipient's body, either as a drug, a drug factory, or an inserted gene.[114]

110. *See, e.g.*, 21 U.S.C.S. § 355 (Law. Co-op. 1997) (establishing FDA regulation of new drugs in interstate commerce). For an activity to be considered purely intrastate, it could not, either alone or in combination with other activities, have a substantial economic effect on interstate commerce or on movement in interstate commerce. *See* United States v. Lopez, 514 U.S. 549, 561 (1995) (possessing firearms in a school zone is not an economic activity that might have a substantial effect on interstate commerce). *But see, e.g.*, Wickard v. Filburn, 317 U.S. 111, 127-28 (1942) (holding that farmer's production of wheat for home consumption could be federally regulated because the cumulative effect of multiple instances of people doing so could be felt in interstate commerce).

111. These could be the consumers or providers as well as components of drugs, biologics, or devices used in the delivery of enhancement services.

112. *See generally* Julie C. Relihan, Note, *Expediting FDA Approval of AIDS Drugs: An International Approach*, 13 B.U. INT'L L.J. 229 (1995) (comparing the FDA drug regulation system to other nations' approaches).

113. The Bureau of Customs enforces FDA restrictions by intercepting unapproved drugs and devices at the borders. This policy has proved controversial in the case of drugs to treat AIDS, which have been brought into the US from abroad and sometimes re-sold through so-called "AIDS clubs." *See* Jon S. Batterman, Note, *Brother Can You Spare a Drug: Should the Experimental Drug Distribution Standards Be Modified in Response to the Needs of Persons with AIDS?*, 19 HOFSTRA L. REV. 191, 193-94 (1990).

114. An argument might be made that the Fifth Amendment's protection against search and seizure prohibits such intrusiveness, although the courts have supported intrusive searches given a reasonable suspicion of an unlawful act. *See, e.g.*, United States v. Himmelwright, 551 F.2d 991 (5th Cir. 1977) (holding strip searches authorized).

F. Drug Enforcement Administration

At first, the notion of regulating genetic enhancements using the authority of the Drug Enforcement Administration ("DEA") under the Controlled Substances Act may sound peculiar, but it might be appropriate on a number of grounds. The Controlled Substances Act is the primary mechanism for regulating drugs that pose a threat to society by their use.[115] The Act creates a system of "schedules" that categorize these products on the basis of comparing their therapeutic value with their potential for abuse.[116] A similar approach might distinguish enhancement and therapeutic uses of genetic technologies. The DEA also has extensive experience with a wide range of practical techniques for restricting access to such products.

Relying on a police regime under a scheme like the Controlled Substances Act to regulate genetic enhancement, however, raises the chilling specter of a government-led "war on genes." Given the intimate contexts in which individuals would obtain genetic enhancements—the realms of reproductive behavior and the patient-physician relationship—the intrusiveness of such a program would be suspect and possibly unconstitutional.[117] The success to date in the War on Drugs is not an encouraging omen for a war on genes.[118] All of the difficulties that have marked that endeavor would be present here: the invasions of privacy, the creation of black markets,[119]

115. *See* 21 U.S.C.S. § 801(6) (Law. Co-op. 1997).

116. *See id.* § 811. Substances are scheduled as follows: Schedule I: high potential for abuse, no currently accepted medical use, lack of accepted safety for use under medical supervision; Schedule II: high potential for abuse, has a currently accepted medical use, abuse may lead to severe psychological or physical dependence; Schedule III: less potential for abuse than Schedule I and II substances, has a currently accepted medical use, abuse may lead to moderate or low physical or high psychological dependence; Schedule IV: low potential for abuse compared to Schedule III substances, has a currently accepted medical use, abuse may lead to limited physical or psychological dependence compared to Schedule III; Schedule V: low potential for abuse compared to Schedule IV, has a currently accepted medical use, may lead to limited physical or psychological dependence compared to Schedule IV. *See id.* § 812.

117. The constitutionality of a "war on genes" would be judged by the nature of the public and private interests at stake and the degree of intrusiveness of the government's actions. If the government could offer a compelling justification for why its actions were necessary to protect the public health and welfare, the courts would be likely to uphold severe regulatory restraints. Similar challenges have failed, for example, in the case of government restrictions on the use of illegal drugs and on sexual behavior that presents a threat to public health. *See, e.g.*, Department of Human Resources v. Smith, 494 U.S. 872, 890 (1990) (rejecting first amendment religious challenge to drug law); Bowers v. Hardwick, 478 U.S. 186, 196 (1986) (upholding Georgia's sodomy statute).

118. *See generally* Doug Bandow, *War on Drugs or War on America?*, 1991 STAN L. & POL'Y REV. 242 (examining the costs and benefits of the drug war, concluding that legalization is the best alternative).

119. A historical analogy would be the availability of illegal abortions prior to *Roe v. Wade*, 410 U.S. 113 (1973). *See, e.g.*, Zad Leavy & Jerome Kummer,

and the inability to seal the borders against the importation of contraband or its purchase abroad.[120] Yet thinking about a drug-enforcement approach to genetic enhancement is an important reminder of the consequences of a highly restrictive attitude toward access to these technologies. If, as some have suggested, we become determined to "ban" genetic enhancement, and to enforce such a prohibition vigorously, it is the model of the War on Drugs that we will be embracing.

G. *Controlling Health Care Professionals Under State or Federal Law*

In contrast to professional self-regulation, in which health care professionals regulate their behavior through internalized or professionally established norms, regulation of genetic enhancement could be handled under state laws that control professional behavior. Chief among these are state licensure laws, the common and statutory laws that govern medical malpractice actions, and general criminal provisions. For example, a state could revoke a physician's license to practice medicine for providing genetic enhancements or a cause of action could be recognized for improper use of enhancement technology. A malpractice action would lie, for example, if a patient suffered adverse physical or emotional effects from an enhancement and could show that the enhancement had been provided in an improper manner (for example, the physician erred unreasonably in the dosage of an enhancement product or in the genetic manipulation of the patient's DNA) or that the physician had failed to obtain the patient's informed consent to the procedure.[121] Finally, the state or federal government could criminalize genetic enhancement. Criminal penalties could be imposed on those who received enhancement, but a more likely approach would be to sanction the providers.

Given the uncertainty and experimental nature of genetic enhancement, malpractice actions are not likely to be a useful regula-

---

Criminal Abortion: Human Hardship and Unyielding Laws, 35 S. CAL. L. REV. 123 (1962) (suggesting that one out of two pregnancies terminate in illegal abortion).

120. For a complete discussion of these difficulties, see MEHLMAN & BOTKIN, *supra* note 46, at 112-21.

121. *See generally* Jeffrey R. Botkin & Maxwell J. Mehlman, *Wrongful Birth: Medical, Legal, and Philosophical Issues*, 22 J. LAW MED. & ETHICS 21 (1994). An action also might be brought by or on behalf of a child who complained that a physician enhanced her without her consent, but, given the presumed benefits from enhancement, such a suit would be likely to fail on the ground that the child was better off as the result of the physician's actions. An analogy would be "wrongful life" actions—suits brought by children claiming that but for the malpractice, the child would not have been born—which the courts generally dismiss. *See, e.g.*, Walker v. Mart, 790 P.2d 735, 741 (Ariz. 1990) (holding that a child born with severe birth defect could not maintain a tort action against physician).

tory tool. There is likely to be little in the way of a standard of care for providing genetic enhancement, at least not when the technology is first being introduced. So long as the health care professional followed the steps required when providing a patient with an experimental treatment, including carefully informing the patient of the inherent uncertainties, the professional is likely to be protected.[122] Moreover, malpractice actions are expensive and, some have argued, highly inefficient techniques for regulating physician behavior.[123] Most importantly, the professional standard of care may have trouble incorporating social concerns such as fairness and cheating. Although, in theory, the standard of care in medical malpractice cases, as in all of tort law, is based on an assessment and comparison of risks and benefits,[124] judges and juries may find it difficult to sanction a physician for acting in her patient's best interest even when doing so creates a threat of social unfairness. Indeed, it may be deemed to be inappropriate for a physician to compromise the care of a patient in order to achieve a societal distributive goal. For example, a physician might be liable for denying a patient a benefit in order to conserve resources for others. For this reason, the Oregon state legislature immunizes physicians from civil liability when they deny Medicaid benefits to patients in reliance on the state's Medicaid rationing program; otherwise, physicians might be liable for malpractice for acting in a way that fell below the standard of care in a particular patient's case.[125]

In order to embed concerns about social justice within the professional standard of care so that physicians might be sanctioned either under licensure laws or tort actions, it would be necessary for a

122. The Department of Health, Education & Welfare, through the NIH, developed three guidelines for human experimentation: (1) protection of rights and welfare of subjects, (2) informed consent requirement, and (3) assessment of risks and potential benefits by a review panel. *See* Karine Morin, *The Standard of Disclosure in Human Subject Experimentation*, 19 J. LEGAL MED. 157, 174 (1998).

123. *See* COMMITTEE TO STUDY MED. PROF'L LIAB. & THE DELIVERY OF OBSTETRICAL CARE, INSTITUTE OF MEDICINE, 1 MEDICAL PROFESSIONAL LIABILITY AND THE DELIVERY OF OBSTETRICAL CARE 54-72 (1989); UNITED STATES DEPT. OF HEALTH AND HUMAN SERVICES, REPORT OF THE TASK FORCE ON MEDICAL LIABILITY AND MALPRACTICE 44 (1987); Harvard Medical Practice Study, Patients, Doctors, and Lawyers: Medical Injury, Malpractice Litigation and Patient Compensation in New York 8-75 (1990); Paul Weiler et al., *Proposal for Medical Liability Reform*, 267 JAMA 2355, 2355 (1992). *But see* Maxwell J. Mehlman, *Bad "Bad Baby" Bills*, 20 AM. J.L. & MED. 129, 136 (1994) (arguing that current system protects most severely injured malpractice victims).

124. *See* United States v. Carroll Towing Co., 159 F.2d 169, 173 (2d Cir. 1947).

125. *See* Maxwell Mehlman, *The Oregon Medicaid Program: Is It Just?*, 1 HEALTH MATRIX 175, 175-76 (1991). An exception would be where the patient needed an organ transplant. There, because of the shortage of transplant organs, the physician might be justified in denying a transplant to one patient in order to maximize the benefit from the organ by giving it to another.

legislature to enact a specific prohibition into law. A legislative initiative also would be needed to criminalize research on or the provision of enhancement services, since there are no existing criminal laws that would achieve this result.

A similar approach is being considered in the case of prohibiting human cloning.[126] Apart from the wisdom of such a goal, questions are being raised about the appropriateness of a legislature in effect trying to "stop science."[127] Critics of a cloning ban argue, for example, that it would have unwanted effects.[128] Due to the difficulty of defining objectionable cloning practices, legislation would be overbroad, inhibiting therapeutic advances that depended on cloning techniques. Similar problems in distinguishing between therapeutic and enhancement uses of genetic technologies, described earlier, would beset legislative efforts to ban genetic enhancement.[129]

1. *Leveling the Playing Field*

The final approach to coping with the societal threats posed by genetic enhancement realistically assumes that it will be impossible to prevent some individuals from enhancing themselves or their children. Even draconian regulatory efforts like a legislative ban or a drug-war-like interdiction program would have only limited success. The question then is: are there means by which society can re-

126. For legislation to outlaw the use of somatic cells in the production of human clones, see, e.g., H.R. 923, 105th Cong. (1997); S. 1599, 105th Cong. (1997); S. 1601, 105th Cong. (1997). For legislation to prohibit the cloning of humans, see, e.g., S. 1574, 105th Cong. (1998); S.B. 8, 1998 Reg. Sess. (Ala. 1998); S.B. 68, 1998 Reg. Sess. (Ala. 1998); S.B. 1344, 1997-98 Reg. Sess. (Cal. 1997); S.B. 1243, 90th Leg., 1997-98 Reg. Sess. (Ill. 1997); A.B. 9116, 221st Leg., 1997 Reg. Sess. (N.Y. 1998); S.B. 5993, 221st Leg., 1997 Reg. Sess. (N.Y. 1998); H.B. 675, 122d Leg., 1997-98 Reg. Sess. (Ohio 1997); S.B. 218, 122d Leg., 1997-98 Reg. Sess. (Ohio 1997). For legislation to prohibit attempts to clone through somatic cell nuclear transfer and the use of Federal funds for such purpose, see, e.g., S. 1602, 105th Cong. (1998); H.B. 2235, 90th Leg., 1997-98 Reg. Sess. (Ill. 1997); A.B. 9183, 221st Leg., 1997 Reg. Sess. (N.Y. 1998). For legislation to prohibit research using cloned cells or tissues, see A.B. 1251, 1997-98 Reg. Sess. (Cal. 1997); H.B. 1237, 1997 Reg. Sess. (Fla. 1997).

127. *See* Charles Krauthammer, *A Special Report on Cloning*, TIME, Mar. 10, 1997, at 60 (stating that "[n]o amount of regulation by the FDA or the NIH or even the FBI will stop . . . [human cloning]").

128. California's attempt to ban human cloning is "so sloppily worded that it prohibits a host of infertility treatments." *Confronting Cloning*, L.A. TIMES, Jan. 31, 1998, Metro Section, at 7. *See also* John A. Robertson, *Human Cloning: Should the United States Legislate Against It?*, A.B.A. J., May 1997, at 81 (discussing briefly the merits of human cloning); John A. Robertson, *Liberty, Identity, and Human Cloning*, 76 TEX. L. REV. 1371, 1376-82 (1998) (discussing the potential benefits of cloning); John A. Robertson, *The Question of Human Cloning*, HASTINGS CTR. REP., Mar.-Apr. 1994, at 6 ("If we ban the immediate steps in order to prevent potentially harmful future applications, infertile couples lose the benefits of the procedure without a clear showing that future harms would necessarily have occurred.").

129. See *supra* text accompanying notes 48-49.

duce the harmful social effects that were described earlier?

A full-scale discussion of this topic is beyond the scope of this Article. However, it is interesting to consider how society has dealt with similar issues in the past. How has society responded to the fact that some people have superior attributes compared with others, attributes that they have developed, inherited, or come upon by chance, and that give them significant advantages?

Curiously, very little has been written about this subject. The literature has focused on society's response to those who are disadvantaged relative to the norm—persons with disabilities, or those who are poor or poorly educated—rather than on those whose attributes are "superior." Yet if one identifies these advantageous traits (such as beauty, size, strength, endurance, intelligence, memory, creativity, knowledge, charm, confidence, energy, experience, reputation, pedigree, socioeconomic status, wealth, and social or political power) and examines society's response to their potential impact in interactions with the unadvantaged, some interesting insights emerge.

In some cases, we ignore the advantages that some people possess. For example, we do not weight performance on college admissions tests according to the IQ of the test taker. Nor do we have basketball leagues restricted to players of "normal" height. In other instances, however, we prohibit people from taking advantage of their superiority. For example, securities trading by people who have "inside information" is illegal.[130] The use of performance-enhancing drugs in many sporting competitions, such as the Olympics, is against the rules.[131] Boxing, but not wrestling, creates com-

130. Although Congress has addressed the issue of insider trading through the Insider Trading and Securities Fraud Enforcement Act of 1988, Pub. L. No. 100-704, 102 Stat. 4677 (1988), and the Insider Trading Sanctions Act of 1984, Pub. L. No. 98-376, 98 Stat. 1264 (1984), there is no statutory definition of insider trading. The courts and the Securities and Exchange Commission ("SEC") have primarily based the prohibition on insider trading on SEC Rule 10b-5, 17 C.F.R. § 240.10b-5 (1998), which prohibits employment of manipulative and deceptive devices. *See In re* Cady, 40 S.E.C. 907, 912 (1961) (stating that "[i]ntimacy demands restraint lest the uninformed be exploited"). The scope of the prohibition was circumscribed in *Chiarella v. United States*, 445 U.S. 222, 233 (1980) (holding that an individual possessing information not available to the public, but who is not a corporate insider, does not violate the prohibition on insider trading in the absence of a relationship between the individual and the seller that gives rise to a special duty). In *United States v. O'Hagan*, 521 U.S. 642, 643 (1997), however, the Court reaffirmed that a person violates the insider trading prohibition "when he misappropriates confidential information for securities trading purposes, in breach of a fiduciary duty owed to the source of the information . . . ." Additionally, SEC Rule 14e-3, 17 C.F.R. § 240.14e-3 (1998), prohibits insider trading in the context of tender offers. For a discussion of an alternative source of a definition of insider trading, see Steve Thel, *Statutory Findings and Insider Trading Regulation*, 50 VAND. L. REV. 1091, 1097-1100 (1997).

131. *See* United States Olympic Committee, *Drug Control Education* (visited

petitive categories based on body weight; featherweights are not made to box against heavyweights.

In still other cases, we permit persons with superior positions to engage in transactions involving the interests of the unadavantaged, but reserve to the unadvantaged the right to undo the transaction if the results seem too unfair. Contract law embodies this principle in the doctrine of unconscionability.[132] Fiduciary law gives this power to beneficiaries when trustees transact business with trust assets.[133]

Yet another approach is to adjust the position of the parties to a transaction to mitigate the effect of superiority. One example is making a person with superior information disclose the information to the other party, such as when sellers of real estate are required to

---

June 6, 1999) <http://www.test.olympic-usa.org/inside/in 1 3 7 1.html> (describing various drugs that are prohibited by the United States Olympic Committee including those that enhance performance such as stimulants and anabolic agents).

132. *See, e.g.*, Williams v. Walker-Thomas Furniture Co., 350 F.2d 445, 449 (D.C. Cir. 1965) (stating that a contract may be unconscionable if there is "an absence of meaningful choice on the part of one of the parties together with contract terms which are unreasonably favorable to the other party."); Jones v. Star Credit Corp., 298 N.Y.S.2d 264, 265-68 (N.Y. Sup. Ct. 1969) (mem.) (holding unconscionable a defendant's sale of a $300.00 freezer for $1234.80, including credit charges, to the plaintiffs, who were welfare recipients); Brooklyn Union Gas Co. v. Jimeniz, 371 N.Y.S.2d 289, 292 (N.Y. Civ. Ct. 1975) (holding as unconscionable a contract written in English only and entered into by the defendant, who spoke and read only Spanish, without the plaintiff's representative explaining the terms to him). Having found a contract to be unconscionable, the court may protect the disadvantaged individual by refusing to enforce the contract, enforcing the contract without the unconscionable clause, or limiting the application of the unconscionable clause so the result is not unconscionable. *See* U.C.C. § 2-302(1) (1998).

133. *See* AUSTIN W. SCOTT & WILLIAM FRATCHER, 1 THE LAW OF TRUSTS § 2.5, at 43 (4th ed. 1987) ("If the fiduciary enters into a transaction with the beneficiary and fails to make a full disclosure of all circumstances known to him affecting the transaction, *or if the transaction is unfair to the beneficiary*, it can be set aside by him.") (emphasis added). Elsewhere, Scott stated: "Where he deals directly with the beneficiaries, the transaction may stand, but only if the trustee makes full disclosure and takes no advantage of his position and the transaction is in all respects fair and reasonable." AUSTIN W. SCOTT, 2 THE LAW OF TRUSTS § 170.25, at 1387 (3d ed. 1967). Scott also stated: "In the case of a purchase by a trustee of the trust property with the consent of the beneficiaries, however, it would seem that if the price is not fair the transaction can be set aside even though the trustee made full disclosure." *Id.* § 496, at 3536; *see also* Alison G. Anderson, *Conflicts of Interest: Efficiency, Fairness and Corporate Structure*, 25 UCLA L. REV. 738, 760 (1978). Anderson noted:

> Where bargaining power is roughly equal, specific fiduciary duties can be waived by the parties on the basis of full disclosure to and consent by the client. Because informational disparities so often mean that bargaining power is unequal, however, all fiduciaries have an unwaivable obligation of fairness toward the other party.

Id. For a discussion of these principles, see Maxwell J. Mehlman, *Fiduciary Contracting Limitations on Bargaining Between Patients and Health Care Providers*, 51 U. PITT. L. REV. 365 (1991).

disclose known defects in the property that the buyer would be hard pressed to discover without unreasonable effort or expense.[134] Another type of adjustment is to handicap the person with superior attributes. Weights are placed in the saddles of lighter jockeys.[135] Strokes are added to the scores of better golfers.[136] Finally, the arms-length nature of a transaction can be eliminated, so that the superior party is forced to "look out for" the interests of the weaker party. Fiduciary rules do this in the case of relationships between parties with disparate power, such as patients and physicians, attorneys and clients, parents and children.[137] Another example is suitability rules in securities offerings, in which the seller must make sure that the buyer possesses sufficient assets that he can afford to lose his investment.[138]

---

134. *See* Ollerman v. O'Rourke Co., 288 N.W.2d 95, 107-08 (Wis. 1979) (stating that vendor had duty to disclose existence of underground well on residential lot); RESTATEMENT (SECOND) OF CONTRACTS § 161(b) (1979).

135. *See* DIAGRAM GROUP, RULES OF THE GAME 258 (1974) (noting that "weights are adjusted to try to give horses an equal chance of winning").

136. *See* Blakney Boggs, *Your Game Handicaps Help Promote Equal Competition*, ORANGE COUNTY REG. (Cal.), Aug. 13, 1998, at D13 (explaining that a handicap "is a way to level out the playing field between golfers of different abilities"); *see also* Greg Wilcox, *See Blue, Tee from the White; Forward Tees Mean More Iron*, L.A. DAILY NEWS, Aug. 6, 1998, at S8 (describing how players are grouped according to their handicaps so that they can compete against golfers of similar skill).

137. *See generally* Dyntel Corp. v. Ebner, 120 F.3d 488, 492 (4th Cir. 1997) (holding that an attorney owes a client a fiduciary duty which comprises meeting the standard of care); Omnitech Int'l, Inc. v. Clorox Co., 11 F.3d 1316, 1331 (5th Cir. 1994) (recognizing the fiduciary relationship between an attorney and a client); *In re* "Agent Orange" Prod. Liab. Litig., 818 F.2d 216, 223 (2d Cir. 1987) (recognizing the fiduciary duty of an attorney to class plaintiffs in class action suit); Pharmacare v. Caremark, 965 F. Supp. 1411, 1419 (D. Haw. 1996) (recognizing fraud violates the fiduciary duty a doctor owes a patient); *In re* Marriage of Honkomp, 381 N.E.2d 881, 882 (Ind. Ct. App. 1978) (holding child support for minor children received by custodial parent in a fiduciary capacity cannot be used to set off individual debts); Ohio Cas. Ins. Corp. v. Mallison, 354 P.2d 800, 802 (Or. 1960) (holding parents owe children a fiduciary duty when entering into a settlement on their behalf); Alexander v. Knight, 177 A.2d 142, 146 (Pa. Super Ct. 1962) (explaining the medical profession stands in a confidential and fiduciary capacity to their patient such that they owe a duty of total care); Gates v. Jensen, 595 P.2d 919, 923 (Wash. 1979) (recognizing that a physician has a fiduciary duty to inform a patient about material facts concerning the patient's body so the patient can make an informed decision).

138. National Association of Securities Dealers Conduct Rule 2310, in relevant part, provides:

> (a) In recommending to a customer the purchase, sale or exchange of any security, a member shall have reasonable grounds for believing that the recommendation is suitable for such customer upon the basis of the facts, if any, disclosed by such customer as to his other security holdings and his financial situation and needs. (b) Prior to the execution of a transaction recommended to a non-institutional customer . . . a member shall make reasonable efforts to obtain information concerning: (1) the customer's financial status; (2) the customer's tax

The question is whether these techniques would be effective to level the playing field in the case of genetic enhancements. Could genetically enhanced people be prohibited from taking advantage of their superior abilities to the disadvantage of "normals"? Could they be handicapped? Should they be made into fiduciaries for the less fortunate, a sort of genetic noblesse oblige?

The answers to these questions depend on several considerations. A key factor is how easy it will be to identify the fact that someone is enhanced. The importance of this factor is demonstrated by the difficulties that detection problems create for efforts to prohibit the use of performance-enhancing drugs in sports.[139] Another crucial consideration is the ratio of societal to personal benefit from allowing an individual to benefit from the enhancements. In sports competitions, for example, it is hard to discern any societal benefit from permitting athletes to use performance-enhancing drugs. But it may be sufficiently advantageous to society for enhanced individuals to be involved in scientific research that they will be permitted to compete on an equal basis with unenhanced persons for scarce research positions or grants.

An example of this is found in the law of torts. In general, people are held to the standard of a "reasonable person" under like circumstances.[140] A failure to behave like a reasonable person, which causes injury to another, subjects the actor to tort liability. This standard is modified, however, in the case of an actor who is physically (but not mentally) disabled.[141] We hold a blind person to the standard of a reasonable *blind* person. If we wanted to impose a

---

> status; (3) the customer's investment objectives; and (4) such other information used or considered to be reasonable by such member . . . in making recommendations to the customer.

National Ass'n of Securites Dealers, *NASD Manual & Notices to Members* (visited June 15, 1999) <http://www.nasdr.com/wbs/NETbos.dll?RefShow?ref=NASD4;&xinfo=../webbos/goodbye.htm>; *see also* Gerald F. Rath & David C. Boch, *Securities Litigation: Planning and Strategies*, SC73 ALI-ABA 191 (1998) (summarizing developments in broker and consumer litigation). The dealer must fulfill the obligation he assumes when he undertakes to counsel a customer; this rule is not limited to situations where comprehensive financial information about the customer is known to the dealer. *See, e.g.*, Erdos v. SEC, 742 F.2d 507, 508 (9th Cir. 1984) (ruling that a dealer has "a duty to act with caution and to make recommendations based on the concrete information that he did have rather than on his speculation . . . ." about a customer's situation); *In re* Gerald M. Greenberg Nat'l Ass'n of Sec. Dealers, 40 S.E.C. 133, 137-38 (1960) (expelling member of National Association of Securities Dealers); *In re* Phillips & Co., 37 S.E.C. 66, 70 (1956) (suspending over-speculative broker).

139. *See, e.g.*, Mark Zeigler, *Illegal Doping is Everywhere Now, and the Culprits are Rarely Caught*, S.D. UNION TRIB., Aug. 17, 1997, at C1 (stating that performance enhancing drugs are "seeping through the sports world like an injectable steroid is absorbed into the blood stream," and the only people who are caught are either "poor or stupid").

140. *See* RESTATEMENT (SECOND) OF TORTS § 283 (1965).

141. *See id.* § 283C.

duty on enhanced individuals to employ their superior traits to avoid accidents, we would not hold them to the standard of a reasonable person, but to the standard of a reasonable *enhanced* person. Thus, a driver whose vision had been enhanced to better than 20/20 would not be held to the standard of a reasonable, unadvantaged individual, but to the standard of a reasonable person with superior vision. If they should have spotted the child running across the road in time to stop the car, even though a person with normal vision would not have seen the child, then, under an enhanced person's standard, they could be liable for failing to stop in time. The enhanced person would be treated much the same way that professionals are treated, that is, held to a higher standard of care than non-professionals.

The Restatement (Second) of Torts appears to take this approach. In section 289, it states "[t]he actor is required to recognize that his conduct involves a risk of causing an invasion of another's interest if a reasonable man would do so while exercising . . . such superior attention, perception, memory, knowledge, intelligence, and judgment as the actor himself has."[142]

There are a few cases in which the courts have held people with superior abilities to a higher standard, but most of these involve professionals.[143] One of the few exceptions is *Fredericks v. Castora*,[144] in which the court held a professional truck driver to the standard of an ordinary driver when he caused an accident driving the family sedan.[145]

What is interesting about tort law in this respect is that a good argument can be made that we should not alter the standard of care

142. *Id.* § 289.

143. In an interesting remark in *Dillenbeck v. Los Angeles*, 446 P.2d 129, 136 n.10 (Cal. 1968), however, the California Supreme Court reasoned that a professional such as an attorney or physician is held to a higher standard of care than a lay person because of the professional's greater expertise, rather than because the professional holds herself out as such: "Essentially, the 'expert' cases flow from the proposition that each person in society is expected to exercise that degree of care which can reasonably be anticipated from him in light of his peculiar attributes, including knowledge, perception, and memory."

144. 360 A.2d 696 (Pa. Super. Ct. 1976).

145. *Id.* at 698. In *Johnston v. United States*, 568 F. Supp. 351, 354 (D. Kan. 1983), a federal court noted that a government contractor cannot hide behind the so-called "contract specification defense"—which protects a contractor from products liability if the contractor follows design specifications—"where the manufacturer has special knowledge or expertise." In *Cervelli v. Graves*, 661 P.2d 1032, 1037 (Wyo. 1983), the court rejected the reasonable person standard in a case involving an accident caused by a professional truck driver, opting instead for an instruction that would permit the jury to consider evidence that the driver "was more skillful than others as a result of his experience as a driver." In *Dillenbeck v. City of Los Angeles*, 446 P.2d 129, 136 (Ca. 1968), a police officer who killed a motorist in the course of a high-speed chase was held to the standard of one who possessed superior knowledge and skill by virtue of his "extensive training and experience."

for an enhanced individual when it comes to avoiding accidents. Instead, we should hold them merely to the standard of a reasonable, unadvantaged person. The reason is that, by doing so, we encourage people to improve their vision, which in itself will avoid accidents, whereas, if we made people with better vision liable under a higher standard, thereby discouraging them from enhancing their vision, we would lose the benefit in terms of accident avoidance. Whether we imposed a higher or normal standard would depend on whether we thought that the benefits from reduced accidents on account of having drivers with better vision outweighed the costs of accidents caused by these drivers when they did not act like someone with improved vision.[146]

CONCLUSION

Although this Article is merely a first stab at the question of how we may regulate genetic enhancements, several points already become clear. The first is that no single method of regulation can accomplish the objectives of assuring safety, efficacy, personal autonomy and minimizing adverse social consequences. Instead, a variety of regulatory mechanisms, public and private, must be brought to bear. In particular, it is important to recognize the limitations of specific regulatory mechanisms. Given the motivation of self-interest, for example, we should not expect personal or professional self-regulation to solve the problems of unfairness or cheating.

Another relatively obvious point is that banning genetic enhancement is unlikely to be completely successful. The allure of enhancement will motivate the creation of a black market, or will lead people to obtain enhancements in other countries that are beyond the reach of our domestic prohibitions. The question then is whether the reduction in enhancement that might be achieved by strict enforcement of a ban is worth the cost in terms of police activity and intrusion into private medical and reproductive behavior.

It follows from the previous point that, in all likelihood, some people will become genetically enhanced. The question, then, is how society should respond. If the number of enhanced individuals is sufficiently small, we may be able to ignore them on the basis that their impact in terms of unfairness and cheating will be minimal.

---

146. A similar analysis might be made of rules that permit a party to a contract to benefit from superior information so long as the result is not too unfair. In this case, the argument would be that, by permitting the party with superior information to capitalize on that information, we give an incentive to create and obtain that information. The societal gain in information, it is reasoned, outweighs the unfairness to the inferior party to the transaction. *See* Anthony Kronman, *Mistake, Disclosure, Information, and the Law of Contracts*, 7 J. LEGAL STUD. 1, 19 n.49 (1978) (noting beneficiary "in effect purchases other party's information").

On the other hand, if a substantial minority of individuals is able to afford enhancements for themselves or their offspring, the risks to society may become too great to disregard. In that case, we will need to reduce the costs to society by leveling the playing fields on which enhanced individuals interact with the unadvantaged.

Balancing Rights: Individuals versus Society

[12]

PUBLIC HEALTH AND PRIVATE LIVES

MARGARET BRAZIER* AND JOHN HARRIS**

I. INTRODUCTION

> The fundamental principle, plain and incontestable, is that every person's body is inviolate.[1]

The common law of England has consistently affirmed a doctrine of bodily integrity which makes no distinction between degrees of violence[2] and prohibits unauthorised touchings. The evolution of the laws of assault and battery into a coherent legal doctrine affirming and protecting patient autonomy in medical treatment is nonetheless of relatively recent origin and remains flawed in its detail. The adoption in *Sidaway* v. *Board of Governors of Bethlem Royal Hospital and the Maudsley Hospital*[3] of the professional standard to govern information disclosure deprives patients on occasion of the information crucial to a maximally autonomous choice.

However, two principles are now crystal clear. First, any treatment involving physical contact with a competent adult must be expressly authorised by her. If a health professional acts without consent (save in emergency), or exceeds the consent given by the patient, he commits a civil battery and a criminal assault.[4] It is no defence that he proves that he acted in what he believed to be the patient's best interests. Secondly, the patient's right to prohibit treatment extends even to life-saving treatment. The state has no right or power to intervene to protect patients from themselves.[5] Lord Donaldson M.R. declared in *Re T*:[6]

---

* Professor of Law, University of Manchester.

** Professor of Bioethics and Applied Philosophy, University of Manchester.

The authors gratefully acknowledge the stimulus and support of the Commission of the European Communities (DGXII) Biomedical and Health Research Programme (BIOMED 2).

We would like to thank John Murphy for his constructive and critical comments on an earlier draft of this paper.

[1] *Collins* v. *Wilcock* [1984] 1 W.L.R. 1172 at 1177 *per* Goff L.J.

[2] Bl. Comm. 3, Bl. Comm. 120. And see *Clerk and Lindsell on Torts* (17th edn.) (1995) at para. 12-01.

[3] [1985] A.C. 871 (H.L.). Though note the glimmer of light in *Smith* v. *Tunbridge Wells H.A.* [1994] 5 Med. L.R. 334.

[4] See *Devi* v. *West Midlands R.H.A.* [1980] 7 C.L. 44.

[5] *Re T (Adult: Refusal of Medical Treatment)* [1992] 4 All E.R. 649 finally laying to rest the long heresy expounded in *Leigh* v. *Gladstone* [1909] 26 T.L.R. 139.

[6] *Ibid.*, at 661.

> The patient's interest consists of his right to self-determination—his right to live his own life how he wishes, even if it will damage his health or lead to his premature death. Society's interest is in upholding the concept that all human life is sacred and that it should be preserved if at all possible. It is well established that in the ultimate the right of the individual is paramount.

It is perhaps ironic that when at last English law catches up with ethical debate and confirms the individual's right to control medical treatment, events are forcing ethicists and health professionals to review the relationship between patients' rights and patients' responsibilities, particularly in the context of infectious diseases.[7] Patient autonomy has more commonly been analyzed by lawyers and philosophers in the context of diseases and conditions which affect that individual patient alone. A woman has a suspicious lump in her breast. What criteria govern the choices which she must make regarding therapy? A Jehovah's Witness traumatically injured in a road accident refuses blood. A person afflicted by multiple disabilities seeks to have all treatment, even feeding, discontinued. The consequences of each potential choice predominantly affect that patient alone. No other person's *physical* health is endangered by a choice to reject treatment.

Traumatic injury, cancer and the neurological diseases have been viewed as the "plagues" of post-war Europe. The *real* plagues, communicable diseases, such as cholera, tuberculosis and the plague itself, have receded in public consciousness. Infectious diseases, those which threatened not only the afflicted patient but the community as a whole, were regarded as of minor import. For most people, infectious diseases equated to influenza and the common cold, or childhood diseases, such as measles, mumps and chickenpox. Catching an infectious disease was nasty but not life-threatening. Vaccination programmes expanded to cover an even greater range of childhood diseases. If someone was unlucky enough to contract "something serious", modern antibiotics offered a cure. The spectre of lethal communicable disease ceased to haunt the nations of Western Europe and the draconian public health measures once commonly invoked to control disease were also largely forgotten. Dogs remained subject to quarantine on entry to the United Kingdom. Human quarantine would be regarded as a violation of civil liberties. Public health became an enterprise largely concerned with studying epidemiology, with public education and prevention of disease. Public health did not directly intrude into

[7] J. Harris and S. Holm, "Is there a Moral Obligation not to infect others?" (1995) 311 *British Medical Journal* 1215.

private lives. Public health barely features as an issue in "medical law" texts or literature in the United Kingdom.[8]

This paper reviews the legal and moral dilemmas posed for society by infectious disease asking how far society should recognise and enforce an obligation not to expose others to infection. The AIDS pandemic was of course the trigger for a re-evaluation of rights and responsibilities in relation to communicable diseases.[9] We shall suggest that in some ways AIDS has obscured rather than clarified the debate. HIV is simply one infectious disease among many. Obligations not to transmit disease should not be determined solely in the context of one disease which provokes so much inflammatory opinion, opinion largely generated not by accurate information concerning the virus itself but by its perceived causes and "victims".

II. THE SPECTRE RETURNS?

We must, or course, acknowledge that the primary cause of revived concern, and intermittent public panic, about communicable diseases is quite obviously the AIDS/HIV pandemic. For the media at least, privacy and autonomy swiftly ceased to have major significance once public health was endangered. The seropositive health worker, the allegedly irresponsible haemophiliac found their names blazoned across the headlines. Frequent calls were made for transmission of HIV to be made a criminal offence, for "dangerous" patients to be locked up.[10] In retrospect, the public health brouhaha generated by HIV can be seen as only the tip of the iceberg of a much more profound dilemma for society. HIV is not a particularly effective infectious agent. It can be transmitted only through direct contact with body fluids. Compared to tuberculosis and cholera, for instance, the threat of contracting HIV recedes in significance. That is not to downgrade the threat of HIV, for while it may be relatively difficult to transmit, many millions of people are infected worldwide and the evidence suggests it is almost inevitably, ultimately, lethal.

---

[8] Contrast the lack of relevant British literature with the extensive jurisprudence and scholarly analysis of public health law elegantly and critically reviewed by L.O. Gostin, "The Americans with Disabilities Act and the Corpus of Anti-Discrimination Law. A Force for Change in the Future of Public Health Legislation" in A. Grubb and M. J. Mehlman (eds.), *Justice and Health Care: Comparative Perspectives* (John Wiley and Sons 1995) at 105–46.

[9] See, J. Montgomery, "Victims or Threats?—The Framing of HIV" [1990] Vol. XII *Liverpool Law Review* 25.

[10] See, for example, the publicity surrounding stories that a young Birmingham haemophiliac who was HIV positive had "deliberately" infected several female lovers: (1992) *The Independent*, 28 June.

What is now clear, however, is that other far more infectious diseases are not solely of historical interest. The incidence of tuberculosis is rising steadily.[11] Patients seropositive for HIV are showing high rates of concurrent TB infection. Such a patient is far more likely to infect others with tuberculosis than HIV. A growing body of evidence also suggests that an increasing number of patients suffering from tuberculosis are resistant to conventional antibiotics. Resistance often arises from earlier failure to complete prescribed courses of treatment. Other infectious diseases, such as diptheria, cholera and typhoid, were never eliminated from the face of the earth. Outbreaks continue to kill thousands of victims in the poorer parts of the world. Increased mobility, and the chaos in parts of the former Communist sector, bring such diseases back to the doorsteps of the European Union.

> The rapid growth of air travel, relaxed immigration controls and emerging infections appearing worldwide mean that we must be as aware of the epidemiology of infection in other countries as we are of events in our own "back yard".[12]

Furthermore any belief that science had overcome communicable disease in this country, or in our European neighbours, was always an illusion. HIV is the sexually transmitted disease every schoolboy hears about. For the past forty years the incidence of other sexually transmitted diseases, such as gonorrhoea, chlamydia, and genital herpes, rose steadily. Women in particular suffered permanent damage to their health and fertility. The "minor" infectious diseases remain with us and are not as minor as first appears. Meningitis kills several children each year. Measles still kills. Chickenpox is simply, and literally, an irritation to most children, but an immunocompromised child can die. Elderly people contracting shingles suffer acutely. Rubella, even today, leads to the birth of damaged infants and very many terminations of pregnancy each year.

III. DRACONIAN LEGISLATION

The erroneous belief that communicable diseases had lost their power is matched by ignorance of the continuation of draconian legislation to control disease. In 1985 news that a magistrate had ordered the detention in hospital of a man suffering from AIDS was greeted with surprise and outrage.[13] Democracies do not generally lock up the sick?

[11] See, the WHO report on the escalation in tuberculosis worldwide: (1996) *The Guardian*, 22 March.

[12] See, the Foreword to E. G. Davies *et al.*, *Manual of Childhood Infections* (British Paediatric Association 1995).

[13] "Detaining Patients with AIDS" (1985) 291 *British Medical Journal* 1102 (Editorial).

The wisdom of coercion in that instance may be questioned. It has never been repeated in relation to patients with HIV or AIDS. Yet there is no doubt that the magistrate acted entirely lawfully.

The Public Health (Control of Diseases) Act 1984 empowers public health officers to act to prevent the spread of disease. The powers conferred by that Act, and the Public Health (Infectious Diseases) Regulations 1988[14] made under it, permit the state to override virtually all individual liberties in the cause of protecting the community. Where a patient is suffering from a notifiable disease (or food poisoning) confidentiality is abrogated.[15] A person knowing that he is suffering from a notifiable disease, or being responsible for a person so suffering, commits a criminal offence if he exposes others to infection in a public place,[16] or if he continues with a trade, business or occupation where he risks exposing others to infection.[17] Notifiable diseases specified under the Act are cholera, plague, relapsing fever and typhus.[18] Other diseases can and are deemed notifiable by regulations made by the Secretary of State for Health or local authorities.[19] This extended list of notifiable diseases includes polio, meningitis, diphtheria, dysentery, most common childhood diseases, rabies and tuberculosis. Neither HIV or AIDS is a notifiable disease.

The 1984 Act provides that if a person is believed to be suffering from a notifiable disease, or to be a carrier of such a disease, a magistrate may order that he be tested for that disease.[20] Where a magistrate is satisfied that a patient with a notifiable disease poses a serious risk of infection to others and his circumstances are such that proper precautions to prevent the spread of disease cannot, or are not, being taken he may order his removal to and detention in a designated hospital.[21] Additional powers are granted to the Secretary of State to make further regulations with a view to the detention of persons with infectious diseases and in particular to police the entry of infected persons at ports and airports.[22]

An individual infected with a communicable disease specified either under the statute itself or the regulations made by the minister thus loses any effective choice in relation to treatment, and, potentially, his/her liberty and his/her privacy. It may well be the case that once

[14] S.I. 1988 No. 1546.

[15] See, 1984 Act, ss. 10–11.

[16] *Ibid.*, s.17.

[17] *Ibid.*, s.19.

[18] See *ibid.*, s.11.

[19] *Supra* n. 14 at Sched. 1.

[20] 1984 Act, ss. 35–6.

[21] *Ibid.*, ss. 37–8.

[22] Extending we believe to imposing quarantine on humans.

detained in hospital he/she can in theory "choose" not to comply with therapeutic treatment, but that is a pretty empty, futile choice. Failure to protect others from the risk of infection he/she poses, exposes him/her to criminal liability. The cholera sufferer, the victim of tuberculosis, even the patient with scarlet fever (or his/her parents) may face the rigours of the criminal law for dissent from medical advice.

The status of AIDS with this framework of draconian legislation is both interesting and instructive. Neither HIV nor AIDS has been designated a notifiable disease in the United Kingdom. The British Government, and the courts,[23] have very deliberately decided that guaranteed confidentiality for patients who suspect that they may be seropositive is crucial to any attempt to control HIV. Patients must not be inhibited from seeking testing and counselling. Yet regulations made under the Public Health (Control of Diseases) Act 1984 do extend to persons suffering from "acquired immune deficiency syndrome" the powers to order the removal of a patient to, and her detention in, hospital.[24] And indeed the power to continue to detain a patient with AIDS in hospital is more extensive than in relation to the other notifiable diseases. Those provisions of the 1984 Act (sections 17 and 19) criminalising conduct exposing others to infection are interestingly not extended to patients with AIDS.

Two features of the public health powers to control AIDS should be noted. First, it seems unlikely that the regulations authorising detention of patients apply to patients with HIV. Only the patient who has developed AIDS is at risk of compulsory "treatment". Secondly, HIV/AIDS finds itself in a half-way house between the coercive powers assumed by the state to control the major communicable diseases and the very different, perhaps more liberal, approach to sexually transmitted disease. The National Health Service (Venereal Diseases) Regulations 1974[25] focus on the creation of a service designed to encourage patients to volunteer for treatment. Confidentiality is strictly enforced and a breach of confidence is justifiable only in the context of contact tracing. No coercive powers to detain patients are provided for, even though most sexually transmitted diseases, unlike AIDS, are readily treatable.

The extent to which the state assumes coercive powers to curtail individual liberty in order to control disease raises deep questions about the extent of personal responsibility and the nature of our harmful contact one with another.

---

[23] See, *X* v. *Y* [1988] 2 All E.R. 648.

[24] Public Health (Infectious Diseases) Regulations 1988, *supra* n. 14.

[25] S.I. 1974 No. 29.

IV. DANGER, MORALITY AND RESPONSIBILITY

> As soon as any part of a person's conduct affects prejudicially the interests of others, society has a jurisdiction over it, and the question whether the general welfare will or will not be promoted by interfering with it, becomes open to discussion.[26]

Mill succinctly sums up the fundamental ground on which a democratic society may properly abrogate the autonomy of its individual members.[27] The range of interests which may be protected against invasion can be the subject of debate. The interest in health and bodily integrity endangered by disease is beyond dispute. The right to life is the core human right. Absent a right to life, all other rights are meaningless. No-one would dispute the right of the state to make laws protecting citizens from violence. The common law, as we have noted, does not differentiate between degrees of violence. We may no more lawfully lightly slap an editor of this Review on the face than we may break his nose. "Trivial" violence is as readily condemned as more obviously injurious conduct for three reasons. First, no contact can be guaranteed as trivial. We may be unaware that the editor has brittle-bone disease and our "gentle" slap smashes his cheekbone. Secondly, the provocation offered by the slap may all too readily escalate the level of violence between us. The editor punches John Harris back, blacking his eye. Margaret Brazier responds by breaking a bottle over the editor's head, and so it develops! Violation of an individual's bodily integrity threatens more than the original participants in the incident; it threatens society. Finally, even the gentle "slap" infringes not just the comfort of the victim but his/her essential liberty as well.

Is there any reason to treat disease differently from violence? A slap affronts dignity. A blow may bruise or even break a bone. The hurt will mend. Communicable diseases, to a greater or lesser extent, can kill and inflict irreversible damage to health. HIV is probably lethal in almost all cases. Cholera kills a percentage of its victims. Meningitis kills and leaves others deaf. Sexually transmitted diseases such as chlamydia can destroy a woman's fertility. The interests of others are prejudicially affected by disease to a greater extent than is the case with much of the overt violence which is the everyday business of the criminal law. Nor should the threat to society as a whole posed by disease be lightly discounted. The highly contagious diseases threaten numbers that even the most notorious serial killer could not dream of. Failure by the state to intervene in the face of an epidemic can trigger

---

[26] Essay *On Liberty* , ch. 1 in M. Warnock (ed.), *Utilitarianism* (Fontana 1972) at 187–8.
[27] *Ibid.*

public disorder. Victims of disease may become victims of violence as happened in the recent outbreak of the plague in Southern India.

The danger to society posed by communicable disease is directly analogous to the danger posed by casual violence. But that is not of itself alone sufficient to justify the draconian powers assumed by governments to control such disease. Mill speaks of a "person's conduct prejudicially" affecting others. He does not mandate prior intervention to control such conduct, he merely concludes that that conduct justifies consideration of whether public welfare will be promoted by intervening via coercive measures to curtail the liberty of the perpetrator.[28] Disease is different from violence in the usual sense of the word. Assuming we are sane, our slapping the editor's face is our voluntary deliberate act. It is truly our conduct which violates his interests. In the majority of instances people do not deliberately and voluntarily spread disease. We may refuse to complete the course of treatment for tuberculosis and by everyday contact infect another twenty colleagues. Unless we deliberately cough in their direction, with express intent to infect a much disliked co-worker, does our conduct directly equate to the deliberate slap?

Perhaps we have conceded too much. While it is true that entering a crowded room knowingly suffering from an infectious disease does not directly equate to the deliberate slap, it may be sufficiently analogous for the moral responsibility for the consequences to be the same. Accepting that in the majority of instances patients do not deliberately and voluntarily spread disease, the crucial question in terms of moral responsibility is what does "deliberately" add to "voluntarily"?

Consider that question in the light of society's experience of HIV/AIDS and the renewed focus that HIV/AIDS offers us on responsibility for communicable diseases.[29] Suppose a new disease emerges, as did HIV, which, like HIV is untreatable but for which the mode of infection comes to copy another existing infectious disease. To take just one possible scenario, imagine for a moment that this new disease followed the transmission mode of say, pulmonary plague.

Pulmonary plague is an airborne infection with an extremely high transmission rate. Although it is a bacterial infection its mode of infection is paralleled by several viral infections including such common viruses as measles and flu. Anybody present in the same house or flat as a victim of one of these diseases will, at least in principle, be infected. Experimental work shows that the inhalation of one single

---

[28] *Ibid.*

[29] See, J. Harris and S. Holm, "If Only AIDS Were Different" (1993) 26(6) *Hastings Center Report* 6–13. In this paper a number of different possible disease models for HIV/AIDS are imagined and the moral and social consequences explored.

plague bacterium belonging to one of the more virulent strains is sufficient to cause a potentially lethal infection. Today plague can be treated with antibiotics and the mortality rate for pulmonary plague has dropped from virtually 100 per cent to approximately 10 per cent. Plague is a relatively short-lasting disease both in its pulmonary and its bubonic form so an isolation and quarantine regime is possible, and has been a main feature of the control of plague epidemics since ancient times.[30]

Now suppose the new disease mimicked the transmission mode of pulmonary plague. What would we say of someone who, knowing they were infected and knowing the infectivity and mode of transmission, deliberately went to work? Would we be much impressed by the supposed distinction between deliberately going to work and deliberately infecting another? Or would moral responsibility be attached to *voluntarily* spreading disease? We are responsible for what we voluntarily bring about, not simply for what we intend, desire or wish to achieve.[31]

Consider society's attitude to drunken driving. The individual who drives with a massive excess of alcohol is held responsible for the harm he causes in an alcohol related accident. That he voluntarily placed others at risk by driving whilst inebriated is sufficient, it need not be demonstrated that he wanted or intended to run down the children in the bus queue. Whether and to what extent we also hold him criminally responsible is of course a further and separate question and one, the answer to which turns on our social policy concerns and to a lesser extent on our theory of punishment. However, the law does frequently punish drunken drivers and so might for related reasons choose to punish those knowingly or recklessly transmitting infectious diseases.

V. CRIMINAL RESPONSIBILITY

The means chosen by society to control violence predominantly revolve around the imposition of criminal responsibility. The criminal law acts retrospectively, and focuses on deliberate conduct in the main. We will be punished if we slap the editor. We will not (once again on the fragile assumption we are both sane) be locked up because we might slap him. We will be punished, if we acted deliber-

---

[30] *Ibid.*

[31] See, J. Harris, *Violence and Responsibility* (Routledge & Kegan Paul 1980) and J. Harris three essays on euthanasia: "Euthanasia and the Value of Life"; "The Philosophical Case Against the Philosophical Case Against Euthanasia", and "Final Thought on Final Acts". Each essay is the subject of a response by John Finnis and all are published in J. Keown (ed.), *Euthanasia Examined: Ethical Clinical and Legal Perspectives* (Cambridge University Press 1995) at 6–22, 36–45 and 56–61.

ately not if we fall against him after too many whiskies at a Christmas party. If we hurt him by negligence, our liberty will not be curtailed, our pockets may be. Responsibility will be normally enforced by the civil not the criminal law.

Control of communicable disease by coercive and anticipatory action within the current legislation on control of disease forces us to ask: why not more readily rely on the criminal law to enforce *individual* responsibility, buttressed where required by civil law? How can you justify "punishing" non-deliberate conduct—locking up the sick? And most importantly is the public welfare promoted by coercive measures to control disease?

The role of the criminal law in the control of communicable disease is complex.[32] Disentangling fundamental questions of ethics and policy from practical difficulty is especially problematic. The common law of England founds its prohibition of personal violence on the concept of assault. Any direct physical contact imposed by A on B constitutes common assault. The Offences Against the Person Act 1861 grades assaults, and fixes punishment, by reference to the degree of harm ensuing from that original assault. So a blow inflicting bruising constitutes assault occasioning actual bodily harm, a stabbing provoking a haemorrhage amounts to causing grievous bodily harm. If there is no contact there is no assault. Breathing tuberculosis laden bacteria in the vicinity of a crowded room of vulnerable elderly people, lending a hated colleague an infected handkerchief is unlikely to constitute assault however evil the motive.[33]

The law's concept of contact remains crude and implausible. There is no doubt that a virus is a physical thing and that it can be projected towards others by many means, including nasally or orally projected airborne droplets, and for that matter, within a poison dart or riding piggy back astride a bullet or a discharge of semen. And, having been projected a virus may also, and non-figuratively, strike home, make palpable physical contact, sometimes with deadly effect. If a would-be murderer chooses a fine aerosol spray laden with cyanide gas, he has not renounced offensive weaponry, nor, if the gas reaches its victim, has he failed to make physical contact. Of course, if someone, knowing that they were infected with the pulmonary plague-mimicking new disease that we imagined above, were to enter a crowded bus they might not *intend* in some narrow sense to infect the other occupants, but they would share the same responsibility for subsequent deaths

[32] See generally, S. Bronitt, "Spreading Disease and the Criminal Law" [1994] Crim. L.R. 21.

[33] Though it would fall within the Law Commission's proposed offence of "causing injury" discussed *infra* at 191.

that would fall to the person who entered such a bus firing randomly a machine gun without taking aim at any particular individual or caring whether anyone or no-one was actually hit.

Much ink has been spent on the criminal law and transmission of HIV. If HIV is transmitted via sexual intercourse, there will of necessity be physical contact. So if a seropositive man fails to warn his female partner of his status deliberately planning to infect her, is her consent to intercourse vitiated, rendering what is done to her an assault, if not rape? The balance of authority in England suggests not.[34] Her consent to the act of intercourse holds good despite her lack of knowledge of the risks attached to intercourse with that man. Suggestions are made that an alternative offence under the Offences Against the Person Act 1861 may be committed, unlawfully administering a noxious thing, *i.e.* infection.[35]

We do not propose to explore further the niceties of law of assault and analogous crimes.[36] No doubt elegant arguments can be formulated to force transmission of disease into the straitjacket of assault or related criminal offences. In practical terms an approach to criminal responsibility and disease founded on the concept of assault is fundamentally flawed. Actual physical contact is irrelevant. The hurt inflicted by disease is not dependent on such conduct. The crimes of assault very necessarily in their proper sphere require that the accuser prove the accused inflicted the harm of which he/she complains. It would be unjust for John Harris to be punished for blacking the editor's eye if it could not be proved that he, and not the editor's disgruntled wife, inflicted the relevant actual bodily harm. Requirements of proof of causation satisfy the needs of justice and are generally pragmatically possible. Proof (whether beyond reasonable doubt or on the balance of probabilities) that X infected Y is much more problematic. The man charged with infecting his lover with HIV will cite her promiscuity as evidence that another was responsible. The parents who believe that their child was infected with tuberculosis by a reckless patient defying medical advice may never be able to prove their hypothesis. True, these are evidential problems which may be contingent upon particular difficulties of identifying say viral strains. In the relatively near future we may be able to track specific vira and establish the source, albeit at considerable cost. We should not, however, in any event establish principles which are hostage to contingent practical problems.

---

[34] *R.* v. *Clarence* (1888) 22 Q.B.D. 23; discussed in *R.* v. *Lineaker* [1995] Q.B. 250 at 258–61 and see, *Hegarty* v. *Shine* (1878) 4 L.R. Ir. 288.

[35] See, ss. 23, 24.

[36] They are elegantly reviewed by Bronitt, *supra* n. 32.

If the criminal law is to play an effective role in the control of disease, the law should seek to punish an offender's fundamental irresponsibility rather than focus exclusively on the outcome of such irresponsibility. Society's interest is in deterring the infected and infectious from creating unjustifiable *risks* to others.

Arthur Miller's play *All My Sons* illustrates poignantly this very point. The Keller family and in particular Steve Keller, who does not appear in the play, were responsible for manufacturing and shipping defective cylinder heads for aircraft in the second world war. Joe Keller admits his part in the killings: "I was the beast; the guy who sold cracked cylinder heads to the Army Air Force; the guy who made twenty-one P-40's crash in Australia". But he does not *feel* himself to be guilty because he pulled no trigger, he only failed to go to work on the relevant day and stop the shipment and thereafter he kept quiet, although he could have recalled the engines. As he says of Steve Keller his "partner in crime": "I know he meant no harm". Neither of them intended or planned the deaths of those pilots. But such excuses do not wash with the next generation of the family. As Ann Keller says of her father "He knowingly shipped out parts that would crash an airplane" and her brother Chris says bluntly "He murdered twenty-one pilots".[37] The crucial issue is not what we directly intend but what we knowingly and voluntarily bring about.[38] This is what makes Steve and Joe Keller murderers in the eyes of their family and in the eyes of every audience. They recklessly and voluntarily endangered the lives of others and their act was complete when the parts were shipped and not recalled before the planes flew.

At the end of the play Joe Keller discovers that his own son, Larry, also a pilot in the war, had committed suicide when he learned of the family complicity in murder. Trying to make Joe and his mother take responsibility, Larry's brother Chris repeats his indictment of his father "Larry didn't kill himself to make you and Dad sorry" and his mother responds "What more can we be?". Chris's answer carries the message of the play: "You can be better. Once and for all you can know that there is a universe of people outside and you're responsible to it, and unless you know that, you threw away your son, because that's why he died".[39]

Interestingly, although the play is concerned to make key characters and its audience face up to their personal responsibilities, it assumes that there will be criminal responsibility for such conduct. Steve is in prison for his part in the deaths. And whether or not imprisonment is

[37] A. Miller, *All My Sons* (Penguin 1961) Act One (p. 117).

[38] See, J. Harris, *Violence and Responsibility* (Routledge and Kegan Paul 1980).

[39] Miller, *supra* n. 37 at Act Three (p. 170).

appropriate, the point about social as well as personal responsibility for reckless endangerment is well taken. In terms of their moral responsibility it does not matter whether or not a particular defective engine caused a crash. The reckless endangerment is what we all have a moral responsibility to prevent and there is clearly a strong public interest in controlling reckless endangerment.

In Scotland the recognition of reckless endangerment as a criminal offence enforces such a policy.[40] In England a patient suffering from certain notifiable diseases may commit an offence under the Public Health (Control of Diseases) Act 1984 if he exposes others to the risk of infection in a public place. That prosecution is a practical reality, and not simply a theoretical possibility, was illustrated in 1994 in *R.* v. *Gaud*.[41] A surgeon suffering from Hepatitis B defied the advice of the General Medical Council and continued to practise. He took measures to evade screening for the disease including substituting patient's blood for his own. It was suspected, but could not be proven, that he had infected patients. He was convicted of causing a public nuisance and gaoled for a year.[42] If the will is present, the means can be found to punish those who spread disease. The common law may not always be logical, but innovative judicial action can often render it flexible.[43] But should we seek to do so?[44]

The arguments for and against the use of the criminal law to promote responsible behaviour by those who risk exposing others to infectious disease are finely balanced. Behaviour such as that of Dr Gaud cannot be distinguished from that, say, of a train driver who consumes several whiskies before embarking on driving an Inter-City express. Few would doubt that he should be punished regardless of whether his inebriated state results in disaster or not. If a seropositive person deliberately embarks on a campaign to infect others, concealing his condition from his several partners, and practising the very opposite of safer sex, his conduct is morally analogous to that of the conventional serial killer. If individuals who endanger others by

[40] See generally, J. K. Mason and A. McCall Smith, *Law and Medical Ethics* (4th edn.) (Butterworths 1994) at 48–9; G. T. Laurie, "AIDS and Criminal Liability under Scottish Law" (1991) 36 *Law Society Scotland* 312.

[41] See, M. Mullholland, "Public Nuisance—a New Use for an Old Tool" (1995) 11 *Professional Negligence* 70.

[42] In an analogous case in Canada an HIV positive blood donor was convicted of committing a public nuisance: *R.* v. *Thornton* [1993] S.C.R. 445; a similar prosecution grounded on infection of sexual partners failed: *R.* v. *Ssenyonga* (1992) 73 C.C.C. 3d 216 (other criminal charges were proceeding).

[43] See, *U.S.* v. *Joseph* (1993) 37 M.J. 392 noted in (1994) 2 Med. L. Rev. 244 (AG).

[44] For a resounding no, to this question see A. Grubb, commentary to *U.S.* v. *Joseph; ibid* 43 at 251.

reckless or deliberate behaviour ought to be accountable to society for what they do, disease, unless it has so distorted judgement to raise questions about the accused's sanity, does not exempt the wrongdoer from the general rule.

However no empirical evidence has suggested other than that the numbers of infected persons who endanger others out of malice or wilful disregard for others are tiny. The number of successful criminal convictions will be low. The role of the criminal law will be largely symbolic. And the symbolism may not be entirely beneficial.[45] The law may prescribe that only the healthworker who quite deliberately conceals her health status and knowingly endangers her patients commits a criminal offence. The law may provide that only on *proof* that an HIV positive Lothario who deliberately risks infecting his several partners, shall he be punished. Nonetheless, the public may come to perceive that any transmission of disease, or at least of HIV, is criminal. Patients suffering from infectious disease will be stigmatised as potential criminals. Such a stigma will deter them from volunteering for screening and treatment.

At a practical level too the role the criminal law can play in control of communicable diseases will be perceived as likely to be minimal. The criminal law operates retrospectively. Its deterrent and protective impact depends on the existence of laws and the possibility of punishment re-inforcing individuals' sense of social responsibility. It cannot be an effective means of controlling a true epidemic. The pre-eminence given in public health laws to measures to restrain infected persons from contact with others, and the relatively low value attached to criminal sanctions, testifies to this fact. Restraining those who pose a real risk to life and health, regardless of their motives or lack thereof, may be seen as a much more pragmatic policy. But can such a crude violation of autonomy be justified?

VI. RESTRAINING THE DANGEROUS

The Public Health (Control of Diseases) Act 1984 in conferring powers to remove persons suffering from certain infectious diseases (including AIDS) to hospital does not address the intent or state of mind of the patient. If there is a serious risk of infection to others and proper precautions cannot be taken to prevent the spread of infection outside hospital, off to a designated hospital the patient may be sent. The patient with, for example, tuberculosis may be too ill to appreci-

[45] See, for example, R. Porter, "History Says No to the Policeman's Response to AIDS" (1986) 293 *British Medical Journal* 1589; P. Old and J. Montgomery, "Law, Coercion and Public Health" (1992) 304 *British Medical Journal* 891.

ate risk to others. The patient with typhus may be a Christian Scientist who scorns the notion of illness. Both may be exemplary characters with no design to harm others. Yet on objective evidence that they might cause harm, and without the protection of the criminal process, they can lose their liberty. Of course they are not alone in facing loss of liberty without proof of crime. The mentally ill patient can be confined to protect others. Tom Campbell and Christopher Heginbotham[46] have attacked such discrimination against mental illness arguing:

> In particular, discrimination occurs when dangerous persons who are not suffering from mental illness are not detained on protectionist grounds although their dangerousness is of a type and degree which would make them liable to detention if they were diagnosed as having a mental illness ...

Patients suffering from certain dangerous communicable diseases are, however, susceptible to detention on just such protectionist grounds. A small sub-category of victims of physical illness find themselves in just the same case as the mentally ill. Are both groups wrongfully deprived of liberty and autonomy?

David Price[47] reviews the arguments for some form of preventive civil detention of those dangerous to others which might include the "critically infectious individual" even though he was not engaged in intentional, reckless or even negligent conduct. The state is entitled to intervene to protect citizens from physical harm.

The implementation and content of powers of civil detention nonetheless concern him. In the context of mental illness Price is concerned to distinguish between compulsory detention to *treat* patients whose disorder is treatable and who are incapable of making autonomous choices for themselves, and those who retain the capacity to make an independent judgement, whose condition may be untreatable, but who nonetheless pose a danger to other. He stresses the primary importance of devising a system for what he describes as "police-powers" to detain the latter category of persons which conform to strict criteria of natural justice. He canvasses how far such "police-powers" can or should be largely incorporated in the criminal justice system. Above all, he rejects a "medical model" of decision-making in relation to mentally ill persons removed from society to protect others. Doctors' business is to treat the sick not to safeguard society. Doctors may generally only treat the sick who want treatment, or whose illness has rendered them incapable of independent judgement.

---

[46] In *Mental Illness, Prejudice, Discrimination and the Law* (Dartmouth 1991) at 98.

[47] D.P.T. Price, "Civil Commitment of the Mentally Ill" (1994) 2 Med. L. Rev. 321 at 347.

Much of Price's argument is difficult to refute, nor would we wish to do so. Liberal democratic societies restrain dangerous conduct by punishing acts endangering others' safety. Individual responsibility is enforced through the deterrent impact on the criminal and civil law. The state intervenes to condemn what people *do* not what they are. Intervention to curtail liberty or autonomy prior to any dangerous tendency manifesting itself in dangerous action needs exceptional justification. If such justification is grounded on disease there are no sound grounds to discriminate between mental and physical illness. What is necessary is to delve further into reasons why risks triggered by disease differ from risks triggered by bad temper, unsocial living conditions or over-indulgence in alcohol, all of which remain exclusively the concern of the criminal justice system operating retrospectively.

Two possible reasons for treating communicable diseases differently suggest themselves. Neither is entirely convincing. First, the relevant disease, physical or mental, may be perceived as so radically increasing the risk that the inherent danger it poses to others will manifest itself in tangible harm to those others that the case is readily distinguishable from other "dangerous tendencies". If X has pulmonary plague and does not submit to isolation he will infect virtually everyone he comes into contact with. The likelihood of even the most violent alcoholic attacking more than one or two people a day is low. Secondly, disease may distort judgement and diminish individual responsibility.[48] Laid low with cholera, Y may no longer appreciate basic requirements of hygiene or be able to assess the danger her habits pose to the rest of her household. She is not deserving of punishment. Deterrence can not affect actions which her disease disables her from understanding. Such arguments are analogous to arguments which can be applied to certain sorts of mental disorder. The patient's illness may increase the risk of dangerous conduct harming others *and* may distort her judgement in relation to the interests of others.

The difficulty with both arguments in the context of communicable diseases is that neither can be applied universally to physical ills any more than mental disorder. Communicable diseases vary widely in their degrees of infectivity and of course in their mode of transmission.[49] It is by no means the case that judgement will always be distorted by such disease thus diminishing personal responsibility. Pulmonary plague, cholera, typhus and meningitis clearly meet both

[48] Justifying the coercive powers enabling the state to detain mentally ill patients, Sir Thomas Bingham M.R. said: "..the very illness which is the cause of danger may deprive the sufferer of the insight necessary to ensure access to proper medical care...": *In re S-C (Mental Patient: Habeas Corpus)* [1996] 2 W.L.R. 146 at 148.

[49] See, L. Gostin, *infra* n. 61 at 130–9.

tests. They create exceptional risk to others and may temporarily disable the patient from exercising responsibility for himself or others.[50] Tuberculosis creates a high risk of infection but will not necessarily distort judgement at the same point in time. HIV and Hepatitis B and C are even more problematic. Infectivity rates are much lower and infection will not be transmitted without some deliberate act on the part of the infected person. Judgement will not be impaired. Similarly persons who are carriers of communicable disease, but suffer no symptoms of disease pose problems for society. Such persons remain capable of making decisions for themselves about the risk they pose to others if they are aware that they are carriers. Is there any better reason to act against such persons prior to establishing that they have committed irresponsible and dangerous acts than to act against the woman of known violent temper? We suggest that there may not be. Yet any recklessly endangering behaviour of the individual who knows that he/she may endanger others by transmitting a disease that can kill or permanently impair others' health is no less morally wrong than that of his/her sister who makes no effort to curb her odious temper. Must we return to the thorny issue of criminal responsibility once again?

VII. CRIMINAL RESPONSIBILITY AGAIN?

Anticipatory intervention to restrain those rendered dangerous by disease requires evidence of the exceptional degree of that danger and of at least some impairment of the individual's ability to exercise personal responsibility for others' safety. Conduct which deliberately or recklessly endangers others is the proper province of the criminal justice system. It is a conclusion we arrive at with some reluctance accepting the concerns expressed earlier about both the practical utility of the criminal law in this context and the symbolic danger of stigmatising disease.

Consider again the case of Dr Gaud.[51] Could it have been just to

[50] Moreover if the disease renders the patient temporarily "incompetent'" he/she can presumably be treated once settled into hospital under the "best interests" doctrine enunciated in *F* v. *West Berkshire H.A.* [1989] 2 All E.R. 545 (H.L.). Note that the Law Commission expressly acknowledges that mental incapacity may be triggered by physical disease; see Law Commission Report No. 23, *Mental Incapacity* (1995) at paras. 3.11–3.13. Being able to treat the patient detained overcomes one of the fundamental objections to the current powers of detention in the Public Health (Control of Diseases) Act 1984 that the Act violates civil liberties "without any saving therapeutic benefit"; see I. Kennedy and A. Grubb, *Medical Law: Text with Materials* (2nd edn.) (Butterworths 1994) at 83–4.

[51] See, *supra* at 83.

allow his irresponsible conduct to go unpunished? Yet could anticipatory action to restrain his "dangerous tendency" have been justified? Had evidence emerged earlier of his status as a Hepatitis B carrier would anyone seriously contend that his liberty could properly have been curtailed because of evidence his character was such he *might* proceed to evade all restrictions on his medical practice and thus endanger patients? Would any rational individual argue that all persons suffering from tuberculosis should be subjected to coercive treatment? Only the most irrational bigot has ever suggested persons with HIV should be subjected to enforced celibacy. In each of these examples the infected individual in question only endangers others if he deliberately acts in a manner calculated to endanger others without regard to their interests or safety. Until he has so acted anticipatory constraint is no more justifiable than in the case of those with other dangerous tendencies. If he does so act, his conduct is equally deserving of punishment as the woman who allows her temper to cause her to lash out at her neighbour, or the driver who permits his fondness for wine to cause him to endanger other road users by driving under the influence of alcohol.

It may be argued that we have concentrated too much of our argument on Dr Gaud. His is an exceptional case in two senses. There is no evidence that other health professionals have acted with similar gross disregard of their patients' welfare. And, infected professionals are themselves an exceptional category of infected, and infectious individuals. Their patients are entirely "at their mercy" unable to protect themselves from the risk posed to them by the doctor or nurse. In society more generally the uninfected person has the ability and the obligation to protect himself. The argument is most often advanced in relation to HIV. The risks of unprotected sexual intercourse are known to all. The primary responsibility to prevent transmission of HIV is to protect oneself by insisting on condom use, a discriminating choice of partners and undertaking cross-examination of such partners about their sexual history before embarking on sexual intercourse. Yet condoms only decrease the risk of transmission of HIV, partners may lie, and equality of bargaining power is not always present between partners. Is a person who deliberately conceals his HIV status, who rejects use of a condom, and adopts a "what the hell" approach to his lover's safety any less morally culpable than Dr Gaud? Outside the context of HIV, can those threatened by other disease protect themselves any more effectively than Dr Gaud's unfortunate patients? How is the passenger on the Manchester to Euston express to know that the woman in the next seat has tuberculosis rather than just a very bad cold?

We are not arguing that it should be a crime to transmit disease only that conduct which quite calculatedly exhibits total disregard for others' health and safety falls within the ambit of criminal law. The essence of the wrong committed by the individual who deliberately exposes others to disease is that of recklessly endangering others. The fact that either no-one else has actually been harmed by contracting the relevant disease, or that it cannot easily be proved that transmission of disease resulted from the accused's reckless conduct should not be relevant. Reckless endangerment should be recognised in its own right as a substantive criminal offence and one well suited, but not confined to, imposing responsibility to transmission of disease.

VIII. REFORMING PUBLIC HEALTH LAWS

We have sought to demonstrate that in an appropriate case even draconian limitations on autonomy imposed by public health laws to control transmission of communicable diseases are justifiable in principle. There is as strong a moral responsibility to protect others from contracting disease as there is to safeguard them from any other violation of bodily integrity. Translating that responsibility into legal principle is more awkward. The current legislation, the Public Health (Control of Diseases) Act 1984 and the 1988 Regulations,[52] go only part of the way to an acceptable solution. The legislation has become to some extent antiquated. Its language is more reminiscent of the Victorian era than our own.[53] In so far as questions of criminal responsibility are pertinent any reform of the law relating to transmission of disease must take account of the Law Commission's proposals for introducing a Criminal Code.[54] Four particular issues need to be addressed:

(1)

> "[N]o adult citizen of the United Kingdom is liable to be confined in any institution against his will, save by the authority of law."

The Master of the Rolls asserted that fundamental principle when construing the provisions of the Mental Health Act 1983 in *In re S-C (Mental Patient: Habeas Corpus)*.[55] Moreover he made it clear that in relation to the detention of the mentally ill, substantive justice must be done and be seen to be done. The state can justify violating the liberty and autonomy of the sick patient, but the process achieving that result must be fair and just. The health care practitioners cannot just "lock up" those perceived to be a danger or a nuisance.

---

[52] See, *supra* n. 14.

[53] For parallels with the USA, see again, L. Gostin, *infra* n. 61 at 105.

[54] Law Commission Report No. 177, *A Criminal Code for England and Wales* (H.M.S.O. 1989); Law Commission Report No. 218, *Legislating the Criminal Code: Offences Against the Person and General Principles* (Cmnd. 2370 H.M.S.O. 1993).

[55] [1996] 2 W.L.R. 146 at 148.

The provisions in sections 35 to 38 relating to medical examination of carriers and detention of sufferers grant extensive, and *ex parte*, powers to magistrates. Theoretically the safeguard of a "legal model" for compulsory intervention against a person's will is thus provided offering, some might contend, better protection than the "medical model" predominant in the Mental Health Act 1983. Realistically a "medical model" is likely to operate with magistrates relying heavily on certificates and evidence offered by doctors. The physically ill, "critically infectious individual", is offered less by way of due process to protect his/her interests than his/her mentally ill sister. The safeguards and procedure, built into the overtly "medical model" of the Mental Health Act 1983 are absent. No review process akin to that provided by Mental Health Review Tribunals exists. Of course, in the context of communicable disease time will be of the essence. There is little utility in a three day hearing in the course of which perhaps many others become infected. However, given the number of circuit judges now available across the jurisdiction, a more senior and experienced judge should be empowered to hear any application for intervention and provisions built into the legislation for review of initial emergency judgments.

(2) The classification of diseases as properly subjects of anticipatory action must be reviewed.[56] The principles we suggest above should govern the legitimacy of imposing any prior restraint on the liberty or autonomy of victims or carriers of disease. There must be evidence that the risk of transmission of disease is exceptionally high and that that disease impairs the individual's judgement and diminishes his responsibility and ability to safeguard others from the danger he presents to them.

(3) Those who endanger others by means of reckless conduct risking transmission of disease should be dealt with by the criminal law. Section 17 of the Public Health (Control of Diseases) Act 1984 already creates a limited offence of exposing others to infection but its remit is limited to notifiable diseases and exposure in public places. Neither limitation is rational. Violence in private is not (at least in principle) treated differently from violence in public nor should disease so be. The core of the wrong done by a person recklessly exposing another to disease is unrelated to the disease.

(4) Such general statements of principle are however much simpler to enunciate than to implement. Consideration needs to be given to whether criminal responsibility for transmission of disease should be embraced within the general criminal law or made the subject of a

[56] Our conclusion on classification of disease reflects those of L. Gostin, *infra* n. 61 reviewing analogous US legislation.

specific "public health" offence. The Law Commission in its proposals for wholesale reform of the criminal law in England barely touched on responsibility for transmitting disease. In a brief reference to disease, it is baldly stated that the proposed new offence of intentionally or recklessly causing injury to another is broad enough to include inflicting illness or disease on another.[57] That statement leaves several issues unresolved. Problems of proof of causation remain. The law can intervene only once the accused's reckless conduct has resulted in injury. Had Dr Gaud been discovered to be endangering patients earlier, his reckless conduct of itself would not be caught by an offence of causing injury. No threshold is set in terms of the nature of diseases triggering criminal liability.[58] The issue of consent is unaddressed. Inflicting more than transient injury remains a criminal offence in England regardless of consent.[59] Whatever the rights and wrongs of such policy in other contexts[60] disregarding consent in the context of sexually transmitted disease would be a nonsense. The wrong is not the transmission of disease *per se* but the violation of the other person's right to control over his/her own body and health.

Our personal preference remains in principle that reckless transmission of disease should be regarded as part and parcel of a wider wrong of recklessly endangering others' safety. We see no moral grounds to distinguish Dr Gaud from the drunken train driver or the employer who flouts health and safety law, in disregard of his workers' safety. Such an approach would meet part of the case against stigmatising disease. The seropositive person who conceals that he is HIV positive from several lovers with whom he engages in unprotected sex is not punished for being HIV positive, nor singled out for unfair treatment. He is punished for his conduct not for his health status. Disease should never result in unjust stigma, but nor, as long as it does not impair a person's mental capacity, should it confer special privileges immunising the individual from responsibility to others.

However we acknowledge that in the absence of support from the Law Commission for such a broad, general offence of "reckless endangerment", the best prospect for reform lies in urgent and radical amendment of the Public Health (Control of Diseases) Act 1984. That course has advantages to recommend it too. Reform of the Act must aim to ensure that a rational pattern of principles can be developed

[57] Law Commission Consultation Paper No. 122, at para. 8.17.

[58] Perhaps no threshold should be set? Passing on a cold may generally be of trivial import but could be fatal to an immunocompromised patient: see S. Bronitt, *supra* n. 32 at 28; and see J. Harris and S. Holm, *supra* n. 29.

[59] *R.* v. *Brown* [1993] 2 W.L.R. 556 (H.L.); see S. Bronitt, *supra* n. 32 at 30–2.

[60] On which see, Law Commission Consultation Paper No. 139, *Consent in the Criminal Law* (H.M.S.O. 1995).

governing both imposing prior restraints on liberty and autonomy and creating criminal responsibility for conduct placing others at risk of disease. It will require that legislators and policy-makers at last address how a modern society can reconcile the right and responsibilities of those who contract communicable diseases, and those who are at risk of so doing. It is an enterprise long overdue and needs to be embarked on, not as a panic response to a new epidemic, nor as a knee jerk response to HIV but in a calm, deliberate manner to anticipate the difficulties that the return of the "real" plagues may pose.

Public health laws in the United Kingdom have attracted little scholarly attention from "medical lawyers" as yet. In comparison with their counterparts in the United States of America, British public health officials have generally eschewed resort to the law. Writing from the USA Larry Gostin[61] invokes the provisions of the Americans with Disabilities Act[62] to argue forcefully for reform of public health law to eliminate unjust discrimination against persons suffering from communicable disease. Our conclusion that the criminal process does have a role to play in the control of communicable disease may at first sight diametrically opposed to Gostin's thesis, re-enforcing discrimination on grounds of disease status. The conflict is much more apparent than real, a matter of language not substance. Gostin acknowledges the right of the state to act to protect its citizens from disease. We endorse the right to be protected from unjust discrimination. What we seek to achieve are laws which strike the proper balance between rights and responsibilities in the context of communicable disease, and which offer all those whose rights are endangered either by violation of their liberty or by a threat to their health, an adequate legal process to protect such rights.

---

[61] See, "The Americans with Disabilities Act and the Corpus of Anti-Discrimination Law: A Force for Change in the Future of Public Health Regulation" in A. Grubb and M. J. Mehlman (eds.), *Justice and Health Care: Comparative Perspectives supra*, n. 8 at 105–46.

[62] The Disability Discrimination Act 1995 includes specifically within its provisions HIV (see s. 1(1) and Sched. 1(8)), although it is not at all clear whether any protection is offered to the seropositive individual who remains asymptomatic: see *ibid.*, Sched. I(4). Other communicable diseases will only even arguably fall within the Act where their effect results in a long term impairment of health (at least 12 months). More importantly even if a patient suffering from such a disease can claim the protection from discrimination afforded by the Act against, for example, employees or education providers, nothing in the Act affects or can affect the state's powers in the Public Health (Control of Diseases) Act 1984 and Regulations. Thus, unlike Gostin, (see, *supra* n. 61) we cannot (at least yet) use anti-discrimination law to prompt the Government into the review we seek in order to implement modern, realistic public health provisions.

Part III
Health Care Resources

Resource Allocation Theory

[13]

McGill Lecture in Jurisprudence and Public Policy

Justice in the Distribution of Health Care

Ronald Dworkin*

In this lecture, Professor Dworkin begins by identifying two questions about justice in the distribution of health care: (1) How much, in the aggregate, should society spend on health? (2) Once established, how should this amount be distributed?

He then examines the ancient *insulation* model of health care distribution, which postulates that health care is chief among all goods and that it is to be distributed in an equal way. He concludes that this model provides no satisfactory answer to either of the two questions. It cannot answer the first, for it would require that society spend all it could on health care until the next dollar would buy no gain in health or life expectancy, something which is manifestly absurd, particularly in our age of ever-expanding medical technology. Nor, he tells us, does the insulation model provide much guidance with the second question, since its egalitarian spirit ultimately leads us to apply notions of efficiency and need which are philosophically controversial and therefore impossible to apply.

By means of a thought experiment, Professor Dworkin then develops an alternative model which he feels does provide an answer to his two questions. He asks us to imagine a society with fair equality in the distribution of resources, in which the public at large has knowledge about the cost and value of medical procedures, but in which no one has any knowledge about the antecedent probability of contracting any particular disease. Moreover, health care is not provided by the government, but, rather, each individual is free to allocate to health care (by purchasing health insurance, for example) as much or as little of his resources as he wishes. Professor Dworkin claims that whatever that society spent on health care would be just — both in the aggregate and in its distribution. Carrying the model through, he discusses its implications for our own society and analyzes possible objections to it. He concludes by stressing the importance of the question of justice in health care and by putting it in its broader political context.

Dans cette conférence, le professeur Dworkin pose d'abord deux questions sur la justice dans la distribution des soins de santé : (1) Combien, en tout, la société doit-elle dépenser pour les soins de santé ? (2) Une fois ce montant établi, comment doit-il être distribué ?

Il examine ensuite l'ancien modèle d'*isolation* des soins de santé. Selon ce modèle, la santé est le plus grand bien qui soit et la distribution des soins de santé doit se faire de façon égale. D'après le professeur Dworkin, ni l'une ni l'autre des deux questions n'est résolue de façon satisfaisante par ce modèle. Le modèle ne répond pas à la première, car il exigerait que la société consacre toutes ses ressources à la santé jusqu'à ce qu'une dépense supplémentaire ne puisse apporter aucune amélioration de la santé ou de l'espérance de vie, conclusion manifestement absurde, surtout dans une société comme la nôtre où la technologie progresse sans cesse. Le modèle d'isolation ne répond pas non plus à la deuxième question, car son approche égalitaire exigerait qu'on tienne compte de facteurs comme l'efficacité et le besoin, lequels sont très controversés et se prêtent donc mal à une application rigoureuse.

Dans le but d'élaborer un modèle qui nous permette de répondre à ses deux questions, le professeur Dworkin nous invite à envisager une situation hypothétique : une société imaginaire où il y a une distribution équitable des ressources, où le public possède des connaissances médicales sur le coût et la valeur des différents traitements possibles, mais où personne ne peut prévoir les chances de contracter telle ou telle maladie. De plus, ce n'est pas le gouvernement qui finance les soins de santé, mais plutôt l'individu, qui est libre de consacrer son argent aux soins de santé (en prenant une assurance, par exemple) comme bon lui semble. Selon le professeur Dworkin, le montant que cette société dépenserait pour les soins de santé serait juste — et dans sa totalité et dans sa distribution. Poussant plus loin son modèle, il en tire des conclusions pour notre société et examine les objections qu'il pourrait susciter. Il termine sa conférence en insistant sur l'importance de la question de la justice en matière de soins de santé et en la situant dans son contexte politique.

* Professor of Jurisprudence, Oxford University; Professor of Law, New York University School of Law.

Professor Dworkin delivered this lecture on March 17, 1993 at the Faculty of Law, McGill University, as the Inaugural Lecture of the McGill Lectures in Jurisprudence and Public Policy.

To be cited as: (1993) 38 McGill L.J. 883
Mode de référence : (1993) 38 R.D. McGill 883

1.

You might think it very odd that, living as I do half the year in Britain and half in the United States, I've come to Canada to talk about justice in the distribution of medical care. In both those countries, the Canadian structure for the distribution of health care is taken by many people to be a model of success. Your Dean mentioned my former colleague at University College, Oxford, who is now my President. Under his administration, and under the supervision of his wife, the United States is now, as you know, engaged in a massive re-examination of health care. Almost every day an article appears in the American press about the Canadian plan, which is widely proposed as a model for Americans to follow. Nevertheless, strains on your system of health care are beginning to become evident. There's talk of rationing, and more people go south of the border to seek medical care. Doctors in negotiation with the provincial authorities claim with greater stridency that they are seriously underpaid. The system, nevertheless, is producing more Canadian doctors than economists think wise. You, too, will face the problems I'll discuss this evening. You too must worry about justice in the distribution of health care when it comes — and I'm sure it will come — to rationing health care explicitly.

Some people, particularly in America now, say there is really no need to ration health care. They agree that medical expense already constitutes an alarming proportion of the American economy, and that, even though America spends that much in the aggregate, forty million Americans are wholly uninsured or without any adequate health care, which is intolerable. But they deny that correcting these deficiencies will require some form of rationing: they say that there is so much waste and inefficiency in the health care system that, if these were eliminated, we could save enough money to insure that everyone had all the medical treatment he needed. We know what they mean. The administrative inefficiency of United States medical insurance companies and carriers is legendary. American doctors' salaries are large and, according to many people, inflated. The average medical salary two years ago in the United States was over $160,000 — the *average*. Nevertheless, a series of recent studies suggests that even if administrative efficiency were greatly improved, and even if doctors' salaries were capped at some reasonable level, rationing of health care would still be inevitable, because by far the biggest cause of the explosion in health care costs (not only in the United States, but, I believe, in Canada as well) is a massive supply of new technology. It isn't that we're paying all that much more for what we formerly bought cheaper; it is that we now have so much more to buy.

Many politicians and some doctors say that much of the new, expensive technology is "unnecessary" or "wasteful" or "inappropriate." But if you look to see what they mean, you find they have in mind techniques that are (as it's often put) "low yield," which is not the same as "no yield." They point, for example, to massive mammography screening of women under the age of fifty, or to the heavy use, in some medical facilities, of magnetic resonance imaging. A society that spends a great deal of money on routine screening or expensive diagnostic equipment may not save *many* more lives than a society that does not. But it will presumably save *some* more lives, and that means that we cannot appeal just to efficiency as an abstract value to justify saving the cost. We cannot recommend eliminating "inappropriate" medical care without deciding what medical care is appropriate, and why, and that, in turn, depends upon how we answer the question: "how much medicine *should* a society provide?"

That question can usefully be divided into two more specific ones. The first is the question of a community's *aggregate* health care budget. Money spent on health care (I include not just acute care but also preventative medicine, care of the chronically sick or disabled, and so forth) is money that might be spent on education, or on economic infrastructure that will produce more jobs. How much of the overall budget should be devoted to health care instead of other plainly valuable projects, like these? The second question, though it's really part of the first, is the question of distribution. Once it's established what a society should spend overall on health care, then it must also be decided who should have that care, and on what basis it should be allocated. Of course, nations struggling with health care costs must resolve many issues beyond these twin questions of justice. There are economic questions — what are reliable predictors of how much a particular health care plan or structure will cost? There are administrative issues: what is the most efficient organization for administering any particular plan? There are medical questions: what is the likely impact of a particular program on morbidity and mortality? Above all, there is the political problem: what plans will a particular democracy in fact be willing to accept and pay for? I don't mean to denigrate the importance of these various problems, or to deny their evident connections with the problems of justice. But I shall concentrate on the latter. To repeat: In all justice, how much should a decent society spend on medical care, broadly described? In all justice, how should that society distribute what it does spend — who should get what? Behind these two questions lies a more explicitly philosophical one. What is the right standard to use in answering these questions? What should we take as our ideal of justice in medical care?

2.

I begin by describing an ancient and attractive ideal that many people instinctively accept, which I shall call the ideal of *insulation*. It has three features. The first argues that health care is, as René Descartes put it, chief among all goods: that the most important thing is life and health and everything else is of minor importance beside it. The second component of the insulation ideal is equality. The ideal supposes that even in a society which is otherwise very inegalitarian — indeed even in a society in which equality is despised as a general political goal — medical care should nevertheless be distributed in an egalitarian way so that no one is denied care he needs simply because of an inability to pay. The third component (it really flows from the other two) is the old principle of rescue, which holds that it is intolerable when people die, though their lives could have been saved, because the necessary resources were withheld on grounds of economy.

This ideal of insulation has exerted great power throughout history. Hospitals have always been paradigm examples of appropriate charities, and religion has, from ancient days, always been associated with them. Contemporary political philosophers — I have Michael Walzer in mind, for example — say that the provision of medicine constitutes a separate sphere of justice, and that in that sphere decency, community, solidarity, and equality must reign. The power of the insulation ideal is so great that people often think that though the administrative, medical, economic and political problems I described are intellectually daunting, the questions of justice are not: that it is clear what the ideal of justice demands in health care, and that our only problem is that we are unwilling to live up to that ideal. That is, I believe, a serious mistake. The crisis in health care includes a crisis in our conception of what a just health care system would be — what answers we should give to the questions of justice I set out. We face that intellectual crisis because it has become clear that the insulation ideal, for all its ancient popularity, is now irrelevant. Consider the first question I posed: the problem of the aggregate expense a decent society will commit to health care, as against competing needs and values. What advice does the ideal of insulation give? It says a society should spend all it can on health care until the next dollar it spends would buy no gain in health or life expectancy at all. Of course no society ever did organize its affairs in that way, any more than any sane individual organizes a plan of life with the goal of making that life as long and as healthy as possible. In past centuries, however, there was not so significant a gap between the rhetoric of the insulation ideal and what it was medically possible for a community to do. It was possible to give lip service to the ideal, and charge social failure to live up to it to collective moral shortfall. But now — when technology continues to produce more and more ways to spend great sums on medical care — it is self-evidently preposterous that a community should treat health as lexicographically prior to all other values. Any community that really tried to do so would secure for its citizens marginally longer lives, perhaps, but these would be lives barely worth living. Once, however, this suggestion of the ancient ideal is rejected as incredible, the ideal has nothing more to say. It has, as it were, no second best or fall-back level of advice. It simply falls silent.

In fact, as a result, philosophers, theorists and medical specialists who nominally subscribe to the ideal of insulation all despair of attacking the first question. After some discussion, they announce that the size of the overall medical budget will be "decided in politics," which is an academic way of saying that abstract considerations of justice have nothing much to contribute to this part of the health-care discussion. I believe that that is a mistake; if I am right, then the dominance of the insulation ideal has been a hindrance, and not just not a positive contribution, to achieving justice in health care.

Now look at the second question, the question of distribution. When the theorists finish saying that politics will set the overall health-care budget, they quickly add that justice will require that that budget, whatever it is, be spent in a fair way. But how does the insulation ideal help us to define a fair distribution? It tells us something negative and undoubtedly important: that how someone is medically treated should not depend, in our society, simply on ability to pay. It tells us that if rationing is necessary, the principle of rationing should not be, as it now largely is in the United States, the pocket book. But we need more positive advice. What should the principle of rationing be, if it is *not* to be money? Once again, the ancient ideal has very little to say. The egalitarian impulse of the ideal seems to recommend that medical care be distributed according to some principle of efficacy and need. And so people committed to the ideal speak about rationing according to cost-effectiveness or according to some principle that requires money to be spent where it will do the most good.

As many of you know, the state of Oregon established a commission some time ago to try to give structure to that idea, to try to describe what rationing health care in accordance with effectiveness would mean. The difficulty, of course, as that commission discovered, is that the concept of doing the "most good" (or, in more academic terms, of maximizing welfare, or utility, or well-being, or happiness, or capability) is systematically and multiply ambiguous. These various terms, when properly used, do not name psychological concepts. Or medical or, in my view, economic ones. They name contested ethical concepts: the proposal that health care money should be spent to do the most good means that it should be distributed in whatever way will make the lives of citizens better lives to have lived, and that goal cannot be restated, without controversy, as the goal of making lives more pleasant, or economically more productive, or socially more beneficial. Whenever you attempt to describe in more detail what making the lives of citizens better actually means, you enter the kind of controversy that it was the promise and hope of the insulated ideal to avoid, and it would be sheer disaster to try to reduce that ideal to something mechanical enough to be measured by a computer. The Oregon commission discovered this. It developed mechanical measures of the cost-effectiveness of various sets of treatment matched to various kinds of disease, typed these metrics into a computer, typed in a great deal of further information, and watched the computer produce a ranking of cost-effectiveness that ranked capping a tooth higher in social priority than appendectomy. It's perfectly true, the computer said, that you will die if you have appendicitis and don't have your appendix removed. But it costs four or five thousand dollars to do that and dentists can cap a great many teeth and prevent a massive amount of toothache if you spend that five thousand dollars on dentistry instead. Well, of course, as soon as that result appeared, the commission saw that its algorithms were hopeless, re-rigged its operational definitions, and produced something at least less implausible than that. But the story indicates the character of the problem I have in mind.

So the old ideal of insulation fails to answer our second question as well as our first. Its proposal, that health care should be distributed according to need, or so as to do the most good, or so as to improve overall welfare, is fatally ambiguous, and becomes evidently unattractive when the ambiguity is resolved by defining success in terms of some utilitarian reading. We have not, after all, settled the question of what justice in health care means, and that philosophical problem stands beside the economic, medical and administrative problems we know we face, and it may be at least equally daunting.

3.

This evening I shall try to construct, at least in very broad outline, an alternate approach to justice in health care, which is based not on the insulation of health care as a separate sphere of justice or activity, but, on the contrary, on the *integration* of health care into competition with other goods. I shall describe an approach that, I believe, is more instructive about the two great issues of justice I named. I can state the central idea in advance: we should aim to make collective, social decisions about the quantity and distribution of health care so as to match, as closely as possible, the decisions that people in the community would make for themselves, one by one, in the appropriate circumstances, if they were looking from youth down the course of their lives and trying to decide what risks were worth running in return for not running other kinds of risks.

At some point (as those of you who have read any political philosophy written after the middle ages know) an imaginary story gets told. My story has the virtue of being less imaginary than some others, but it will nevertheless require you to exercise your imagination. Suppose that your community were to develop and change in the following three ways.

First, *per impossibile*, suppose it developed into a society in which the economic system provided "fair equality" in the distribution of resources. I mean that government recognized its inevitable responsibility to choose amongst economic and tax structures, and chose a structure that treated all members of the society with equal concern. I have my own idea about what that means in practice, and I've tried to spell this out in a series of articles.[1] I said (this is a very crude summary) that an economic structure treats all members of the community with equal concern when it divides resources equally, measured by the opportunity costs of each person owning a particular resource, and then leaves each member free in principle to spend those resources designing a life that each believes appropriate. That conception of equality will not make people equal in the amount of money or goods each has at any particular time; still less will it mean that everyone will lead the same kind of life. Some people will have invested and some people will have consumed. Some will have spent early and some will have saved for late. The result will nevertheless be egalitarian, because the choices people will have made will answer to their own conceptions of what life is right for them.

These are my views about what a just economic system would be like, but I offer it only by way of illustration. You may — you probably do — have a different conception of what economic structures genuinely treat all people with equal concern; if so, your view of how that community would have changed, in order to meet my first condition, will be different from mine. That does not matter for the present exercise: I merely ask you to assume that it has changed, in whatever way you think justice and equal concern require.

Second, imagine that your community is also different in that all the information that might be called, roughly, state-of-the-art knowledge about the value

[1]The central article, for purposes of this lecture, is *What is Equality? Part II*, which appeared in Philosophy and Public Affairs, Fall 1981.

and cost and side-effects of particular medical procedures — everything, in other words, that very good doctors know — is known generally by the public at large as well.

Third, imagine that no one in your community — including insurance companies — has any information available about the *antecedent* probability of any particular person contracting any particular disease or infirmity that he or she does not evidently already have. No one would be in a position to say, of himself or anyone else, that that person is more or less likely to contract sickle-cell anemia, or diabetes, or to be the victim of violence in the street, than any other person. So no information exists about how likely it is that young blacks, as distinguished from people generally, will die in violent fights, for example.[2]

The changes I am asking you to imagine in your community are heroic. But they are not, I think, beyond the reach of imagining, and I am not inviting you to imagine other changes. Indeed, I am asking you not to: I want you to assume that your preferences and ethical convictions, and those of other members of your community, have remained constant in spite of these changes. Very well. Suppose that your community is indeed changed in those three ways, and then also suppose that health care is simply left to individual market decisions — in as free a market as we can imagine. Medical treatment is not provided by the government for anyone, as it is for everyone here and for some people in America. Nor are there any government subsidies for health care — in particular, the premiums people pay for health care insurance are not, as they are now in the United States, tax-deductible. If people choose to purchase such insurance, they do so as they buy anything else: out of post-tax funds.

What kind of health care arrangements would develop in such a community? How much of its aggregate resources would end up devoted to health care? How would medical treatment in fact be distributed among its members? Well, of course, it is hard to say; indeed it is impossible to say with any precision, though I shall offer you some speculations in a moment. But I'm anxious to make two claims in advance of any such speculation, to show you why the question of what such a society would do is important. The first is that *whatever* the society I've just described spends as its total health-care budget, which means simply the aggregate of what individuals spend, would be the just and appropriate expense for that society. The second is that *however* health care is distributed in that society would be a just distribution of health care for that society. I must qualify those two dramatic claims to some degree, but the qualifications I need are not major, and I'll relegate them to a footnote.[3] So I shall

[2]I am ignoring an important issue that I will have to consider in a subsequent full presentation of this material. Is it right, in the hypothetical exercise I am constructing, to exclude information relating risk of disease to voluntarily chosen behaviour? Should insurance companies be in a position to charge cigarette smokers or mountain climbers higher premiums, for example? If so, then what counts as voluntary behaviour? Should sexual behaviour of a particular kind be treated as voluntary for this purpose? Should insurance companies be able to charge active male homosexuals higher premiums because they are more likely to contract Aids?

[3]Some paternalistic interference with individual decisions about health care insurance, particularly those people make early in their lives, might be necessary out of fairness to people who might

proceed on the flat assumptions just stated: nothing that society does, by way of health care arrangements, is open to objection on grounds of justice, though of course what it does might be questionable or objectionable in many other ways.

If so, then it is indeed important to consider what health care arrangements our society would make if it were changed in the ways I described, because, as I shall argue, what they would do through independent decisions can serve as a guide to what we should do, in whatever way we can, to improve justice in our own circumstances. So speculation seems worthwhile. It seems likely that even though the members of the imagined community — our community transformed — would perhaps begin by making individual insurance decisions, they would soon develop, through these individual decisions, collective institutions and arrangements; it also seems likely that progressively more and more people would join those collective arrangements. They would develop very large cooperative insurance plans, or very large health maintenance organizations which provide stipulated categories of medical care for a stipulated advance contract price, or both, for example. As such plans became larger, and more efficient, it would become progressively more and more expensive, relatively, for people to make wholly personalized, individual medical arrangements for themselves, and progressively fewer and fewer people would do so. (Remember that in this society wealth is much more equally distributed than it is in our society now, and though some people are relatively rich there, they are mainly people who have decided to concentrate on saving.) So the number of people who could and would turn their back on the economies of scale and administration of the collective provisions will be few, and, as the process continues, fewer still. The result of the process might very well be something functionally very close to the single, comprehensive health care provision scheme that you have reached here in Canada. Large insurance cooperatives or health maintenance organizations might negotiate a basic scheme of provision that would be much the same for everyone. If so, however, the community would probably also develop a secondary insurance market: people would be free to negotiate specialized insurance in *addition* to that basic insurance package. What form that secondary market would take, and how large a market it would be, would, of course, depend on factors we cannot sensibly predict. But even in a much more egalitarian society, some people would be able and willing to make provision for queue-jumping, or elective cosmetic surgery, or other benefits that the basic provision made available through general collective schemes would not provide. (In a more egalitarian society, the cost of some of these special benefits might well be lower than it is now — since doctors' salaries, for example, would presumably be lower, specialized services might be available at lower cost.)

We need not dwell on the character of that secondary market: it is more important to consider the basic, standardized coverage packages which I'm assuming that the large cooperative institutions would provide. What would be the character of those packages? Well, of course, that would depend upon the

make imprudent insurance decisions when young. And some constraints and requirements might be necessary in the interests of justice toward later generations.

mix of preferences and convictions. But we can speculate with some confidence about what would *not* be covered in such a plan. Some private insurance decisions would be plainly irrational in the imagined community: they would be what the economists might call *dominant* mistakes, by which I mean they would be mistakes, even in retrospect, no matter what happened in the future, including the worst. I'll give you one or two examples: they are extreme, but of course they would be, given the claim I've just made about them.

Almost no one would purchase insurance that would provide life-sustaining equipment once he had fallen into a persistent vegetative state, for example. That would be a dominant mistake: the substantial sum spent year-by-year in insurance premiums to provide that coverage would be at the expense of training or experience or culture or investment or jobs that would have enhanced real life. Even someone who lived only a few months after purchasing the insurance before he fell into a vegetative state would have made, in retrospect, a mistake, giving up resources that could have made his short remaining conscious life better to buy a longer unconsciousness. My second suggestion might seem more controversial. I suggest that almost no one would purchase insurance providing for expensive medical intervention, even of a life-saving character, after he entered the late stages of Alzheimer's disease or other forms of irreversible dementia. Almost everyone would regard that decision, too, as a dominant mistake, because the money spent on premiums for such insurance would have been better spent, no matter what happens, making life before dementia — life in earnest — more worth while.

Now I come to a further suggestion, more controversial still. In most developed countries, a major fraction of medical expense — in the United States it approaches forty percent of the health care budget — is spent on people in the last six months of their lives. Of course, doctors don't always know whether a particular patient will die within a few months no matter how much is spent on his care. But in many cases, sadly, they can say, with considerable confidence, that he will. I believe that if people reflected on the value of buying insurance that would keep them alive, by heroic medical intervention, four or five more months, in the condition in which most such patients undergoing that intervention live, compared with the value the premiums necessary to purchase that insurance could add to their earlier lives if spent in other ways, they would decide that buying that kind of insurance was not a wise investment. That is not to say, of course, that most people would not want those additional months, no matter in what state or condition they spent them. Many people want to remain alive as long as possible, provided they remain conscious and alert, and provided the pain is not too great. My point is rather that they would not want those additional months at the cost of the sacrifices in their earlier, vigorous life that would be necessary if they had to make that choice. They would think the money better spent, earlier, on job-training or education or investment or on something else that would benefit their lives as a whole more than just taking on a few months of very limited life at the end. I cannot quite make the claim here that I made about persistent vegetative state or advanced-stage Alzheimer's disease: that purchasing insurance for costly procedures extending life a few months would be a dominant mistake. We can imagine circumstances — someone falls fatally ill the day after buying a policy providing for such care — in which, in retrospect, the decision to buy it turned out to be a good one. But most people would agree, I think, that in the circumstances we are imagining — in which, remember, no one knows he is more likely than anyone else to contract a disease not already evident — that decision would be an *antecedent* mistake.

How much further can we go down this road? How much more insurance can we be reasonably confident people would not buy in the circumstances we are imagining? I'm not sure, and anyway have no time to explore other examples now. But I do want to raise, at least, one further issue which, as I suggested to you earlier, is already of crucial importance and will become even more critical in the next decades. How far would people in the imagined community make provision for access to the ultra-expensive medical equipment now in use, or which is being developed, or is still over the horizon?

I came here from attending a meeting at the Harvard Medical School in which new advances in technology were being described. You ain't seen nothin' yet. I've already mentioned advances in diagnostic radiology: expensive magnetic resonance imaging, for example. Much of the talk at this meeting was about molecular biology: about, for example, promising research into treating cancer by creating monoclonal antibodies specific for each patient, from the patient's own genetic material, at stupendous cost, and new, very expensive, blood tests that marginally — very marginally — improve the accuracy of a diagnosis of heart disease. Each of these examples illustrates, though in different ways, how technology might come to be regarded as "low yield" relative to its large cost. Both would undoubtedly save some lives. But at a cost, in development and production, that might seem very high when we consider how a community might use the funds in other ways that would enhance the economy and provide more jobs and a higher standard of living for more people.

Would people in the imagined society, ultimately deciding for themselves how to allocate their resources, provide for expensive and/or speculative technology? People informed and reflective might make distinctions along the following lines. They might pay to provide life-saving techniques for diseases that tend to occur relatively early in life, particularly when these techniques have a high probability of success. But they might not spend to insure for technology that is very speculative, even though it will save some lives, or for technology whose main results benefit people in relatively old age. Paying all our lives to secure the latter kind of technology, if we need it, might seem a poor decision when it means that we run a higher risk than we need to run of unemployment or an otherwise less satisfactory life. I won't pursue these speculations further. I hope I've given you some idea of the kind of choices that people in the conditions we're imagining would have to make, and of how they might be tempted to make them.

4.

Do you resist my claim that whatever such a society spent, through collective institutions governed by individual decisions of this character, would be just, and that the distribution of health care such a society achieved would also be just? You will not, if you accept a conception of social justice that assigns individuals responsibility for making the ethical choices for their own lives against a background of competent information and a fair initial distribution of resources. If you accept that vision of a just society, then you will accept my claim — though, as I said, you may well have a different conception of what a fair initial distribution of resources would be like, and how unjustified inequalities should be remedied, than I do — in which case your understanding of the conditions I described will be correspondingly different from mine.

So I will assume that you do agree with my main claim: that whatever our imagined society achieves, by way of health care arrangements, cannot be faulted on grounds of justice. I suggested, earlier, that we might therefore make practical, political use, for our own communities, of at least our less speculative conclusions about what people in the imaginary community would provide for themselves. There is a natural way in which we might be tempted to do this. Almost all government-sponsored or supervised health schemes now in existence, and almost all of those that have been proposed as vehicles of reform in the United States, define a basic health-care package of benefits that must be made available, at responsible cost, to everyone, and supplied without charge to those who cannot pay that responsible cost themselves. We might use our speculations about the imaginary society to help us to define what should be in that basic package, and what that responsible cost should be.

In one way, at least, the imaginary story might be helpful for countries, like the United States, who have not settled on a particular structure for health care reform. As I said, many people in America believe we should follow your example in constructing a single-payer arrangement in which government, not private insurance firms or health care providers, decides what medicine to offer and at what price. But others think the United States should adopt what is called a scheme of "managed competition," in which private insurers compete to offer a basic package stipulated by government, and government supervises their performances and premium structures. As of this evening, at least, most commentators predict that a managed competition scheme will be adopted, primarily, they say, because it is better suited to the political culture of the United States than a single-payer scheme would be. But our imaginary story might be helpful in guiding the choice between the two forms of scheme, in the following way. The decision might turn, among other things including suitability to the political culture, on the degree of confidence we have in our speculations about what people would choose in the imaginary community. If we were reasonably confident that we knew roughly what such people would buy — what the dominant collective arrangements they would reach would provide — then that would argue for trying to set in place a single-payer system like yours or like the National Health Service in Britain. Government can more effectively guarantee people what it is persuaded justice demands that they have if it is free to provide it itself, in some such way. To the degree we are uncertain about what people in the imaginary world would decide, however, that argues for a scheme of managed competition with enough flexibility to allow different people to choose different packages all meeting a common stipulated standard. The choices that actual people make among such schemes would provide a self-regulating mechanism that would bring us closer to the just distribution of the imagined world.

But of course whether the United States ultimately chooses a single-payer scheme like yours or, as seems more likely, a scheme that includes private competition, is more likely to depend on considerations other than justice. Nor, I think, is justice decisive of that issue one way or the other. Both types of scheme include the idea of a basic package (or set of such packages) of insurance made available to all, and the main issues of justice consolidate in the question of what should be in that basic package or set of packages. That is the question, as I suggested, that is most directly responsive to the exercise I've been imagining. I offered you reasons for thinking that certain kinds of insurance or health organization contractual provision would be rare in the community we imagined, and that, I now submit, is a good reason why that kind of provision should *not* be part of the basic package that will be the heart of any reform in the United States and any readjustments here in Canada. Since those are expensive provisions, this is an important result. But it is a negative one, and the exercise must be conducted on the other side as well. I have little doubt that people in the imagined community would insist on provision for standard prenatal care, for example, and on the kinds of primary medical care, including relatively inexpensive routine examinations and inoculations that poor people in the United States so conspicuously lack. It follows, from the argument I have been making, that these are essential elements in the basic package that any responsible health care reform would establish.

5.

I have been exploring ways in which practical health care administration and reform could be guided by the exercise I hold out: trying to imagine what health care people in the imaginary circumstances I described would provide, out of their own pockets, for themselves. It is past time, however, for me to consider the drawbacks and pitfalls of my overall argument. One danger is evident: my suggestions about how people would behave in the imaginary society are speculative, and even though some of these speculations seem very plausible, we cannot test them by asking how everyone actually behaves in communities as they are now constituted. Resources are unjustly distributed among us: Canada is not as bad in this respect as is the United States, but even Canada is very far from ideal justice in economic distribution. We obviously don't have a society in which people enjoy state-of-the-art information about medicine. On the contrary, people's medical ignorance is often cited as one reason why medical expenses continue to rise. And, of course, our insurance companies do know that risks are higher among certain groups within the community than others, and the curse of experiential rather than community rating for premiums has dogged attempts to make commercial medical insurance fair.

But it doesn't follow that our speculation about what people would want under very different, and fairer, circumstances must remain just speculation. The choices Americans of average income make about their employee insurance package in wage negotiations, for example, can offer some guidance. And research and publicity can provide better guidance. Not only government but private organizations — large medical schools, for example — could help design a few sample paradigm insurance protocols representing different insurance strategies. Some of these would provide for catastrophic care or transplant surgery in circumstances in which others denied it, for example. The protocols could be accompanied by the medical information of the kind that is crucially missing from public awareness now: by some realistic expert opinion of the expected consequences for mortality and morbidity from a public commitment to each protocol, together with, for each, some estimate of its total cost and consequent macro-economic effect. If information of that sort were put into the public domain, and challenged and debated there, the resulting discussion would be at least minimally informative about how much people value what kind of care, and might be very informative. When we think of the kind of opinions that pollsters examine now, and that feature on television discussion shows and radio phone-ins, we might welcome a shift to the kind of discussion I'm now imagining.

A second difficulty is potentially much graver, however, at least conceptually. I've imagined a utopian (in some respects) society and I've then suggested that we set out to copy one feature of that utopian society: the provision it would make for medical care. An economist will remind me that, when the first best is impossible, the second best is not always achieved by mimicking the first best *partially*. That may, indeed, make matters worse than the *status quo*, and it is not difficult to see this possibility as a threat to my argument. Suppose, for example, that we decide that if our community were just, and different in the other ways I imagined, the standard medical package nearly everyone would purchase through collective insurance arrangements would include a particular set of benefits. If we decide, therefore, that that set of benefits should make up the basic package that must be made available to everyone in our own community, some relatively low-income people may end up paying a higher share of their actual income for medical care (for themselves and, through taxes, for others) than they would have chosen to pay in a just society. Or, to put the matter the other way around, they may have less left over for other expenses than they would have chosen in those circumstances. That may not seem, particularly to them, an improvement in justice.

I do not want to minimize the problem this hypothetical example illustrates. But the possibility that the test of justice I propose *might* produce unjust results is not, in itself, a sufficient argument against accepting that test; someone who objects must show a strong likelihood that the result would in *fact* be worse, from the point of view of justice, than using some other defensible standard for designing the basic package of protection. This is not a question of who has the burden of proof. If it is true that if our economic structure were just, everyone would be able to and nearly everyone would purchase a particular medical provision, that supplies a very strong even if not decisive argument that our structure would be closer to a just one if we made sure that everyone had that provision now. We should act on that strong argument unless we have some positive reason, not just the bare possibility, that it is mistaken.

It is true, however, as the example I just gave demonstrates, that the new model of health care provision and distribution I am proposing will work more dependably as the community's tax system grows more just. If relatively low-paid workers pay much more than their fair share of taxes, because the tax structure is insufficiently progressive to be fair, then any governmental program that relies on the redistribution of tax proceeds to improve justice for those with scarcely any income at all will be compromised for that reason. It will involve an unjustified transfer to the worst-off group from the almost-worst-off-group. That reflection provides a strong reason why tax reform must be at the centre of any general campaign to improve social justice. It would be ironic and disappointing, however, if the point were stood on its head, and if those who resisted redistribution to the very poor were able to point to imperfections in the tax structure as justification for doing nothing, and retaining their own privileges under the *status quo*.

We must next consider a very different kind of issue, which I must not evade, though my views on that issue, I fear, will disappoint many of you. Suppose that everything I've been describing as possible came to pass. Suppose that, after the right kinds of collective consultation, after meetings and discussions and polls and electronic politics and all the rest, we settled on a particular basic program of medical care that we collectively thought government should, in one way or another, make available to everyone. That basic package, as my earlier argument suggests, will not include some treatment that rich people are now in a position to buy for themselves. I said earlier, for example, that the test I proposed would very likely rule out ultra-expensive marginal diagnostics or extraordinarily costly treatments that have some but very little prospects for success. Some people in Canada and America now have the money to buy health care that would be excluded from the basic package. They have the money to buy a liver transplant when the odds are very small but nevertheless real that the procedure would save their lives. In England, people are standardly denied even renal dialysis on the National Health Service when they are sixty-five. So people of that age die if they cannot afford to pay for dialysis themselves.

If we adopted the kind of scheme that I'm describing, in our admittedly imperfect society, and took no steps to forbid people buying more expensive care than the basic package provides, some people would have better medical care — some people would live longer and healthier lives — only because they had more money. In most cases, since the basic economic structure would continue to be unjust, because they unjustly had more money. Should we therefore take steps to prohibit or constrain the private market in medicine? Should that be part of any respectable campaign to improve justice in health care? Of course, we couldn't actually abolish the private market in health care altogether: we would end by producing back street dialysis. But should we do what we can, aiming to prevent anyone from buying better medical care than the basic package provides, so far as that is possible?

The insulation model of medical justice I began by describing, if taken seriously, would insist that we should, and I believe many people here this evening would agree. Solidarity is compromised, they think, when some people can live while others die only because the former have more money. That seems to me the wrong answer, however. The spirit of the argument I have been making suggests that no one can complain *on grounds of justice* that he has less of something that someone else does, so long as he has all he would have if society were overall just. And, of course, in the circumstances we are now considering, people whose basic provision does not include liver transplants, and cannot afford to buy such an operation for themselves, are by hypothesis not denied what they would have if economic justice were perfect.

Some of you will hate that argument, as I said: you will think it intolerable. May I remind you, however, that the hypothetical inequality in medical care I'm now considering is, in one important respect, relatively benign compared to other inequalities in our society. If health care were rationed in the way we are contemplating, then everyone would have at least the medical care he would have in a just society, and that would not be true in most other departments of resource allocation. In education, employment, culture, recreation, travel, experience and a host of other goods and opportunities that for most of us make up the value of being alive, the poor would continue to have much less than they would if we had reformed not just health care but our economic and social life more generally. If we somehow manage to succeed in providing the poor with the medical care that justice requires, it would be perverse, given that a rich man can spend on more comfortable housing or better education for his children, not to allow him to spend on more expensive health care. We would do better to put an excise tax on special health care, and use the proceeds of that excise tax to improve public education, or the economic infrastructure, or to reduce public debt that blights employment prospects, or in some other ways that would make the community distinctly more egalitarian.

6.

I will offer you no final summary of my somewhat discursive remarks; I shall try, instead, to broaden the argument in closing it. I began by criticizing the insulation model, as I called it, and you may think I've been undermining that criticism in the last part of the lecture. I've been arguing how we might make our communities better in just one respect, and that goal seems to assume, with the insulation model, that health care is special, "chief" among goods. But my special interest in medical care is largely practical. Medicine is now a problem for people so high up in the economic scale — well up into the middle, fat part of the economic diamond where the votes are. People generally, not just the poor, agree that government should take a larger role in structuring, controlling and financing the provision of health care. We can seize on this opportunity to make the distribution of health care more just as well as more efficient.

But if America does make new progress in that direction, as Canada already has, then the lesson might be of more general political importance. For one thing, it might teach us that the bad press the ideal of equality has had for some time is unjustified. There is a rap against equality: that accepting equality as an ideal, even one among others, means levelling down and requiring everyone to live the same kind of life. But the conception of equality I've been relying on has quite the opposite character: it is dynamic and sensitive to people's differing convictions about how to live.

I end with this further observation: the question of health-care reform in America, including politically acceptable and fair health-care rationing, is ideologically leveraged. If we find, after all the fuss, that politically we can't do much to make the distribution of medical care more just, in spite of the apparent present opportunities to do so, then a pessimistic conclusion may be irresistible: we may abandon hope for any more widespread or general democratic concern for social justice. But if we do now make substantial and recognizable political progress in this one urgent matter, we may learn more, from the experience, about what justice itself is like, and we might find it to our taste, so that we can steadily, bit by bit, incrementally, fight the same battle in other areas. So the war against injustice in medicine that you have been fighting so well here, and that we are about to take on in America, is indeed a crucial one. Health might not be more important than anything else — but the fight for justice in health might well be.

[14]

Symbols, Rationality, and Justice: Rationing Health Care

Daniel Callahan*

Proposals to ration health care in the United States meet a number of objections, symbolic and literal. Nonetheless, an acceptance of the idea of rationing is a necessary first step toward universal health insurance. It must be understood that universal health care requires an acceptance of rationing, and that such an acceptance must precede enactment of a program, if it is to be economically sound and politically feasible. Commentators have argued that reform of the health care system should come before any effort to ration. On the contrary, rationing and reform cannot be separated. The former is the key to the latter, just as rationing is the key to universal health insurance.

One of the most important domestic tasks before the United States is to put in place a just and universal health care plan. Most people seem to believe, however, that such a plan would obviate the need for rationing health care, indeed that it is an alternative to rationing. This Article argues that universal health care is neither feasible nor plausible without health care rationing. This contention is based not on some theory of just health care but on the experience of other countries that have some form of universal health insurance already in place. Each provides a decent level of health care. None provide all the health care that people might want, nor necessarily provide it in the way in which they would most like to have it.[1]

Why do these countries set such limits? Because early on they came to recognize what might be called the economic iron law of universal health care plans: to be affordable they must be limited. If you want universal coverage, then be prepared to ration. If you are not prepared to ration, abandon all hopes of an affordable plan of universal coverage. To these general propositions, good for all countries and

* Director and Co-founder, The Hastings Center, Briarcliff Manor, New York; Ph.D., 1965, Harvard University.

[1] *See* Mark Pauly et al., *A Plan for "Responsible National Health Insurance"*, HEALTH AFF., Spring 1991, at 5, 20-21 (comparing experiences of the United States, the United Kingdom and Canada).

times, must be added a specifically American point: if we ever hope to persuade American politicians to enact a plan of universal coverage, then we must show them in advance how such a plan will control costs and how it will have built into it the ingredients to keep it from breaking the bank.

It is hard to say such things in the United States. Any discussion of the possibility of rationing health care in this country begins under a cloud. Symbolically, the very idea seems to offend a nicely tinted picture of ourselves as a rich, powerful nation, one that can afford to do whatever it takes to do whatever we want.[2] A nation that can put a man on the moon, that can afford Desert Storm and that can afford the S & L bailout is a nation that does not have to stint on health care. Especially for liberals, for whom the idea of universal health care has long been a high goal, any embrace of rationing seems a great betrayal. Since the main motive of the push for national health insurance has been coverage for the poor, the prospect of rationing care for that same group seems particularly offensive. It would seem to build into a program for the poor precisely those features that have so long burdened them: limits on what they can receive, while the more affluent can buy whatever care they want. As a symbol, then, rationing has nothing at all going for it. It seems, in fact, the perfect negative symbol of a weak and unjust society.

A strong and generous society must, however, be realistic if it is to do what needs doing. In case anyone addicted to symbols has not noticed, we have yet to enact universal health insurance in this country, and that failure comes at the end of at least forty years of trying. It is at best naive, at worst obstructionist, to continue invoking some idealized picture of ourselves to justify a failure to do what can be done, in a way it can be done, and to put in place something better than we now have. We can have universal health care in this country, but only if we can convince legislators and the American public that it is sensible and affordable. The only way to make such a case is to build an acceptance of rationing into it. What is now a negative symbol must be turned into one that is powerful and forthright: we can get what we need if we are prepared, in the process, to restrain ourselves. Rationing should be understood as a symbol of reasoning and restraint.[3] So understood, it can have great power, showing that we are concerned enough about the

---

[2] *See, e.g.*, Robert J. Blendon, *The Public's View of the Future of Health Care*, 259 JAMA 3587 (1988); Cindy Jajich-Toth & Burns W. Roper, *Americans' Views on Health Care: A Study in Contradictions*, HEALTH AFF., Winter 1990, at 149.

[3] *Cf.* David C. Hadorn, *Emerging Parallels in the American Health Care and Legal-Judicial Systems*, 18 AM J.L. & MED. 73, 85 ("The problem of rationing merely is another instance of the need to balance individual welfare and public good.").

poor to pursue reasonable policies. However wonderfully symbolic, an anti-rationing policy is not reasonable.

There are other, more literal objections to rationing. It has often been taken for granted that health care rationing would positively harm the poor,[4] and that it would also represent a precipitate abandonment of efforts to control costs and eliminate waste.[5] It need not do any of those things. On the contrary, rationing is likely the only way in which we can improve care for the poor and manage our health care system in a more efficient manner. This Article's argument, therefore, is strong and direct. Both as a symbol, and as a way of organizing the health care system, rationing represents the most promising route available to us. Or, put somewhat differently, so long as it builds a method of rationing into it, the United States can have, and can afford, a solid, decent and just health care system.

In this Article, "rationing" means an action undertaken when there is: (a) a recognition that resources are limited, and (b) when faced with scarcity, a method that must be devised to allocate fairly and reasonably those resources. Rationing is the effort to distribute equitably scarce resources. This definition is consistent with much common usage.[6]

Rationing may be understood in a hard and a soft sense. The hard sense is that of the lifeboat at sea, where a limited amount of fresh water must be shared. In that case a method of distribution must be devised that accepts the fact that there will be no more water. The limits are absolute.

The soft sense of rationing is the kind that we confront with health care, and just about everything else, in the United States. The limits to resources are not absolute. We could, if we chose to do so, spend far more on health care. We could go from 12% of our GNP[7] to 20%. We could, for that matter, declare superb health care to be the main goal of American society, and the delivery of health care our main industry.

---

[4] *See, e.g.*, Joan Beck, *Oregon Health Plan Faces the Reality of Care Rationing*, CHI. TRIB., Mar. 2, 1992, at C15; Spencer Rich, *Advocates for the Poor Hit Oregon Health Plan: Governor Vows to Prevent Inadequate Care*, WASH. POST, Sept. 17, 1991, at A3.

[5] *See, e.g.*, David Lauter & Edwin Chen, *Health Care For All: Three Plans Compete*, L.A. TIMES, Nov. 11, 1991, at A1.

[6] *See* Kai N. Lee, *Salmon, Science and the Law in the Columbia Basin*, 21 ENVTL. L. 745, 776-77 (1991) ("[In] rationing lifesaving medical care . . . societies must attempt to make allocations in ways that preserve the moral foundations of social collaboration."); Pascal Fletcher, *Feeding Family Food Basket is Frustrating Chore in Cuba*, REUTER LIBR. REP., Sept. 30, 1991, BC cycle ("The authorities say the rationing system is the only way to ensure a fair distribution of scarce resources.").

[7] *See* GEORGE J. ANNAS ET AL., AMERICAN HEALTH LAW 121 (1990) (11.1% of GNP in 1987); Roberrt D. Ray, *Health Tax Credits? A Sickly Idea: Here's A Plan That Won't Do Anything to Make the System Work*, WASH. POST, Jan. 26, 1992, at C5 (13% of GNP in 1991).

That is not likely to happen, and for a good reason. There are practical political constraints on how much money can be spent on health care. Limits are imposed by an unwillingness to pay higher taxes, to increase the burden of employers to provide health care, or to pay personally out of our own pockets. Public opinion polls time and again show that Americans, however high their aspirations for good care, are not willing to pay an unlimited amount to have it or to put up with the restrictions that it might entail.[8] There are, as politicians know all too well, limits to a public willingness to tolerate tax increases, both across-the-board and for health care. For their part, employers cannot afford to jeopardize the overall fiscal soundness of their businesses by readily tolerating constant cost escalations. The Hastings Center[9] has had to put up with average increases of 25% per year for the past three years, and that is not atypical. Neither the Hastings Center nor more affluent organizations can afford to continue that pattern.

Limits are further imposed by common sense. We ought not to spend excessively on health care. We do so spend only at the cost of other important recipients of limited resources. We need a good educational system, good parks and roads, good welfare and poverty programs, good industrial research and development policies. Health is not the only human good. Despite the great hand-wringing about the state of our health care system, for the most part American citizens already have a high and adequate level of general health. No special national gain adheres in increasing average life expectancy, or in trying to conquer each and every human disease. It would be nice, but it is not an imperative goal for the overall well-being of the country. Only a nation that over-values health could think we need more of it.

This Article speaks primarily about the health status of middle-class white people, those who can expect, on average, to live a long life, well into old age. But what is true of this group is not true of everyone. The most immediate pressing problem is whether we can bring to the poor and deprived the same benefits now available to the rest of us.

This Article proposes the following ideal for the American health care system. Every American should be guaranteed a decently adequate, affordable level of health care. The poor, in particular, should be provided such care. The goal would be universal access to decent care. The achievement of that goal will require significant government expenditures; the government should provide the base guarantee for the poor. Beyond that, a combination of employer and personal contributions can provide the remainder of the needed money for everyone

---

[8] Robert J. Blendon, *supra* note 2, at 3588-90; Cindy Jajich-Toth & Burns W. Roper, *supra* note 2, at 153.

[9] Daniel Callahan, Director.

else.[10]

Such a system would not make economic sense without some form of rationing, at least in its public government programs and its private employer programs. Why rationing? Because the government would be foolish to promise an unlimited system of health care, one devised independently of the costs of that system. No country on earth, including one with the most generous system, has done that. The government cannot say, in effect, that it will pay whatever it costs to give you the most advanced health care. It cannot promise to pay for every technological advance, however efficacious and however expensive. It cannot promise to help all of us live as long as we choose, regardless of what private hopes we might have. It cannot promise to jeopardize other important societal needs in the pursuit of improved health. It cannot promise to conduct an unending struggle against mortality.

The American Congress has a long memory. It can recall how it was assured, in 1972, that the kidney dialysis program would cost no more than $250 million per year in its fourth year of operation or thereafter.[11] It now costs over $3 billion per year.[12] Congress can recall when it put Medicare in place in 1965,[13] assured that the costs would be manageable. Those costs now are expected to bankrupt the Medicare Trust Fund within the next decade.[14] In neither case were any methods conceived or developed to keep the costs under control; they were not thought to be needed. With memories of this kind, Congress cannot be expected to initiate major new entitlement programs that do not show, in advance, how the costs are to be managed. Blank checks will not be issued. The estimate of the Pepper Commission in 1990, the major bipartisan congressional effort to formulate a response to the problem of indigent and long-term care, was a cost of an additional $69.6 billion per year for decent coverage.[15] That estimate was for the first year. Nothing was said about the second year; the Commission knew better than to do that.

In short, both because no nation on earth, not even the United States, can promise unbounded health care regardless of the cost, and because Congress will not pay for such health care, some system of limits must be put in place. I call such a system a "rationing." It is ration-

[10] This Article does not address the details of that kind of system.

[11] 118 CONG. REC. 33,004 (daily ed. Sept. 30, 1972) (statement of Senator Hartke in sponsoring the end-stage renal disease section of the Social Security Amendments of 1972).

[12] *See* GEORGE J. ANNAS ET AL., *supra* note 7, at 890.

[13] Health Insurance for the Aged Act, Pub. L. No. 89-97, 79 Stat. 290 (1965) (codified as amended at 42 U.S.C.A. §§ 401-426 (West 1991)).

[14] John Holahan & John L. Palmer, *Medicare's Fiscal Problems: An Imperative for Reform*, 13 J. HEALTH POL., POL'Y & L. 53, 77 (1988).

[15] THE PEPPER COMM'N: UNITED STATES BIPARTISAN COMM. ON COMPREHENSIVE HEALTH CARE, 101ST CONG., 2D SESS., A CALL FOR ACTION 17 (S. Print 1990).

ing in the worst sense if it is capricious and discriminatory, as is our present method of using ability-to-pay as a way of limiting costs. But it can be rationing in the best sense of the term if, in response to the need for limits, a fair and reasonable way is developed to set and maintain these limits.

But of course, for symbolic and practical reasons, every possible rationale, every conceivable evasion, is being developed to avoid the need for rationing. If we could just organize our present system better, it is said, we could have all the necessary health care we want.[16] If we could simply wring the waste, inefficiency and excess bureaucratic and malpractice costs out of the system, we would not even have to think about rationing.[17] The basis for this faith in efficiency is not groundless. We know that our administrative costs are high, approximately 20% of all costs (in comparison with approximately 10% in Canada).[18] We know that a huge amount of money is spent in response to malpractice problems and on our present system of tort compensation.[19] These costs are not incurred in other countries.[20] We know that we waste billions of dollars on untested or misused technologies.[21] We know that most other developed countries can show as good or better mortality and morbidity outcomes for considerably less money per capita[22] and for a smaller percentage of their GNP.[23] It is not, in a word, hard to show that we could get much better value for the money that we do spend and probably even could get as good or better an outcome for less money.

Nonetheless, we are profoundly mistaken in believing that we should not move to open and conscious rationing *until* we have wrung all of that waste out of the system. This is a version of what this Article

[16] *See Administration Health Care Proposals: Hearings Before the House Ways and Means Comm.*, 102d Cong., 2d Sess. (1992) (statement of Dr. Louis Sullivan, Secretary of Health and Human Services) ("Indeed, one of our principles is to increase the efficiencies in our system because of my belief that we already have enough dollars in the system, but we're not spending them wisely."), *reprinted in* FED. NEWS SERV., Feb. 20, 1992.

[17] *See* Amitai Etzioni, *Health Care Rationing: A Critical Evaluation*, HEALTH AFF., Summer 1991, at 88-95.

[18] Steffie Woolhandler & David U. Himmelstein, *The Deteriorating Administrative Efficiency of the U.S. Health Care System*, 324 NEW ENG. J. MED. 1253, 1255 (1991).

[19] *See* Leonard S. Weiss, *Finding the Remedies for Ills in Health Care: They Don't Come Easy, but They Do Exist*, NEWSDAY, Mar. 5, 1992, at 97 (defensive medicine adds more than $18 billion to health care costs).

[20] *Cf.* Frank A. Sloan & Randall R. Bobvjerg, *in Medical Malpractice: Crises, Response and Effects*, HEALTH INS. ASS'N OF AMERICA, RESEARCH BULLETIN 43 (1989) ("Price rises for liability coverage and heightened fears of litigation with its many uninsured costs have surely affected the climate of American medical practice.").

[21] INSTITUTE OF MEDICINE, ASSESSING MEDICAL TECHNOLOGIES 211-27 (1985).

[22] *See* George J. Schieber & Jean-Pierre Poullier, *International Health Spending: Issues and Trends*, HEALTH AFF., Spring 1991, at 106, 114 exhibit 6.

[23] *Id.* at 110 exhibit 2.

calls the "best of all possible worlds fallacy": if we could just organize ourselves more efficiently, we could have all the necessary and affordable health care we want.

Why am I skeptical, and why do I call that a fallacy? Mainly because I have heard the same refrain again and again, for well over a decade now. Yet during that time, and despite a variety of highly touted cost containment programs, nothing has worked to any substantial degree to control costs or to bring much greater efficiency into the system. We have tried DRGs,[24] managed care,[25] HMOs[26] and competition.[27] No attempt has had any striking success, although some evidence shows that Medicare cost increases are being controlled.[28] The most that we can say is that costs might have been higher without these alternative health care plans. Overall health care costs continue to increase at two to three times the rate of inflation in general, and have risen even more sharply over the past three years.[29] Why should we expect some great shift in the historical pattern? Why, if we have failed for years in controlling costs, should we expect a transformation — the equivalent of a religious conversion experience — of the national character and of the present system?

It is a fallacy to conclude that because there is room for great savings, which there is, it therefore follows that we will have, and can get, those savings. On the contrary, one can conclude only that the surest prescription to maintain the unfair and costly status quo is to continue talking about all the money that we can save simply by eliminating waste, malpractice excess and bureaucracy. This is a method that surely has worked well toward that end so far. Nothing changes and there is no prospect of any immediate change.

Why? We do not know how to eliminate waste in behavioral practice (even if we do in economic theory). In fact, we make things all the harder to change by posing the elimination of waste as an alternative to

---

[24] Diagnosis-related group, which is a Medicaid payment plan under which hospitals receive a lump sum payment on the basis of discharge diagnosis, without regard to actual treatment provided. *See* GEORGE J. ANNAS ET AL., *supra* note 7, at 215-16, 234-48.

[25] Under a managed care system, the patient chooses, or is assigned to, a primary care provider who then controls the patient's access to hospitals and specialists. Under most plans, the provider's income decreases if the provider approves expensive specialists or hospital care. *Id.* at 784.

[26] Under a health maintenance organization system, the patient pays a fixed sum and the organization promises to provide a defined package of inpatient and outpatient services. Doctors may be paid as salaried employees or on a fee-for-service basis. *Id.* at 774-75.

[27] *See* DANIEL CALLAHAN, WHAT KIND OF LIFE: THE LIMITS OF MEDICAL PROGRESS 76 (1990).

[28] *Id.* at 76-77. *See also* Sandra Christensen, *Did 1980s Legislation Slow Medicare Spending*, HEALTH AFF., Summer 1991, at 135.

[29] *See* Stuart M. Butler, *Coming to Terms on Health Care*, N.Y. TIMES, Jan. 28, 1990, at C13; Robert Pear, *Social Security Benefits to Go Up 3.7%*, N.Y. TIMES, Oct. 18, 1991, at A10.

rationing. On the contrary, we will eliminate waste only by rationing. Only if we understand that we must live within restraints, and take the steps consistent with that recognition, can we contain costs. To be undertaken seriously, cost containment must be understood as another form of rationing. Responsible cost containment means saying "no" to some things that physicians, patients and administrators want. Serious cost containment means establishing practice guidelines and making them stick. Serious cost containment means the setting of priorities.

The issue before us is not a matter of cost containment *or* rationing. Both are necessary. They should be thought of as two sides of the same coin, not as alternatives. The experience of the European countries should sober those who think cost containment will make unlimited beneficial care available. Those countries — which have already in place most of the reforms that are desired in the United States — are beginning to feel the strain.[30] They have managed to control costs, but at the price of limiting services and requiring long waiting times for many procedures.[31] With the same demographic forces at work in those countries as here (that is, with an aging population), with an increase in high technology medicine, and with rising patient demands, these countries will be forced, as will we, into even more rationing in the future. They are quietly beginning their own rationing discussion — and are immensely curious to see how ours progresses.

The main concern about rationing in the United States is that the burden will fall upon the poor.[32] That is a serious problem. How can it be avoided? The overriding requirement is that this country have national health insurance and, with it, an adequate baseline of care. Inevitably, this baseline will have to be set at a level lower than the richest people can set their baseline. Rich people can hire limousines to get to their medical treatment, and helicopters to take them from their resort villas to daily psychoanalysis. Rich Americans can fly to Switzerland to use experimental treatments not available here. Rich people can seek out the very best specialists in the country and use them rather than their local doctors. No conceivable government program could offer benefits of this kind to everyone. No private employee benefit program could offer them either.

Why should that matter anyway? What does matter is not whether the rich do better than the poor, but how well the poor do. The crucial issue is whether the baseline of care for the poor is set high enough to eliminate the most serious disparities between rich and poor. It could

---

30 *See Yesterday's Mirage: Why Britain's NHS Needs Competition*, THE ECONOMIST, Apr. 28, 1984, at 26 [hereinafter *Yesterday's Mirage*]; *see also* DANIEL CALLAHAN, *supra* note 27, at 88-89.

31 *See Yesterday's Mirage*, *supra* note 30, at 26-30.

32 *See* GEORGE J. ANNAS ET AL., *supra* note 7, at 70-74, 104-06.

not eliminate all of them. It would take a totalitarian state to keep the rich and powerful from the health care that they want. The communist countries of Eastern Europe, as well as the Soviet Union, had the pretense of a single-tier, egalitarian system. The reality was that powerful party members got care not available to others, and that ordinary citizens had to bribe their way through the system to get good care. A democratic society would not even attempt to impose a single-tier system. It would invite corruption and evasion. But a democratic society would try to make certain that the poor have decent health care.

Yet if decent care is not the same as maximal care, how can the former be determined? It will, by definition, be rationed care. A fair system of rationing will have to set some priorities. If not everything can be made available to everyone, what is comparatively more or less important? The Oregon initiative is of great national importance. Using a combination of technical and economic considerations, and tempering them with expressed public values, that state has set up a system of priorities.[33] The Oregon legislators determined that it is better to provide health care coverage to everyone falling below the federal poverty line than to eliminate some people altogether in order to give virtually unlimited care to those who qualify. To make the new system possible, Oregon plans to limit services by means of its priority list.[34] The plan will also mandate that small businesses provide health insurance or pay into a pool that would make that insurance available to all employed persons.[35] The long-term goal is a system of universal health care in Oregon.

As the Oregon planners recognized, any process of rationing health care will have to find a way to balance medical judgment, economic possibilities, and public values. Yet it took some years to gain that insight. When the Medicaid program was established by Congress in 1965 to provide health care for the poor,[36] it specified that the indigent were to receive care that was "medically necessary."[37] Congress did not, unfortunately (but perhaps deliberately) specify what that term meant or what means would be appropriate to make such a determination. It may have presumed that a purely medical standard of medical necessity could be determined.

[33] *See* Charles J. Dougherty, *Setting Health Care Priorities: Oregon's Next Steps*, HASTINGS CENTER REP., May-June 1991, at special supp. 1-16; Sara Rosenbaum, *Mothers and Children Last: The Oregon Medicaid Experiment*, 18 AM. J.L. & MED. 97 (1992).

[34] Sara Rosenbaum, *supra* note 33, at 104.

[35] Act effective July 1, 1989, ch. 836, 1989 OR. LAWS 836 (codified as amended in scattered subsections of OR. REV. STAT. § 414 (1989)).

[36] Pub. L. No. 89-97, § 1901, 79 Stat. 343 (1965) (codified as amended at 42 U.S.C.A. §§ 1396a-1396u (West 1992)).

[37] *Id.*

If that is what Congress believed, it was wrong. As the intervening years have demonstrated well, it has turned out to be impossible to specify a purely scientific standard of medical "need," the basic concept that lies behind the idea of that which is "medically necessary." The problem is that "need" admits of no precise definition, ranging as it does over mental and physical needs, life-saving and life-enhancing needs. It is a notion, moreover, that is subject to different interpretations, open to the changed possibilities provided by technological developments, and subject to different valuative interpretations. Thus although "medically necessary" and meeting health care "needs" have about them the ring of objectivity, they turn out to be flexible and malleable concepts. They combine both a descriptive and a normative content. They are at once scientific and moral concepts. This was not so obvious in 1965.

As time has gone on, it has been possible to trace a steady enrichment of our understanding of the ingredients necessary to specify a decent minimum of adequate health care.[38] Such care must include, in some plausible way, first, some reference to medical need; it must be rooted in commonly accepted notions of what people characteristically look for in health care. Yet, for all the above-mentioned reasons, it cannot use such a standard exclusively. Inevitably, many questions about the extent of those needs and the various evaluations required to deal with the borderline cases[39] will arise. Second, therefore, a decent minimum of average health care must include judgments about the efficacy of available treatments to meet those needs; that is, what works and what does not work? A consideration of efficacy will, however, force a third set of considerations — that of the relative costs and benefits of different treatments. What will it cost to provide different benefits and is there a good return on the money spent?

Next a decision will have to be made. If not everything can be afforded, what treatments and benefits are relatively more or less important? At this point, it should be abundantly clear that this question and those that preceded it require a central political component to be properly answered. Because these questions address fact and value, and the weighing of costs and benefits, they transcend a technical level. The questions call for collective judgment, judgment of a kind that will combine both expert and lay opinion. Thus, the fourth consideration is that a political process will have to be devised.

---

[38] CHARLES J. DOUGHERTY, *supra* note 33, at special supp. 3-4. *See also* Daniel Callahan, *Medical Futility, Medical Necessity: The Problem Without A Name*, HASTINGS CENTER REP., July-Aug. 1991, at 30.

[39] For example, coronary artery bypass surgery for an elderly person, or resuscitation efforts with a very low birthweight baby.

Since the political process almost certainly will encounter resource limitations, a question will then be raised: what is relatively more or less important in the provision of health care? The setting of priorities, then, will be a fifth consideration. How might that best be done? The state of Oregon has devised one method to do this,[40] and perhaps one could imagine others. Whatever other possible ways they might use to set priorities, however, other states would be wise in following the lead of Oregon in organizing community discussion of health care policy prior to the more formal political process of priority setting. Thus, the sixth consideration is the importance in giving the public not only a chance to express its opinions and preferences on priorities, but also a chance to become educated on the issues.

In a sharp attack on the Oregon approach to rationing and priority-setting, one of our most astute health care analysts, Lawrence D. Brown, wrote that "rationing has been elevated to the pantheon of fashionable solutions — competition, managed care, prudent purchasing, and more — that policymakers intermittently embrace as all-American answers to uncontrollable health care costs."[41] He then goes on to say that

> [v]iewed in cross-national context, Oregon's contribution is mainly to show that, at least today in the United States, rationing is not a profound but a spurious issue. . . . The United States should worry less about rationing and more about constructing a rational policy framework whose watchwords are budgeting, planning, regulation, and negotiation. If the polity has declined to make those hard choices, rationing cannot save it from itself. American policymakers have not earned the right to ration health care, and the very policies that would earn it would eliminate much of the need to exercise it.[42]

Dr. Brown is wrong. First, rationing has not been proposed as one more solution to be put alongside competition or managed care, but as a strikingly different kind of proposal. The other approaches were all designed to control costs within the present system of health care, not to change the system altogether. For many, in fact, they were meant as ways of avoiding rationing, as rationing is a generically different kind of approach. Second, what Dr. Brown proposes is perfectly sensible, but it *also* is fashionable. For what has been more common of late than to call for "a rational policy framework," and the national health insurance that would embody it? It is the best solution, and even those of us

[40] OR. REV. STAT. § 414.720 (1991).

[41] Lawrence D. Brown, *The National Politics of Oregon's Rationing Plan*, HEALTH AFF., Summer 1991, at 46-47.

[42] *Id.* at 50.

who support rationing would prefer such a framework as our starting point in an ideal world. But Dr. Brown neglects to mention that there has been no national progress of any significance toward that goal. There has been neither the political will for such a framework nor, in the face of budget deficits, any serious, politically potent constituency for it.

Third, the real genius of the Oregon initiative is that it starts with a recognition of limits as the first step toward a comprehensive health care system.[43] Its organizers say that in the present American political climate, the best way to get to Dr. Brown's goal of "budget, planning, and negotiation" is to concede at the very outset that rationing is necessary, and that the setting of priorities is the most sensible way of effecting it.[44] It is striking that none of the major national universal health care plans that have been proposed make any serious provision for controlling their costs. The Oregon plan takes limitation as its *point of departure* and then works from there.[45]

In effect, the Oregon plan stands Dr. Brown's approach on its head. Dr. Brown says that "American policymakers have not earned the right to ration health care, and the very policies that would earn it would eliminate much of the need to exercise it."[46] The organizers of Oregon's plan, by contrast, say that only by a willingness to embrace rationing — the orderly, equitable allocation of scarce resources — can we make progress toward universal health care, not the other way around.[47] They also say, moreover, that it is high time we stop talking about how a better, more rational system would obviate the need for rationing.[48] No universal health care system could avoid some degree of rationing. In any case, we are still far from significant national reforms, and the need now is to find a good starting point. In the absence of the will, leadership and public support necessary for national health insurance, Oregon is actually taking some real steps in that direction. The other states and the federal government are just talking.

The animus against rationing in the United States, symbolically

---

[43] *See* Daniel Callahan, *Ethics and Priority Setting in Oregon*, HEALTH AFF., Summer 1991, at 78-87.

[44] *See Oregon Medicaid Rationing Experiment: Hearings Before the Subcomm. on Health and the Environment of the House Comm. on Energy and Commerce*, 102d Cong., 1st Sess. 19 (1991) [hereinafter *Hearings on Oregon Rationing*] (statement of Jean I. Thorne, Director, Medical Assistance Programs, Dep't of Human Resources); *id.* at 83 (testimony of Tina Castanares, Oregon Health Servs. Comm.).

[45] *See id.* at 65 (testimony of Rep. Les AuCoin) ("Oregon's health plan is a program of expansion, not of limits.").

[46] Lawrence D. Brown, *supra* note 41, at 50.

[47] *See Hearings on Oregon Rationing*, *supra* note 44, at 157, 160 (statement of Sisters of Providence in Oregon).

[48] *See id.* at 151 (statement of Peter O. Kohler, M.D., President, Oregon Health Sciences University); *id.* at 157 (statement of Sisters of Providence of Oregon).

and literally, expresses in one sense some of our most admirable values. Those are our touching faith in the power of efficiency, our commitment to egalitarianism, and our reluctance officially to pick upon the poor to test our social schemes. Rationing is thought to offend all of those values and thus is rejected.

We deceive ourselves. Serious efficiency would require the equivalent of rationing, and that is why we have not achieved it. Our egalitarianism is more rhetorical than it is real. We tolerate a radically inegalitarian health care system as a day-to-day affair but then rail against anyone — in the name of perfection — who would accept some degree of inequality as the first step on the way to a genuinely fair system. Although we carry out social experiments with the poor all of the time, including the crazy mess that is our Medicaid system, we rail at efforts to bring some sensible priorities and planning into that system, as Oregon is trying to do.

The usual approach to American problems is to say that since we are such a powerful and rich nation, we can afford nothing less than the best: the most lavish health care system and, with reform, the fairest and most efficient as well. So we reject any notion of limits, boundaries or self-restrictions. We live with our dreams. We should give them up and put realism and sobriety in their place. An acceptance of rationing would be a good place to begin. In fact, if we want national health insurance, it is likely to be the only feasible place to begin.

[15]

NORMAN DANIELS
& JAMES SABIN

Limits to Health Care: Fair Procedures, Democratic Deliberation, and the Legitimacy Problem for Insurers

I. Introduction

Millions of Americans are finding out that when they are ill, neither they nor their physicians may have the authority to make decisions about their own well-being. Unlike the earlier era of "unmanaged" insurance, at present considerable authority rests with managed care organizations (MCOs),other insurers, and, more indirectly, with large employers who, in trying to reduce benefit costs, force intense competition among MCOs and other providers. This shift of authority from the patient to private organizations raises important questions about the fairness and legitimacy of decisions that limit medical care, since they fundamentally affect our well-being.

There is a political irony in this shift. During the Clinton Administration's effort to reform health care in 1993, many Americans were influenced by a $15 million insurer-sponsored television ad campaign featuring a middle-class couple, Harry and Louise, who lamented the prospect of "big government" taking away their choices about physicians and treatments. With the failure of reform, "big business" has more often been making these decisions for us. Anyone who worries about the bureaucrat in Washington setting limits on what the doctor can do should be just as concerned about vesting that authority in private, increasingly for-profit institutions.

This article draws on research that is funded by grants from the National Science Foundation, the Retirement Research Foundation, the Greenwall Foundation, the Robert Wood Johnson Foundation, and the Harvard Pilgrim Health Foundation. We also wish to acknowledge the invaluable assistance of Susann Wilkinson, research associate for this project, as well as the cooperation of many people at our collaborating sites.

This shift in authority highlights a special problem of making acceptable moral decisions about medical limit-setting. Shortly, we shall locate that problem where three inadequate ways of addressing it—standard insurance-market solutions, some familiar types of philosophical inquiry, and purely procedural accounts of public alternatives—converge. We shall also propose a solution to it. First, however, we want to specify the type of limit-setting decision on which we shall focus.

Through their coverage decisions, managed care organizations (MCOs) and other insurers limit access to some beneficial medical services,[1] including those for new technologies.[2] Though some patients may be able to afford these services without insurance coverage, and some may get access to them through sponsored clinical trials, many will not be able to receive promising but unproven technologies. The coverage decisions of MCOs or other insurers (hereafter just "MCOs")[3] thus effectively restrict access to treatment for many patients. The decision-making power of the MCO, even if it only affects payment for a procedure, can greatly impact a subscriber's life and quality of life.

Why or when should a patient or clinician who thinks an uncovered service is appropriate or even "medically necessary" accept as legitimate the limit-setting decisions of a MCO?[4] In what follows, we shall refer to this problem as the "legitimacy problem." Since limit-setting decisions affect the well-being of patients in fundamental ways, they are moral

1. Medical insurance traditionally excludes beneficial nonmedical services (e.g., dental, home supports); it also arbitrarily limits beneficial mental health services (e.g., 10 not 20 therapy sessions, or 30 not 35 hospital days). The use of guidelines, utilization review, and systematic technology assessment arguably limits some beneficial services at the margin, including cases when a patient or clinician has good reason to object to the limits.

2. Decisions about new technologies are only the tip of the limit-setting iceberg. Much of what is said about these decisions can be generalized to other, explicit limit-setting decisions, including practice guidelines approved by MCOs. Despite their importance, we will not discuss the discretionary, limit-setting decisions of practitioners who limit care because they are responding to economic incentives to reduce treatment.

3. Since even "unmanaged" indemnity insurers manage coverage for new technologies, lumping them together is less problematic than it might otherwise be.

4. The term "medical necessity" is partly intended to confer legitimacy on some decisions about limiting our obligations to provide medical assistance. See Norman Daniels and James E. Sabin, "When Is Home Care Medically Necessary?" *Hastings Center Report* 21, no. 4 (July–August 1991): 37–38, and James E. Sabin and Norman Daniels, "Determining 'Medical Necessity' in Mental Health Practice: A Study of Clinical Reasoning and a Proposal for Insurance Policy," *Hastings Center Report* 24, no. 6 (November–December 1994): 5–13.

decisions that involve important issues of distributive justice. The legitimacy problem asks why, and under what conditions, authority over these matters should be placed in the hands of private organizations, such as MCOs.

We can pose a parallel question and problem, the fairness problem: *When does a patient or clinician who thinks an uncovered service appropriate or even medically necessary have sufficient reason to accept as fair the limit-setting decisions of a managed care organization?*

To illustrate this fairness problem, consider some quite different kinds of reasons that might underlie a limit-setting decision not to provide coverage for a particular treatment. Suppose patients who want the treatment, or clinicians who think the treatment is appropriate for their patients, are given reasons for denying it such as these: "The treatment is expensive, and providing it for similar cases would make it hard to produce an adequate return to investors," or "If we provided this treatment we could not support a competitive CEO salary," or "We could provide this treatment only by cutting into bonuses paid to clinicians or by scrimping on marketing costs," or "We can offer this only by losing some of the competitive edge on premiums we charge to employers." Patients would not—and should not—find these reasons persuasive even if they believed them to be factually correct. As stated, they only show that what is to the patients' disadvantage works to others' advantage. These reasons would and should persuade only people who also believe that the system which appealed to these reasons was making the patient no worse off than anyone need be in alternative, feasible systems. Vague assurances about the "efficiency" of competition do not suffice to show that. (We return in greater detail to the "business" of medicine later.)

In contrast, other reasons for setting limits on access to the treatment provide more plausible grounds to accept the decision as fair: "This expensive treatment is not yet proven to be safe and effective, and the organization is not obligated to cover unproven therapies when (as in this case) doing so would undercut its ability to provide proven therapies to others," or "This therapy serves less important needs than some other therapy that cannot be offered under budget constraints if this one is," or "There is a much more cost-effective way to provide the same outcomes than covering this treatment." We shall discuss these reasons more fully in Section IV. Here they are intended to illustrate the point that some grounds for setting limits to care will be (and should be) viewed as reasonable and fair, while others will not be without substantial further argument.

The legitimacy and fairness problems are distinct. A legitimate authority can act unfairly, e.g., a public-school teacher may grade students in a gender- or race-biased manner, or a legislatively mandated insurance benefit package might be biased in favor of physical health services and against mental health services. Conversely, an illegitimate authority can deliver fair decisions, e.g., a street-gang leader may force one gang member to compensate another for a past wrong. Still, they are related. We may reasonably accept something as a legitimate authority only if it abides by a procedure or process or even substantive constraints (for example, Constitutional protections) that we consider generally fair. If it abandons the fair procedure, it may lose its legitimacy. Similarly, in contexts where an authority that claims no legitimacy employs a fair procedure, especially where there may be prior disagreement about what counts as a fair outcome, we may accept the outcome as fair.

In Section II we begin to locate the legitimacy and fairness problems more precisely. Limit-setting by private insurers, it might be thought, is no different from other decisions made by product and service providers in other markets. Limits are legitimized and fair when consumers "consent" to purchase products involving them at fair market prices. We argue that this consensual model fails in our health care system and, further, that we have a social obligation to ensure that the private sector of our health care system delivers health care fairly, an obligation that we cannot discharge unless MCOs are more publicly accountable than typical businesses.

A second strategy for dispelling the legitimacy and fairness problems would be to seek clear, compelling principles governing fair limit-setting from moral philosophy. Using such principles, anyone—MCO administrators, clinicians, plan enrollees—could establish what were acceptable limits and no special issue of legitimacy would trouble us. In Section III we argue that coverage decisions for new technologies raise moral issues about which there is currently no clear consensus and that, even if some lines of moral inquiry produced answers persuasive to some, we should not expect consensus on them in a pluralist society. The combined failures of a straightforward market solution and a market solution supplemented by moral consensus might push us toward thinking public, democratic procedures offered the only acceptable way to address these moral issues. Our lack of confidence in this third strategy (see Section IV) completes our effort to locate our problem. Leery of purely proceduralist solutions to moral questions, and believing that institutions with the responsibility for delivering care may be better situated and informed to make limit-setting decisions, we propose a solution that realistically remains within the framework of our existing health care system.

We argue that decision-procedures for limit setting in MCOs must have certain general features if they are to qualify as legitimate and fair (Section IV). One key feature is the provision of publicly accessible reasons, that is, a public rationale, for decisions. A second is that the rationale must constitute a reasonable construal of how to meet the medical needs of a covered population under acceptable resource constraints. A third key feature is that there be mechanisms for considering challenges to decisions that are made and for revisiting those decisions in light of counter-arguments. Our claim is normative: these features should count toward viewing these procedures as fair and legitimate. We also believe that if these features are instituted, over time people will come to view the procedures as fair and legitimate. A point we shall return to later is that our account is compatible with the idea of "deliberative democracy," an appealing approach to the justification of democratic procedures quite generally. Specifically, our account extends elements of a deliberative democratic account to nonpublic institutions. We hope to make the rationale for our account plausible independently of appeal to a more general theory, however, and we make no attempt to derive our account from that theory or justify its more controversial features.

Though we raise a problem that might seem to be limited to medical ethics, it is really a problem in political philosophy of wider interest and importance. Like medical insurers, many institutions in our society—public and nonpublic, political and nonpolitical—make morally controversial decisions that affect our well-being in fundamental ways. What conditions should constrain the making of those decisions if they are to be acceptable to those affected by them? An answer to the problem we raise here throws light on this broader class of moral decisions made in a wide variety of institutions.

Solving the legitimacy and fairness problems for limit-setting decisions is only part of what makes a health care system just overall.[5] Without eliminating financial and other barriers to care, e.g., through universial insurance coverage, no system will be just overall. Nevertheless, the kinds of accountability required to address the legitimacy and fairness problems must be part of any universal coverage system, whether a British national health service, a Canadian single payer, or a mixed system, as in Germany or as envisioned in the failed Clinton reforms.

II. Why Question the Legitimacy of Limits Set by MCOs?

Trust vs. Legitimacy

Cynicism surrounds the interactions of subscribers (patients) and MCOs, including disputes about the denials of new (and unproven) technologies. Although contract language universally excludes coverage for "experimental" or "unproven" treatments, disagreements arise about how reasonable it is to exclude an experimental treatment, especially when it represents a "last chance" for survival or significant improvement in quality of life. Often, patients, practitioners, and the wider public firmly believe that MCOs hide behind a "hard line" about new therapies primarily to cut costs and to produce a good "bottom line," not because they believe the therapy is not "appropriate" treatment.

One reason the climate of suspicion and mutual cynicism sustains itself is that many limit-setting decisions are made outside the public view. In the more entrepreneurial MCO cultures, decision-making about limits is seen as "proprietary," on the model of "trade secrets." The argument is that the techniques for producing efficient delivery and efficient limit setting are a form of intellectual property and constitute one of the valued assets of a well-functioning MCO. To expose the decisions and the process to public scrutiny would be to lose proprietary control of the intellectual and organizational assets that are key to retaining a competitive edge.

The situation described so far shows that trust of MCOs is clearly lacking, but lack of trust is not the same thing as lack of legitimacy. We often

5. For discussion of a ten-dimensional matrix for assessing the fairness of reforms, or of a system, see Norman Daniels, Donald Light, and Ronald Caplan, *Benchmarks of Fairness for Health Care Reform* (New York: Oxford University Press, 1996).

fail to trust legitimate authorities. We often insist that they earn our trust, because trust does not automatically come with authority.

The Car Purchase Analogy

The claim that there is no problem of legitimacy—even if there is a problem of trust—is put forcefully in the following argument, which we shall call the *car purchase analogy*. As long as there is clear coverage language in subscriber contracts, there is no special problem of "legitimacy" facing MCOs who make limit-setting decisions any more than there is a problem of "legitimacy" facing automobile manufacturers when they make decisions regarding product features and design. If a car manufacturer makes cost-cutting decisions that affect the quality of a product, the market provides a mechanism for putting a price on that decision and allowing consumers to match their preferences with the price of products. Although some safety features of automobiles are mandated by law, and although consumer protection legislation provides some further defense against some indefensible behaviors by car manufacturers, we already have similar protections in the case of health care through insurance law and tort litigation. Beyond that, the market—for cars or health insurance—provides an efficient mechanism for matching consumer preferences to market share. Accordingly, if consumers do not like the limit-setting decisions of a medical insurer, they are free to purchase other medical insurance that better meets their preferences for services. The obligation of the insurer, like the auto manufacturer, is to be honest and forthright about the features of the product, eschewing deception. There is no further obligation to provide access to a process of decision-making to make sure it meets some standard of fairness that really plays no role in a market economy.

A Failed Analogy

The car purchase analogy aims to show that consumer choices in a market for medical insurance confer legitimacy since they involve consent. The analogy fails for three main reasons. First, uncertainty is a much greater factor in markets for medical insurance than it is in markets for autos.[6] With cars, we have a good idea just what our needs are: we know how many passengers we will have to carry, what kinds of commuting

6. Kenneth Arrow, "Uncertainty and the Welfare Economics of Medical Care," *American Economic Review* 53 (1963): 941–73.

or cargo carrying we will do, and what our style of driving is. We also have reasonably good information about outcomes: *Consumer Reports* or its equivalent tells us which cars get what kinds of mileage under what conditions, which have better safety records, which have better service records (with detailed ratings for different aspects of the car), and which have higher customer satisfaction and resale value. We have much greater trouble anticipating our needs for health care if we have no obvious history of problems, and if we do have such a history, we may be excluded from purchasing insurance, that is, from shopping around, because of medical underwriting practices of insurers. We also have not yet developed an adequate technology for reporting on the quality of MCOs through good measures of outcomes, though new measurement techniques are being developed.

Features of the design of our health care system also undercut the car purchase analogy. Most Americans receive their health insurance through their employers, who select their employees' health plans. We do not buy our private cars through fleet purchases made by our employers. The assertion that people can consent with their purchases to the limits that insurers impose on them has no grip on the actual situation of most insured Americans, who cannot practically "vote with their dollars" even if (in theory) that would constitute consent. If they are lucky enough to have insurance at all, it comes with the job, and the only choice they have is to change jobs, if they can. If, however, they try to exercise choice by changing jobs or seeking their own insurance coverage, perhaps in awareness of some special medical needs they have, they might then be shut out from insurance, or might have to pay much more for it, by the medical underwriting rules of insurers. Nor should we say that we "consent" to the terms of the medical insurance policy because we "consent" to having our employer select our insurance coverage for us. Although some employers may seek a plan that produces good value for money, it would be naive to think that an employer's interest in containing costs always can be translated without controversy into an employee's interest in accepting compromises in coverage. The employer is not the employee's fiduciary agent.

Justice, Health Care, and Accountability

The car purchase analogy fails for a deeper, moral reason as well: We have a widely recognized social obligation to meet people's medical needs,[7] within reasonable resource constraints, but we do not have a social obligation to meet people's preferences or needs for autos. Although we might admit that people have a need for transportation, and that the need for automobiles is increased by social decisions that lead to inadequate public transportation, individual transportation needs are generally viewed as an individual responsibility, one that people can budget for out of a decent minimum income. For example, where the inability to afford a car means that some jobs are inaccessible to some people, the view is still widely held that people can and should make appropriate adjustments. They should move closer to transportation that makes the job accessible, or take a different job, or decide that the job is "not worth it" if it does not enable the purchase of a car. After all, an older car that meets basic employment transportation needs is not expensive (in the U.S.). The idea that people have only a liberty right to a car—they are free to buy one if they can—and not a positive right to a car—no one has an obligation to provide them with the means to buy a car—seems to be universal among industrialized societies.[8]

Just as universal is the belief that we have social obligations to meet medical needs. For the sake of specificity, consider one way to ground such a claim. On this view, our social obligation to meet medical needs follows from a more general obligation, namely, our obligation to assure people *fair equality of opportunity*. Health care makes a distinctive but limited contribution to assuring fair equality of opportunity by aiming to keep people functioning as closely to normal as possible.[9] The point

7. Despite the failure of the Clinton effort at universal coverage and the recent elimination of entitlement status to Medicaid, survey evidence still points to widespread support for universal coverage in the U.S., and we should be wary of drawing inferences about the decline of support from the complex political events involved in welfare reform and the failure of health care reform. See Daniels, Light, and Caplan, *Benchmarks of Fairness for Health Care Reform*, Chapter 2.

8. A possible exception might be people with physical disabilities, though we generally see our obligation to them as requiring that existing transportation for others be accessible to them.

9. Formal equality of opportunity (careers open to talents) prohibits legal or quasi-legal barriers to access to jobs and offices. Equality of fair opportunity corrects for socially induced disadvantages in the development of talents and skills that result from social practices such as racism, sexism, or significant inequalities in family background. See John Rawls, *A Theory of Justice* (Cambridge, Mass.: Harvard University Press, 1971), pp. 65ff. By subsuming health care under the fair equality of opportunity principle, Daniels extends Rawls' principle and theory. See Norman Daniels, *Just Health Care* (New York: Cambridge University Press, 1985), Chapter 3.

is that disease and disability restrict the range of opportunities that would otherwise be open to healthy people, whereas health care protects that range of opportunities. Since health care is not the only important social good, and since resources are limited, we must discharge our obligation to keep people functioning normally within reasonable resource constraints, aiming to protect a defined population with varied needs as best we can.

This characterization of our obligation to meet health care needs makes it clear that limit-setting decisions are themselves a requirement of justice, since we cannot meet all legitimate needs with limited resources and rapidly improving technologies. This implies that, *properly done*, the limit-setting decisions of MCOs may further, not oppose, the interests of justice. These limit-setting decisions, however, involve important issues of distributive justice. Both winners and losers from those decisions have some legitimate or principled claim to assistance. Because matters of distributive justice are at issue, however, the limit-setting decisions and the grounds for them must be publicly accessible.

This publicity and accountability requirement holds whether the decisions are made by public agencies managing a public insurance scheme or by private corporations to which society delegates the responsibility for organizing both the delivery and reimbursement of services. Regardless of the mechanism for organizing and reimbursing these services, justice requires that they be distributed fairly, and *there is no way to assure that outcome without requiring that limit-setting decisions and their rationales be public and be challengeable by those affected by them.*

Consider an objection to this point about accountability. Justice requires the fair distribution of health care resources, and in a mixed public and private system, this requires a careful and explicit division and delegation of responsibilities. In our system, private corporations organizing and delivering health care have not been delegated specific obligations requiring them to deliver health care fairly and accountably. Without such a specification of responsibility, we cannot say that private corporations have an obligation to behave differently with regard to health care than they do with regard to automobiles. Without specifying their obligations for accountability, we cannot say they violate them.[10]

10. Daniels argues that the fact that we have social obligations to provide universal coverage for medical needs does not imply that individual physicians have some specific

313 *Limits to Health Care*

The objection misses the point. True, a mixed public and private system that aims at the just distribution of health care must delegate responsibilities and assign explicit obligations. We are not, however, trying to assign blame to health plans for failure to meet a previously, socially specified obligation, since no such specification was made. Instead, we are trying to show what the socially specified obligations of private corporations should be in order for us to be assured that health care is fairly distributed. We focus on reform, on what ought to be, not on blame, on what ought to have been.

Where private organizations distribute a fundamental good on society's behalf, as in the case of health care, simply behaving like a responsible corporation that meets high but ordinary ethical standards is not enough. By itself, that standard is insufficient to assure justice. In a just system with mixed public and private institutions, even the private institutions must be publicly accountable and provide rationales for decisions that affect the distribution of health care.

Critics of Publicity

This requirement of publicity is not without its critics. Public limit-setting decisions have their costs: they involve openly favoring some claims against others, possibly in life-or-death situations, and we can expect losers—whoever they are—to have little to lose by fighting the decision. So one claim is that public decision-making will be infeasible. The costs of publicity may also include threatening some public values. In a celebrated book, Calabrese and Bobbit argue that the costs may include eroding public values, such as the sanctity of life, and that somewhat more indirect methods of decision-making might accomplish the same distribution but without the public costs.[11] In effect, the argument is that nonpublic rationing methods are sometimes morally superior to public ones, when we weigh all costs and benefits.

set of obligations to treat all needy patients (Daniels, *Just Health Care*, pp. 115–19). Similarly, insurers who legally exclude high-risk patients from coverage are not to be blamed for violating an obligation of justice, even if the exclusion of these patients is unjust (see Norman Daniels, *Seeking Fair Treatment: From the AIDS Epidemic to National Health Care Reform* (New York: Oxford University Press, 1995), Chapter 4). The obligation here is society's, not the corporations'. But the social obligation means that collective action must be taken to specify the obligations of individual practitioners and corporations, modifying "business as usual" if that is needed to produce just outcomes.

11. Guido Calabrese and Philip Bobbit, *Tragic Choices* (New York: Norton, 1978); see also Jon Elster, *Local Justice: How Institutions Allocate Scarce Goods and Necessary Burdens* (New York: Russell Sage, 1992).

These objections deserve a more careful reply than can be given here, but enough has been said to offer an adequate response. To the charge that publicity is infeasible there is the reply that nonpublicity is also infeasible for reasons we have already cited. It does not work. The public is too suspicious, especially of private organizations, and especially of for-profit ones. As a result, all decisions are viewed with skepticism and opposed through litigation or even legislation. Whereas nonpublicity has been tried and failed, however, publicity has not been seriously attempted.

To the charge that nonpublicity is morally preferable to publicity because it better preserves certain public values, the reply must be that nonpublicity seems to undercut the public sense that fairness obtains in the system. The cynicism and suspicion we noted earlier must be weighed against the alternative scenario. If publicity obtains and it establishes a necessary condition for public acceptance of limit setting, provided it is done fairly (and legitimately), then the social fabric is better protected than through nonpublicity. Again, whereas nonpublicity has been tried and failed (as a solution to the fairness and legitimacy problems), little effort has been made to see what effects publicity produces.

What would it mean to say that publicity "worked" whereas nonpublicity for limit-setting decisions "failed"? We can recast this as the following question: Under what conditions should the public begin to view MCOs as a legitimate locus for making limit-setting decisions? We answer this question in Section IV.

III. Moral Disagreements and the Need for Fair Procedures

Comparative vs. Noncomparative Decisions

Currently, MCOs make decisions to provide coverage for new technologies *noncomparatively*, that is, solely by considering whether or not there is adequate evidence that a new technology meets reasonable criteria for safety and efficacy and whether there are other social, legal, or market reasons for covering it. In effect, only one new technology is on the table for consideration at a time. Decision-makers judge only whether the new technology is at least as good as the standard alternative for the same condition. In a more resource-constrained environment, for example, where a budget restricts the introduction of new treatments, *comparative* decisions would be necessary. Decision-makers would have to compare several new technologies aimed at treating quite different conditions with each other, evaluating their respective "opportunity costs" by asking what the next-best use of limited resources would be for each.

Both kinds of coverage decision involve moral considerations about which there is considerable disagreement. The noncomparative decisions raise disagreements about issues with which we are more familiar, though they remain difficult. The comparative ones MCOs may someday make raise moral problems that we have even less idea how to solve. Both kinds of problem must be resolved in real time. The need to resolve these disagreements requires an appeal to fair procedures.

Noncomparative Decisions: Moral Disagreement and the Case of Last Chance Therapies

To illustrate the kind of moral controversy raised by current, noncomparative coverage decisions, consider the highly visible, politicized controversy surrounding coverage for high-dose chemotherapy with bone marrow transplant for advanced breast cancer. Assume, for the sake of argument, that the therapy remains unproven ("investigational") despite legislative mandates in some states requiring provision of the treatment and despite some lawsuits holding MCOs liable for not providing it. Specifically, assume that the kind of criteria used by the Medical Advisory Panel (MAP) of the national Technology Evaluation Center of Blue Cross/ Blue Shield, calling for scientific evidence of a net benefit, are not met.[12]

Strong moral arguments with different conclusions about coverage

12. The MAP criteria are as follows:

a. The technology must have final approval from the appropriate government regulatory body.

b. The scientific evidence must permit conclusions concerning the effect of the technology on health outcomes.

c. The technology must improve the net health outcome.

d. The technology must be as beneficial as any established alternative.

e. The improvement must be attainable outside the investigational settings.

MAP does not make coverage decisions, however; MCOs do. A South African study (WR. Bezwoda, L. Seymour, RD. Dansey, "High-dose Chemotherapy with Hematopoietic Rescue as Primary Treatment for Metastatic Breast Cancer: A Randomized Trial," *Journal of Clinical Oncology* 13 [1995]: 2483–89), the only published randomized clinical trial available as of mid-1966, used as its control a regimen of standard chemotherapy that was inferior in outcomes to the conventional therapy that would standardly be available in the U.S.

can still be made. Two arguments against coverage, or for supporting coverage only for those in approved clinical trials, might go like this: (1) MCOs will undermine the generation of a public good if they approve coverage outside clinical trials, since too many people will fail to register for trials if they have the option of receiving the unproven therapy (rather than only a fifty-percent chance of receiving it in a randomized control trial);[13] (2) in addition, MCOs must protect the reasonable rationing principle, embodied in contract language, which says there is no obligation to offer unproven or investigational treatments, since protecting that principle is a way to assure overall better use of resources in producing medical benefits for all covered patients.

Both of these arguments rest on patient-centered values and reasons, though they address the needs of a population of patients, not just those requesting this treatment. Even patients or clinicians who wanted the therapy would have to agree that these kinds of considerations are weighty and reasonable, even if they did not agree with the specific coverage decision. Of course, the patients or clinicians might still think these are not the real reasons for denial and that the MCO is simply hiding behind them to postpone having to cover expensive new treatments. Leaving the issue of trust aside, however, these arguments must be addressed.

Despite these arguments, some MCOs, such as Aetna (in a 1991 program that may have been modified after its purchase of US Health Care) and Kaiser-Permanente of Northern California, have adopted an alternative approach to "last chance" therapies of this sort. They allow patients who want an unproven therapy to bring their requests before a panel of medical specialists, or before a medical director's committee, for review. If the panel or committee still rejects the request, they can appeal to a panel of experts that is independent of the MCO, thus avoiding the appearance of any conflict of interest in the decision-making. (In the original Aetna plan, medical directors who said "no" to a last-chance request triggered an external review.) The MCO agrees to abide by the decision of a majority of the outside panel.

For these MCOs, the real issue is to make sure the patient fully under-

and elsewhere. Consequently, it should not persuade us of the superior efficacy of the high-dose regimen. Using the same criteria, Blue Shield of Northern California judged the therapy "investigational" even after the national MAP voted the opposite.

13. See Norman Daniels, *Seeking Fair Treatment*, Chapter 5.

stands the risks and benefits, given the uncertainty about the procedure. In practice, MCOs using such a process report that once there is no blanket denial of coverage, a better discussion can take place with patients. The use of an independent panel is also obviously intended to counter distrust and to disarm the suspicion that a denial is tainted by a conflict of interest. Patients who had been adamant about wanting an experimental procedure may then feel freer to decide about its risks and benefits for them and often decide it is not for them after all.

The "last chance" policy might simply be dismissed as a cost-benefit calculation made by the MCO. Put cynically, it is better to pay for a few treatments than face lawsuits, any one of which would be more costly than several treatments. The "last chance" policy can also be defended—and is by some MCOs that adopt it—on more explicitly moral grounds.

A moral defense of the policy recognizes the fundamental importance in a medical system of "shared decision-making" between patients and clinicians about risk-taking. If a "last chance" (unproven) therapy is viewed by some acknowledged experts as the most appropriate treatment for the patient, and if the patient understands the risks as presented by parties on all sides, then organizations have no better option than to rely on the informed decision of the patient and her clinician. This is not the same as saying that a patient can be granted just any last wish regarding treatment: there must be some basis in evidence and expert view that the therapy is not quackery. Under those conditions, refusing to provide coverage fails to acknowledge the obligation not to impose paternalistically on the choices of desperately ill patients with few options.

The MCO still remains a guardian of shared resources, but, on this view, because the patient's need is so urgent in these life-and-death situations, the obligation to seek a climate of shared decision-making is given greater weight than the obligation to conserve resources. To see the point, suppose a patient made a claim for a non-last-chance treatment that was still investigational. She might then be told, "we are not giving you the treatment because we are devoting resources to those for whom the unproven treatment is really a last chance; their needs are more urgent than yours." The disappointed member would still have to recognize the force of the reason behind the denial. A proponent of the strategy might also say that taking a hard line against last-chance therapies is so likely to lead to a waste of resources in the legal and political climate surrounding MCOs that the more efficient way to respect resources is to be more lenient toward last-chance therapies.

Both positions—holding the line and adopting a last-chance policy—can be defended by plausible moral arguments. This appears to be a matter about which reasonable moral agents can and do disagree. In fact, the reasons that are advanced to support each position can be tied to comprehensive moral views. For example, one such view might give more weight to guarding collective resources and maximizing health benefits for a community. Another may give more weight to respect for individual autonomy. Each, however, recognizes the relevance of the reasons to which the other gives priority, since in other contexts, these factors also count as reasons. Since disputes about such moral issues must be resolved in real time, a fair procedure must be adopted for resolving them. Of course, it remains to be seen just what counts as a fair procedure for resolving this kind of dispute in this sort of institution.

Moral Controversy and Unsolved Rationing Problems

With continuing pressures to lower premiums in a highly competitive environment, it may become necessary for MCOs to examine the relative importance of new technologies, that is, to make comparative judgments about their opportunity costs and to pursue some methodology for establishing priorities among types of services covered. (Some uses of cost-effectiveness analysis purport to provide a technology for examining opportunity costs, but there are moral objections to the adequacy of that technology for this general purpose.[14]) In effect, on this scenario, MCOs will have to follow the state of Oregon's lead from the early 1990s. The Oregon Health Services Commission (OHSC) was charged with establishing priorities among covered services for the new Oregon Health Plan, which was to cover all Medicaid patients and state employees as well.

Setting priorities among services that provide different sorts of benefits to different groups of patients will involve taking a stand on a family

14. See Marthe Gold, Joanna Siegel, Louise Russell, and Milton Weinstein, *Cost-Effectiveness in Health and Medicine* (New York: Oxford University Press, 1966), Chapter 1. Also see Norman Daniels, "Rationing Fairly: Programmatic Considerations," *Bioethics* 7 (1993): 223–33, reprinted in Norman Daniels, *Justice and Justification: Reflective Equilibrium in Theory and Practice* (Cambridge: Cambridge University Press, 1996), pp. 317–27.

of unsolved rationing problems.[15] These problems share these features: (a) they arise when a scarce resource is "lumpy" in the sense that it cannot be divided to meet the needs of those who could benefit from it; (b) those competing for it can legitimately claim they are owed it in principle, e.g., because they all have a legitimate medical need that it could in part satisfy; (c) the general principles of distributive justice that give us some guidance about the fair allocation of health care services are too indeterminate to tell us how to establish priorities among claimants; and (d) in part because of (c), there will be moral disagreements about how to establish priorities among claimants in order to ration these services. Since these disputes also will require practical resolution, MCOs will have to develop fair procedures for addressing them of just the sort they already need for noncomparative coverage decisions about new technologies.

Priorities Problem. To illustrate the kind of moral controversy that surrounds these unsolved rationing problems, consider first what we shall call the "priorities problem": How much priority should we give to treating the sickest or most disabled patients? To start with, imagine two extreme positions. The Maximin position ("maximize the minimum") says that we should give complete priority to treating the worst-off patients. The Maximize position says that we should give priority to whatever treatment produces the greatest net health benefit (or greatest net health benefit per dollar spent), regardless of which patients we treat. Suppose comparable resources could be invested in Technology A or in B, but the resources are "lumpy" (we cannot introduce some A and some B) and we can only afford one of A or B in our MCO budget. The Maximin position would settle the matter by determining whether patients treated by A are worse off before treatment than patients treated by B. If so, we introduce A; if patients treated by B are worse off, we introduce B. If the two sets of patients are equally badly off, we can break the tie by considering whom we can provide the most benefit. The Maximize position chooses between A and B solely by reference to which produces greatest net benefit.

In practice, most people are likely to reject both extreme positions.[16]

15. See Daniels, "Rationing Fairly," pp. 223–33.

16. The claim is based on observations over several years of how audiences of students and medical personal vote on hypothetical cases of this sort. Eric Nord has reported variations in attitudes toward priorities of this sort between different groups of students and

If the benefits A and B produce are nearly equal, but patients needing A start off much worse than patients needing B, most people seem to believe we should introduce A.[17] They prefer to provide A even if they know we could produce somewhat more net health benefit by introducing B. But if the net benefit produced by A is very small, or if B produces significantly more net benefit, then most people will overcome their concern to give priority to the worst off and will prefer to introduce B to A. Some people who would give priority to patients needing A temper their preference if those patients end up faring much better than patients needing B. In all situations where groups of students or health professionals have been informally polled on these cases, there is considerable disagreement: a definite but very small minority are inclined to be maximizers and a definite but very small minority are inclined to be maximiners. Most people fall in between, and they vary considerably in how much benefit they are willing to sacrifice in order to give priority to worse-off patients.

Disputants about these hypotheticals are quite willing to back their conclusions with reasons. Some will say, for example, "although patients needing B are being asked to forgo a significant benefit, I simply cannot turn my back on patients needing A, since they are so badly off." In response, someone else will say, "I hate to abandon A, but I simply cannot expect B to sacrifice a much greater benefit just because A starts off so poorly."

We might hope, faced with this kind of complexity, that a very careful examination of hypothetical cases might reveal some convergence on a

professionals. See Eric Nord, "The Relevance of Health State After Treatment in Prioritising between Different Patients," *Journal of Medical Ethics* 19 (1993): 37–42. There is some cross-national evidence that people are not straight maximizers in Eric Nord, Jeff Richardson, Andrew Street, Helga Kuhse, and Peter Singer, "Maximizing Health Benefits vs Egalitarianism: An Australian Survey of Health Issues," *Social Science and Medicine* 41, no. 10 (1995): 1429–37.

17. A distinct minority of students and health professionals would argue as follows: if helping the less-sick patient actually returns her to a level of functioning that permits her to work and carry out other social activities, whereas helping the sicker patient does not accomplish this outcome, then it is more important to help the healthier patient. Some holding this view reason that the healthier patient will then return more to society, but others justify their view by saying the healthier patient is likely to be happier than the sicker one, focusing only on the relative well-being of the patients, not on their social contribution.

complex set of underlying principles.[18] This hope, however, may be unrealistic. The weightings that different people give to different moral concerns, such as helping the worst off versus not sacrificing achievable medical benefits, probably depend on how these moral concerns fit within wider moral conceptions people hold. If so, there is good reason to think these disagreements will be a persistent feature of the situation. Indeed, some of the kinds of theoretical devices we might appeal to, such as forcing people to choose an allocation scheme from behind a veil of ignorance, are themselves the focus of considerable dispute. Is it reasonable, for example, for such people to gamble on their likelihood of being one type of patient or the other, or must they somehow identify with each category of patients and refuse to gamble?[19]

Two other types of rationing problems, which we cannot discuss here, also suggest we are not straight maximizers, though we lack principled characterizations of acceptable solutions. The Fair Chances / Best Outcomes Problem asks, Should we give all who might benefit some chance at a resource, or should we give the resource to those who get the best outcome? The Aggregation problem asks, When do lesser benefits to many outweigh greater benefits to a few?

Moral Controversy and Fair Procedures

The best outcomes/fair chances, priorities, and aggregation problems may turn out to have principled solutions on which consensus can be established. Our claim here is not that they are unsolvable but only that they are unsolved now and that we have no real prospect of arriving at solutions that would be publicly acceptable in the foreseeable future. Our skepticism about any rapid solution in part rests on the fact that these are all problems on which there is moral disagreement. Such dis-

18. Frances Kamm suggests this may be true. Her brilliant discussion of cases often points to less disagreement than we find in thinking about them with students or public audiences. See Frances Kamm, *Morality and Mortality*, Volume 1: *Death and Whom to Save From It* (New York: Oxford University Press, 1993). For some concerns about her methods, see Norman Daniels, "Kamm's Moral Methods" forthcoming in *Philosophy and Phenomenological Research*.

19. See Daniels, "Rationing Fairly," pp. 226–27; Kamm, *Morality and Mortality*, Chapter 12; and T. M. Scanlon, "Contractualism and Utilitarianism," in Amartya Sen and Bernard Williams, *Utilitarianism and Beyond* (Cambridge: Cambridge University Press, 1982), pp. 103–28.

agreement emerges quickly in class or group settings where hypothetical cases are discussed in detail. Eric Nord has found that different subgroups of the Norwegian population, for example, those who identified themselves as members of different political parties, tend to have systematically different responses to these problems.[20] When the Swedish government set up a commission to select principles for establishing priorities in its health care system, the commission gave great weight to helping the sickest or most disabled individuals, probably more weight than other societies considering the same question (or many of my students) would give.

Even if there are principled solutions that philosophical investigation may eventually uncover, there is considerable disagreement now about how to solve these problems. Typically, for example, a minority will be willing to give significant priority to the sickest patients, trading away much more significant benefits to those who are less sick in order to obtain some benefits for the sickest (as was the Swedish commission), but the majority is not. These commitments support two distinct criteria for ranking (or rationing) various kinds of treatments that might be applied to the very sick or the mildly sick. Each group is willing to provide reasons for its belief about the correct solution. How should we decide among policies when there is this kind of disagreement in underlying moral commitment?

We recast the question posed at the end of Section II so that it explicitly reflects the concern about moral controversy discussed in this section: under what conditions should the public come to view MCOs as a legitimate locus for making limit-setting decisions, given the moral controversies they involve? That is, under what conditions should they be viewed as an appropriate or acceptable authority for resolving these sorts of moral questions, at least for purposes of establishing public policy?

IV. Reason-Giving and Fair Procedures

Four Conditions

If the following four conditions were satisfied, we would take a giant step toward solving the problems of distrust, legitimacy, and fairness that face MCOs:

20. Personal communication and presentation at the Stockholm Conference on Priorities in Health Care, October 17, 1996.

1. Decisions regarding coverage for new technologies (and other limit-setting decisions) and their rationales must be publicly accessible.
2. The rationales for coverage decisions should aim to provide a *reasonable* construal of how the organization should provide "value for money" in meeting the varied health needs of a defined population under reasonable resource constraints. Specifically, a construal will be "reasonable" if it appeals to reasons and principles that are accepted as relevant by people who are disposed to finding terms of cooperation that are mutually justifiable.
3. There is a mechanism for challenge and dispute resolution regarding limit-setting decisions, including the opportunity for revising decisions in light of further evidence or arguments.
4. There is either voluntary or public regulation of the process to ensure that conditions 1–3 are met.

These four conditions capture the essential elements in achieving legitimate and fair coverage decisions about new treatments. (To cover limit-setting more broadly, they would have to include accountability about clinician-incentive arrangements, guidelines, and decisions about implementing all of these.) Condition 1 requires openness or publicity, that is, transparency about reasons for a decision. Condition 2 involves some constraints on the kinds of reasons that can play a role in the rationale: it recognizes the fundamental interest all parties have in finding a justification all can accept as reasonable. Conditions 3 and 4 provide mechanisms for connecting deliberation and decisions within MCOs to a broader deliberative process, that is, for making them accountable to the results of a wider deliberation about what fairness requires.[21]

Before developing a case for these conditions in turn, it is worth discussing their collective effect and joint rationale. The guiding idea behind them is to convert private MCO solutions to problems of limit setting into part of a larger public deliberation about a major, unsolved

21. These conditions were developed independently but fit reasonably well with the principles of publicity, reciprocity, and accountability governing democratic deliberation cited by Amy Gutmann and Dennis Thompson, *Democracy and Disagreement* (Cambridge, Mass.: Harvard University Press, 1996). For reservations about their account, see Norman Daniels, "Enabling Democratic Deliberation," Pacific Division of the American Philosophical Association, March 28, 1997.

public policy problem. This problem, how to use limited resources to protect fairly the health of a population with varied needs, is made progressively more difficult by the successes of medical science and technology. In the U.S., it is especially difficult because our system enrolls people among competing insurers, rather than among politically meaningful cooperative ventures, such as districts or provinces, which must share various resources to solve common problems.

If the U.S. had a publicly financed health care system, as in Canada, Great Britain, and many European countries, Americans might think that the way to address this problem is to do what the Netherlands and Sweden have done, namely, form public commissions to frame general principles to be followed in setting priorities among health needs and services. There is good reason to believe, however, that general principles of distributive justice and general characterizations of the goals of medicine[22] cannot really address the problems of setting priorities in ways that satisfy our moral concerns in particular cases, or so we suggested in the previous section (see also Section VI). Rather, we must agree on how to make the practical decisions about limits that arise at various levels within both purely public and mixed public and private delivery systems. Oregon had to face this problem of reconciling general approaches with the difficulties involved in particular decisions. It developed a public process, but it had to revise its methodology several times, shifting, for example, away from cost-effectiveness rankings, to rankings by categories of benefits, to much more subtle adjustments and deliberations about their appropriateness. It is unclear whether any general principles really characterize the process or outcomes that resulted in the Oregon procedure. In many cases, the process ended up with commissioners making fairly specific choices in response to arguments and evidence about the rankings of particular services.

Since the U.S. health care system is a mixed public and private one, key decisions will be made by private institutions that reimburse and organize the delivery of services for specific groups of patients. The four conditions we describe convert those otherwise private and localized decisions into part of a larger public deliberation about acceptable solu-

22. See Hastings Center, "Goals of Medicine: Setting New Priorities," in *Hastings Center Report* 26:6 (November–December, 1966): S1–S28, Special Supplement; see also Norman Daniels, "Justice, Fair Procedures, and the Goals of Medicine," *Hastings Center Report* 26:6 (November–December 1966): 10–12.

tions to these problems of setting limits. There are reasons to believe that keeping the focus of problem solving within delivery systems may yield more coherent and defensible practices in the end than proclamations by public commissions—provided these delivery systems are properly connected to a broader public deliberation and provided the results of that deliberation can modify or constrain the decisions made within particular elements of the delivery system. If met, these conditions help these private institutions to enable or empower a more focused public deliberation that involves broader democratic institutions. They may indeed be a model for how solutions should be approached even in public systems. The broader public deliberation we envision here is not necessarily an organized democratic procedure, though it could include the deliberation underlying public regulation of the health care system. Rather, it may take place in various forms in an array of institutions, spilling over into legislative politics only under some circumstances.[23]

For private health care institutions to acquire legitimacy for their limit-setting decisions they must see themselves, and be seen by others, as contributors to a broader deliberative process that they constructively embrace. The four conditions contribute to solving the legitimacy and fairness problems by placing MCOs visibly in that role. By embracing these conditions and the way in which they connect internal decisions to broader, public deliberation, many of these organizations would reach beyond the dominant perceptions they have of their own organizational and (in many cases) "corporate" culture, for it makes them accountable to more than their own boards of directors and in more ways than they are accountable to stockholders (if they have them). In an intensely competitive environment, embracing these conditions may be easier for associations of organizations than for individual MCOs, though there may also be demonstrable market value to having a visible record of commitment to patient-oriented decision-making.

Condition 1: Publicly Accessible Rationales

The first condition requires that rationales for decisions, e.g., about coverage for new technologies, be publicly accessible, that is, to clinicians,

23. See Joshua Cohen and Charles Sobel, "Directly Deliberative Polyarchy," *European Law Journal* (forthcoming), for a discussion of the value of democratic deliberation in decentralized institutions that converges with points we make here.

patients, and would-be subscribers. To see what this condition means in practice, consider how one leading MCO disseminated its coverage decision for biosynthetic growth hormone (in 1993). In a Medical Director's Letter distributed to all clinicians, the policy stated that growth hormone treatment would be covered (for those with a contractual drug benefit) only for children with growth hormone deficiency or Turner's syndrome. No explanation was offered for the restrictions in coverage to the categories of patients noted. We compared this coverage statement to those made by several other MCOs: they placed similar coverage restrictions on growth hormone treatment and also failed to say why.

Why insist that the rationale for limitations on coverage, and not simply the decisions themselves, be made public, for example, in an instrument such as the Medical Director's Letter? The point of offering the rationale is made clearer when we imagine the parents of a child projected to have very short stature who want the treatment but whose child does not fit the patient-selection criteria. What can be said to them that would make the limitation seem nonarbitrary and based on reasons that take into account the patients' welfare?

When the committee of the MCO charged with making a coverage decision originally made its decision, it deliberated quite carefully about two reasons for the restrictions, drawing on literature reviews and expert opinions. First, growth hormone therapy had not been shown to be effective in increasing ultimate adult height in short children who were not deficient in growth hormone. Second, apart from the hormone's effectiveness, the committee considered that while extreme short stature may be disadvantageous, without growth hormone deficiency it should not be considered an illness and therefore is not eligible for "treatment" in the insurance benefit package.

A failure to be clear about these reasons in either coverage committee minutes or the disseminated coverage decision has important consequences. The first reason has obvious relevance for anxious parents, but if efficacy were later demonstrated, and the second reason were not explicit and explicitly defended, then it might seem that coverage would have to be provided. The distinction between treatments for disease or disability and therapies that enhance otherwise normal traits is crucial in other coverage decisions, and so ought to be explicitly defended. For example, it is central in decisions about coverage for donor oocyte IVF for post-menopausal women and in restrictions on breast reduction surgery. Consequently, explicitness about the underlying reasoning can demonstrate the coherence and consistency of an overall policy toward coverage. It can demonstrate a commitment to the even-handed appeal to reasons and principles, so that relevant similarities and differences in particular cases are recognized and attended to.

Analogy to Case Law. One important effect of making public the reasons for coverage decisions is that, over time, the pattern of such decisions will resemble a type of "case law." The virtues of a case-law model will help us see that the benefits of the publicity requirements of Condition 1 are both internal to MCOs committed to it, leading to more efficient, coherent, and fairer decisions over time, and external, since the emerging "case law" will strengthen broader public deliberation and contribute to the perceived legitimacy of the decision-makers.

One important requirement of fairness is that similar cases be dealt with similarly and that differential treatment requires relevant reasons. A body of case law establishes the presumption that if some individuals have been treated one way because they fall under a reasonable interpretation of the relevant principles, then similar individuals should be treated the same way in subsequent cases. The earlier decision reflects a *commitment* to act on the cited reasons and principles in future similar cases. There is a presumption of respect for the weight of earlier, reason-based deliberation about a case.

There are two ways to rebut this presumption that a subsequent case should be treated similarly to an earlier one. The least disruptive rebuttal involves showing that the new case differs in relevant and important ways from the earlier one, justifying different treatment. A much more disruptive rebuttal would involve rejecting the reasons or principles embodied in the earlier case. Sometimes such a revision of past policy is justifiable and required. The respect for past commitments embodied in case-law does not mean that past errors of judgments cannot be corrected with due deliberation. Case-law does not imply past infallibility, but it does imply giving careful consideration to why earlier decision-makers would have made the choices they did. Since treating a new case differently from a (similar) old one thus involves acknowledging a change and perhaps an earlier error in policy, the case-law model demands a clear rationale and new avowal of principles and commitments in order to avoid the appearance of inconsistency or deliberate unfairness in treatment.

Case-law thus involves a form of institutional reflective equilibrium. The considered judgments reflected in past decisions constitute relatively fixed points that can be revised only with careful deliberation and good reasons. Overall, there is a commitment to coherence in the giving of reasons—decisions must fit with each other in a plausible reason- and principle-mediated way. Through its reasoning in cases, an institution exhibits its moral commitments in a relatively transparent way.

A commitment to the transparency that case-law requires improves the quality of decision-making. An organization whose practice requires it to articulate explicit reasons for its decisions becomes focused in its decision-making. It might, for example, develop a "checklist" of key features of coverage decisions, such as the specification of patient-selection criteria, and relevant reasons for those criteria, such as the limits of evidence from clinical trials or the range of patients for whom risk-benefit ratios are acceptable. The committee deliberating about coverage is better able to notice the relationship between one decision and others it has made or will have to make. It may become more sensitive to the ways in which the reasons or principles it often invokes sometimes conflict. Then it must engage in a difficult deliberation about how to resolve the conflict and articulate the reasons for the particular resolution.[24]

The disciplined search for coherent reasons embodied in such a case-law approach leads to fairer decisions over time for two reasons. First, formal requirements of fairness are better met since there is consistent treatment of similar cases. Second, the discipline involved in specifying the appropriate reasons and making sure they really bear on the case promotes thoughtful evaluation of these reasons and their foundations within our thinking. To the extent that we are then better able to discover flaws in our moral reasoning, we are more likely to reach fair decisions.

If the process improves formally and substantively the fairness of decisions, then over time people will understand better the moral commit-

24. Frederick Schauer notes that "decisionmakers themselves are unlikely to fully apprehend and appreciate this function [that reason-giving increases discipline], for most decisionmakers underestimate the need for external quality control of their own decisions. But when institutional designers have grounds for believing that decisions will systematically be the product of bias, self-interest, insufficient reflection, or simply excess haste, requiring decisionmakers to give reasons may counteract some of these tendencies." Frederick Shauer, "Giving Reasons," *Stanford Law Review* 47, no. 4 (1995): 633–59, at 657.

ments of the institutions making these decisions. If an institution is committed to arriving at fair decisions in a publicly accountable way, then people should acknowledge that commitment to acting fairly, and, we may suppose, they will over time come to see the institution as acting (more) fairly. Only by being explicit about reasons will it be possible for MCOs to demonstrate that the solutions they adopt to coverage under resource constraints reflect a pattern of reasons and principles that all affected by those decisions must take seriously.

Condition 2: Constraints on Rationales

The second condition imposes two important constraints on the rationales that are made publicly accessible. Specifically, the rationales for coverage decisions should aim to provide (a) a *reasonable* construal of (b) how the organization (or society) should provide "value for money" in meeting the varied health needs of a defined population under reasonable resource constraints. Both constraints need explanation.

Providers and patients alike may be considered to pursue the *common or public good* of meeting the varied needs of the population of patients within reasonable resource contraints. This goal is avowed in mission statements and marketing by many MCOs, whether they are for-profit or not. It is avowed by the clinicians engaged in treatment, who have professional obligations to pursue their patients' best interests. Finally, it is avowed by patients seeking care, who want their needs met but also want a cooperative scheme that provides affordable, nonwasteful care.

It is not enough simply to specify the goal of the cooperative enterprise. Reasoning about that goal must also meet certain conditions. Specifically, a construal of the goal will be "reasonable" only if it appeals to reasons, including values and principles, that *are accepted as relevant* by people who are disposed to finding mutually justifiable terms of cooperation. We need to see why this further constraint on reasoning is necessary to be more specific about what it means.

We can begin by asking why reason-giving is appropriate or even demanded in some legal contexts but not others. For example, no reasons are given when juries give verdicts, when state supreme courts refuse review, when trial judges rule on objections, or zoning authorities refuse to grant variances. In his discussion of this question (the examples are his), Schauer notes that giving reasons (viewed as general rules under which cases are subsumed) is a way to show respect for persons and to "open a conversation" rather than to forestall one: "Announcing an outcome without giving a reason is consistent with the exercise of authority. . . . But when decisionmakers expect voluntary compliance, or when they expect respect for decisions because the decisions are right rather than because they emanate from an authoritative source, then giving reasons becomes a way to bring the subject of the decision into the enterprise."[25]

Since MCOs cannot claim to be an authoritative source—their legitimacy and the fairness of their decision-making is exactly what is at issue—to achieve acceptance and compliance, they must bring the subject of the decision "into the enterprise." The "conversation" the MCO has must be with others who have diverse moral perspectives on the issues under discussion. Consequently, the giving of reasons must itself respect the moral diversity of those affected by the decisions. Not just any kind of moral reason, compelling as it might be to the decision-maker (or the patient), will command recognition of its appropriateness or relevance from those affected by the decision. The reasons offered by decision-makers must be the types of reasons those affected by the decisions can recognize as relevant and appropriate for the purpose of justifying decisions to all who are affected by them.

How the Constraints Limit Reasons. Perhaps the most widely used criteria in MCO technology assessment are those adopted by the Blue Cross/Blue Shield MAP (see note 12) as well as by other commercial technology assessment organizations and many MCOs. Each of them involves a publicly accessible method of reasoning. Thus it is easy to establish that a technology has final approval from appropriate regulatory bodies or to establish that controlled clinical trials have been run and show some net health benefit. Adequately trained reviewers can usually readily agree on the quality of the evidence produced by the available studies or expert panels. Showing that the treatment involves a net benefit to patients and that there is at least as much net benefit as an alternative therapy also involves publicly accessible methods of reasoning, though some further elements of judgment that include evaluation are also involved. There might be some disagreement, for example, about the relative importance of the benefits and risks that attend the

25. Schauer, "Giving Reasons," p. 658.

treatment, but then it will be clear just what is at issue. Nevertheless, these criteria are ones that all must accept as relevant and appropriate—if not sufficient—for making decisions about the inclusion of new technologies in benefit packages.

To see their appropriateness more clearly, contrast these criteria with a reason that a religious patient (or clinician) might offer to justify a claim that a treatment be covered. Imagine that her religion requires her to pursue every avenue for survival and that some technology that fails to meet the MAP criteria nevertheless might turn out, she believes, to be the occasion for a miraculous cure. Compelling though this reasoning might be to the patient, it has no relevance at all for those who lack the appropriate faith. The patient (or clinician) advancing it must recognize that she cannot expect those who do not share her faith to give weight to this type of reason or to consider it relevant to the deliberation. In contrast, even this religious patient—as opposed, say, to a Christian Scientist—will recognize the relevance of the MAP criteria that bear on establishing the net benefit of the treatment. She is seeking a form of justification that all involved can see is relevant to the common good they pursue, the meeting of patient needs under resource constraints. People whose religious beliefs preclude pursuit of standard medical treatments would not be involved in offering or seeking justification about the inclusion of treatments within the benefit package. They would avoid the cooperative endeavor altogether.

This appeal to the miraculous should be distinguished from disagreements about how to address uncertainty, as in the moral controversy regarding "last chance" therapies that we discussed in Section III. There we argued that there is more than one "reasonable" way to manage uncertainty, reflecting more than one way of weighing the importance of the stewardship of scarce resources, the generation of public goods, and the meeting of urgent patient needs. Consequently, MCOs might decide these matters differently and yet each be fair in what it concludes.

In our discussion of the importance of reason-giving (required by Condition 1), we argued that an MCO deciding to cover growth hormone treatment only for patients with growth hormone deficiency should provide an explicit rationale for that decision. In this case, the rationale restricts the goal of meeting patients' needs to the treatment of disease and disability and excludes the enhancement of otherwise normal conditions. This reason for excluding some therapies and limiting the use of others is controversial. Many may accept it as characterizing a reasonable limit on the goals of medical coverage, but others may argue that the goals of medical treatment should be broader.[26] For example, they might think that "normal" conditions still impose some competitive disadvantage, and if we have medical interventions that could ameliorate these disadvantages, we should use them. If we defend the treatment of disease and disability because doing so protects opportunity, then, they claim, we are committed to protecting opportunity by eliminating normal disadvantages as well.

Still, proponents on both sides of this dispute can recognize that reasonable people might disagree about the specific requirements of a principle protecting opportunity. Both sides of the dispute about the scope of the goals of medicine nevertheless must recognize the relevance and appropriateness of the kind of reason offered by the other, even if they disagree with the interpretation of the principle or the applications to which it is put.

Once MCOs begin to make comparative decisions about new technologies, the perception that the decision-making process produces winners and losers will become clearer. Patients who need treatments for which coverage is denied will legitimately complain that they are made worse off by the decision than others whose coverage decisions were favorable. What weight should we give to patients' complaints that they are made worse off than other patients by an unfavorable decision?

Clearly, any decision to cover a technology benefits some people, just as any decision to exclude a technology from coverage disadvantages other people (unless the technology would have been harmful to use). Every (comparative) decision will make some people better off and some worse off than they would be as a result of some other set of coverage decisions. Because comparative coverage decisions always advantage some and disadvantage others, mere advantage or disadvantage is not a relevant reason in debates about coverage.

There are, however, two sorts of reasons concerning relative advantage or disadvantage that all must consider relevant. First, if a coverage

26. See Daniels, *Justice and Justification*, Chapters 10 and 11; also Norman Daniels, "Growth Hormone Therapy for Short Stature: Can We Support the Treatment/Enhancement Distinction?" *Growth: Genetics and Hormones* 8, suppl. 1 (1992): 46–48.

decision disadvantages one patient more than others similar in all relevant ways, then this is a reason based on disadvantage that all must agree is relevant, since it violates formal requirements of justice that *similar* cases be treated similarly, as noted in our discussion of case-law. It points to morally objectionable arbitrariness in the outcome. In contrast, if the decision involves an appeal to (say) a lottery for purposes of patient selection, then there is a relevant difference in the winners and losers, namely, that they won or lost the lottery.

Second, if a coverage decision disadvantages someone (and others like him) more than anyone need be disadvantaged under alternatives available, then this too is a reason that all must consider relevant. Whereas the mere fact of being disadvantaged relative to others is a necessary feature of these situations, being disadvantaged more than anyone need be is not a necessary feature of the situation. It is the basis for a complaint that each person would want to be able to make were they to turn out to be the person so severely disadvantaged. Therefore, it is a reason that meets the constraints of Condition 2.

The Case of Costs: Cost Effectiveness. How should we view as a reason for excluding coverage the claim that a treatment "costs too much"?

A first point to note, surprising in the context of current distrust of MCOs, is that we saw little explicit discussion of costs in the context of technology assessment in our study of MCOs (though we did not examine drug formulary decisions, where there is evidence that costs play a more explicit role). Costs (or cost-effectiveness) are not included in the MAP criteria. Of course, a concern about overall magnitude of costs is likely to put a new technology on the agenda of an organization, but the decision-making process we observed involved little explicit discussion of costs. We even saw "expert panels" avoid explicit requests to consider "costs relative to benefits" (for example, in evaluating lung-volume-reduction surgery for chronic pulmonary disease), and we saw one committee decide to cover a very expensive drug (alglucerase) even for those not covered by a drug benefit.

There are strong reasons for MCOs to be leery of claiming that a beneficial technology is "too costly" in the current climate of public distrust. Saying that a new technology is "too costly" invites a demand for clarification, both internally to patients and clinicians and externally to would-be enrollees and the public at large. Some clarifications would be widely acceptable, but many others would not. For example, if there were an alternative technology for treating the same condition that had comparable net medical benefits but were less expensive, then "being too costly" should readily be accepted as a reason for rejecting the more expensive one. Presumably, all would accept avoiding unnecessary costs as a relevant reason.

Outside that simple case—same outcomes at lower cost—clarification of the claim that some technology is "too expensive" begins to enter controversial terrain. For example, if slightly greater net benefits were possible, especially in the form of decreased risk of death, but only with a much more expensive technology, there is considerable risk to being criticized for putting so direct a price on the value of life. The case of streptokinase and tissue plasminogen activator (TPA), used in dissolving clots in emergency treatment of coronary infarcts, is relevant. TPA, the much more expensive drug, has slightly better outcomes. The more expensive drug is more widely used in the U.S. than in Canada, where it was deemed cost-ineffective. More generally, though an MCO would rely on a properly conducted cost-effectiveness study to compare different strategies for treating or preventing the same condition, it currently would have little use for "league tables" ranking treatments for cost-effectiveness across wide disparities in the conditions involved.

A common sentiment revealed in our interviews with medical directors and managers in MCOs, especially those involved in technology assessment, is that it is a "societal" decision, not simply an MCO decision, to determine when producing a significant medical benefit is not "cost-worthy." Similarly, comparative decisions—that is, those comparing technologies for treating different conditions (see Section III)—would also involve judgments that they view as societal, not simply organizational. In the absence of some social consensus, perhaps the result of some public commission charged with making such decisions, MCOs are leery of being labeled as "rationers" of new, beneficial technologies (even if they attend to cost-effectiveness in their less visible forumlaries). Nor do they relish the idea of defending such rationing in the courts.

Ironically, one of the bugaboos underlying opposition to national health care reform was that it would lead to national agencies making rationing decisions. Better, some insisted, to leave rationing to the implicit workings of the market. But, because they fear being labeled as rationers, MCOs resist the hard choices involved in comparative decision-making about new technologies. The result is the continued rapid dissemination of new technologies, raising costs and ultimately making the need for comparative decision-making greater. The problem has the structure of a many-persons prisoners dilemma.[27]

Despite the fact that MCOs do not make widespread appeals to relative cost-effectiveness or to opportunity costs, such reasons, appropriately supported, would meet Condition 2. If people share the goal of meeting the varied medical needs of a population covered by limited resources, and they share a commitment to justifying limitations by reference to reasons all can consider appropriate and relevant, then they will be interested in a reason that says a particular technology falls below some defensible threshold of cost-effectiveness or relative cost-worthiness. Not meeting the needs of those for whom the only treatment was marginally effective but quite costly would not be making the affected population of patients worse off than anyone need be, for under reasonable constraints on resources, there will always be some patients who find that there is no cost-worthy treatment for their condition. The (heavy) burden, in these cases, is to establish the factual presuppositions that underlie giving such a reason. We have to show that the resources are limited in a reasonable way, that the costs and effects are as claimed, and that the comparison class of competing technologies that we would approve all are superior in the ways claimed, and that there are no special reasons of distributive fairness that override these considerations.

The Case of Costs: Competitive Markets. Saying that a technology is "too costly" might also be clarified in a quite different way: it may ultimately refer to the competitive economic situation of the MCO, not to relative medical cost-effectiveness. To remain competitive, the MCO must provide a reasonable return to investors (if it is for-profit); it must be able to invest capital in a way that helps it retain market share. We may even be told that high CEO salaries are needed to attract talented leadership that in turn keeps the organization competitive. Are reasons such as these simply disguised ways of saying that the decision advan-

27. See Norman Daniels, "Justice and the Dissemination of Big Ticket Technologies," in Deborah Mathieu, *Organ Substitution Technology: Ethical, Legal, and Public Policy Issues* (Boulder: Westview, 1988), pp.211–20.

tages some and disadvantages others, claims that by themselves we argued did not meet the requirements of Condition 2?

The answer to this question is complex. To support reasons that refer in this way to the competitive position of the MCO would require providing information that the MCO often is not willing to reveal for quite defensible business reasons. Similarly, supporting arguments for those reasons would often depend on economic and strategic judgments that require special experience and training to make. Finally, these reasons ultimately depend for their credibility on a much deeper and more fundamental fact about the design of the system, namely, the claim that a system involving competition in this sort of market will produce efficiencies that work to the advantage of all who have medical needs.

Our point is not that these reasons are in principle the type that cannot be supported, but that providing support for them requires information that is often not available, that is hard to understand when it is available, and that ultimately depends on fundamental moral and political judgments about the feasibility of quite different alternative systems for delivering health care. These are deeply contested and contestable issues. These reasons are likely to fuel further disagreement, not resolve it. Indeed they are likely to spark disagreement at each step about whether or not they really are just claims about advantage or disadvantage of the sort we are not considering reasonable by Condition 2. By itself that consequence is not sufficient to reject these kinds of reasons in light of Condition 2. Instead, it shows that we may find ourselves with intractable disagreements about whether the kinds of reasons being advanced are in principle relevant and appropriate. That is part of what we hoped could be avoided by introducing Condition 2, so this is not a welcome outcome. Therefore, we expect MCOs to be reluctant to rest their case for limit setting on these sorts of reasons.

Remark on the Connection to "Democratic Deliberation"

The points we have been making about the need for the constraints on reasons involved in Condition 2 are analogous to claims that lie at the heart of a philosophical debate about how to understand the legitimacy of democratic procedures themselves.[28] The reasons for our constraints

28. See Joshua Cohen, "Deliberative Democracy" (unpublished 1996 ms); Joshua Cohen, "Procedure and Substance in Deliberative Democracy," in Seyla Benhabib, ed., *Democracy and Difference: Changing Boundaries of the Political* (Princeton University

may be clarified if we consider briefly that more foundational debate about the nature of democratic legitimacy. In pointing to the way in which our account is compatible with aspects of the theory of democratic deliberation (and extends that theory to nonpublic institutions), we nevertheless do not derive our account from any particular version of that theory, nor do we endorse some of the controversial implications of that theory.

What gives majority (or plurality) rule its legitimacy as a procedure for resolving moral disputes about public policy and the design of institutions? One prominent answer, which Joshua Cohen refers to as the "aggregative" conception of democracy,[29] holds that the procedure is fair and acquires legitimacy simply because it counts everyone's interests equally in the voting process: each counts for one, not more or less. Adult persons are presumed to be the best judges of their own interests and can present and advance them in the political process.

Something important seems to be left out of this proceduralist view of the virtues of aggregation through voting. It allows us to compel people to abide by a majority rule, even where there are fundamental moral disagreements, simply by aggregating the voters' *preferences*, whatever they may be.[30] If we had a large group and the option of buying only one flavor of ice cream, vanilla or chocolate, we might settle the dispute by voting. We might think that aggregating preferences through the mechanism of voting was a way to achieve the greatest net satisfaction of preferences. If most people prefer chocolate, then we get the greatest aggregate satisfaction of preferences by buying chocolate. Everyone's interests are counted, including those who prefer vanilla, since the frustration of the vanilla lovers is offset by the greater pleasure of the chocolate lovers.

Abiding by a majority decision that compels people to act in ways that

---

Press, 1996), pp. 95–119; Joshua Cohen, "Pluralism and Proceduralism," *Chicago-Kent Law Review* 69, no. 3 (1994): 589–618; John Rawls, *Political Liberalism* (New York: Columbia University Press, 1993); Cass Sunstein, *The Partial Constitution* (Cambridge, Mass.: Harvard University Press, 1993).

29. We here follow Joshua Cohen, "Deliberative Democracy," p. 14.

30. Cohen notes that an aggregative view might arguably be extended to give some protection from outcomes that involved discrimination against those who are targets of stereotyping or hostility, e.g., against people with disabilities or racial minorities. A process that allowed simple aggregation of those preferences arguably does not give people equal consideration and so violates its own rationale. Cohen, "Deliberative Democracy," p. 15.

counter their fundamental beliefs about what is morally right is not simply like frustrating a taste for vanilla ice cream, however. Even a craving for vanilla is not to be assimilated to a moral conviction. Settling moral disputes simply by aggregating preferences seems to ignore some fundamental differences between the nature of values and commitments to them and tastes or preferences.

The aggregative conception seems insensitive to how we ideally would like to resolve moral disputes, namely through argument and deliberation. We expect people to offer reasons and arguments for their moral views, and we hope that the better arguments will prove persuasive. We want to be shown what is right by appeal to reasons that we consider convincing. If a good moral argument persuades us that our original belief about what is right is in fact incorrect, we may be chagrined, but we are (or should be) grateful as well. We have been spared doing what is wrong. It is more important to end up knowing what is right and doing it, given our motivation to act in ways that we can justify morally, than it is to get our way. This helps to explain why we are not satisfied in cases of moral disagreement simply to be told, "a majority of people think otherwise." The problem is not that the majority will simply keep us from getting our way (as it would be if we preferred vanilla), but that majorities can be morally wrong and may make us do the wrong thing. In addition, they may be moved by reasons that minorities cannot even accept as relevant to resolving the dispute.

The aggregative account fails as an account of the legitimacy of a democratic procedure because it ignores the way in which the search for reasons we can agree on plays a central role in our deliberations about what is right. A deliberative account of how a procedure such as majority rule acquires legitimacy depends on emphasizing the deliberative process that may conclude in a vote. Specifically, it imposes some constraints on the kinds of reasons that can play a role in that deliberation. Not just any preferences or grounds for preferences will do. Reasons must reflect the fact that all parties to a decision are viewed as seeking terms of fair cooperation that all can accept as reasonable. Where their well-being or fundamental liberties or other matters of fundamental value are involved and at risk, people should not be expected to accept binding terms of cooperation that rest on reasons they cannot view as acceptable types of reasons. For example, reasons that rest on matters of religious faith will not meet this condition. Reasonable people differ in their religious, philosophical, and moral views, and yet we must seek terms of fair cooperation that rest on justifications acceptable to all.

Suppose that a deliberation appeals only to reasons that all can recognize as acceptable or relevant kinds of reasons, but that consensus about an outcome is still not achieved. To settle the practical matter, we rely on a majority vote. What can be said in favor of reliance on this voting procedure that could not be said on the purely proceduralist view?

On the deliberative view, the minority can at least assure itself that *the preference of the majority rests on the kind of reason that even the minority must acknowledge appropriately plays a role in the deliberation.* The minority is not being compelled to do something for reasons it thinks irrelevant or inappropriate—even if it does not accept the weight or balance given to various considerations by the majority. In contrast, on the aggregative view, the minority has to accept that it loses only because more people prefer an alternative, for whatever reasons. Although majority rules in both cases, the further restriction in the deliberative case to reasons all must acknowledge as appropriate reduces the plausibility of claiming that the majority exercises brute power of preference.

The constraints on reasons that are involved in Condition 2 have a similar effect, even though the decision-making procedure is not a democratic one since it takes place in a privately controlled managed care organization. If the organization shows through the pattern of reasoning (the "case law") reflected in its public reason-giving (Condition 1) that its decisions rest on the kinds of reasons all can consider relevant to deciding how to meet varied patient needs under reasonable resource constraints (Condition 2), then even those who disagree with the specific decisions made should acknowledge they are reasonable decisions that are arguably aimed at producing fair outcomes. If all affected by these decisions should acknowledge that much, then they are well on their way toward recognizing the legitimacy of the decision-making process.

In what follows we consider conditions further aimed at making the decision-making process publicly accountable and responsive to wider public deliberation. More to the point, the combination of Conditions 1–4 means that wider public deliberation is enhanced by the contribution made by those engaged in decision-making within delivery organizations weighing the merits of new technologies and setting limits to their use and the use of other treatments. It is in this sense that our Conditions 1–4 provide a way of engaging nondemocratic institutions in a process of wider public deliberation that is fully compatible with the requirements of "democratic deliberation."

Condition 3: Dispute Resolution Procedures

How may a decision concerning coverage of a new technology (or other limit setting decision) be challenged by those affected by it? Typically, internal dispute resolution procedures in MCOs range from informal complaints to ombudsmen, to more formal grievance procedures with well-defined stages of appeal, to final appeals to panels to medical directors or other last-step internal procedures. Where these mechanisms fail, patients and even practitioners may choose the threat of litigation or legislative remedies to their complaints. Because these external routes are costly to MCOs, it is in their interest to provide effective internal mechanisms. In fact, National Committee on Quality Assurance (NCQA) regulations require MCOs to establish appeals and dispute resolution mechanisms.

MCO dispute resolution procedures play two quite distinct roles, one internal to the decision-making process and the other linking it to broader social mechanisms for addressing these issues. Where the patients or clinicians use these procedures to challenge a decision, and the results of the challenge lead effectively to reconsidering the decision on its merits, the decision-making process is made iterative in a way that broadens the input of information and argument. Parties that may have been excluded from the decision-making process and whose views may not have been clearly heard or understood find a voice, even if after the original fact, through these mechanisms. Whether specific decisions are actually changed or not, if the arguments raised by these appeals lead to honest reconsideration of the original decision on its merits, they have an important effect on the overall legitimacy of the decision-making process and on its likelihood of achieving fair outcomes.

A dispute resolution mechanism that provides a "feedback" route into the decision-making process engages a broader segment of those affected by the decision in the process of deliberation, even if they are placed in the adversarial role of aggrieved parties. Because the reasons involved in the original decision are publicly accessible (Condition 1), and because they are constrained to focus in a reasonable way on meeting the health needs of the insured population (Condition 2), those affected by the decisions are given an opportunity to reopen the deliberation, even if they are not fully empowered to participate in the decision-making. Of course this does not mean that every grievance leads to a reconsideration of the decision by the original committee responsible for it. It does, however, mean that good arguments that plausibly challenge the original decision are provided a visible and public route back into the policy formulation process. The MCO decision-making process is thus enriched by the new resources for argument the grievance process brings to bear. Conversely, those affected adversely by the original decision are compelled to engage in the process of constrained reason-giving that informed the original decision. This task is instructive for all involved. That is, the grievance and reconsideration become part of the process through which the broader social deliberation about the problem of limits takes place. The mechanism enables and enhances that broader social process.

A well-developed internal dispute resolution mechanism might reduce the degree to which patients or clinicians adversely affected by decisions seek external authorities or institutions to pursue their interests. Even if the courts or legislature are pursued, however, the fact that there is a robust internal dispute resolution mechanism can lead to improved external deliberation. This is especially true if the courts come to expect a robust internal mechanism and take up issues only when there is reason to think internal mechanisms have somehow failed.

The courts are ill equipped to deliberate about the issues of limit-setting, especially about the more technical matters involved in assessing efficacy and safety. Court procedures, for example, bring opposing "experts" to bear, and they leave the final decision up to those with no expertise about the technical matters, whether judges or juries. This may simply not be the best way to deliberate about these matters, despite its appearance of a "democratic" input through the opinion of peers. If, however, a healthy deliberative process, including an exchange of reasons and information in the grievance process, has already taken place, then a court deliberation about the matter may itself involve better deliberation about the merits.

Earlier we pointed out that the constraints on reasons we propose are similar to those invoked by the theory of democratic deliberation when its advocates attempt to explain the legitimacy of appeals to democratic procedures in general. Although we focused there on explaining the legitimacy of voting procedures when they are seen as the culmination of democratic deliberation, we should not be misled into thinking that only large, public votes are at issue, or that the deliberative process requires direct, grass-roots participation, a la town-meeting democracy. Much of our democratic process takes place in decentralized procedures in which those affected by decision-making often do not participate. This is true not only of representative legislative bodies, but in executive and legislative branch agencies. What is crucial is that the heart of that process involve democratic deliberation.

Similarly, the fact that direct participation in decision-making by enrollees or many clinicians is not a feature of private organizations, such as MCOs, does not mean that the deliberative process is not key to addressing the issues of fairness and legitimacy. (We obviously do not oppose consumer participation in decision-making, but we think it neither necessary nor sufficient to solve the legitimacy problem.) The dispute resolution mechanisms we are discussing serve to connect those affected by decisions to the deliberative process, and whether this connection follows or precedes the original deliberation is not crucial. The dispute resolution mechanisms do not empower enrollees or clinicians to participate directly in the decision-making bodies. Nor does that happen in many public democratic processes. But it does empower them to play a more effective role in the larger social deliberation about the issues, including in those public institutions that may help to regulate MCOs or otherwise constrain their acts. The mechanisms we describe thus play a role in assuring broader accountability of private organizations, such as MCOs, to those who are affected by limit-setting decisions.

Condition 4: Voluntary or Public Regulation

There are private regulatory mechanisms that might suffice to ensure the MCOs abide by the constraints involved in Conditions 1–3. For example, NCQA regulations currently require that organizations have some procedure for assessing new technologies. These regulations, however, do not specify what features the process of technology assessment should have. Were Conditions 1–3 incorporated into those NCQA guidelines, then an important private regulatory process would come into play. Employers and others seeking to do business only with accredited MCOs would then be assured that they were doing business with organizations that were actively addressing the fairness and legitimacy problems MCOs now face.

Failure to adopt Conditions 1–3 voluntarily, or through the nonlegal coercive force of sanctions from private associations, could set the stage for public regulation. Currently, many state legislatures are considering or passing regulations governing the behavior of MCOs and other insurers, including restrictions on "gag" orders or other constraints on what physicians may say to patients. Our analysis of how to solve the legitimacy and fairness problems is neutral between public or voluntary private enforcement of the conditions we outline. Either would suffice to establish the kind of accountability that is necessary where fundamental issues of fairness are involved, provided that the process meets the four conditions. Either can facilitate a broader public deliberation about meeting the needs of a covered population by connecting private, organizational deliberation about these controversial matters to whatever broader public discussion is also taking place. The broader public discussion could be prompted by dissatisfaction with the results of the now publicly accessible decisions made by MCOs, or it could simply endorse those decisions and incorporate some of their elements within publicly administered health delivery systems.

MCO deliberation that meets the four conditions does not *substitute for* any public democratic process (or democratic process constrained by constitutional restrictions). Rather, it *facilitates* that process. The four conditions compel MCOs to contribute their deliberative capacities to whatever broader public deliberation is conducted through democratic institutions, formally or informally. The arrangements required by the four conditions provide connective tissue to, not a replacement for, broader democratic processes. Ultimately, these broader processes have authority and responsibility for guaranteeing the fairness of limit-setting decisions.

V. Meeting the Four Conditions in Practice

Building on Current Practices

In our study of several leading MCOs, we have found some practices that already embody aspects of these conditions, at least in some contexts, and we have found some willingness to improve practices to meet them. For example, when we observed that one organization's published policy statements did not include rationales for coverage decisions that reflected their careful reasoning, the organization improved its practice. Despite the importance we attach to making rationales publicly available in such documents, however, it is even more important that reasons be explicit when patients share in the decision-making about new treatments. That, in turn, means that clinicians must be very clear about the rationales behind limits on coverage for these treatments, since they have ultimate responsibility for sharing decision-making with patients.

One interesting finding in our study is that organizations are much clearer about the importance of providing clinicians with rationales for limits involved in "practice guidelines" than they are in the case of coverage decisions for new treatments. They know that clinicians will not modify their traditional practices to conform to such guidelines (which are presumably based on good evidence about outcomes) unless they are given good reasons for the features of the guideline.

Those patients (and clinicians) who are apparently most resistant to limits on new-technology use are those who face life-threatening conditions and who have run out of promising lines of treatment from standard therapies. In these cases, as we suggested earlier in our discussion of strategies for last-chance therapies, the limits set by the organization are widely perceived either to be cost-driven or overly paternalistic. To the desperately ill patient, the organization may appear to be denying a "last chance" just to save money, hiding behind contract language that excludes coverage for investigational procedures or drugs. Alternatively, if it is insisting on its own view of acceptable risk-benefit ratios (medical appropriateness), it may appear overly paternalistic. Why not, the patient insists, let the patient decide what risks to take when her life is at stake?

Reason-giving assumes special importance in these highly charged situations, and one practice we observed in a large MCO is exemplary of the role reasons can play in arriving at acceptable policy. This MCO adopted the policy that it would cover a variety of still-investigational high-dose chemotherapy regimens using stem-cell transplants, but only for patients who enrolled in a clinical trial. The problem for some patients wanting such treatments is that there is no suitable clinical trial whose protocols they meet. Would the MCO cover a transplant for them anyway?

The transplant coordinator for this MCO has the task of addressing these patients' demands. Her strategy involves engaging the patient in reason-giving aimed at producing new policy. She points out that the patient has an interest in the organization's making systematic, reasonable, and consistent decisions about how to treat different classes of patients, since ad hoc decisions would open the door to special treatment of some patients over others. She urges the patient to offer reasons why his case should be seen as representative of a class of cases that warrants coverage, given the goal of generating knowledge about these treatments. He might, for example, show that his exclusion from the existing protocols is really only incidental and does not reflect an important fact about his case. Leaving him out might then seem arbitrary (remember our discussion of consistency in case law). Or he might be able to show that his case is clearly different from that examined in existing protocols, but nevertheless there is no reason not to develop a trial for such cases. He might insist that if his exclusion is just bad luck about what is locally available, he should be covered.

In the last-chance strategy described in Section III, an outside medical ombudsman was invoked to disarm concerns about conflict of interest. In this MCO, the transplant coordinator viewed her failure to reach an agreement with a patient as evidence that the process of discussion and deliberation about the case had not been adequately carried out. She claims that she has never had a case of a patient with whom no agreement could be reached without litigation. In every case, the patient discovers through more careful deliberation that the desired treatment is, after all, not really appropriate, or some provision is made to expand coverage policy to include cases of this sort, or by mutual agreement an alternative treatment course is pursued because all come to see it as preferable.

A cynical gloss on this example might be that patients are worn down until they back off from their demands. We have no access to the specific cases that could provide evidence for or against that interpretation. If the reports of the organization and interviews with relevant personnel are accepted, however, the practice gives weight to the idea that reason-giving by organizations and an honest effort to involve patients and clinicians in the practice of connecting their own cases to relevant reasons bears fruit even in the most highly charged of contexts.

Reason-giving about policies regarding coverage bears fruit for an MCO beyond what derives from the impact on patients and clinicians. We interviewed one administrator in an MCO who was responsible for revising contract language regarding coverage to reflect up-to-date clinical practice. The most difficult part of this administrator's job, she claimed, was understanding the rationale behind coverage decisions. Without a clear grasp of that rationale, she found it exceedingly difficult to draft a contract that reflected a coherent basis for existing practices. Too often, she insisted, coverage decisions were announced in a way that did not provide sufficient rationales. From this administrator's perspective, an important goal of the organization was to write a contract that reflects a coherent and defensible way of thinking about meeting patient needs in a population. Since all organizations must reconcile contract language with the particulars of decisions about cases and about new technologies, clarity and accountability of reasoning about new technologies are to the organization's advantage in articulating its approach, both internally and externally. Of course, this assumes that its approach is intended to be justifiable to all involved.

Objections to Reason-Giving. Fear of litigation and exposure in the media are the most common objections to our proposal that organizations be more explicit and accountable about their reasonsfor limit-setting decisions regarding new technologies. Specifically, there is a concern that being explicit about reasons "opened the door to attack" from dissatisfied patients and their lawyers or reporters. In part, the fear was that the organization would be laying out its grounds for its defense, exposing itself to rebuttal by expert witnesses or to "gaming" regarding insurance coverage.

The objection and any reply to it both suffer from being speculative. There is simply no evidence that not disclosing reasons protects an organization against litigation, or that giving them opens it up to more, or more successful, litigation. Nor is there evidence that providing sound reasons for decisions makes an organization more susceptible to bad press. Our reply regarding the courts rests on this contention: the courts will be less likely to want to substitute their substantive decisions about providing new technologies if they see that MCOs use robust, careful deliberative procedures and base their conclusions on reasonable arguments which appeal to the evidence produced in the evaluative process. The best defense against the charge that the organization is negligent in providing contractually promised care is to show that the reasons for limiting access to the care are weighty and appropriate and that decisions were actually based on them. We have some evidence from other kinds of cases, including termination-of-treatment decisions involving careful ethical consultation, that courts will give some deference to developed procedures used in medical contexts. Since the courts are notoriously bad places in which to carry out technical assessments of evidence, the courts themselves have good reason not to intrude into decisions about which technologies have met some reasonable standard of evidence regarding their safety, efficacy, and medical appropriateness.

If we are right that MCOs will begin to address the legitimacy and fairness problems by demonstrating to enrollees and clinicians that they base decisions on a concern for meeting the needs of patients in a covered population under reasonable resource constraints (our Conditions 1 and 2), then the distrust of MCOs may diminish, and with it, the inclination to resolve all disputes by litigation. This point too is speculative: there is no direct evidence. But the fear underlying the objection, that giving reasons will increase litigation (or successful litigation) is just as speculative. Moreover, the current strategy does not work to the satisfaction of anyone: either MCOs or the public.

Regulative Strategies

Ultimately, there is a coordination problem here. If all organizations agreed, either through voluntary self-regulation or through publicly imposed regulation, to a practice in which reason-giving was explicit, the risk to any one organization from the change would be reduced. Facing uncertainty, each might reasonably fear being the first to give reasons in an already litigious climate. The effect of such universal reluctance may be that all are actually worse off, for all then actually face more litigation, not less. If coordinated reason-giving led to less litigation and more trust, then all would benefit from cooperation with the conditions we propose. We believe all are worse off from not cooperating in this way. We also think that organizations can use their openness about reasons in order to gain some competitive advantage. But even if we are wrong about the latter point, there is all the more reason to seek self- or public regulation along the lines of the conditions we propose.[31]

In view of these remarks about the fears of accountability and the public-goods problem created by those fears, it is important to seek cooperation around a regulative strategy. A first step would be to expand the NCQA requirements on procedures for making technology assessments. Currently, these are described only in the most minimal way. Expanding the requirements so that they call for a procedure as publicly accountable as the one we propose would accomplish much of what we want without recourse to public regulation through legislation or through mandates by state insurance regulators. The advantage of the NCQA regulations is that they avoid the limits on state regulation of insurance imposed by the federal legislation known as ERISA. Where state regulation of MCOs is attempted, we would urge *process focused* efforts, not mandates about specific coverage decisions. A reasonable model for regulating process is the Friedman-Knowles Act in California, which calls for an external review of denials of last-chance therapies along the models of the strategy discussed in Section III.

VI. The Legitimacy and Fairness Problems in Public Systems

The legitimacy and fairness problems that face our private health delivery organizations, such as MCOs, have their analogues in public systems such as the British National Health Service in Great Britain or the Canadian systems. At one level, the legitimacy problem has a clearer answer: in a publicly administered and financed system, public agencies that make limit-setting decisions have a legitimacy that is easier to identify than the legitimacy that we might attach to private delivery institutions in our mixed system. Nevertheless, much of what we have said here about explicit reason-giving and accountability, as well as about mechanisms for appeal and dispute resolution, carries over to these public systems as well.

In Section IV, we suggested that national commissions concerned with articulating "principles" governing priorities in health care, such as

31. If organizations that put reasons forward (call them ice breakers) actually benefited, then the coordination problem we describe comes from a misestimate of what self-interested action calls for. It is the misestimate that sets up the public-goods problem (the many-person prisoners dilemma) informally described in the text. If organizations that act as ice breakers when others fail to do so actually do worse, then we have a true many-persons prisoners dilemma.

those established by the Dutch, the Norwegians, the Danes, and the Swedes in recent years, do not readily resolve the problems we have been discussing. Very abstract principles, such as those the Danes and the Norwegians articulated in their first attempts to address the problem of setting priorities and limits to health care, lead to considerable controversy in their application. Indeed, it may seem easier to articulate and agree to quite general principles in the context of a commission than to determine what those principles really mean in practice when specific decisions about limiting access to new technologies or other treatments are involved.

At a recent international conference on priorities in health care, Danish and Norwegian members of current commissions on the ethics of limit setting reported dissatisfaction with their earlier efforts for just this reason. Their current efforts focus more on establishing processes for decision-making about specific cases than on developing support for an ordered set of principles. One Danish participant said, "We found that all the hard work remained of justifying limits set in particular instances and that vague appeals to commission-sanctioned principles did not suffice to persuade people about particular cases."

The development should not be understood as a rejection of an attempt to get social agreement on general principles. Rather, it is a recognition that specific decisions need justification, and too little effort—or process—was in place to legitimize specific decisions. Indeed, even in a public system not driven by competition or profit, suspicion would arise that specific limit-setting decisions were being driven too much by cost considerations and too little by specific argument about how this decision fit with the task of meeting the health care needs of a population under reasonable resource constraints.

Just as limiting access to certain high-cost transplant technologies has been the focus of the most visible opposition to limit-setting in the U.S., so too these have been the most highly charged decisions in publicly administered systems. Norway, Great Britain, and New Zealand, for example, have all experienced widely publicized cases of individuals being denied access to a transplant, followed by extensive legal and political efforts to pressure local administrators to modify their decisions. We cannot here discuss these cases in detail,[32] but a common element emerges in all of them. The public has usually not been given a clear

32. Detailed presentations of these cases took place at the Stockholm Conference on Priorities in Health Care, October 1996.

statement of the reasons underlying these decisions and there is no specific track record of similar decisions to provide a "case law" argument showing consistent treatment around a coherent set of reasons. To be sure, the authorities making these decisions may well have deliberated about them in ways that invoked appropriate reasons which all should consider relevant, had they the chance to think about them. But the practice in these publicly administered systems is just what it is in our privately administered system. Reason-giving is not standard practice and public accountability—and trust—suffers.

We believe that the conditions we describe for addressing the legitimacy and fairness problems apply to public as well as nonpublic delivery institutions. All must engage in a process of establishing their credentials for fair decision-making about such fundamental matters every time they make such a decision. Whether in public or mixed systems, establishing the accountability of decision-makers to those affected by their decisions is the only way to show, over time, that arguably fair decisions are being made and that those making them have established a procedure we should view as legitimate. This is not to say that public participation is an essential ingredient of the process in either public or mixed systems, but the accountability to the public in both cases is necessary to facilitate broader democratic processes that regulate the system.

Property Rights in Health Care Resources

[16]

Can Patents Deter Innovation? The Anticommons in Biomedical Research

Michael A. Heller and Rebecca S. Eisenberg

The "tragedy of the commons" metaphor helps explain why people overuse shared resources. However, the recent proliferation of intellectual property rights in biomedical research suggests a different tragedy, an "anticommons" in which people underuse scarce resources because too many owners can block each other. Privatization of biomedical research must be more carefully deployed to sustain both upstream research and downstream product development. Otherwise, more intellectual property rights may lead paradoxically to fewer useful products for improving human health.

Thirty years ago in *Science*, Garrett Hardin introduced the metaphor "tragedy of the commons" (*1*) to help explain overpopulation, air pollution, and species extinction. People often overuse resources they own in common because they have no incentive to conserve. Today, Hardin's metaphor is central to debates in economics, law, and science and is a powerful justification for privatizing commons property (*2*). Although the metaphor highlights the cost of overuse when governments allow too many people to use a scarce resource, it overlooks the possibility of underuse when governments give too many people rights to exclude others. Privatization can solve one tragedy but cause another (*3*).

Since Hardin's article appeared, biomedical research has been moving from a commons model toward a privatization model (*4*). Under the commons model, the federal government sponsored premarket or "upstream" research and encouraged broad dissemination of results in the public domain. Unpatented biomedical discoveries were freely incorporated in "downstream" products for diagnosing and treating disease. In 1980, in an effort to promote commercial development of new technologies, Congress began encouraging universities and other institutions to patent discoveries arising from federally supported research and development and to transfer their technology to the private sector (*5*). Supporters applaud the resulting increase in patent filings and private investment (*6*), whereas critics fear deterioration in the culture of upstream research (*7*). Building on Heller's theory of anticommons property (*3*), this article identifies an unintended and paradoxical consequence of biomedical privatization: A proliferation of intellectual property rights upstream may be stifling life-saving innovations further downstream in the course of research and product development.

The authors are at the University of Michigan Law School, Ann Arbor, MI 48109-1215, USA. E-mail: mheller@umich.edu; rse@umich.edu

The Tragedy of the Anticommons

Anticommons property can best be understood as the mirror image of commons property (*3, 8*). A resource is prone to overuse in a tragedy of the commons when too many owners each have a privilege to use a given resource and no one has a right to exclude another (*9*). By contrast, a resource is prone to underuse in a "tragedy of the anticommons" when multiple owners each have a right to exclude others from a scarce resource and no one has an effective privilege of use. In theory, in a world of costless transactions, people could always avoid commons or anticommons tragedies by trading their rights (*10*). In practice, however, avoiding tragedy requires overcoming transaction costs, strategic behaviors, and cognitive biases of participants (*11*), with success more likely within close-knit communities than among hostile strangers (*12–14*). Once an anticommons emerges, collecting rights into usable private property is often brutal and slow (*15*).

Privatization in postsocialist economies starkly illustrates how anticommons property can emerge and persist (*3*). One promise of the transition to a free market was that new entrepreneurs would fill stores that socialist rule had left bare. Yet after several years of reform, many privatized storefronts remained empty, while flimsy metal kiosks, stocked full of goods, mushroomed on the streets. Why did the new merchants not come in from the cold? One reason was that transition governments often failed to endow any individual with a bundle of rights that represents full ownership. Instead, fragmented rights were distributed to various socialist-era stakeholders, including private or quasi-private enterprises, workers' collectives, privatization agencies, and local, regional, and federal governments. No one could set up shop without first collecting rights from each of the other owners.

Privatization of upstream biomedical research in the United States may create anticommons property that is less visible than empty storefronts but even more economically and socially costly. In this setting, privatization takes the form of intellectual property claims to the sorts of research results that, in an earlier era, would have been made freely available in the public domain. Responding to a shift in U.S. government policy (*4*) in the past two decades, research institutions such as the National Institutes of Health (NIH) and major universities have created technology transfer offices to patent and license their discoveries. At the same time, commercial biotechnology firms have emerged in research and development (R&D) niches somewhere between the proverbial "fundamental" research of academic laboratories and the targeted product development of pharmaceutical firms (*7*). Today, upstream research in the biomedical sciences is increasingly likely to be "private" in one or more senses of the term—supported by private funds, carried out in a private institution, or privately appropriated through patents, trade secrecy, or agreements that restrict the use of materials and data.

In biomedical research, as in postsocialist transition, privatization holds both promises and risks. Patents and other forms of intellectual property protection for upstream discoveries may fortify incentives to undertake risky research projects and could result in a more equitable distribution of profits across all stages of R&D. But privatization can go astray when too many owners hold rights in previous discoveries that constitute obstacles to future research (*16*). Upstream patent rights, initially offered to help attract further private investment, are increasingly regarded as entitlements by those who do research with public funds. A researcher who may have felt entitled to coauthorship or a citation in an earlier era may now feel entitled to be a coinventor on a patent or to receive a royalty under a material transfer agreement. The result has been a spiral of overlapping patent claims in the hands of different owners, reaching ever further upstream in the course of biomedical research. Researchers and their institutions may resent restrictions on access to the patented discoveries of others, yet nobody wants to be the last one left dedicating findings to the public domain.

The problem we identify is distinct from the routine underuse inherent in any well-functioning patent system. By conferring monopolies in discoveries, patents necessarily increase prices and restrict use—a cost society pays to motivate invention and disclosure. The tragedy of the anticommons refers to the more complex obstacles that arise when a user needs access to multiple patented inputs to create a single useful product. Each upstream patent allows its owner to set up another tollbooth on the road to product development, adding to the cost and slowing the pace of downstream biomedical innovation.

How a Biomedical Anticommons May Arise

Current examples in biomedical research demonstrate two mechanisms by which a government might inadvertently create an anticommons: either by creating too many concurrent fragments of intellectual property rights in potential future products or by permitting too many upstream patent owners to stack licenses on top of the future discoveries of downstream users.

Concurrent fragments. The anticommons model provides one way of understanding a widespread intuition that issuing patents on gene fragments makes little sense. Throughout the 1980s, patents on genes generally corresponded closely to foreseeable commercial products, such as therapeutic proteins or diagnostic tests for recognized genetic diseases (*17*). Then, in 1991, NIH pointed the way toward patenting anonymous gene fragments with its notorious patent applications on expressed sequence tags (ESTs) (*18*). NIH subsequently abandoned these patent applications and now takes a more hostile position toward patenting ESTs and raw genomic DNA sequences (*19*). Meanwhile, private firms have stepped in where NIH left off, filing patent applications on newly identified DNA sequences, including gene fragments, before identifying a corresponding gene, protein, biological function, or potential commercial product. The Patent and Trademark Office (PTO), in examining these claims (*20*), could create or avoid an anticommons.

Although a database of gene fragments is a useful resource for discovery, defining property rights around isolated gene fragments seems at the outset unlikely to track socially useful bundles of property rights in future commercial products. Foreseeable commercial products, such as therapeutic proteins or genetic diagnostic tests, are more likely to require the use of multiple fragments. A proliferation of patents on individual fragments held by different owners seems inevitably to require costly future transactions to bundle licenses together before a firm can have an effective right to develop these products (*21*).

> The editors have asked selected members of the scientific community to respond to the Policy commentary by J. J. Doll and the Review by M. A. Heller and R. S. Eisenberg. Their remarks are available at www.sciencemag.org/feature/data/980465.shl

Patents on receptors useful for screening potential pharmaceutical products demonstrate another potential "concurrent fragment" anticommons in biomedical research. To learn as much as possible about the therapeutic effects and side effects of potential products at the preclinical stage, firms want to screen products against all known members of relevant receptor families. But if these receptors are patented and controlled by different owners, gathering the necessary licenses may be difficult or impossible. A recent search of the Lexis patent database disclosed more than 100 issued U.S. patents with the term "adrenergic receptor" in the claim language. Such a proliferation of claims presents a daunting bargaining challenge. Unable to procure a complete set of licenses, firms choose between diverting resources to less promising projects with fewer licensing obstacles or proceeding to animal and then clinical testing on the basis of incomplete information. More thorough in vitro screening could avoid premature clinical testing that exposes patients to unnecessary risks.

Long delays between the filing and issuance of biotechnology patents aggravate the problem of concurrent fragments. During this period of pendency, there is substantial uncertainty as to the scope of patent rights that will ultimately issue. Although U.S. patent law does not recognize enforceable rights in pending patent applications, firms and universities typically enter into license agreements before the issuance of patents, and firms raise capital on the basis of the inchoate rights preserved by patent filings. In effect, each potential patent creates a specter of rights that may be larger than the actual rights, if any, eventually conferred by the PTO. Worked into the calculations of both risk-taking investors and risk-averse product developers, these overlapping patent filings may compound the obstacles to developing new products.

Stacking licenses. The use of reach-through license agreements (RTLAs) on patented research tools illustrates another path by which an anticommons may emerge. As we use the term, an RTLA gives the owner of a patented invention, used in upstream stages of research, rights in subsequent downstream discoveries. Such rights may take the form of a royalty on sales that result from use of the upstream research tool, an exclusive or nonexclusive license on future discoveries, or an option to acquire such a license. In principle, RTLAs offer advantages to both patent holders and researchers. They permit researchers with limited funds to use patented research tools right away and defer payment until the research yields valuable results. Patent holders may also prefer a chance at larger payoffs from sales of downstream products rather than certain, but smaller, upfront fees. In practice, RTLAs may lead to an anticommons as upstream owners stack overlapping and inconsistent claims on potential downstream products. In effect, the use of RTLAs gives each upstream patent owner a continuing right to be present at the bargaining table as a research project moves downstream toward product development.

So far, RTLAs have had a mixed reception as a mechanism for licensing upstream biomedical research patents, but they appear to be becoming more prevalent. When Cetus Corporation initially proposed RTLAs on any products developed through the use of the polymerase chain reaction (PCR) in research, they met strong resistance from downstream users concerned with developing commercial products (*22*). Later, Hoffmann–La Roche acquired the rights to PCR and offered licenses that do not include reach-through obligations (*23*). The resulting pay-as-you-go approach increases the upfront cost of a license to use PCR, but it decreases the likelihood of an anticommons emerging.

More recently, some universities and other nonprofit research institutions have balked at terms DuPont Corporation has offered for licenses to use patented oncomouse (*24*) and cre-lox (*25*) technologies, although others have acquiesced to the license terms (*26*). These patents cover genetically engineered mice useful in research that could result in products falling outside the scope of the patent claims. DuPont has offered noncommercial research licenses and sublicenses on terms that seem to require licensees to return to DuPont for further approval before any new discoveries or materials resulting from the use of licensed mice are passed along to others or used for commercial purposes (*27*). DuPont thereby gains the right to participate in future negotiations to develop commercial products that fall outside the scope of their patent claims. In effect, the license terms permit

DuPont to leverage its proprietary position in upstream research tools into a broad veto right over downstream research and product development.

As RTLAs to use patented research tools multiply, researchers will face increasing difficulties conveying clear title to firms that might develop future discoveries. If a particularly valuable commercial product is in view, downstream product developers might be motivated and able to reach agreements with multiple holders of RTLAs. But if the prospects for success are more uncertain or the expected commercial value is small, the parties may fail to bargain past the anticommons.

Transition or Tragedy?

Is a biomedical anticommons likely to endure once it emerges? Recent empirical literature suggests that communities of intellectual property owners who deal with each other on a recurring basis have sometimes developed institutions to reduce transaction costs of bundling multiple licenses (*28*). For example, in the music industry, copyright collectives have evolved to facilitate licensing transactions so that broadcasters and other producers may readily obtain permission to use numerous copyrighted works held by different owners. Similarly, in the automobile, aircraft manufacturing, and synthetic rubber industries, patent pools have emerged, sometimes with the help of government, when licenses under multiple patent rights have been necessary to develop important new products (*28*). When the background legal rules threaten to waste resources, people often rearrange rights sensibly and create order through private arrangements (*12–14*). Perhaps some of the problems caused by proliferating upstream patent rights in biomedical research will recede as licensors and licensees gain experience with intellectual property rights and institutions evolve to help owners and users reach agreements. The short-term costs from delayed development of new treatments for disease may be worth incurring if fragmented privatization allows upstream research to pay its own way and helps to ensure its long-run viability. Patent barriers to product development may be a transitional phenomenon rather than an enduring tragedy.

On the other hand, there may be reasons to fear that a patent anticommons could prove more intractable in biomedical research than in other settings. Because patents matter more to the pharmaceutical and biotechnology industries than to other industries, firms in these industries may be less willing to participate in patent pools that undermine the gains from exclusivity (*29*). Moreover, the lack of substitutes for certain biomedical discoveries (such as patented genes or receptors) may increase the leverage of some patent holders, thereby aggravating holdout problems. Rivals may not be able to invent around patents in research aimed at understanding the genetic bases of diseases as they occur in nature.

More generally, three structural concerns caution against uncritical reliance on markets and norms to avoid a biomedical anticommons tragedy: the transaction costs of rearranging entitlements, heterogeneous interests of owners, and cognitive biases among researchers.

Transaction costs of bundling rights. High transaction costs may be an enduring impediment to efficient bundling of intellectual property rights in biomedical research. First, many upstream patent owners are public institutions with limited resources for absorbing transaction costs and limited competence in fast-paced, market-oriented bargaining. Second, the rights involved cover a diverse set of techniques, reagents, DNA sequences, and instruments. Difficulties in comparing the values of these patents will likely impede development of a standard distribution scheme. Third, the heterogeneity of interests and resources among public and private patent owners may complicate the emergence of standard license terms, requiring costly case-by-case negotiations. Fourth, licensing transaction costs are likely to arise early in the course of R&D when the outcome of a project is uncertain, the potential gains are speculative, and it is not yet clear that the value of downstream products justifies the trouble of overcoming the anticommons.

Even when upstream owners see potential gains from cooperation and are motivated to devise mechanisms for reducing transaction costs, they may be deterred by other legal constraints, such as antitrust laws. Patent pools have been a target of antitrust scrutiny in the past (*30*), which may explain why few, if any, such pools exist today. Although antitrust law may be less hostile to patent pools today than it was in 1975 when a consent decree dismantled the aircraft patent pool (*31*), the antitrust climate changes from one administration to the next (*32*). Even a remote prospect of facing treble damages and an injunction may give firms pause about entering into such agreements.

Heterogeneous interests of rights holders. Intellectual property rights in upstream biomedical research belong to a large, diverse group of owners in the public and private sectors with divergent institutional agendas. Sometimes heterogeneity of interests can facilitate mutually agreeable allocations (you take the credit, I'll take the money) (*33, 34*), but in this setting, there are reasons to fear that owners will have conflicting agendas that make it difficult to reach agreement. For example, a politically accountable government agency such as NIH may further its public health mission by using its intellectual property rights to ensure widespread availability of new therapeutic products at reasonable prices. When NIH sought to establish its co-ownership of patent rights held by Burroughs-Wellcome on the use of azidothymidine (AZT) to treat the human immunodeficiency virus (HIV) (*35*), its purpose was to lower the price of AZT and promote public health rather than simply to maximize its financial return. By contrast, a private firm is more likely to use intellectual property to maintain a lucrative product monopoly that rewards shareholders and funds future product development. When owners have conflicting goals and each can deploy its rights to block the strategies of the others, they may not be able to reach an agreement that leaves enough private value for downstream developers to bring products to the market.

A more subtle conflict in agendas arises between owners that pursue end-product development and those that focus primarily on upstream research. The goal of end-product development may be better served by making patented research tools widely available on a nonexclusive basis, whereas the goal of procuring upstream research funding may be better served by offering exclusive licenses to sponsors or research partners. Differences among patent owners in their tolerance for transaction costs may further complicate the emergence of informal licensing norms. Universities may be ill equipped to handle multiple transactions for acquiring licenses to use research tools. Delays in negotiating multiple agreements to use patented processes, reagents, and gene fragments could stifle the creative give-and-take of academic research. Yet academic researchers who fail to adopt new discoveries and instead rely on obsolete public domain technologies may find themselves losing grant competitions. Large corporations with substantial legal departments may have considerably greater resources for negotiating licenses on a case-by-case basis than public sector institutions or small start-up firms. This asymmetry may make it difficult to identify mutually advantageous cross-licensing arrangements. Patent owners are also likely to differ in the time frames they can tolerate for recouping current investments in transaction costs.

Owners are also likely to differ in their willingness and ability to infringe the patents of others, resulting in asymmetrical motivations to negotiate cross-licenses. Use of a patented invention in an academic laboratory or a small start-up firm may be inconspicuous, at least if not described in a publication or at a scientific meeting. Patent owners may be more reluctant to sue public sector investigators than they are to sue private firms. Differences in institutional cultures may make academic laboratories and biotechnology firms more tolerant of patent infringement than large pharmaceutical firms. Owners who do not feel vulnerable to infringement liability may be less motivated to enter into reasonable cross-licenses than owners who worry more about being sued.

Cognitive biases. People consistently overestimate the likelihood that very low probability events of high salience will occur (*36*). For example, many travelers overestimate the danger of an airplane crash relative to the hazards of other modes of transportation. We suspect that a similar bias is likely to cause owners of upstream biomedical research patents to overvalue their discoveries. Imagine that one of a set of 50 upstream inventions will likely be the key to identifying an important new drug, the rest of the set will have no practical use, and a downstream product developer is willing to pay $10 million for the set. Given the assumption that no owner knows ex ante which invention will be the key, a rational owner should be willing to sell her patent for the probabilistic value of $200,000. However, if each owner overestimates the likelihood that her patent will be the key, then each will demand more than the probabilistic value, the upstream owners collectively will demand more than the aggregate market value of their inputs, the downstream user will decline the offers, and the new drug will not be developed. Individuals trained in deterministic rather than probabilistic disciplines are particularly likely to succumb to this sort of error (*37*).

A related "attribution bias" suggests that people systematically overvalue their assets and disparage the claims of their opponents when in competition with others (*38*). We suspect that the attribution bias is pervasive among scientists because it is likely adaptive for the research enterprise as a whole. Overcommitment by individuals to particular research approaches ensures that no hypothesis is dismissed too quickly, and skepticism toward rivals' claims ensures that they are not too readily accepted. But this bias can interfere with clear-headed bargaining, leading owners to overvalue their own patents, undervalue others' patents, and reject reasonable offers. Institutional ownership could mitigate these biases, but technology transfer offices rely on scientists to evaluate their discoveries. When two or more patent owners each hope to dominate the product market, the history of biotechnology patent litigation suggests a likelihood that bargaining will fail (*39*).

Conclusion

Like the transition to free markets in post-socialist economies, the privatization of biomedical research offers both promises and risks. It promises to spur private investment but risks creating a tragedy of the anticommons through a proliferation of fragmented and overlapping intellectual property rights. An anticommons in biomedical research may be more likely to endure than in other areas of intellectual property because of the high transaction costs of bargaining, heterogeneous interests among owners, and cognitive biases of researchers. Privatization must be more carefully deployed if it is to serve the public goals of biomedical research. Policy-makers should seek to ensure coherent boundaries of upstream patents and to minimize restrictive licensing practices that interfere with downstream product development. Otherwise, more upstream rights may lead paradoxically to fewer useful products for improving human health.

REFERENCES AND NOTES

1. G. Hardin, *Science* **162**, 1243 (1968).
2. H. Demsetz, *Am. Econ. Rev.* **57**, 347 (1967).
3. M. Heller, *Harvard Law Rev.* **111**, 621 (1998).
4. R. Eisenberg, *Va. Law Rev.* **82**, 1663 (1996).
5. 35 U.S.C.A. §§ 200-11 (West 1984 and Suppl. 1992).
6. Senate Committee on the Judiciary, Subcommittee on Patents, Copyrights, and Trademarks, *The Bayh-Dole Act, A Review of Patent Issues in Federally Funded Research: Hearings on Pub. L. No. 96-517*, 103d Cong., 2nd sess., 1–2 (1994).
7. M. Kenney, *Biotechnology: The University-Industrial Complex* (Yale Univ. Press, New Haven, CT, 1986).
8. F. Michelman, *Nomos* **24**, 3 (1982).
9. W. N. Hohfeld, *Fundamental Legal Conceptions as Applied in Judicial Reasoning and Other Legal Essays* (Yale Univ. Press, New Haven, CT, 1923). This work introduced the now standard vocabulary of "privileges of use" and "rights of exclusion."
10. R. Coase, *J. Law Econ.* **3**, 1 (1960).
11. ______, *The Firm, The Market and The Law* (Univ. of Chicago Press, Chicago, 1988), p. 174. "The world of zero transaction costs has often been described as a Coasian world. Nothing could be further from the truth. It is the world of modern economic theory, one which I was hoping to persuade economists to leave."
12. R. C. Ellickson, *Order Without Law: How Neighbors Settle Disputes* (Harvard Univ. Press, Cambridge, MA, 1991).
13. E. Ostrom, *Governing the Commons: The Evolution of Institutions for Collective Action* (Cambridge Univ. Press, Cambridge, UK, 1990).
14. C. Rose, *Univ. Chicago Law Rev.* **53**, 711 (1986).
15. D. Baird, R. Gertner, R. Picker, *Game Theory and the Law* (Harvard Univ. Press, Cambridge, MA, 1994).
16. R. Merton, *The Sociology of Science* (Univ. of Chicago Press, Chicago, 1973).
17. R. Eisenberg, *Emory Law J.* **39**, 721 (1990).
18. R. Eisenberg and R. Merges, *AIPLA Q. J.* **23**, 1 (1995).
19. National Human Genome Research Institute (NHGRI), Policy on availability and patenting of human genomic DNA sequence produced by NHGRI pilot projects (funded under RFA 95-005) (NHGRI, Bethesda, MD, 1996).
20. U.S. Patent and Trademark Office, *BNA Pat. Trademark Copyright J.* **52**, 732 (1996).
21. R. Merges and R. Nelson, *Columbia Law Rev.* **90**, 839 (1990).
22. "Cetus to exact royalties from PCR sales; probe absolves convicted rapist," *Biotechnology Newswatch* **8**, 7 (5 September 1988).
23. National Research Council, *Intellectual Property Rights and Research Tools in Molecular Biology* (National Academy Press, Washington, DC, 1997).
24. Harvard University, U.S. Patent 4,736,866, 1988; U.S. Patent 5,087,571, 1988. DuPont, as research sponsor, holds an exclusive license under these patents.
25. DuPont, U.S. Patent 4,959,317, 1990.
26. Non-commercial research license agreement between E. I. DuPont de Nemours and Company and Howard Hughes Medical Institute (24 June 1996) (on file with authors).
27. This interpretation requires careful parsing of inartfully drafted licenses, on file with the authors.
28. R. Merges, *Calif. Law Rev.* **84**, 1293 (1996).
29. R. Levin, A. Klevorick, R. Nelson, S. Winter, *Brookings Pap. Econ. Activ.* **1987**, 783 (1987).
30. G. Bittlingmayer, *J. Law Econ.* **31**, 227 (1988).
31. *U.S.* v. *Manufacturers Aircraft Assn.*, 1975 U.S. Dist. LEXIS 15333; 1976-1 Trade Cas. (CCH) ¶ 60,810 (S.D.N.Y. 1975).
32. J. Gould and J. Langenfeld, *IDEA J. Law Technol.* **37**, 449 (1997).
33. G. D. Libecap, *Contracting for Property Rights* (Cambridge Univ. Press, Cambridge, UK, 1989).
34. D. Fundenberg and E. Maskin, *Econometrica* **54**, 533 (1986).
35. *Burroughs-Wellcome* v. *Barr Laboratories*, 40 F. 3d 1223 (Fed. Cir. 1994).
36. A. Tversky and D. Kahneman, *J. Risk Uncertainty* **5**, 297 (1992).
37. D. Lehman, R. Lempert, R. Nisbett, *Am. Psychol.* **43**, 431 (1988).
38. L. Ross and C. A. Anderson, in *Judgment under Uncertainty: Heuristics and Biases*, D. Kahneman *et al.*, Eds. (Cambridge Univ. Press, Cambridge, UK, 1982), pp. 129–152.
39. *Amgen* v. *Chugai Pharmaceutical Co.*, 927 F. 2d 1200 (Fed. Cir. 1991) (erythropoietin); *Scripps Clinic & Research Found.* v. *Genentech*, 927 F. 2d 1565 (Fed. Cir. 1991) (factor VIII:C); *Genentech* v. *Wellcome Found.*, 29 F. 2d 1555 (Fed. Cir. 1994) (tissue plasminogen activator); *Hormone Research Found.* v. *Genentech*, 904 F. 2d 1558 (Fed. Cir. 1990) (human growth hormone); *Genentech* v. *Eli Lilly & Co.*, 998 F. 2d 931 (Fed. Cir. 1993) (human growth hormone); *Bio-Technology General* v. *Genentech*, 80 F. 3d 1553 (Fed. Cir. 1996) (human growth hormone); *Genentech* v. *Novo Nordisk*, 108 F. 3d 1361 (Fed. Cir. 1997) (human growth hormone); *Genentech* v. *Chiron*, 112 F. 3d 495 (Fed. Cir. 1997) (insulin-like growth factor); *Regents of the Univ. of Calif.* v. *Eli Lilly*, 119 F. 3d 1559 (Fed. Cir. 1997).

40. Supported by the Cook Endowment at the University of Michigan Law School and the Office of Health and Environmental Research of the U.S. Department of Energy. We thank I. Cockburn, F. Collins, R. Cook-Deegan, S. Cullen, R. Ellickson, P. Goldstein, D. Hanahan, E. Jordan, K. Paigen, R. Nelson, N. Netanel, E. Posner, H. Varmus, anonymous reviewers for *Science*, and workshop participants at the National Bureau of Economic Research and the University of Michigan, Stanford University, and George Washington University law schools for reading and commenting on earlier versions of this manuscript.

[17]

Human Tissue: Rights in the Body and Its Parts

GERALD DWORKIN AND IAN KENNEDY*

Society has entered into an exciting, though uncertain, age of biotechnology and genetic engineering. Medical procedures which were pure science fiction a generation ago are a reality today: human or animal body parts are being used for transplantation into other humans or animals with ever increasing frequency and ingenuity; animals and humans are being genetically modified; and gene therapy, although in its infancy, shows great promise. All this is occurring under the arc lights of the media which avidly publicize the ethical dilemmas to which these activities give rise.[1]

Inevitably, rational discussion of many of the ethical issues tends to be clouded by emotive reactions. Rational discussion is also clouded by the uncertain state of the law: uncertain both because many of these matters have not yet been considered properly by Parliament or the courts and also because there is frequently a lack of consensus as to whether and, if so how, existing law ought to be reformulated to cope with new issues.

One such area of uncertainty concerns the rights which may exist over the whole or parts of the human body.

The terms "human tissue" or "biological material" are used to describe every aspect of a person's being, ranging from body waste (such as urine, faeces, hair, nail clippings), to a list representing an atlas of the human body; for example, blood, skin, bone, bone marrow, organs such as the cornea, liver, heart and kidneys, amputated limbs, fetal tissue, the placenta and other accompanying fluid and membranes (*i.e.* the contents of the uterus, other than the fetus resulting from pregnancy), fetal tissue, semen, ova. Such tissues will often be removed from the body during surgery or an autopsy.

The destination and use of human tissue removed from the body varies. Some body or clinical waste ordinarily will be destroyed, discarded or otherwise disposed of immediately; some material may be used for medical purposes, for the therapeutic benefit of the patient who was the source of the material or, for example in transplantation situations, for the medical benefit of another; some may be used for

---

* School of Law, King's College, London.

[1] For a consideration of the ethical issues, see the Clothier Report of the Committee on the Ethics of Gene Therapy (Cmnd. 1788 1992).

medical research or teaching; some may be stored in tissue banks (or archived for record or other purposes); and in some cases, the body material may be used for non-medical purposes: for example, in research and development of non-therapeutic cosmetic products.

What property rights exist in such tissue? For example, what is the precise legal nature of the transaction when biological materials are supplied to an academic or commercial researcher? Can the human body or its parts be the subject of "ownership" and, if so, what does that imply?

Until recently, such issues were not often raised and seemed to be of little or no practical significance.[2] The situation has changed. A number of matters have given rise to public concern: for example, the purported sale of organs from living donors; disputes between spouses as to who owns their frozen embryos; and who own or should be entitled to the commercial profits from products developed from human cell lines. Therefore, it has become more pressing to examine the legal basis of activities involving human body materials in medical and research practice, even though, in some of these cases, those involved might find it surprising, or indeed ludicrous, to do so. What are the legal rights of those who provide and those who acquire such material?

It is often stated that there are no property rights in the human body, reflecting an evident reluctance to regard the body in such a distasteful way. The English common law has never got to grips properly with this issue: many of the relevant common law authorities are ancient and of little real value in modern situations. In law, rights may be classified as simply "personal"; others may be much stronger and categorized as "proprietary". The law also uses other related terminology, such as "possessory" rights, "possession" and "custody". As every lawyer knows, however, such terminology is imprecise and is often applied in different senses in different legal contexts.

If the meaning of terms such as "property" and "ownership" are so imprecise, why bother to ask whether any particular subject matter, the body or its parts, is or is not capable of being property, or is capable of

[2] The limited literature in academic journals has multiplied recently. For early discussions, see B. Dickens, "The Control of Living Body Materials" (1977) 27 *University of Toronto Law Journal* 142; and P. Matthews, "Whose Body? People as Property" [1983] C.L.P. 193. For more recent discussions, see R. Magnusson, "The Recognition of Proprietary Rights in Human Tissue in Common Law Jurisdictions" (1992) 18 *Melbourne University Law Review* 601; S. Perley, "From Control Over One's Body to Control Over One's Body Parts: Extending the Doctrine of Informed Consent" (1992) 67 *New York University Law Review* 335; B. Dickens, "Living Tissue and Organ Donors and Property Law: More on *Moore*" (1992) 8 *Journal of Contemporary Health Law and Policy* 73; and E. Scowen, "The Human Body—Whose Property and Whose Profit? (1990) 1 *Dispatches* 1 (Centre of Medical Law and Ethics).

being owned? Why not simply identify the rights which attach to any particular subject-matter and proceed from there? Unfortunately, the law is not entirely logical. In some cases, the courts may have to determine whether or not something is property because it is only when that matter is settled that particular legal consequences flow: for example, the precise causes of action available, against whom, and the rights to trace the destination of the property when considering remedies. Thus, there is a circular analysis: property does not exist unless certain rights normally attach to it; but it may not be possible to determine whether those rights are attached to that subject-matter without first determining whether the subject-matter is property! It is beyond the scope of this paper to explore the finer, philosophical, aspects of the concept of property. However, it will be seen that it does become a matter of some importance to decide whether rights in the body and in body parts are, or should be, regarded by the law as personal or proprietary.

In recent years, several countries have introduced legislative measures dealing with *specific issues* (for example the sale of organs for transplantation) but there is now greater interest in addressing the problems from a broader perspective. Several national committees are preparing general reports: for example, the Office of Technology Assessment in the USA, the Health Council of the Netherlands, the French National Bioethics Committee, the Australian Health Ethics Committee and a Working Group of the Nuffield Council on Bioethics in the United Kingdom. Further, a bill was introduced in France this year to regulate the use of human tissue, organ transplants, and assisted procreation.

The purpose of this paper is to identify some of the ethical and legal issues which are being raised. National laws differ in detail. This paper will be concerned primarily with UK law. It should serve to indicate the legal and social trends which are developing.

The issues may differ depending upon whether we are dealing with rights in the whole body or in its parts, or whether we are dealing with a person's rights in his or her own body or in another's body or parts of it.

I. RIGHTS IN THE WHOLE BODY

A. *During a Person's Life*

One matter which is beyond question, whatever the position may have been when slavery flourished within the law, is that there are *no longer* any property rights over another *living* human being.[3]

[3] Thus, however onerous the duties of some employees may be, employers have no property rights over them. They are contracts for personal services and employers cannot ordinarily obtain specific performance of those contractual obligations.

B. Rights of the Deceased in His/Her Own Body After Death?

The common law position is the same after death. There are many dicta going back through the centuries proclaiming that there can be no property in a corpse.[4] Thus, where a person by will had directed that his body should be cremated after death, it was held that such a request, though it might be honoured in practice, could not be imposed as a legal obligation upon his executors since he lacked any property rights in his body.[5]

C. Rights of Third Parties in Corpses

Nor do any third parties acquire any property interests in a corpse. At most, there are obligations on the next of kin or others in possession of a body to dispose of it decently[6] and it may be a criminal offence at common law to neglect to carry out these duties or in any other way interfere with a corpse. Modern writers maintain that such well established rules survive and limit the modern law of theft (which involves the taking of property), at least to the extent that there could be no theft of a buried corpse.[7]

D. Changing Characteristics

The situation appears to change, however, after a period of time. If the law did not recognize any property rights in a cadaver, or in body parts, problems could arise at a later stage about the status of any physical material which remains. Thus, if the law is not prepared to recognize property rights in skeletons possessed by medical institutions or students, or in the embalmed body of Jeremy Bentham (which has been taken from University College London from time to time by enterprising students from other colleges), or in Egyptian mummies, then those who take them may not be committing any theft, nor, possibly, any legally redressible wrong against those from whom they have been taken.[8]

The common law has occasionally grappled with this situation. If, after some time, the characteristics of the body, or the body parts, have changed in some way so that one is no longer concerned with a corpse

---

[4] *E.g.* "There can be no property in a dead corpse" (2 East PC 652); "Our law recognises no property in a corpse" (*R.* v. *Sharpe* Dears. & B. 160 at 163); "Though the heir has a property in the monuments and escutcheons of his ancestors, yet he has none in their bodies or ashes" (2 Bl.Com. 429).

[5] *Williams* v. *Williams* (1882) Ch.D. 659.

[6] *Cf.* Anatomy Act 1984, s.5(3).

[7] E. Griew, *Theft Acts 1968 and 1978* (6th edn. 1990).

[8] Whilst a plaintiff who is not the owner of property may sue others for interfering with "possessory" rights, actions ordinarily would not be available if what has been taken is not regarded as "property".

awaiting burial, the law *may* look upon it as property and confer upon owners the usual rights to protect it from interference and to deal with it commercially. Thus, in *Doodeward* v. *Spence*[9] an Australian court appears to have held that a still-born two-headed fetus,[10] which had been preserved with spirits in a bottle by the doctor some 40 years earlier, was now an item of property in the hands of its present owner. In that case it was said that

> "... when a person has by the lawful exercise of work or skill so dealt with a human body or part of a human body in his lawful possession that it has acquired some attributes differentiating it from a mere corpse awaiting burial, he acquires a right to retain possession of it, at least as against any person not entitled to have it delivered to him for the purposes of burial..."[11]

In this case it was said that work and skill had been bestowed by the plaintiff's predecessor in title upon the body and it had acquired actual pecuniary value.

E. Outraging Public Decency

Attitudes to property issues may well be affected by the particular circumstances of a case, especially by any sense of outrage that may be felt about the case. Strictly speaking, it should be possible to separate questions as to the *existence of property* and title from any indecent or otherwise unacceptable *use* made of such property. Thus, in *Doodeward* v. *Spence* itself, the police had successfully prosecuted the owner for outraging public decency; yet the owner was held to be entitled to the return of the body. In a more recent English decision,[12] defendants

---

[9] (1908) C.L.R. 406. The precise ratio of the case is by no means clear, however.

[10] The legal status of the fetus is uncertain. The Polkinghorne Report (*Review of the Guidance on the Research Use of Fetuses and Fetal Material* (Cmnd. 762 1989), which focused more upon the need to obtain the mother's consent to research, rather than any property rights in the dead fetus or fetal material, states that 'while in the uterus the fetus is not a legal person. If the fetus is born and lives *ex utero*, even if only for a short time, it then becomes a legal person and the general law applicable to children applies. The consequence ... is that in considering the use for transplantation or research of tissue from fetuses whose death occurs *in utero*, the provisions of the Human Tissue Act 1961 relating to consent are not relevant, since they refer to removal of tissue from deceased persons. It may be that no consent is required in law." (Paras, 3.8 and 3.9). But the same *moral* obligations to "decently dispose" of the fetus would appear to apply: the Report differentiates between the fetus, which has the potential for development into a fully-formed human being and so is entitled to respect, and other fetal material (or "contents of the uterus") *i.e.* the placenta, fluid and membranes, which has no such potential.

[11] (1908) 6 C.L.R. 406 at 414, *per* Griffith C.J.

[12] *R.* v. *Gibson* [1991] 1 All E.R. 439.

who had exhibited in a commercial art gallery "human earrings" made out of freeze-dried human fetuses were successfully convicted of the common law offence of outraging public decency. Yet the Court of Appeal does not appear to have cast any doubt on the property or other rights of the owners of the earrings.[13]

If, ordinarily, there is only a duty to bury a body upon death, it is not always clear what authority exists for preserving the body, or the body parts, until that uncertain point in time when the relevant material is acknowledged to have ripened into property. Presumably, possession originally is vested in a relative, or medical institution, or doctor. In the fetal earrings trial, it had been stated that the fetuses of three to four months' gestation "had been obtained legally from a London college professor", although no further explanation of this appears.[14] In *Doodeward* v. *Spence* Higgins J. observed that "... sundry contraventions of the strict law as to dead bodies are winked at in the interests of medical science, and also for the practical reasons that no one can identify the bones or parts, and that no one is interested in putting the law in motion. Probably some amendment of the Anatomy Act may be required to meet modern conditions."[15]

These remarks, although made in Australia in 1908, may be relevant to the United Kingdom in 1993. The Anatomy Act 1984 does provide that after the anatomical examination is concluded, and subject to the same consents and power to object as applies to the examination itself, it is lawful to have possession in accordance with the given authority of parts (or any specified parts) of a body.[16] It is doubtful whether this right would entitle the lawful possessor to do whatever he liked with the body, give it away or sell it, before it acquired property characteristics; however, in practice, property rights are being exercised over body parts.

F. Special Legislation

The need to obtain and use cadavers for teaching and research and, more recently, for transplantation, resulted in specific legislation for such purposes.

---

[13] In the nineteenth century there was a flourishing trade in New Zealand and elsewhere in preserved and tattooed Maori heads. Although this practice was declared illegal by the Governor of New South Wales in 1831, its legality was not challenged elsewhere. Indeed, proceedings were instituted in 1989 by the Maori Council in New Zealand, supported by the New Zealand Government, to halt the proposed sale of such a preserved head at a London auction. However, the head was withdrawn from the auction and the matter settled prior to trial.

[14] *The Independent*, 10 February 1989.

[15] (1908) 6 C.L.R. 406 at 423.

[16] Anatomy Act 1984, s.6.

The Anatomy Act[17] has already been referred to: although it makes provision for the use of bodies of deceased persons, and parts of such bodies, it is narrowly defined and subject to very strict controls. It empowers a person, prior to death, or a person "lawfully in possession" of a body after death (who has no reason to believe that the deceased or surviving relative has expressed any objection) to give effective directions for the "anatomical examination"[18] of a body after death. Such examinations must be carried out on licensed premises by licensed persons.

The Anatomy Act 1984 does provide that after the anatomical examination is concluded, and subject to the same consents and power to object as applies to the examination itself, it is lawful to have possession in accordance with the given authority of parts (or any specified parts) of a body.[19]

The Human Tissue Act 1961[20] which is the source of the authority to use parts of bodies of deceased persons for transplantation purposes, extends more widely to include "therapeutic purposes ... medical education or research". However, similar permission is required either from the deceased prior to death or the person "lawfully in possession" of the body, and the removal of the body part has to be effected by a fully registered medical practitioner.[21]

The problem with legislation based upon the need for prior permission is that the number of organs made available in this way does not match the pressing demands which exist. An efficient and practical way of meeting the demand would be to have a "contracting-out" system. This would allow the medical authorities to use the organs from cadavers *unless* they had specified in advance that they objected to such use and, possibly, that such objection is noted on some public register.

This is a highly controversial proposal and many countries have been reluctant to introduce such a provision in the face of opposition from a significant part of the population; other countries have placed the need of sick patients first and have introduced contracting-out provisions.[22]

---

[17] The original Anatomy Act 1832, which was a reaction to the evils of body-snatching and the scandal of Burke and Hare, has been replaced by the Anatomy Act 1984.

[18] "Anatomical examination" means the examination by dissection of a body for purposes of teaching or studying, or researching into, morphology; and where parts of a body are separated in the course of its anatomical examination, such examination includes the examination by dissection of the parts for those purposes": Anatomy Act 1984, s.1(1).

[19] Anatomy Act 1984, s.6; Anatomy Regulations 1988 (S.I. 1988 No. 44), Reg. 4.

[20] Replacing, and widening, the Corneal Grafting Act 1952.

[21] *R.* v. *Lennox-Wright* [1973] Crim. L.R. 529.

[22] See *Guiding Principles on Human Organ Transplantation* (World Health Organisation 1991).

Whatever view is taken on problems of supply, these Acts provide little support for the existence of property rights in the cadaver, or parts of it: references are to persons "lawfully in possession" of the body and the emphasis is centred far more on the issue of donor consent.[23]

II. RIGHTS IN PARTS OF THE BODY

A. *Personal Rights and the Importance of Consent*

We all have strong *personal rights* in our own bodies and its component parts, at least before they are removed. Cardozo J. expressed the principle in a frequently cited passage: "Every human being of adult years and sound mind has a right to determine what shall be done with his body; and a surgeon who performs an operation without his patient's consent commits an assault, for which he is liable in damages."[24]

We are all protected by the criminal and the civil law from uninvited attacks or physical intrusions from others. In many cases, however, provided consent has been given, tissue may be removed from a person's body quite legitimately; otherwise surgery would be unlawful.

B. *Limitations Upon the Power to Consent*

Consent is not the only determinant, however. There are some situations where Parliament has felt it necessary to prohibit or restrict the freedom of individuals to consent to particular types of physical interference with the body: for example, abortion, the tattooing of minors, and female circumscision.[25] From time to time, campaigns are waged for legislation to control or prohibit controversial procedures: for example, fetal tissue transplantation research. Fears were expressed in the USA and in the United Kingdom that some women might be encouraged or influenced to abort fetuses to provide tissue for research or transplantation. In the United Kingdom, the Polkinghorne Report led to a Code of Practice being introduced to regulate fetal tissue research activity.[26]

Even in the absence of legislation, the courts sometimes feel compelled, in extreme cases, to step in paternalistically and override the

---

[23] However, there is an intriguing, open-ended, provision in the section dealing with the removal of body parts that "nothing [therein] shall be construed as rendering unlawful any *dealing* with, or with any part of, the body of a deceased person which is lawful apart from [the] Act": Human Tissue Act 1961 s.1(8).

[24] *Schloendorff* v. *Society of New York Hospital* (1914) 105 N.E. 92.

[25] Abortion Act 1967 (as amended); Tattooing of Minors Act 1969; and Prohibition of Female Circumcision Act 1985.

[26] *Review of the Guidance on the Research Use of Fetuses and Fetal Material* (Cmnd. 762 1989).

consent of the individual. Thus, in the days of Coke, a person was convicted of a criminal offence when he amputated another's hand, so that he was in a better position to beg, notwithstanding that consent had been given.[27] This readiness to disregard consent has been endorsed much more recently. In one case, Lord Lane C.J. stated that: "... It is not in the public interest that people should try to cause or should cause each other actual bodily harm for no good reason ... [However nothing] ... is intended to cast doubt on the accepted legality of [*inter alia*] ... *reasonable surgical interference* [which] ... can be justified as ... needed in the public interest..."[28] Lord Lane later developed this point further when he said:

> There are ... certain circumstances in which the law does not permit a defendant to rely ... on the victim's consent. The victim's consent to being killed would provide no excuse for the killer. Where the assault to which consent is given involves permanent injury or maiming—e.g. the severing of a limb—there is no dispute that the victim's consent is immaterial.

Even where there is no permanent injury, Lord Lane adopted a textbook comment that:[29]

> ... even the most complete consent, by the most competent person, will not suffice to legalise an assault which there are public grounds for prohibiting. This consent is no defence, criminally, for any assault that involves some extreme and causeless injury to life, limb or health; ... nor for any assault likely to cause bodily harm (whether extreme or not) and not justified by good reason, *e.g.* sport, lawful chastisement, *etc.*

He then reserved the right of judicial supervision by emphasizing that it was necessary to decide what may be "good reason".[30]

This flexibility is necessary, if, in the absence of appropriate legislation, the courts are to keep up with medical progress. The legality of live organ transplantation demonstrates this. The very first transplants, insofar as they could not be categorized as therapeutic from the point of view of the donor, were questionable—there was no judicial authority

---

[27] R. v. *Wright* (1603).

[28] *Attorney-General's Reference (No. 6 of 1980)* [1981] Q.B. 715..See also *R.* v. *Brown* [1993] 2 All E.R. 75 at 90, *per* Lord Jauncey.

[29] *Kenny's Outline of Criminal Law* (19th edn. 1966).

[30] *R.* v. *Brown* [1992] 2 All E.R. 552 (C.A.); affirmed by a majority of the House of Lords [1993] 2 All E.R. 75. Consent to sado-masochistic acts was not an operative consent.

to establish whether there was sufficient "just cause" to provide a defence. It was certainly arguable that a person did not have the legal power to consent to such an operation if it was not performed for his own therapeutic benefit. However, as transplantation of organs from live donors became accepted medical practice, it became clear (almost by default) that such recognized medical practices are not unlawful. It is possible that other interventions and removal of tissue, if not therapeutic, might be regarded as reprehensible and so unlawful: the courts have to weigh up the risks and benefits very carefully. "The dividing line between permissible and prohibited tissue loss remains a matter of public policy, as judicially determined, but public policy evolves over a course of time and can be adapted to accommodate biotechnical developments and changing social priorities and recognition of the limits of self-sacrifice."[31]

C. Are There "Property Rights" in Body Materials?

The power to consent to physically intrusive activity suggests that we have some control over what others may do to our bodies. Does control mean that, save for those cases where there are statutory or common law limitations, we can authorize the taking and use of parts of our body, either gratuitously or for reward? Can human tissue become a commodity? If so, then the *personal* rights we have in our own body in some respects broaden into *property* rights.

Some body material, for example hair once removed from the body, appears always to have been regarded as property: nobody would question a person's right to sell it; and the criminal law would treat the stealing of hair as theft of property. There are other examples of successful convictions for the theft of urine and blood.[32] There is also legislative recognition that there can be transactions in human body materials: for example, the supply and disposal of blood in the National Health Service;[33] and there are European Community provisions for the exchange and transportation of substances of human

---

[31] B. Dickens, "The Control of Living Body Materials" (1977) *University of Toronto Law Journal* 142 at 165.

[32] *R.* v. *Welsh* [1974] R.T.R. 478; *R.* v. *Rothery* [1976] R.T.R. 550. See Smith, "Stealing the Body and its Parts" [1976] Crim. L.R. 622.

[33] National Health Service Act, s.25: "Where the Secretary of State has acquired –

(a) supplies of human blood for the purposes of any service under this Act, or

(b) any part of a human body for the purpose of, or in the course of providing, any such service, or

(c) supplies of any other substances or preparations not readily obtainable,

he may arrange to make such supplies or that part available (on such terms, including terms as to charges, as he thinks fit) to any person."

origin.[34] There has been slightly greater hesitation in acknowledging property in various kinds of reproductive material[35] although property type disputes have begun to appear in some parts of the world. One example was of frozen embryos held in store: what are the rights of the persons who produced or possessed the embryos: family rights as if the embryos were persons or, if the embryos are simply tissue, rights as co-owners of property, whatever such rights may be? There is an understandable reluctance to treat embryos out of the womb as property.[36] The Human Fertilisation and Embryology Act 1990, which provided a new code of law dealing with the control and supervision of research involving human embryos and the licensing of certain types of assisted conception using the new reproductive technologies, could have resolved the issue. However, the property question was sidestepped. The Act imposes severe constraints upon those who have possession of embryos in relation to their storage and use; yet, arguably, a sufficient number of core rights are retained to satisfy the test of property.[37] Nor

---

[34] The Council of Ministers of the Council of Europe in furtherance of Res.(78)29 adopted Recommendation R(79)5 calling upon Member States to facilitate the *international exchange and transportation of specific* substances of human origin; to ensure the exchange of information on the demand for and availability of the substances and to exempt the substances and their containers from all duties and taxes on import and export.

[35] "Blood and sperm banks must surely be protected by the law of theft. Nor need the status of 'property' be denied to parts of living donors removed for transplantation or even removed for *in vitro* fertilization. The case of an ovum fertilized *in vitro* is, to say the least, more doubtful." (E. Griew, *The Theft Act 1968 & 1978* (6th ed. 1990) at para 2–18).

[36] In a US decision, *Del Zio* v. *Manhattan's Columbia Presbyterian Medical Center* (1978), where a medical department, without consent, had destroyed the contents of a test-tube containing a couple's fertilized egg, the Court favoured a personal remedy for severe emotional distress rather than a claim for tortious destruction of property. In the recent, much publicized, decision in *Davis* v. *Davis* (1992) 842 S.W. 2d 605, the Supreme Court of Tennessee refused to categorize embryos as persons or property. They occupied an "interim category". See Grubb (1993) 1 Med.L.R. 273 Similar views have been expressed in the UK: "Until now, the law has never had to consider the existence of embryos outside the mother's uterus. The existence of such embryos raises potentially difficult problems as to ownership. The concept of ownership of human embryos seems to us to be undesirable. We recommend that legislation be enacted to ensure that there is no right of ownership in a human embryo" (*Report of the (Warnock) Committee of Inquiry into Fertilisation and Embryology* (Cmnd 9314 1984), paras. 10–11); "It is wrong to try to define a human embryo in terms of established legal definitions which are plainly inapplicable to human embryos. Why must an embryo be one or the other? Why cannot it be just an embryo?" *per* Lord Hailsham (H.L. Deb. 6 Feb. 1990, col. 751).

[37] See *Belfast Corp.* v. *OD Cars* [1960] A.C. 490; D. Morgan and R. Lee, *Human Fertilisation and Embryology Act 1990* (Blackstone 1991) at 31–32; I. Kennedy and A. Grubb, *Medical Law Text and Materials* (Butterworths 1989) at 682.

has any other recent, related, legislation concerned itself directly with the question whether human tissue was or should be regarded as property in law.[38]

Thus, apart from prohibited acts, there appears to be nothing at common law, apart from vague arguments as to immorality and public policy, which would prevent courts from regarding parts of the body, or at least most parts of the body, in the same way as other forms of personal property, once the parts have been removed from the body.

D. The "Non-Commercial" Transfer of Rights in Human Tissue

The analysis so far has been highly theoretical. What difference should it make whether, in law, property rights do or do not exist in human body materials if, and as long as, those who acquire, use or dispose of them do so with the express or tacit agreement of the persons who are the source of the material? One reason is that, should the law regard rights in human tissue as property rights, issues relating to ownership and title could affect all those who directly or indirectly acquire such tissue.

The first situation to explore is the standard medical scenario: in the course of treatment, human tissue is removed from the body and destroyed. The lay, and common sense, analysis is that since the patient has consented to the treatment, that suffices to give legitimacy to the entire procedure.[39] A comparable legal analysis would be that although property does not come into existence until the tissue is removed, the consent to removal ensures that, upon removal, the property becomes vested *in the person removing it.*

However, there is a more technical legal analysis. There is a general principle that *legal* title to property cannot be transferred until it comes into existence; at the most, a purported transfer of future property may take effect as a contract to transfer the title once the property is created.[40] Thus, the title must vest, in the first instance albeit

[38] For example, the Surrogacy Arrangements Act 1985, which outlawed commercial surrogacy contracts and other arrangements, was not directly concerned with rights in reproductive material as such. The Human Organ Transplants Act 1989, discussed *infra*, also did not address the property issue.

[39] In *Browning* v. *Norton Children's Hospital* (1974) 504 S.W. 2d 713 (Ky) it was said that "when one consents to and authorises an operation while a patient in a hospital (absent any specific reservation, demand or objection to some normal procedure) he then and thereby in effect accepts all the rules, regulations, and the modus operandi of that hospital" as to disposal of surgically removed tissue.

[40] A rare statutory exception to that rule applies to copyright where it is possible to assign future works so that the legal title vests in the assignee at the moment the copyright work comes into existence: Copyright, Designs and Patents Act 1988, s.91.

momentarily,[41] in the patient. Assuming that the hospital authority is not acting as agent for the patient, the title must then pass in some way from the patient to the hospital authority, presumably by way of a gift. A donation of personal property takes effect when there is a transfer of possession of the property coupled with an intention to make the gift. Here, the intention could be express (for example, in a consent form which specifically refers to this) or, in most cases, implied.

Another analysis would be to rely upon the doctrine of abandonment. Although this doctrine has not been used to any great extent in English law, there is little question that it exists,[42] and there is no reason why English courts should not follow American judicial comments regarding the abandonment of waste materials from operations.[43] Thus, any property interest in the removed tissue passes from the patient to the medical authorities.

Should the analysis be any different if the human tissue which is removed from the body is not destroyed but retained by the medical authorities for the purposes of, say, teaching or research? It is submitted that, at common law, in most cases where a patient has consented to

---

[41] The concept of *scintilla temporis*, namely, the moment of time in which title must first vest in a transferor if he is to have any right to pass a legal interest to the transferee is well known, albeit losing favour, in English law. In *Abbey National BS* v. *Cann* [1990] 1 All E.R. 1085 at 1099–1100 Lord Oliver said: "As a matter of legal theory ... a person cannot [deal with] a legal estate that he does not have ... Nevertheless [this case] flies in the face of reality. The reality is that [the two transactions here] ... are not only precisely simultaneous but indissolubly bound together ... The *scintilla temporis* is no more than a legal artifice."

[42] *Halsbury's Laws of England* (4th edn.), vol. 35 para.1125. There are occasional references to abandonment in case law stretching through the centuries. See, for example, Chitty J. in *Elwes* v. *Brigg Gas Co.* (1886) 33 Ch.D. 562 (a case concerning the ownership or possession of an ancient boat dug up when excavations were taking place): "obviously the right of the original owner could not be established; it had for centuries been lost or barred, even supposing that the property had not been abandoned when the boat was first left on the spot where it was found"; *Cumberland* v. *Ireland* [1946] K.B. 264 (a case concerning the abandonment of "rubbish"). *Hibbert* v. *McKiernan* [1948] 2 K.B. 142 (a case of lost golf balls). It would appear that courts, in cases where property is clearly valuable, would not apply a presumption of abandonment lightly. There is also some reluctance to find that there can be abandonment without the title automatically vesting in another person. For example, it was said in *Hayne's Case* (1614) 12 Co. Rep. 113 that: "A man cannot relinquish the property he hath to his goods unless they be vested in another"; *cf. R.* v. *Small* (1987) 86 Crim. App. Rep. 170; [1987] Crim. L.R. 777.

[43] "By the force of social custom, we hold that when a person does nothing and says nothing to indicate an intent to assert his right of ownership, possession or control over such material, the only rational inference is that he intends to abandon the material": *Venner* v. *State of Maryland* (1976) 354 A. 2d 483 at 498.

medical procedures without more, the presumption of abandonment of all property or other rights in the removed tissue could apply, leaving the patient with no further legal interest in the material, whatever may subsequently be done to it. Whilst the recipients of the tissue may be bound by ethical and professional constraints as to its acquisition and use,[44] they are not subject to any continuing legal control by the patient.

However, a patient's consent to particular uses may be required or sought expressly in advance. Patients might react to such requests in a number of ways: some, probably very few, might refuse consent to anything but destruction; most are likely to indicate that it matters not whether the tissue is destroyed or used for other medical or medical-related purposes; some might say that they agree to its use for such purposes but not, for example, for anything which affects their social or religious sensibilities or which is in some other way offensive to them, or, possibly, not for any commercial purposes. In law, such reactions may modify the nature of the abandonment or gift which has taken place. A donor is free to reserve a right to revoke a gift or to impose conditions upon a donee, provided they are not illegal or contrary to public policy.[45]

The closest statutory analogy can be found in the Human Fertilisation and Embryology Act 1990 which contains detailed, mandatory, provisions relating to the nature of conditional consents to use gametes

---

[44] See, for example, the Polkinghorne Report (*Review of the Guidance on the Research Use of Fetuses and Fetal Material* (Cmnd. 762 1989)) and the resulting Code of Practice on the Use of Fetuses and Fetal Material in Research and Treatment; *Guidelines on the Practice of Ethics Committees in Medical Research involving Human Subjects* (2nd edn.) (Royal College of Physicians 1990) at para.13.20 (Use of Discarded Tissues for Research); *Responsibility in Investigations on Human Participants and Material and on Personal Information (No. 9: Human Material)* (Medical Research Council 1992).

[45] *E.g. Parkinson* v. *College of Ambulances* [1925] 2 K.B. 1. It is less clear whether a patient would be able to impose a condition preventing the sale of the tissue: a general condition against alienation of donated property is inconsistent with the nature of an absolute gift and is said, albeit controversially (see Glanville Williams, "The Doctrine of Repugnancy" (1943) 59 L.R. 343), to be repugnant. However, limited conditions against alienation, such as that the tissue may be sold for use in the National Health Service only, arguably may be acceptable.

US courts have acknowledged the right of a person to reserve interests in their tissue: "It is not unknown for a person to assert a continuing right of ownership, dominion or control, for good reason, or no reason, over such things as excrement, fluid waste, secretions, hair, fingernails, toenails, blood and organs or other parts of the body, whether their separation from the body is intentional, accidental or merely the result of normal body functions": *Venner* v. *State of Maryland* (1976) 354 A. 2d 483 at 498.

or embryos for treatment, research, storage etc., and to the variation and withdrawal of such consents.[46]

It is also possible to argue that, even in the absence of express conditions, an implied condition as to use may arise in some situations where there are written or other clear indications (for example, in a Code of Practice) specifying the uses to which tissue should be put. However, the courts have sometimes emphasized that the mere motive behind a donation by itself cannot control the future application or destination of the property unless the donor's purpose can be construed as a condition. It would appear, therefore, that a patient, at least in theory, has the legal right to specify expressly what may be done with the tissue, or, more realistically, what may not be done with it.

E. Sale of Body Materials?

If it is acknowledged, in law, that human tissue is property, then in principle it should be possible for it to be transferred not only by way of gift but also by sale. Can a person sell his tissue to medical researchers; can a hospital sell its tissue to commercial research companies? Medical students have long bought and sold whole or parts of the human skeleton; the sale of hair is a long standing and accepted practice: few would seek to challenge the legality of such transactions. Modest payments are made to blood and semen donors (although these are often regarded as compensation for expenses incurred and the time involved). In some countries there are organizations which acquire human organs and other tissue and supply them to researchers on a commercial basis.[47]

From an ethical standpoint, however, commercial dealings with human tissue have always been looked upon with unease. Objections range from those who simply find it ethically degrading to those who fear that commercialization can lead to abusive practices: improper exploitation of the human source of the material, poorer quality tissue, etc.[48]

---

[46] Section 12 and Schedule 3. Another statutory analogy can be found in the Copyright, Designs and Patents Act 1988, s.87, where the "moral" rights in copyright works (*i.e.* the legally enforceable, but unassignable, rights of authors and directors to be acknowledged as such and their right to prevent the works being subjected to "derogatory treatment") may be waived, conditionally or unconditionally, in relation to specific or existing or future works; and the waiver may be expressed to be subject to revocation. Such a waiver, which may be in writing or informal, is presumed to extend to licensees and successors in title in the absence of a contrary intention.

[47] *E.g.* International Institute for the Advancement of Medicine (Keystone Skin Bank) and Human Biologics Inc. (USA). There have been recent proposals to set up a research human tissue bank in the UK.

[48] For the powerful and influential case against the commercialization of blood, see R. Titmuss, *The Gift Relationship* (1970).

It was the publicity given to cases where poor persons were being induced to sell their organs for transplantation purposes that led to the introduction of the Human Organ Transplants Act 1989. It is now a criminal offence to make or receive any payment for organs removed from a dead or living person intended for transplantation into another person, whether in the UK or elsewhere.[49] The definition of "organ" is "any part of a human body consisting of a structured arrangement of tissues which, if wholly removed, cannot be replicated by the body".[50] Thus, the Act applies only to certain types of body material as opposed to the Human Tissue Act 1961 (concerning the use of cadavers) which refers to "the body or any specified part".

The Human Organ Transplants Act 1989 was introduced hastily, in response to public concern focused on particular abuses. It is an open question whether the legislation should have gone further and dealt with the commercialization of all, or most other, kinds of human tissue.[51] Whilst there is scope for abuse, it is not likely to be as great, and there are ethical arguments both for and against such an extension.

Another important consideration, which can only be mentioned in passing, is that when there is a transfer of tissue, whether by the patient or some later transferee, there may be potential civil liability on the transferor: in tort, should the tissue turn out to be defective and cause injury; and in contract, where implied conditions that the tissue is of merchantability quality and fit for its purpose may arise.[52]

F. The Moore Case: Is it a Property Issue?

The significance of determining that a person's right to control the destiny of tissue removed from his body is not simply personal but proprietary can be illustrated by looking at the unusual fact situation, and legal analysis, in *Moore* v. *University of California*.[53]

Moore had a form of leukaemia and was a patient at a university hospital. His spleen was unusual and interesting to the doctor and his medical research colleagues. A cell line was created from one of his

---

[49] The Act also prohibits the removal of an organ from a living person for transplantation into another person with whom there is no genetic relationship without the approval of the Unrelated Live Transplant Regulatory Authority.

[50] Human Organ Transplants Act 1989, s.7(2).

[51] See, for example, the Human Tissue Act 1982 (Victoria, Australia) ss. 38 and 39 which prohibits the sale of all tissue. A 1993 French bill (not yet enacted) proposes that no remuneration may be given to the donor of parts, of blood or of products of his body.

[52] For example, under legislation such as the Consumer Protection Act 1987, the Supply of Goods and Services Act 1982. There is considerable US litigation dealing with cases of the supply of contaminated blood. Sadly, there are now several examples of contaminated blood causing AIDS, including cases in the United Kingdom.

[53] (1990) 793 P. 2d 479 (Cal. Sup. Ct.). The legal debate turned upon *alleged* facts.

cells, patented and licensed to several pharmaceutical and biotechnical firms.

Moore had never been told about the unique properties or the commercial value of his cells, nor was he aware of the research being undertaken and of the commercial negotiations that were taking place. Indeed, it was alleged that, when he made a series of visits to the hospital after his spleen was removed, for the purposes of providing samples of blood and bodily substances, he was given the impression that this was for therapeutic purposes whereas in fact it was for research and commercial purposes.

When proceedings were brought against the defendants, the Supreme Court of California considered two types of possible action:[54] first, a *personal* action based upon the failure to obtain informed consent and the breach of the doctor's fiduciary duty to disclose material facts to a patient and, secondly, a *proprietary* action alleging that the patient's rights in his body tissue had been unlawfully converted to the defendants' use.

The majority of the Supreme Court decided in favour of Moore on personal rather than proprietary grounds: the Court refused to strike out his claim based on breach of duty and remanded it for trial. It is submitted that the analysis of the majority of the Court is less satisfactory than that of the minority, which is more likely to be consistent with the, admittedly uncertain, present state of UK law.

The personal action was upheld by relying upon the overlapping concepts of informed consent and the fiduciary obligation to disclose relevant information to the plaintiff. The vast majority of US jurisdictions oblige a doctor to disclose to a patient all those medical facts which might influence a patient in deciding whether or not to undergo a medical procedure. Here, the Court extended his duty of disclosure beyond matters relating to the risks involved in the medical procedures to matters relating to the doctor's *research* or *economic* interests. An alternative way of putting this was to say that "the existence of a motivation for a medical procedure unrelated to the patient's health is a *potential conflict of interest* and a fact which is material to the patient's decision". Thus, the patient's consent was not informed and there was also a breach of the doctor's fiduciary duty.

In English law, it is less likely that a patient would ordinarily have a personal cause of action against the doctor on the same grounds. The doctrine of consent to medical procedures is not so favourable to patients. It is doctor-based and concentrates on what reasonable

---

[54] These had been narrowed down from the 13 causes of action originally alleged by the plaintiff.

doctors in the particular circumstances, and in the light of medical practice, might tell a patient rather than on what a reasonable patient would expect to be told. Similarly, there would be difficulty at present in relying upon a breach of a fiduciary relationship since, perhaps inexplicably, English law appears not to regard the doctor-patient relationship as having a fiduciary character as such.[55] It may be, perhaps, that on the very special and extreme facts of this case, a court might regard the deliberate failure to disclose and the deceit involved in the subsequent hospital visits as sufficient to ground an action in negligence (although there would be problems in determining the nature of any damage causally connected to the breach of duty or the measure of any such damage) or under some equitable principle relating to "fraud, duress or undue influence", or even as giving rise to an action in battery, if the original consent would have been gained through fraud or misrepresentation. This is a matter which will be mentioned later in this paper.

The majority of the Supreme Court decided that the plaintiff must be satisfied with a personal remedy and rejected the proprietary action. The arguments of the scientific community that research and development in biotechnology would be slowed down and otherwise hampered if persons were to have proprietary rights in their own tissue weighed heavily with the court: "*unencumbered* access to human tissue for research is essential to progress and public health; ... these sources must remain unencumbered, and medical researchers be free to both combine these materials with tissue taken from others, and dispose of the tissues, without answering to the person from whom the tissue was taken ... [If the] plaintiff is permitted to have decision making authority and a financial interest in the cell-line, he would then have the unlimited power to inhibit medical research that could potentially benefit humanity. He could conceivably go from institution to institution seeking the highest bid and, if dissatisfied, claim the right simply to prohibit the research entirely."[56]

Thus, the primary reason for the Court's approach was one of public policy and all the subsidiary arguments employed were designed simply to add weight to this factor. Even in terms of American law, the reasons employed, as the dissenting opinions of Broussard and Mosk JJ. demonstrate, are challengeable.

First, it was argued that since the case was novel and no previous decision had applied the conversion remedy to human tissue, it would

[55] *Sidaway* v. *Bethlem Royal Hospital* [1985] 1 All E.R. 643 H.L. *Cf. McInerney* v. *MacDonald* (1992) 93 D.L.R. (4th) 415 (Supreme Court of Canada); (1993) 1 Med. L.Rev. 126.

[56] See the comments in the court below: (1988) 51 Cal.App. 3d 1230 (Cal. C.A.).

be wrong for the Court to extend the law. It would have been just as valid, however, to regard tissue as personal property and simply accept that conversion should apply here as in all other property cases.

Secondly, it was maintained that in an important policy matter of this kind any extension of the law is best left for the legislature. The simple response is that, however desirable legislative consideration of this matter may be, where a court is called upon to determine a tortious dispute, it has traditionally exercised its jurisdiction to develop the law on a case-by-case basis.

The third approach was to look at the trend of related Californian legislation (for example, that dealing with the disposal of tissue and organs for transplantation) to see whether any clear policy could be discerned. The majority found, implicit in this legislation, a clear policy against persons having proprietary control over their tissue. The minority, however, disputed this.

A fourth point, emphasized by one judge, was the immorality of Moore seeking recognition of a right to *sell* his body tissue *for profit*: "the ramifications of recognising and enforcing a property interest in body tissues are not known, but are greatly feared ... [as was] the effect on human dignity of a marketplace in human body parts [and] the impact upon research and development of competitive bidding for such materials." Whilst the issue of commercializing human tissue is an important general matter ripe for legislative consideration, it is less obvious that the court should take action on this matter unless it was convinced that there was an overwhelming case for it to exercise its controversial paternalistic jurisdiction to ban unacceptable conduct in the public interest. In any event, it has been pointed out that, whilst it is arguable as a matter of policy or morality that a court may ban or restrict any person from profiting from the fortuitous value that adheres in a part of the human body, this decision does not do that: it simply bars Moore, the source of the cells, from obtaining the benefit of the cells' value but permits the doctor, who obtained the cells from Moore by allegedly improper means, and others, to retain and exploit the full economic value of their "ill-gotten" gains free of their ordinary common law liability for conversion.

It was this fear that Moore might be able to use the conversion argument to extend his remedy as far as the revenue obtained from the exploitation of the patents that led the Court additionally to disclaim any causal relationship between his cells and the patented cell line and products derived from it. Even though there was no apparent significant difference between the cells and the cell line, the Court regarded them as both *factually* and *legally* distinct. The majority concluded that the patent somehow cut off all Moore's rights; even though Moore was not claiming that he was solely entitled to the patent which had been based upon his cells but merely to some share in the commercial exploitation of the patent or products which were derived from his cells.

A fifth consideration concentrated upon the position of third parties. In particular, it was feared that a conversion remedy, which was not linked to fault, would impose liability on all those into whose hands the cells might come, whether or not the particular defendants participated in, or knew of, the inadequate disclosures that violated the patient's right to make an informed decision. In the absence of any provision safeguarding the bona fide innocent user of tissue, there is certainly a risk of liability, but this risk exists when people acquire any property from those without proper title. Those who acquire property have to be alert as to the organizations from who they obtain their material and it is likely that the fears expressed have been considerably overestimated.

Lastly, the majority of the Court concluded that not only was the conversion remedy undesirable but, in any event, it was unnecessary since Moore's *personal* remedy for breach of fiduciary duty and the failure to obtain informed consent was sufficient to protect him. To Moore, that must have seemed a curious conclusion. It was not clear what compensation Moore would have been entitled to on the basis of the personal remedy: the Court did not see fit to discuss this issue. Does an action for negligence in this context extend beyond any possible physical damage (and there was none) to any emotional distress or other personal injury to cover also the loss of any profits from the exploitation of the patent? Had Moore been informed of all the facts he might still have given his unconditional consent and he would have suffered no loss; alternatively, had he objected, there would have been no relevant exploitation of his cells and no damage; alternatively, he might have given his consent on terms that he shared in the profits and was entitled to compensation for that.

On the other hand, putting aside the limitations inherent in a negligence action, an action for breach of fiduciary duty is grounded in equity and, as will be discussed later, provides the opportunity to seek an account of profits or other restitutionary benefits. Thus, although this appears to have been the assumption, it is by no means clear that Moore would have been entitled to less than he would have been entitled to under a proprietary action. The majority of the Supreme Court may have been right that Moore would not suffer by having to rely on an action for breach of fiduciary duty, even though they assumed that this action would not threaten the research community. Arguably, however, it would be difficult to bring an action against *third parties* on the basis of the personal rather than the proprietary remedy, which would be important for all those defendants other than the doctor treating Moore.

G. Would Moore Have Succeeded Under English Law?

Moore might have a greater chance of success under English law were he to pursue the conversion-proprietary claim rather than the personal action. Conversion (or trover) lies where a defendant carries out some wrongful act or interference with the dominion or control of goods in the possession of another.[57] On the basis of the earlier analysis, there is no reason to suppose that, *prima facie*, human tissue would not be regarded as "goods". For example, Halsbury states that "trover may ... lie for human tissue or for human remains".[58]

Thus, an English common law approach to the *Moore* case could proceed on the following lines. Moore's personal right to physical security ensures that nobody may take tissue from his body without appropriate prior consent. At this stage, at the most, Moore might have an inchoate right of property in his tissue which would become a full property right once it has been removed from his body. Prior to removal Moore could have expressly (for example, in an appropriately worded consent form) abandoned any material removed from his body or transferred the property to the hospital or medical authorities for destruction or for specific or general research or other purposes. It would also have been possible, though extremely unusual, for such an express transfer of any human tissue (other than an "organ" within the meaning of the Human Organ Transplants Act 1989) to be by way of sale for some monetary or other consideration. In the absence of any express provision, it is likely that Moore's standard consent to medical treatment would carry with it an implied abandonment of discarded human tissue. Accordingly, the medical authorities would then be free to assume total property rights over the tissue without any further legal obligation to refer back, or be accountable to, Moore. In most circumstances, the mere fact that the physician failed to disclose any research or economic potential of discarded tissue is unlikely to affect the analysis: the norm of implied abandonment is likely to prevail. Thus, in the vast majority of situations, though a conversion action is technically feasible, it would not be sustainable.

The situation is likely to be different, however, in two cases. First, where the patient, or other person from whom tissue is removed, expressly addresses the question of what will, or should, happen to the tissue after its removal. On the argument advanced earlier, he would have a right to control the future of the removed tissue. In those

---

[57] Today, the action is subsumed within the broader category of "wrongful interference with goods" in the Torts (Interference with Goods) Act 1977, but the principles of law, subject to the express provisions of the Act, are broadly the same.

[58] *Halsbury's Laws of England* (4th edn.) vol. 45 para. 1421.

circumstances, it is for the medical authorities to decide whether to accept the terms upon which it is to receive the tissue. If it acts inconsistently with the donor's wishes, then, *prima facie*, there is an action for conversion.

Secondly, the fact situation may be extreme. Simply to know that patients' tissue may be used for research (even *sold* to laboratories) and that in some rare cases it could have unique and valuable economic potential should not in itself be sufficient to impose an obligation upon a physician to disclose such a matter to the patient. There would have to be some element of deception. *Moore* was argued as a case of blatant deception prior to the removal of the relevant tissue. In such unusual circumstances, it is likely that the failure to disclose known information about commercial potential could be regarded as so important to the patient's decision to undergo the medical procedures as to affect the validity of Moore's consent and so justify an action against the physician for *trespass*.[59] In any event, it is likely that an English court would be prepared to employ equitable principles in support of the patient: Moore surely must come somewhere within the equitable principles relating to "fraud, duress or undue influence" to receive the support of equity. Moore would have the right to avoid the transaction and be free to pursue a conversion action, in addition to any other cause of action that may be available.

Given that, adopting an English law analysis, Moore would have one or several causes of action, it next becomes appropriate to consider the remedies to which he might be entitled.

Damages are likely to be very difficult to assess. At one extreme, he would be entitled to the normal measure of damages for conversion, which would be the value of the "goods" *at the time of the conversion*, together with any consequential and non-remote damage. This would be unlikely to satisfy Moore: the value of his cells was negligible until they were transformed by the defendants' skill into a patented cell line and its various products. At the other extreme, he might claim some or all of the profits from the exploitation of the patent and its products, which could be regarded as the improved products of Moore's cells. In some cases of conversion, where the value of the converted goods has risen by the time of the judgment, the latter date can be used for

[59] For a full discussion of this issue, see I. Kennedy and A. Grubb, *Medical Law: Text and Materials* (Butterworths 1989) at 137–43 citing, *inter alia*, Laskin C.J. in *Reibl* v. *Hughes* (1980) 114 D.L.R. (3d) 1; Sir John Donaldson M.R. and Dunn L.J., at Court of Appeal level, in *Sidaway* v. *Bethlem Royal Hospital* [1984] 1 All E.R. 1018 and in *Freeman* v. *Home Office (No. 2)* [1984] 1 All E.R. 1036. It is of interest to note that Moore alleged that had he been informed of the true situation, he would not have agreed to the removal of his spleen.

valuation. The case law suggests that there is no hard and fast rule: it is not possible "... to attempt to lay down any rule which is intended to be of any universal application as to the date by reference to which the value of the goods is to be assessed. The method of valuation and the date of valuation will depend on the circumstances".[60]

Thus, the measure of damage is anyone's guess, as also would be the extent to which the work of the defendants in improving the cell-line could be taken into account in reducing the amount of compensation due to Moore. Whilst the Torts (Interference with Goods) Act 1977, section 6 provides that an allowance may be made to a defendant for any increase in the value of the goods due to expenditure or work on them by a defendant who acted in the mistaken but honest belief that he had a good title to the goods, the physician in the *Moore* case would not be able to rely upon that provision, although those who later used the tissue for research and development might well be able to do so.[61]

An alternative to damages would be to seek equitable remedies such as delivery up or an account of profits or some similar equitable principle: there is considerable scope, although not in this paper, for developing arguments based upon constructive trust, unjust enrichment, and the like.

There are many examples of defendants being ordered to disgorge their profits, or a major part of them, although none appears to be directly comparable to the Moore situation. For example, in one very old and unusual case, the plaintiff was the father of baby Siamese twins who had given custody of them to the defendant who agreed to main-

---

[60] *I.B.L* v. *Coussens* [1991] 2 All E.R. 133 at 139 *per* Neill L.J. See also *B.B.M.B. Finance* v. *Eda Holdings* [1991] 2 All E.R. 129 (P.C.). There is also a slim argument that Moore might have proprietary rights in the material containing his cells, *although not in any patents* (Patents Act 1977, s.7): ownership of property may be acquired by "confusion or intermixture" if the materials, when mixed, are indistinguishable. *Halsbury's Laws of England* (4th edn.) vol. 35 para. 1139. *cf. Indian Oil Co.* v. *Greenstone Shipping* [1988] Q.B. 345.

[61] It is interesting to compare this provision with the well-known American case of *Wetherbee* v. *Green* (1871) 22 Mich. 311. The defendant had manufactured hoops from timber wrongfully taken from the plaintiff's land. The value of the timber at the time it was cut was $25 and the value of hoops at the date of the trial was $700. The Court held that where the defendant had acted in good faith, the innocent improver was entitled to keep the benefit of the improvement; it was felt that it would have been unjust to have given the plaintiff a remedy beyond the value of the goods prior to the conversion. On the other hand, had the defendant "committed the wrong recklessly, wilfully or maliciously, and under circumstances presenting elements of aggravation" the plaintiff would have been entitled to greater damages. Such a rule, although in some respects similar to s.6 of the English Act, is much more generous to the plaintiff in cases of fraud and arguably, therefore, a conversion remedy in the USA would have left Moore in a very favoured position.

tain the father and his family during the babies' lives, and to pay one eighth of the proceeds of displaying them. The twins died after one month and the defendant then embalmed their bodies and continued to exhibit them. The plaintiff brought equitable proceedings and the Court ordered that the bodies should be buried and that the defendant should account to the plaintiff for all the money obtained from the wrongful exploitation of these bodies.[62]

More recent authorities demonstrate that those who obtain patents as the result of unlawful acts may be ordered to hold the patent on trust for the person who had been wronged,[63] that some wrongdoers may be ordered by courts of equity to account for *all* the profits gained from their wrongful conduct,[64] and, to demonstrate the continuing flexibility of equity, even in cases of undue influence where restitution would ordinarily be ordered, the courts have been prepared to permit wrongdoers to retain a *reasonable* sum for the efforts involved in making profits.[65]

An English court has sufficient scope to provide a robust and common sense answer to the *Moore* case: which, on these facts should provide him with something akin to a royalty for using unique property of his in circumstances where he should not be regarded as having abandoned his rights.

H. Intellectual Property Rights in the Human Body and Parts Thereof

In recent years, a new dimension has been introduced into the general debates. If it is accepted that the law does at present recognize some scope for property rights in parts of the human body, is there any further scope for *patenting* "inventions" involving human subject-matter?

A patent provides a legal monopoly to an inventor to exploit the patented invention for a certain number of years. Those who are involved in biotechnology and in genetic engineering and who are concerned with manipulating tissue and genetic materials understandably maintain that their innovative developments should be capable of

---

[62] *Herring* v. *Walround* (1682) 22 E.R. 870. Cited in Matthews, "Whose Body? People as Property" [1983] C.L.P. 193 at 220.

[63] *Seager* v. *Copydex* [1967] R.P.C. 349; [1967]2 All E.R. 415. In this case, unlike *Moore*, the patent was the direct result of using the plaintiff's confidential information. No major additional skill and labour was involved in preparing the invention and the product for commercialization.

[64] *E.g. Franklin* v. *Giddins* [1978] Qd. R. 72 (Australia); *L.A.C. Minerals* v. *International Corona Resources* [1990] F.S.R. 441 (Canada); *Normalec* v. *Britton* [1983] F.S.R. 318 (UK).

[65] *O'Sullivan* v. *Management Agency* [1985] 3 All E.R. 351.

being protected by patents in just the same way as any other industrial innovation; if not, there will be less incentive for researchers and industry to research and invest in these areas. In practice, patents are routinely and increasingly being granted for inventive developments involving the use of human tissue or cell lines derived from human tissue.[66]

The problem, however, is that there has always been some unease about the legitimacy of patenting life forms. In 1980 it was thought that the US Supreme Court had given the green light in the USA in a famous case where it accepted that a newly developed micro-organism (which could eat up oil slicks) was patentable subject-matter.[67] In its view, "anything under the sun" apart from human beings, was patentable provided it otherwise met the statutory criteria. That green light turned to amber when, in the course of that decade, attempts to obtain patents for higher animal life forms met with bitter criticism from those groups who both oppose the type of research which involves engineering of new life forms as well as, by way of fall-back position, the patenting of any such inventive developments.[68] The campaigns, so far, have been concerned primarily with animal life forms, but the developments are highly pertinent to the patenting of human materials.

There are some who adopt a fundamentalist attitude and deny that there should be property rights in any life forms. This sweeping approach quite clearly is untenable. Property rights in animals have always been accepted: I can enlist the aid of the law in preventing others from taking my animals away or to obtain redress if they have been taken: title to animals passes when they are bought, sold or given away.

Just as vocal are those who oppose the creation of special rights in any newly developed form of animals. Thus the United States policy of allowing patents for newly developed micro-organisms,[69] for sterile oysters[70] and for the Harvard Oncomouse (a mouse with cancer inducing traits which was bred for cancer research) is still being resisted by strong pressure groups. They maintain that the patenting of animals reflects an inappropriate sense of human control over animal life and an underestimation of the value of non-human life: *patenting* animal life is the first step towards a decline in belief in the sanctity and dignity of

---

[66] For example, in the *Moore* case itself no objection was raised to the patenting of inventions involving the use of a human cell line.

[67] *Diamond* v. *Chakrabarty* (1980) 447 U.S. 303.

[68] In each session of Congress since 1987, "moratorium" bills have been introduced designed to halt the patenting of life forms and the commercialization of genetically engineered animals pending full consideration of all the "ethical, environmental and economic considerations" involved.

[69] *Diamond* v. *Chakrabarty* (1980) 447 U.S. 303.

[70] *ex parte Allen* 2 U.S.P.Q.2d 1425 (1987).

life. Thus, campaigners such as Rifkin argue that "the patenting of animals really gives people a sense that we are talking about reducing life to the status of the manufactured commodity".

Then there is the Frankenstein complex: ownership rights are being conferred on new life forms which scientists should not be producing. Fears were expressed by US Senators in the following ways: "To permit the patenting of just one animal will effectively eliminate all constraints ... against genetically altering all other animals including human beings ... Once life forms are protected, then there will be no stopping the types of life which can be patented, and we will soon be patenting human beings"; and, "We've approved the patenting of plants in 1930, seeds in 1970, microbes in 1980, and now we've moved to considering patenting animals ... next is human beings ..."

In response to such concerns, the US Patent and Trademarks Office issued a Notice stating that "a claim directed to or including within its scope a human being will not be considered patentable subject-matter ... The grant of a limited, but exclusive property right in a human being is prohibited by the Constitution" and legislative attempts, so far unsuccessful, have been made in recent years to amend the US patent law to provide that human beings do not represent patentable subject-matter. As will be seen in relation to the European draft Biotechnology Directive, there is an inherent ambiguity in such pronouncements. As genetic engineering develops, the boundary to be drawn, *in patent law*, between acceptable and unacceptable human genetic innovation will have to be worked out.

Opposition to intermeddling with life forms as such is centuries too late and accordingly irrational. *Natural* cross-breeding has taken place since the beginning of civilization. The real fear is of the new biotechnological and genetic engineering techniques, which increase the range of opportunities for developing new life forms, whether of micro-organisms, organisms, animals or man: these may result, for example, in viruses or insects whose capacity to cause untold damage in the world may be unforeseen or animals or humans with qualities or forms which society regards as unacceptable.

All the concerns expressed in the USA have been echoed forcefully in Europe. There has been a two-pronged assault on the European patent system: first, by taking advantage of the opportunity presented by the current European Community's review of biotechnology and the patent system; and, secondly, by reawakening the long-dormant "ordre public" and "morality" provisions in the patent legislation itself.

One of the underlying objectives of the EC Draft Directive on Biotechnology was to strengthen patent rights relating to biotechnological developments so that European industry is not placed at a disadvantage *vis-à-vis* its US and Japanese competitors. It attempted to clarify patent policy. Thus, Article 2 specified that "A subject-matter of an invention shall not be considered unpatentable for the reason only that it is composed of living matter"; and Article 7 that "An invention concerning a biological material[71] shall not be considered a discovery or lacking in novelty [and so not capable of being patented] for the reason only tnat, although not known, it formed part of an existing material."[72]

Clear and rousing statements of this kind sounded alarm bells amongst those lobbying against manipulation of, and control over, living material. The commercial objectives of the Draft Directive became overshadowed by the ethical debate and the European Parliament, on grounds of public policy and morality, was persuaded[73] to introduce various qualifications relating to living material.

One amendment provides that, "in the light of the general principle that the ownership of human beings is prohibited ... the human body or parts of the human body [shall not be patentable] *per se*". This exclusion, at face value, would be a major blow to the pharmaceutical and biotechnology industries. Such a broad exclusion is not intended by the Commission which wishes to preserve such patenting opportunities. The key lies in the words "*per se*". If they are construed to exclude from patentability only human tissue in its natural form, which has not been the subject of any technical intervention, few if any innovative developments which have presently patentable will be excluded in the future.[74]

How the precise wording of the final form of the Directive will be expressed remains to be seen. Any further amendments, instead of strengthening patent law in relation to inventions involving human material, could severely threaten the existing scope of patentable subject-matter.

---

[71] Now defined in draft Article 2.2 as "any self-replicating living matter and any matter capable of being replicated through a biological system or by any indirect means".

[72] Presumably, this means that if biological material is isolated from other biological material and an invention satisfying the patentability conditions results, then there is no prima facie bar to patentability.

[73] October 1992.

[74] "Parts of the human body" *per se* means parts of the human body as found inside the human body. [It is necessary to avoid] all possible ambiguity with respect to the position of certain products or parts of the human body which are already covered by patents granted in connection with the development of medicinal products *e.g.* a human lymphoblastoid cell line, a recombinant DNA molecule capable of inducing the expression in a unicellular host of a polypeptide displaying the immunological or biological activity of human B-interferon; a human hepatocyte culture process; the molecular cloning and characterization of a gene sequence coding for human relaxin; a method for producing human antibody; and a process for producing a human protein of therapeutic value.

The second line of attack concentrated on the existing mechanisms in the patent laws of most European countries. The European Patent Convention, Article 53[75] provides that "European patents shall not be granted in respect of ... inventions the publication or exploitation of which would be contrary to *ordre public* or morality..." Thus, in the controversial *Harvand Onco-mouse* decision[76] a patent application for a transgenic non-human mammalian animal whose germcells and somatic cells contained an activated oncogene sequence was found to be ethically acceptable: transgenic mice to be used for cancer experiments were useful to mankind; the animals presented no risk to the environment and the invention contributed to the reduction of overall animal suffering since the number of such animals required was smaller than the number of conventional animals which would otherwise be used. However, a later decision rejected a European patent application for a transgenic mouse used for testing in the field of cosmetics: the benefit for mankind was not sufficient![77]

No one doubts that there should be ethical controls over the genetic manipulation of life forms, whether animal or human. Such controls, as for all research, should be exercised when the research protocols are being drawn up. The introduction of such ethical considerations into the patent system is more questionable: if the initial research is unethical, no question of patents should arise; if it is acceptable, there is no reason why innovation and investment in such activity should be treated differently to any other area of innovation. Whether inappropriate or not, it must be remembered that all these issues relate to whether the "owners" of such genetically engineered animals are entitled, *in addition to their basic ownership rights in them*, to additional monopoly rights for a number of years to prevent others from producing similar animals.

It seems quite clear, however, that the injection of ethical considerations into the legal question of what is patentable means that there will be more opposition to, and more examination of, the ethical factors affecting applications for patents for inventions using human materials. Article 53 will be prayed in aid much more frequently. There may also be more express provisions requiring the law to be tempered by ethical considerations. For example, the draft Biotechnology Directive provides that "processes for modifying the genetic identity of the human

[75] This provision is mirrored in the national law of all Member countries of the European Patent Convention.

[76] "Onco-mouse/HARVARD" [1990] E.P.O.R. 4; [1990] E.P.O.R. 501.

[77] Upjohn Company/Transgenic mice for the analysis of hair growth [1991].

body for a non-therapeutic purpose *which is contrary to the dignity of man*" shall be unpatentable.[78]

III. CONCLUSIONS

The conclusions to be drawn from this brief survey can only be general.

There is little doubt that the nature of rights in, and control over, tissue is now becoming of increasing importance and potential controversy. Consensus and clarification are required.

A societal consensus is required as to what can, or should, be done with human tissue (which may vary of course depending on the type of tissue involved); what patients or other donors of tissue should be told at the time that tissue is taken from their bodies, whether and what type of control they should be entitled to have over the destination of their tissue; and whether it should be possible for financial benefits to be sought from those who take and use such material for research or commercial purposes.

Professional guidance must be provided in the form of Codes of Practice and these should set out clear procedures as well as indicating the boundaries of acceptable practice.

Finally, the law is likely to be in need of clarification in a way which is consistent with such accepted practices. The forthcoming Report of the Nuffield Council on Bioethics should be considered carefully. It is imperative, however, to remember that whatever changes do take place, they should be balanced against the clear desirability of research and development, including that carried out by commercial organizations, designed to benefit society.

---

[78] Article 2.3(b).

Legislative and Judicial Approaches to Resource Allocation

[18]

Resource Allocation in the National Health Service

Christopher Newdick†

I. INTRODUCTION

In the United Kingdom, how does the National Health Service (NHS or the Service) respond to the pressures imposed on it by patients, doctors and the government? What techniques for distributing resources have been adopted for managing these pressures? Part I of this Article explains the administrative evolution of the NHS. Part II discusses the legal framework surrounding the allocation of resources throughout the different tiers of the NHS: (1) from the Secretary of State for Health to health authorities, (2) from health authorities to hospitals and general practitioners (GPs), and (3) from doctors to patients. Part III comments on the case for a standing committee to advise the government on matters of resource allocation within the NHS. It also considers the legal, political, and managerial contributions to the debate and, in particular, comments on the future of the traditional notion of clinical freedom.

II. ADMINISTRATIVE DEVELOPMENT OF THE NHS[1]

Section A describes the culture that developed within the NHS, Section B discusses the pressure for reform that developed during the 1980s, and Section C reviews the system of the "internal market" for health that was introduced in 1990. These comments serve as an introduction to the legal issues that arise in Part III.

A. EVOLUTION OF CULTURE OF THE NHS

The National Health Service Act of 1946 created the NHS which commenced operation in 1948. NHS's most profound commitment was that the service it provided should be "comprehensive" in the sense that it should be available to everyone, to meet all their needs, whenever it was required to do so. The White Paper of 1944 on which the Service was based described this objective as follows:

> The proposed service must be 'comprehensive' in two senses—first,

---

† Christopher Newdick is a barrister and Reader in Health Law at the University of Reading, U.K. He is a member of the Department of Health's Medicines Commission which advises the government on the licensing of pharmaceutical products.

1 See RUDOLPH KLEIN, THE NEW POLITICS OF THE N.H.S. (3d ed. 1995), for the most authoritative account of the development of the NHS by a social scientist.

> that it is available to all people and, second, that it covers all necessary forms of health care. . . . The service designed to achieve it must cover the whole field of medical advice and attention, at home, in the consulting room, in the hospital or the sanatorium, or wherever else is appropriate—from the personal or family doctor to the specialists and consultants of all kinds, from the care of minor ailments to the care of major diseases and disabilities. It must include ancillary services of nursing, of midwifery and of the other things which ought to go with medical care. It must ensure that everyone can be sure of a general medical advisor to consult as and when the need arises, and then that everyone can get access—beyond the general medical advisor—to more specialised branches of medicine or surgery.[2]

Toward the end of the Second World War "rationing" was commonplace, but the idea meant sharing resources fairly among all. The thought that those with genuine needs might be denied care contradicted the noble principle on which the service was based. But only three years after coming into operation, demand for care so exceeded expectation that statutory provision was made to charge patients for prescriptions and spectacles.[3] As a result, the first Secretary of State responsible for the health service, Mr. Aneurin Bevan, resigned from office. He regarded the measure as a betrayal of the principles on which the Service was founded.[4] This began a consistent story of providing exceptional service for the victims of accidents and emergencies; generally, a very good service for patients in urgent need of care; but less consistent service for others who often found themselves on long waiting lists. Surprisingly, as this Article will describe, it was not until 1980 that the promise of a "comprehensive" service was first used by a patient to found a claim to NHS resources, although the number and variety of claims has increased ever since.[5]

In addition, an important characteristic of the service in 1948 was its commitment to clinical discretion.[6] Patients were entitled to expect that managers would always defer to the judgment of the medical profession in matters of clinical care.[7] This counsel of "professional perfectionism" contained two important factors. First, "[f]rom the doctor's point of view, this implied that he should be free to carry out his professional imperative of doing his utmost for the individual patient without regard to the cost."[8] Second, the commitment extended well beyond decisions concerning individual patients.[9] Even today, but to a far greater extent fifty years ago, there were no effective measures by which performance in the NHS could be measured, no reliable yardstick against which individual patient's needs could be assessed, and no means of gauging the quality of care that hospitals were providing. As a result, doctors also made decisions concerning the allocation of resources within hospitals. "Lacking independent criteria of their own, policy-makers were forced to fall back

---

[2] MINISTRY OF HEALTH, A NATIONAL HEALTH SERVICE, 1944, Cmd. 6502, *reprinted in* RUDOLPH KLEIN, THE POLITICS OF THE NATIONAL HEALTH SERVICE 10 n.10 (1983).

[3] *See* MICHAEL FOOT, 2 ANEURIN BEVAN ch. 8 (1973).

[4] *See id.*

[5] The modern legislation is contained in the National Health Service Act of 1977, discussed *infra* Part III.A.1.

[6] *See* KLEIN, *supra* note 1, at 33.

[7] *See id.*

[8] *Id.* at 33.

[9] *See id.*

on the [medical] professional view of what services were needed and how quality should be assessed."[10] The relative impotence of managers during this period was compounded by scarce resources.

> The paradox of the financial stringency was that [while] it led to tighter control over the total budgets available to health authorities, it also weakened the centre's ability to use incentives to persuade the periphery to follow national policies: the Ministry of Health could neither command nor bribe.[11]

Thus, the medical profession, rather than administrators or managers, assumed a dominant role in decisions concerning the management of resources,[12] a predominance which endured until the reforms introduced in 1990.

The combined effect of these characteristics was to foster expectations that exceeded the capacity of the Service, and to create a system of management that was slow to react and difficult to control. The NHS had explained the objectives it intended to achieve, but could not settle on the means by which they were to be attained.

B. PRESSURE FOR REFORM

During the 1980s a number of cases exposed the dissatisfaction the public was beginning to feel with the NHS. One in particular, *R. v. Central Birmingham Health Authority, ex parte Collier*, which is considered below, concerned a four-year-old boy who, despite being put at the top of the doctor's list of clinical priorities, could not be admitted to the hospital for a hole in the heart operation.[13] The unease provoked by the case prompted Prime Minister Thatcher to announce that she had committed herself to reforming the financial administration of the Service. The subsequent reforms were much influenced by an American commentator, Professor Alain Enthoven, who had made a number of telling observations about the management of NHS finances.[14]

First, he observed that the old formula by which money was allocated by the central government to the local health authorities for distribution to hospitals discouraged efficiency.[15] Although the formula was adjusted from time to time, it rested on the principle that the needs of an area could be assessed solely by reference to the profile of its population, taking account of factors such as age, social class, morbidity and mortality.[16] However, the formula paid no attention to the efficiency with which the population was treated in the hospital. Thus, the most efficient hospitals may have been penalized in the sense that they would tend to treat patients more effectively and more quickly, but inevitably exhaust their fixed revenue allocations before the end of the financial year. In this case, they were forced to turn patients

---

[10] *Id.* at 42.

[11] *Id.* at 47. As he puts it, "[t]he captain shouted his orders: the crew went on as before." *Id.* at 69.

[12] *See* STEPHEN HARRISON ET AL., JUST MANAGING: POWER AND CULTURE IN THE NATIONAL HEALTH SERVICE 26 (1992).

[13] Eng. C.A. Jan. 6, 1988 (LEXIS, Enggen Library, Cases file).

[14] *See* ALAIN C. ENTHOVEN, REFLECTIONS ON THE MANAGEMENT OF THE NATIONAL HEALTH SERVICE—AN AMERICAN LOOKS AT INCENTIVES TO EFFICIENCY IN HEALTH SERVICES MANAGEMENT IN THE UK 13–15 (1985).

[15] *See id.*

[16] *See id.* at 13, 34–37.

294 AMERICAN JOURNAL OF LAW & MEDICINE VOL. XXIII NOS. 2&3 1997

away and close hospital wards until the following financial year. By contrast, the less efficient hospital, which treated fewer patients, could keep all its beds open or transfer "surplus" patients to hospitals in other areas. Thus, Enthoven observed in 1985 that the system contained no serious incentives to guide the NHS in the direction of better quality care and service at reduced cost.[17]

> In fact, the structure of the NHS contains perverse incentives. For example, a [health authority] that develops an excellent service in some specialty that attracts more referrals is likely to get more work without getting more resources to do it. A [health authority] that does a poor job will 'export' patients and have less work, but not correspondingly less resources, for its reward . . .; management and consultants in [an authority] risk weakening the case for a new hospital wing they have been campaigning for by solving their waiting list problem by referring patients to other districts with excess capacity . . .; [and] GPs have weak or no incentives to reduce referrals. They have neither the incentives nor the resources to make extra efforts to keep people out of hospital.[18]

The solution proposed to this "efficiency trap" was to introduce a system that rewarded those hospitals able to manage their resources most effectively by enabling them to raise revenue according to the numbers of patients treated and the quality of care provided.[19] By contrast, those that operated below the requisite standards would have to improve or lose revenue.[20] This idea of contract funding provided a central foundation for the internal market.

C. Mechanism of the Internal Market

The incentive to become more sensitive to the relative costs and benefits of providing care was created by a system, referred to as the *internal market*, which divided itself into purchasers and providers.[21] The purchasers are Health Authorities and GP Fund-holders, to whom money is allocated annually by the Secretary of State.[22] The providers are hospitals, now called NHS Trust hospitals, that must generate their income by providing services to purchasers of the right nature, quality and price. In this way, in theory, the best hospitals generate the most revenue by attracting the most patients. Thus, they, rather than the less efficient provider, can expand for the benefit of patients. The energy that propels the system is the NHS contract.[23] NHS contracts enable providers to negotiate with purchasers regarding the details of the quantity and quality of the services to be provided to patients and their cost. In a recent survey, hospitals were reported to work with around thirty contracts,[24] but this number fluctuates according to the number of GP fund-holding practices in the area

---

[17] *See id.* at 13.
[18] *Id.* at 13–15.
[19] *See id.* at 38–42.
[20] *See id.*
[21] *See* National Health Service and Community Care Act of 1990, § 4 (Eng.).
[22] *See id.* § 97A, *amended by* Health Services Act of 1995 (Eng.).
[23] *See id.* § 4.
[24] *See* John Appleby, Developing Contracts—A National Survey 10 (1994).

with whom the hospital must contract.[25] For the present, contracts are typically negotiated on the basis of large groups of patients, for a lump sum, to be renegotiated approximately every two or three years. Contracts may provide for the sum to be increased or decreased, depending on the performance of the provider at the end of a specified period.

Three comments should be made about the system of NHS contracts. First, although the system may prove beneficial, it carries its own significant management transaction costs, in particular, with respect to GP fund-holding practices. Considerable time and energy is required from health authority managers in agreeing to the sum to be allotted to fund-holders. No specific formula exists by which such a sum is calculated and much hard bargaining occurs during negotiations.[26]

Second, the system may be suitable for arranging care for large groups of patients because prices can be set according to aggregates.[27] Thus, in theory diagnostic-related groups are able to accommodate those whose treatment is unexpectedly prolonged and expensive, by including those whose discharge from the hospital is unexpectedly speedy and inexpensive. But the system may be insufficiently flexible when small numbers are involved. Cystic fibrosis, for example, demands hi-tech, high-cost, but low-volume, specialist care. Many hospitals might have limited experience in its treatment and insufficient expertise to offer adequate care. It is inappropriate either for them to have to estimate the average cost of caring for such a patient, or for the system to encourage hospitals to compete against one another to do so.[28] The government has accepted, therefore, that in areas of this nature health authorities should liaise with one another in order to agree which hospitals should be funded to become the centers of excellence. This demonstrates the view that an unregulated market cannot provide an adequate health service and that there are circumstances where collaboration is more important than competition.[29]

Finally, in addition to these structural reforms, an ideological challenge to the prevailing deference to medical authority existed in the allocation of hospital resources. In 1983, a small group with a record of success in commerce was appointed to advise and make recommendations regarding the management of NHS.[30] Its major observation, contained in the *Griffiths Report*, was the limited managerial supervision of resources in the NHS:

> The NHS does not have the profit motive, but it is, of course, enormously concerned with control of expenditure. Surprisingly, however,

[25] Fund-holding practices are allocated specific sums of money each year to spend for the benefit of their patients in the manner the fund-holders think most suitable. *See* National Health Service and Community Care Act of 1990, §§ 14, 15 (Eng.).

[26] Also, much paperwork is generated by hospitals having to invoice fund-holders for services provided to patients. Indeed, some hospitals have failed to issue invoices and lost their entitlement to income. At present, there is concern whether the additional efficiency savings generated by the internal market are greater than the transaction costs associated with its management. *See* AUDIT COMM'N, WHAT THE DOCTOR ORDERED—A STUDY OF GP FUNDHOLDERS IN ENGLAND AND WALES ¶¶ 78, 86 (HMSO 1996).

[27] *See* CLINICAL SERVICES ADVISORY GROUP, CYSTIC FIBROSIS (HMSO, 1993) [hereinafter CYSTIC FIBROSIS]; *see also* CLINICAL SERVICES ADVISORY GROUP, NEONATAL INTENSIVE CARE (HMSO, 1993) [hereinafter NEONATAL INTENSIVE CARE].

[28] *See* CYSTIC FIBROSIS, *supra* note 27; *see also* NEONATAL INTENSIVE CARE, *supra* note 27.

[29] *See* DEPARTMENT OF HEALTH, GOVERNMENT RESPONSE TO THE REPORTS OF THE CLINICAL STANDARDS ADVISORY GROUP (1993).

[30] *See* DEPARTMENT OF HEALTH, THE GRIFFITHS REPORT, NHS MANAGEMENT INQUIRY 10 (1983).

> it still lacks any real continuous evaluation of its performance against criteria . . . . Rarely are precise management objectives set; there is little measurement of health output; clinical evaluation of particular practices is by no means common and economic evaluation of those practices is extremely rare. Nor can the NHS display [the] effectiveness with which it is meeting the needs and expectations of the people it serves. Businessmen have a keen sense of how well they are looking after their customers. Whether the NHS is meeting the needs of the patient, and the community, and can prove that it is doing so, is open to question.[31]

The report recommended a management structure for the NHS in which the creation of policy at the national level would clearly be distinguished from the responsibility for its implementation and operation.[32] At each level of operation, managers should set specific responsibilities and targets and be held accountable for them.[33] The recommendations of the Report were introduced into practice without the need for legislation and, of course, brought clinicians and managers into more direct conflict with one another.

III. RESOURCE ALLOCATIONS IN THE NHS[34]

From this consideration of the political and administrative development of the control of NHS resources, Part III considers the legal principles on which allocations are made throughout the different tiers of the Service. Section A discusses allocations by the Secretary of State for Health to health authorities, Section B, allocations by health authorities to hospitals and doctors, and Section C, allocations by doctors to patients.

A. ALLOCATIONS BY THE SECRETARY OF STATE

The following considers (1) the duty imposed on the Secretary of State to allocate resources, (2) the nature of the duty, and (3) the power to charge for some services.

1. The Duty to Allocate Resources

The National Health Service Act of 1977 imposes on the Secretary of State for Health a duty to pay to each health authority sums attributable to (1) the payment of remuneration of those who provide services under the Act and (2) the reimbursement of expenses of persons providing services thereto.[35] It is also the duty of the Secretary of State

> to pay in respect of each financial year to each Health Authority sums not exceeding the amount allotted for that year by the Secretary of State to the Health Authority towards meeting the expenditure of the

---

31 *Id.*

32 *See id.*

33 *See id.*

34 *See generally* CHRISTOPHER NEWDICK, WHO SHOULD WE TREAT? LAW, PATIENTS AND RESOURCES IN THE N.H.S. 204–12 (1995).

35 National Health Service Act 1977, § 97(1)–(2), *substituted by* Health Authorities Act 1995, §§ 2(1), 8 (Eng.).

> Health Authority which . . . is attributable to the performance by the Health Authority of their functions in that year.[36]

Correspondingly, it is the duty of each health authority to perform its functions in a manner that does not exceed its income[37] and to pay to GP fund-holding practices an "allotted sum" representing the fund for which they have accepted responsibility.[38]

The distribution of NHS resources to Health Authorities, i.e., "purchasers" of health care, is calculated on the basis of a weighted capitation formula[39] which assesses health needs according to: (1) the projected size of the population concerned; (2) the numbers of elderly people in the population; (3) the health needs of the population, distinguishing between general, acute and psychiatric care and morbidity and mortality ratios; and (4) an allowance to allow for local market forces with respect to the cost of labor and the higher costs of the London Regions.[40] It is difficult to conceive of circumstances in which the formula for allocating funds could be successfully challenged, for example, by a health authority that considered it had received inadequate funding.

An analogous issue arose concerning expenditure guidance issued by the Secretary of State for the Environment to Local Authorities, which was challenged for being *Wednesbury* unreasonable, i.e., so unreasonable that no reasonable person addressing himself to the issue in question could have come to such a decision. Lord Scarman dealt with the claim as follows:

> we are being asked to review the exercise by the Secretary of State of an administrative discretion which inevitably requires political judgment on his part . . . . I cannot accept that it is constitutionally appropriate, save in very exceptional circumstances, for the courts to intervene on the ground of 'unreasonableness' to quash guidance framed by the Secretary of State and by necessary implication approved by the House of Commons, the guidance being concerned with the limits of public expenditure by local authorities and the incidence of the tax burden as between taxpayers and ratepayers . . . these are matters of political judgment for him and for the House of Commons. They are not matters for the judges.[41]

Unsurprisingly, therefore, for practical purposes the level of resources invested in health by the central government is beyond the supervision of the courts.

Such stark legal commentary may not satisfy those who observe that the United Kingdom spends only six percent of its gross domestic product on health care, which is small by comparison to other wealthy nations.[42] It ranks twentieth; only Spain, Portugal, Turkey and Greece spend less.[43] On the other hand, direct comparisons

---

[36] *See id.* § 97(3).

[37] *See id.* § 97A.

[38] *See* National Health Service and Community Care Act of 1990, § 15(1), *amended by* Health Authorities Act 1995, § 2(1).

[39] *See* NATIONAL HEALTH SERVICE EXECUTIVE, HOSPITAL AND COMMUNITY HEALTH SERVICES RESOURCE ALLOCATION: WEIGHTED CAPITATION FORMULA (1944).

[40] *See id.*

[41] R. v. Secretary of State for the Environment, *ex parte* Nottinghamshire County Council [1986] App. Cas. 240, at 247; *see also* R. v. Secretary of State for the Environment, *ex parte* Hammersmith and Fulham London Borough Council [1991] 1 App. Cas. 521.

[42] *See* OFFICE OF HEALTH ECONOMICS, COMPENDIUM OF HEALTH STATISTICS (8th ed. 1992).

[43] *See id.*

between nations are notoriously difficult. For example, although the United States spends the most per capita on health care, a larger portion of that sum is devoted to the payment of its medical staff than is the case in the United Kingdom.[44] On a comparative scale taking these transaction costs into account, the United States moves from first to eighth place, and the United Kingdom rises from twentieth to thirteenth place.[45] The problem with comparisons of this nature is that they measure quantity rather than quality; hence they have to be treated with great caution. Though many would agree that the NHS would benefit from additional resources, the issue of how much it requires defies objective analysis.

2. Nature of the Duty

A number of general statutory duties are imposed on the Secretary of State, the most broad-ranging of which is contained in Section 3 of the National Health Service Act of 1977, which provides that

> it is the Secretary of State's duty to provide . . . to such extent as he considers necessary to meet all reasonable requirements . . . hospital accommodation, . . . medical, dental, and ambulance services; . . . such facilities for the prevention of illness, the care of persons suffering from illness and the after-care of persons who have suffered from illness as he considers appropriate as part of the health service; [and] such other services as are required for the diagnosis and treatment of illness.[46]

In addition to this statutory duty, there are two major statements of Department of Health policy. The first is contained in *The Health of the Nation,* which introduces targets for the reduction of levels of specific areas of disease, i.e., coronary heart disease and stroke, cancers, mental illness, HIV, AIDS and accidents.[47] The clear emphasis of these targets is preventive, rather than curative, much of which comes from educational programs aimed at susceptible communities. The second restatement of NHS policy is included in *The Patient's Charter,* which promises that "*every* citizen has the following National Health Service Rights: [*inter alia*] to receive health care on the basis of clinical need, regardless of ability to pay. . . no later than [eighteen months] from the day when your consultant places you on a waiting list."[48]

Are these duties and undertakings capable of being enforced by individual patients? The first claim of this nature arose in *R v. Secretary of State for Social Services, ex parte Hincks.*[49] Plans for a new orthopedic unit in the City of Birmingham had been approved by the Secretary of State in 1971, postponed in 1973 and even-

---

[44] *See* JOHN APPLEBY, FINANCING HEALTH CARE IN THE 1990'S, at 73 (1992); D. Parkin, *Comparing Health Service Efficiency Across Countries, in* PROVIDING HEALTH CARE: THE ECONOMICS OF ALTERNATIVE SYSTEMS OF FINANCE AND DELIVERY 179 (A. McGuire et al. eds., 1991).

[45] *See* APPLEBY, *supra* note 44, at 73; Parkin, *supra* note 44, at 179.

[46] National Health Service Act of 1977, § 3 (Eng.).

[47] DEPARTMENT OF HEALTH, THE HEALTH OF THE NATION (1992)

[48] DEPARTMENT OF HEALTH, THE PATIENT'S CHARTER 8–10 (1991). The waiting period was reduced to 18 months in 1995. This initiative has had a dramatic effect on reducing overall waiting times, but there is a suspicion that some urgent cases have had to be postponed in order to include nonurgent treatments within the deadline.

[49] 1 B.M.L.R. 93 (Eng. C.A. 1980), *available in* LEXIS, Enggen Library, Cases File.

tually abandoned in 1978.[50] It was alleged that the Secretary of State had failed in his duty to provide a "comprehensive health service" under Section 3 of the National Health Service Act of 1977.[51] The court of appeal decided, however, that Section 3 cannot be interpreted to impose an absolute duty to provide services, irrespective of economic decisions taken at the national level.[52] The provision has to be read subject to the implied qualification that the Secretary of State's duty was "to meet all reasonable requirements such as can be provided within the resources available,"[53] which "must be determined in the light of current Government economic policy."[54] Thus, with respect to the Secretary of State, the courts are extremely reluctant to involve themselves in determining priorities between competing claims for resources. And, as we shall see when we consider the actions against health authorities and their refusals to offer care, the consistency with which applications of this kind have been rejected suggests that the "duty" imposed by Section 3 is more in the nature of an aspiration or a target, and that only the most extreme case has even the remotest chance of success.

3. Charging for Services

As a general rule under the 1977 Act, all services to NHS patients "shall be free of charge,"[55] whether they are provided in the hospital or in the community. However, consistent with the controversial decision of 1951, the 1977 Act permits charges to be imposed in specific circumstances, the most general of which are (1) prescription charges for medicines and (2) charges for dental treatment.[56] Both powers have been exercised subject to a number of exceptions, so that children continue to receive such services free of charge, as do retired people and those on state support.[57] With respect to prescription medicines,[58] there is a standard charge of around £5 ($10.00) for each prescription. For many, this is not an undue burden. They are happy to make an additional contribution to the NHS. However, for those on long-term medication, perhaps involving more than one medicine and lasting many years, the cumulative costs may be high and it is not clear why such a disproportionate burden should fall on them alone. However, because around eighty percent of all prescriptions are exempt from charges (e.g., with respect to children and those receiving state support), a very small number of people have to pay relatively large sums for the medication. It is also curious to note that the cost to the government of the majority of medicines dispensed is less than the standard prescription charge,[59] so that the minority who pay are in effect obliged to make an additional payment to the NHS, over and above the actual cost of the medicine.

---

[50] *See id.*

[51] *See id.* at 94.

[52] *See id.*

[53] *Id.* at 95 (per Lord Denning M.R.).

[54] *Id.* at 97 (per Bridge L.J.).

[55] *See* National Health Service Act of 1977, § 1(2) (Eng.).

[56] *See id.* §§ 77–78.

[57] *See id.*

[58] Medicines are categorized as follows: (i) prescription only, i.e., only to be provided on a doctor's instruction, (ii) pharmacy medicine, i.e., only to be dispensed by a pharmacist without the need for a doctor's prescription, and (iii) general sales list, i.e., may be supplied without restriction.

[59] Priority Setting in the NHS: The NHS Drug Budget ¶ 878 [HC80-VII, Session 1993–1994].

Slightly different considerations apply to dental treatment. The charges depend on the extent of the treatment given, but they are not significantly less than the full value of the care provided.[60] Thus, around seventy-five percent of the dental costs to the NHS are recovered in charges.[61] In addition, many dental practitioners have simply withdrawn their services from the NHS because the rates of remuneration are considered so low. Accordingly, there has been a steady increase in the number of dentists who only offer care privately, with the additional level of fees which that entails. The reality, therefore, is that for those who are not prepared to travel long-distances to visit an NHS dentist, dental care is simply not available under the NHS. Recall that under Section 3 of the 1977 Act "it is the Secretary of State's duty to provide . . . dental . . . services."[62] Given the scarcity of the dental services, there must be concern that, in some regions, the Secretary of State is failing in his duty to provide a "comprehensive" dental service.

Adult dental services are more expendable than other NHS services and it would be sensible to abandon this area of care to the private practitioner. One of the recommendations of the enquiry of the Dutch government into *Choices in Health Care* was that, other than for children, this aspect of health provision ought to be the responsibility of the individual rather than the state.[63] However, the principle of charging for services prompts two comments. First, the government might succeed in raising additional revenue from patients and provide further support for the system. Equally, setting off the administrative costs involved with collection and exempting certain categories of less wealthy patient, the gain could be extremely small.[64] Second, charges would inevitably have the most deterrent effect on less wealthy people, who generally require more health care than the more affluent sections of the community. To set charges too high would tend to increase ill health and ultimately create unwanted implications for other budgets within the welfare system, such as social security and unemployment.[65] Clearly, such an effect would be counterproductive.

B. ALLOCATIONS BY HEALTH AUTHORITIES

Other than under Section 3 of the 1977 Act, there is no statement of "essential" or "core" services that ought to be available within the NHS. This gives health authorities considerable discretion in deciding how to allocate the resources voted to them by the Department of Health. They do so by means of NHS contracts with providers, i.e. hospitals, for particular categories of patient services. The health authority's responsibility is to assess the health care needs of its population, to set priorities within those set by the government, and to negotiate and enter into NHS contracts with suitable hospital providers.

Contracts provide a very visible way of knowing whether services have been excluded from patients. For the present, however, NHS contracts have not led to

---

60 *See* OFFICE OF HEALTH ECONOMICS, *supra* note 42.

61 *See id.*

62 National Health Service Act of 1977, § 3 (Eng.).

63 MINISTRY OF WELFARE, HEALTH AND CULTURAL AFFAIRS (The Netherlands), CHOICES IN HEALTH CARE 90 (1992).

64 This may be why NHS patients do not pay "hotel" charges involved with staying in hospital; they would be too expensive to collect. *See* KLEIN, *supra* note 1, at 35.

65 *See* S. WANDSWORTH ET AL., INSTITUTE FOR PUBLIC POLICY RESEARCH, CAN WE AFFORD THE NHS? 19–23 (1996).

dramatic changes of practice between hospitals and health authorities.[66] There is a high degree of stability in terms of purchasers' behavior because in practice they operate under constraints.[67] For example, (1) many hospital providers are effectively monopolies, so that, unless health authorities wish to send their patients to distant hospitals, they are obliged to contract with their local provider; (2) there is considerable lack of data and information to support significant changes in providers; (3) the unrestricted application of market forces could force hospitals out of business and cause unacceptable instability in the system; and (4) many patients have a sense of loyalty to a local provider.[68] Overall purchasing patterns, therefore, have not been radically affected, but there remains the question of individual patients for whom treatment is refused. What mechanism exists for such a refusal to be challenged? The following considers the reactions of the courts to the various circumstances in which resources have been implicated in the denial or provision of inadequate care.

1. Insufficient Resources and Judicial Review

The courts have reserved the right to review the decisions of managers and administrators if they are *Wednesbury* unreasonable. Lord Diplock has described the power of review as follows:

> It applies to a decision which is so outrageous in its defiance of logic or of accepted moral standards that no sensible person who had applied his mind to the question to be decided could have arrived at it. Whether a decision falls within this category is a question that judges by their training and experience should be well equipped to answer, or else there would be something badly wrong with our judicial system.[69]

But this power of review has yet to be exercised in matters concerning the allocation of NHS resources. In *R v. Secretary of State, ex parte Walker*, the health authority was satisfied that a premature baby required a heart operation.[70] The authority was unable to perform the procedure due to a decision not to staff all of the intensive care units in its neonatal ward.[71] The plaintiff alleged that her baby had been denied the surgical care the hospital acknowledged he needed.[72] Rejecting the application for an order that the operation be performed, the Master of the Rolls, Sir John Donaldson, said

> It is not for this court, or indeed any court, to substitute its own judgment for the judgment of those who are responsible for the allocation of resources. This court could only intervene where it was satisfied that there was a prima facie case, not only of failing to allocate resources in the way in which others would think that resources should be allocated, but of a failure to allocate resources to an extent which was *Wednesbury* . . . unreasonable.[73]

---

66 *See* APPLEBY, *supra* note 24, at 11.
67 *See id.*
68 *See id.*
69 Council of Civil Service Unions v. Minister for the Civil Service, [1985] App. Cas. 374, 410.
70 3 B.M.L.R. 32 (Eng. C.A. 1987), *available in* LEXIS, Enggen Library, Cases File.
71 *See id.*
72 *See id.*
73 *Id.*

302 AMERICAN JOURNAL OF LAW & MEDICINE VOL. XXIII NOS. 2&3 1997

Note that in *Walker*, there was no immediate danger to the baby and that, had an emergency arisen, the operation would have been performed.[74] What is the position when facilities are not made available to patients whose health will be damaged, or whose lives are put in danger, as a result?

This was the issue in *ex parte Collier*, which concerned a four year old boy suffering from a hole in the heart.[75] In September 1987, his consultant said that "he desperately needed open heart surgery" and placed the boy at the top of the waiting list, expecting that intensive care facilities would be made available by the hospital within a month.[76] By January 1988, the operation had been arranged, then canceled on three occasions and had still not been carried out because no intensive care bed could be made available.[77] The court of appeal was invited to order that, because the boy would probably die unless the operation was performed, the operation should be carried out.[78] It said, however, that:

> even assuming that [the evidence] does establish that there is immediate danger to health, it seems to me that the legal principles to be applied do not differ from the case of *Re Walker*. This court is in no position to judge the allocation of resources by this particular health authority . . . there is no suggestion here that the hospital authority have behaved in a way which is deserving of condemnation or criticism. What is suggested is that somehow more resources should be made available to enable the hospital authorities to ensure that the treatment is immediately given.[79]

Understandably, the courts must be extremely careful before becoming involved in telling hospital managers which cases should take priority. During litigation on behalf of an individual patient, who will speak for the large numbers of patients who are not party to the dispute but who could be affected by its outcome, or for those particular patients whose operations will have to be canceled if someone else is treated first? Subsequently, the point was made in the court of appeal, by Lord Justice Balcombe, who said

> I would stress the absolute undesirability of the court making an order which may have the effect of compelling a doctor or health authority to make available scarce resources (both human and material) to a particular child, without knowing whether or not there are other patients to whom those resources might more advantageously be devoted.[80]

Nevertheless, the case of *Collier* concerned a child who, as everyone agreed, was in need of common, if not routine, life-saving cardiac surgery. Despite being placed top of the waiting list by his responsible doctor, the hospital was unable to make facilities available. How could this have happened? On what system of priorities was such an apparently meritorious patient considered so much less urgent

[74] *See id.* at 34.

[75] Eng. C.A. Jan. 6, 1988 (LEXIS, Enggen Library, Cases File).

[76] *See id.*

[77] *See id.*

[78] *See id.*

[79] *Id.*

[80] Re J, 4 All E.R. 614, 625 (Eng. C.A. 1992). But in *Airedale NHS Trust v. Bland*, 1 All E.R. 821, 879 (H.L. 1993), Lord Browne-Wilkinson stated that "it is not legitimate for a judge in reaching a view as to what is for the benefit of the one individual whose life is in issue to take into account the wider practical issues as to allocation of limited financial resources."

than other cases demanding care and attention? Was the nursing staff attending to other patients in greater need of care? Was there a temporary shortage of staff owing to sickness? Could the operation not have been performed in another hospital? Was it impossible to borrow nursing staff from elsewhere? The astonishing thing about the case is that no one seemed to know exactly why intensive care facilities could not be made available to the patient. Counsel for the boy accepted that he simply did not know why the surgery had been canceled; as he said, "it may be good reason or bad reason."[81] And, in the absence of an explanation, Lord Justice Ralph Gibson commented, somewhat forlornly, "[n]o doubt the health authority would welcome the opportunity to deal with such matters so that they could explain what they are doing and what their problems are."[82]

One feels great sympathy for the case and all the reliable opinion polls suggest that the public, doctors and health service managers all believe that such cases ought to be top of the list of priorities.[83] Indeed, subsequent NHS guidelines issued by the Department of Health specify that, for patients with recognized clinical needs, "it is not acceptable for a purchaser to refuse authorization [for treatment] solely on the grounds of the proposed cost of the treatment in relation to the contracted services."[84] Given these factors, is it acceptable for the courts simply to shut their eyes in the face of such an application? In another context, Lord Denning has said that in some cases the failure to furnish a reason may incline the court to find that there are no sufficient reasons, and thereby declare the decision unreasonable.[85] Arguably, such an approach should be adopted in cases as distressing as *Collier*, both for the reassurance of the patient and the public.

2. Insufficient Resources and Negligence

A very different question arises in connection with the provision of inadequate care. The considerable unwillingness of the courts to intervene in cases of failure to provide care, i.e., an omission to act, is not matched when patients receive substandard care, i.e., a negligent act. The issue of insufficient resources leading to inadequate care was raised in *Bull v. Devon Area Health Authority* which concerned the system by which the hospital staffed its obstetrics wards.[86] The system failed to provide a consultant to deal with an emergency case.[87]

---

[81] *Collier*, Eng. C.A. Jan. 6, 1988 (LEXIS, Enggen Library, Cases File).

[82] *Id.*

[83] *See* Ann Bowling, *Health Care Rationing: The Public's Debate*, 312 BRITISH MED. J. 670 (1996).

[84] NATIONAL HEALTH SERVICE EXECUTIVE, GUIDANCE ON EXTRA CONTRACTUAL REFERRALS ¶ 51 (1993).

[85] *See* Secretary of State for Employment v. A.S.L.E.F., 2 Q.B. 455, 493 (1972). In *R v. Cambridge HA, ex parte B*, 2 All E.R. 129 (1995) (discussed *infra*), in an unreported judgment, Justice Laws expressed sympathy for the proposition that the courts should be sure that good reasons really do explain why treatment of needy patients cannot be provided. He said:

> merely to point to the fact that resources are finite tells one nothing about the wisdom, or . . . the legality of a decision to withhold funding in a particular case. . . . Where the question is whether the life of a 10 year-old child might be saved, by however slim a chance, the responsible Authority must do more than toll the bell of tight resources. They must explain the priorities that have led them to decline to fund the treatment.

Id. But these comments were not endorsed by the court of appeal.

[86] Eng. C.A. Feb. 2, 1989 (LEXIS, Intlaw Library, UKCase File).

[87] *See id.*

304 AMERICAN JOURNAL OF LAW & MEDICINE VOL. XXIII NOS. 2&3 1997

The defendant's hospital was located on two sites and the responsible doctor was unable to travel from one site to the other with sufficient speed to deal properly with the complicated delivery of a second twin.[88] As a result, a baby suffered cerebral palsy and spastic quadriplegia.[89] The defendants argued that limited resources precluded their ability to offer an "ideal" solution, one that might have been appropriate to a centre of excellence; "[t]hey could not be expected to do more than their limited best, allocating their limited resources as favourably as possible."[90] The defendant's experts refused to accept that there was anything wrong with the system, or that the standards in the hospital compared unfavourably with those that existed in other split-site hospitals.[91] As one expert stated, "it was 'par for the course.'"[92]

Lord Justice Mustill, however, rejected this defense based on scarce resources.[93] With reference to this defense, he said:

> it is not necessarily an answer to allegations of unsafety that there were insufficient resources to enable the administrators to do everything which they would like to do. I do not for a moment suggest that public medicine is precisely analogous to other public services, but there is perhaps a danger in assuming that it is completely sui generis, and that it is necessarily a complete defence to say that even if the system in any hospital was unsatisfactory, it was no more unsatisfactory than those in force elsewhere.[94]

Thus, the court was able to examine the system's adequacy of providing obstetric care. It described the system as being so delicately balanced that it was "obviously operating on a knife edge"[95] because it could only provide an acceptable level of care if it was operated with supreme efficiency.[96] The doctors knew that the mother was expecting twins, that any undue delay between the delivery of each would be very dangerous, and that she would probably need skilled assistance. According to its own standards, the hospital ought to have been able to provide care within a maximum of twenty minutes. But, as a result of a failure in the system, the mother had to wait over an hour.[97] Thus, the failure to provide her with the prompt care she needed was attributable to "the negligence of the defendants in implementing an unreliable and essentially unsatisfactory system for calling for the registrar"[98] and the defendants were held liable for the deficiency in its system of management.[99]

One is struck by the different reactions of the courts to applications for judicial review on the one hand and actions in negligence on the other. Given that both might be based on scarce resources, why should those who have been denied care be so unsuccessful in their applications (as in *Collier*), whereas those who have received inadequate care be encouraged to claim compensation (as in *Bull v. Devon Health*

---

[88] *See id.*
[89] *See id.*
[90] *Id.* (per Mustill L.J., representing the gist of the defence).
[91] *See id.*
[92] *See id.*
[93] *See id.*
[94] *Id.*
[95] *See id.* (per Slade L.J.).
[96] *See id.* (per Dillon L.J.).
[97] *See id.*
[98] *Id.*
[99] *See id.*

Authority)? Of course, the fact of personal injury is a distinguishing factor, but as *Collier* itself demonstrates, a refusal of care may be equally catastrophic. Some may consider that a common response ought to be achieved by both and that, if evidence of reasonable systems of caring for patients can be adduced in negligence cases, the same should apply to applications for judicial review of decisions to deny care, particularly those as extreme as *Collier*.[100]

3. Long-Term Care and "Ageism": Who Is a "Patient"?

In the United Kingdom, a crucial distinction exists between those who are considered "patients" within the NHS and those who are cared for in the community as "residents" in nursing homes and therefore are the responsibility of local governmental social service authorities.[101] As indicated, NHS care is generally provided free of charge.[102] Community care, on the other hand, is chargeable to the patient and many residents of nursing homes have to sell their homes to pay the charges.[103] The burden imposed on hospitals by long-term care patients, in terms of the beds which cannot be made available to earn revenue from further NHS contracts, has led some health authorities to adopt policies that exclude cases of chronic illness from NHS care. Such policies are clearly driven by resources.

Obviously, the burden we impose on the system in the later years of our lives is likely to increase, and some health authorities have sought to reduce the extent of services provided to elderly patients. This issue was considered by the Health Service Ombudsman in the case of a man who suffered a stroke and serious brain damage in 1989.[104] In 1991, when he was fifty five, the hospital in which he had been receiving treatment told his wife that his condition had stabilized, there was nothing more that could be done for him and that the bed was needed for other patients.[105] Nevertheless, his care required a medical bed in a nursing home because he continued to need nursing care.[106] He was discharged into a private nursing home which was able to provide the needed care at a net cost (deducting social security benefits) of £6,000 per year.[107] His wife complained to the Ombudsman that because he

---

[100] A recent decision of the House of Lords, however, may have the opposite effect. *Stovin v. Wise* considered the liability in negligence of a local authority for failing to exercise its statutory discretion to keep its roads safe, which failure led to a motor accident. *See* 3 All E.R. 801 (1996). Denying the existence of a duty of care to the plaintiff, Lord Hoffman said that

> the minimum pre-conditions for basing a duty of care upon the existence of a statutory power, if it can be done at all, are, first, that it would in the circumstances have been irrational not to have exercised the power, so that there was in effect a public law duty to act, and secondly, that there are exceptional grounds for holding that the policy of the statute requires compensation to be paid to persons who suffer loss because the power was not exercised.

Id. at 828. One such ground is where the statute creates expectations in the community on which a party relies on the public authority. *See id.* at 829. This appears to have a restrictive impact on the court of appeal's reasoning in *Bull*. Its effect on the liabilities of NHS Trust hospitals has yet to be assessed.

[101] *See* National Health Service Act of 1977 (Eng.); National Assistance Act of 1948 (Eng.).

[102] *See* National Health Service Act of 1977, § 1(2).

[103] *See* National Assistance Act of 1948, § 22(1).

[104] *See* HEALTH SERVICE COMMISSIONER, SECOND REPORT FOR SESSION 1993–94, Case No. 197 (failure to provide long-term NHS care for a brain-damaged patient).

[105] *See id.*

[106] *See id.*

[107] *See id.*

needed such intensive nursing care, he met the criteria for care either in an NHS hospital or in a nursing home paid for by the health authority.[108]

The health authority replied to the complaint saying that it could not meet every need.[109] Its policy mandated shorter inpatient stays so that continuing care was provided in the community.[110] For this reason, the authority provided no long stay hospital beds, nor did it have contractual arrangements under which such care could be provided by a nursing home.[111] It said that were it obliged to provide such care, it would soon become financially overstretched.[112] The chief executive of the NHS Management Executive maintained that the duty to provide care on clinical grounds was always subject to the duty to remain within available resources and, accordingly, to distinguish among patients.[113] The Ombudsman condemned the policy:

> The patient was a highly dependent patient in hospital . . .; and yet, when he no longer needed care in an acute ward but manifestly still needed what the National Health Service is there to provide, they regarded themselves as having no scope for continuing to discharge their responsibilities to him because their policy was to make no provision for continuing care. . . . In my opinion the failure to make available long-term care within the NHS for this patient was unreasonable and constitutes a failure in the service provided by the Health Authority.[114]

Thus, the complaint was upheld and the health authority agreed to reimburse the complainant her out-of-pocket expenses including the private nursing home fees and to pay for the future cost of his care.[115]

The adjudication had considerable impact within the NHS. New Health Service Guidelines[116] were introduced by the Department of Health in 1995, and they indicated that those with "specialist" nursing requirements are "patients" and should not be discharged from the hospital.[117] This guidance is welcome for providing some, though limited, clarification as to the duties of health authorities toward those with long-term needs. But, in common with many other developed nations, the proportion of elderly people in the community will increase relative to those who are in work and on whom they depend. The United Kingdom has yet to resolve the problems for health care resources that is posed by the increasing proportion of elderly people.[118]

---

[108] *See id.*

[109] *See id.*

[110] *See id.*

[111] *See id.*

[112] *See id.*

[113] *See id.* ¶ 18.

[114] *Id.* ¶ 22.

[115] The court of appeal appears to have taken a similar view in *White v. Chief Adjudication Officer*, 17 B.M.L.R. 68 (1994).

[116] *See* NATIONAL HEALTH SERVICE EXECUTIVE, NHS RESPONSIBILITIES FOR MEETING CONTINUING HEALTH CARE NEEDS, HSG (1995). Health Service Guidelines have no direct legal force; they are administrative measures designed to assist the operation of the Service.

[117] *See* Christopher Newdick, *Patients, or Residents?: Long-Term Care in the Welfare State*, 4 MED. L. REV. 144 (1996).

[118] *See id.*

4. "Luxury" Care

A related matter concerns the care that might provide benefit to patients, but is considered too peripheral to the objectives of the NHS to deserve treatment (though, of course, the patient may purchase the operation privately). For example, some health authorities have expressly excluded from their NHS contracts treatment for tattoo removal, gender realignment,[119] vasectomy and sterilization operations, and cosmetic surgery, unless there are exceptional reasons why such treatment should be provided. In theory, of course, one is inclined to accept the idea that some medical treatment commands such a low priority that it should not be paid for by the NHS. The difficulty is in knowing where and how to draw the line.

The issue arose in *R.. v. Sheffield H.A. ex parte Seale*,[120] in which the plaintiff was refused in vitro fertilization treatment because she was thirty-seven. The upper age limit set for such procedures by Sheffield H.A. was thirty-five.[121] She alleged that the policy was illegal because it was contrary to Section 3 of the National Health Service Act of 1977, and because it was irrational for failing to consider her own particular clinical circumstances.[122] As to the allegation of illegality, Justice Auld held that the extent to which such a service was provided was within the discretion of the health authority:

> it is not arguable . . . that [the H.A.] is bound, simply because it has undertaken to provide such a service, to provide it on demand to any individual patient for whom it may work, regardless of financial and other constraints upon the authority. In my view it is clear that if the Secretary of State has not limited or given directions as to the way in which such a service, once undertaken, should be provided, the authority providing it is entitled to form a view as to those circumstances and when they justify provision and when they do not.[123]

Further, the court held that the age limit was not irrational or absurd for failing to consider the clinical circumstances of each individual case:

> [A] clinical decision on a case by case basis is clearly desirable and, in cases of critical illness, a necessary approach. However, it is reasonable, or at least not *Wednesbury* unreasonable . . . of an authority to look at the matter in the context of the financial resources available to it and the many other services for which it responsible. I cannot say that it is absurd for this authority . . . to take [35] as an appropriate criterion when balancing the need for such provision against its ability to provide it.[124]

Although the application was refused on its merits, the case distinguishes between "critical," and other, illnesses.[125] If critical illness necessitates an individual clinical decision of the case, the *Wednesbury* test of managerial reasonableness is

[119] For differing conclusions on whether transexual surgery is medically "necessary," compare *Rush v. Parham*, 625 F.2d 1150 (5th Cir. 1980), with *Pinneke v. Preiser*, 623 F.2d 546 (8th Cir. 1980).

[120] (1995) 25 B.M.L.R. 1 (Eng. C.A.).

[121] *See id.*

[122] *See id.*

[123] *Id.* at 3.

[124] *Id.*

[125] *See id.*

308 AMERICAN JOURNAL OF LAW & MEDICINE VOL. XXIII NOS. 2&3 1997

presumably limited to other areas of elective or optional health care. Note how uncomfortably this approach to clinical merits sits with *Collier*. This case is useful on its own facts for identifying that some care may fall into a category in which a clinical assessment is necessary. It says nothing, however, about the components of such a decision, who is responsible for making it, or where the line should be drawn.

The issues provoked by peripheral or luxury treatment will become more pressing, yet litigation based on Section 3 of the 1977 Act is obviously unable to offer a systematic response to this matter. Assuming that a comprehensive health service cannot include all the procedures that patients want, it would be helpful to develop guidelines to assist local policy-makers. As the House of Commons Health Committee has said:

> We are concerned that at present these decisions are taken by purchasers in the absence of any firm lead from the Department [of Health]. For example, how much discretion should reside with individual purchasers? What rights do individuals have to challenge these decisions? What values and criteria should purchasers use to assess the limits of local provision? . . . We recommend that the Department set out clearly the framework within which purchasers will be expected to define the local package of services, and set out the criteria by which these decisions may be scrutinised, debated and, if needs be, challenged by individuals.[126]

In the absence of such criteria, different health authorities have taken differing views as to the extent of their obligations, so that, at times, the system appears to be more of a *federal* than a *national* health service.

5. "Undeserving" Patients

An issue yet to reach the courts concerns patients considered undeserving of treatment because they are the authors of their own illness. For example, some doctors have advocated the exclusion of smokers from cardiac surgery.[127] One doctor had difficulty deciding whether to offer a second artificial heart valve to an intravenous drug abuser who destroyed both his own heart and the first replacement valve by his persistent drug abuse.[128] The Department of Health has made only one comment on the matter. It considers that "patients . . . need to accept that they have responsibilities as well as rights, not only in their use of services but also in taking care of their own health so limited resources can be used effectively."[129]

However, it goes no further and does not suggest excluding patients from care on this ground. The difficulty with the notion of "deserts" is the need to make a nonclinical judgment. Many people expose themselves to avoidable health risks that do not attract criticism, such as playing contact sports that damage their muscles and bones, or working in a high-pressure environment and damaging their hearts or psychological stability. This suggests that the distinctions that would have to be drawn

---

126 Priority Setting in the NHS: Purchasing ¶ 113 (H.C. 134-I, Session 1994–95).

127 *See* M. Underwood & J. Bailey, *Coronary Bypass Surgery Should Not be Offered to Smokers*, 306 BRIT. MED. J. 1047 (1993).

128 *See* TROYEN A. BRENNAN, JUST DOCTORING: MEDICAL ETHICS IN THE LIBERAL STATE 176 (1991).

129 NATIONAL HEALTH SERVICE EXECUTIVE, PRIMARY CARE: THE FUTURE ¶ 9.2 (1996).

before patients could be deemed "undeserving" are so invidious, and have so little connection with *clinical* judgment, that doctors should not make them.

Also, the class or environment in which people grow up may have a direct influence on smoking, eating and drinking habits.[130] It would be unfair to heap further misfortune on an individual by denying him or her health care, when the original illness or disease has arisen by virtue of the unfavorable environment in which they live. And what about their dependents? Who really suffers when a bread-winner is no longer able to work or a person with an infectious disease is denied access to care? Such a policy would be so inconsistent, so random, and so unfair to innocent parties that it ought to be discouraged. On the other hand, for those whose life-styles make (or have made) the likelihood of clinical success so small that the risk of the procedure cannot be justified by the limited benefits expected from it, such a purely *clinical* decision to deny treatment may be justified.

C. ALLOCATIONS BY DOCTORS

The common law has always been reluctant to criticize a doctor for exercising responsible clinical discretion. The now famous *Bolam* test of medical malpractice holds that

> [a] doctor is not guilty of negligence if he has acted in accordance with a practice accepted as proper by a responsible body of medical men skilled in that particular art . . . a doctor is not negligent if he is acting in accordance with such a practice merely because there is a body of opinion that takes a contrary view.[131]

This test has been applied to the clinical matters of diagnosis, prognosis, the techniques adopted for caring for the patient, and, to a lesser extent, the disclosure of information.[132] Should it extend to discretion as to the allocation of scarce resources? The question arises because of developments in pharmaceutical and medical technology that enable considerable sums of money to be devoted to very few patients.

In a publicly funded system, can the notion of clinical freedom survive? One commentator has said

> the gap between what medical technology makes possible and what [we] can afford is going to widen steadily and inexorably . . . I suspect that in 20 years time our successors will look back on the early 1990's as the age of innocence, or perhaps even as the age of naivety, when people . . . thought that with two or three extra billion pounds, a bit more attention to clinical effectiveness and the elimination of treatments of unproven value we would be able to afford all the treatments that the country and its population needed and wanted. Sadly, that's pie in the sky.[133]

[130] *See* M. Whitehead, *The Health Divide*, *in* INEQUALITIES IN HEALTH 3055 (1988).

[131] Bolam v. Friern Hospital Management Committee, 2 All E.R. 118, 122 (1957). Modern law confirms that the courts must remain the ultimate arbiters of what is "responsible," and be capable of condemning opinion despite the support of other doctors. *See, e.g.*, Bouchta Swindon H.A., 7 MED. L. REV. 62 (1996).

[132] *See generally* MICHAEL JONES, MEDICAL NEGLIGENCE (1991).

[133] R. Kendall, *Improving Clinical Effectiveness—The Future*, *in* CLINICAL EFFECTIVENESS: FROM GUIDELINES TO COST EFFECTIVE PRACTICE 138 (M. Deighan & S. Hitch eds., 1995).

310 AMERICAN JOURNAL OF LAW & MEDICINE VOL. XXIII NOS. 2&3 1997

This implies either that doctors will have their clinical freedom restricted or that their commitment to promote the interests of individuals will be abandoned to be replaced by the more recondite objectives of managers, economists, and politicians. "In a management culture, individual interests are subordinated to the whole or collective. The role is an essentially collectivist one, emphasizing strategic planning, establishing the corporate mission and goals of the organization."[134] This tension between the "macro-" and the "micro-" goals of health care systems provides one of the most pressing problems in the whole of medical law and ethics and the following comments make no claim to resolve them. Instead, they concentrate on a number of particular areas of practice in which the issue has been addressed as a means of explaining the character of the discussion in the United Kingdom. They consider (1) clinical freedom and futile care, (2) managing marginal treatment and (3) evidence-based medicine and clinical guidelines.

1. Clinical Discretion and Futile Care

Futile care is discussed as a means of introducing the more general powers of doctors and managers to withdraw treatment from, or refuse to offer treatment to, patients. Traditionally, the medical profession has always committed itself to the Hippocratic notion of clinical freedom. "I will follow that system of regimen which, according to my ability and judgment, I consider for the benefit of my patients,"[135] which, in the language of the World Health Organisation's Declaration of Geneva means "the health of my patient shall be my first consideration."[136] The General Medical Council, which exercises statutory control over the medical profession in the United Kingdom, "endorses the principle that a doctor should always seek to give priority to the investigation and treatment of patients solely on the basis of clinical need."[137] To what extent does this freedom permit treatment to be withdrawn from a patient on the basis that it is futile?

The matter was considered by the House of Lords in *Airedale NHS Trust v. Bland*, in which a twenty one year-old patient, Anthony Bland, suffered anoxia (oxygen starvation) after being crushed in 1989.[138] By 1992 he was in a persistent vegetative state and had no prospects of regaining consciousness.[139] The hospital sought a declaration that it would be lawful to discontinue artificial feeding, hydration and other medical treatment in order for him to "end his life and die peacefully with the greatest dignity and the least of pain and distress."[140] The House of Lords decided that there is no absolute obligation to keep patients alive regardless of their condition and prospects of recovery.[141] In extreme cases, reasonable doctors are entitled to believe that it is no longer in the patient's best interests that treatment be

134 D. Hunter, *Doctors as Managers: Poachers Turned Gamekeepers*, 35 SOC. SCI. & MED. 557, 562 (1992).

135 *See* BRITISH MEDICAL ASS'N, MEDICAL ETHICS TODAY—ITS PRACTICE AND PHILOSOPHY app. (1993).

136 *See id.*

137 GENERAL MEDICAL COUNCIL (LONDON), CONTRACTUAL ARRANGEMENTS IN HEALTH CARE: PROFESSIONAL RESPONSIBILITIES IN RELATION TO THE CLINICAL NEEDS OF PATIENTS ¶ 8 (1992).

138 Airedale NHS Trust v. Bland, 1 All E.R. 821 (1993).

139 *See id.*

140 *Id.* at 824. Note that "the question is not whether it is in the best interests of the patient that he should die. The question is whether it is in the best interests of the patient that his life should be prolonged by the continuance of this form of medical treatment or care." *Id.* at 869 (per Lord Goff).

141 *See id.*

continued.[142] In these circumstances, treatment may be withdrawn in the full knowledge that the consequence of doing so will be the patient's death.[143] Lord Goff said:

> I cannot see that medical treatment is appropriate or requisite simply to prolong a patient's life when such treatment has no therapeutic purpose of any kind, as where it is futile because the patient is unconscious and there is no prospect of any improvement in his condition. . . . It is the futility of the treatment which justifies its termination.[144]

Lord Keith confirmed the legitimacy of responsible *clinical* discretion in such cases:

> [A] medical practitioner is under no duty to continue to treat such a patient where a large body of informed and responsible medical opinion is to the effect that no benefit would be conferred by continuance. Existence in a vegetative state with no prospects of recovery is by that opinion regarded as not being a benefit, and that, if not unarguably correct, at least forms a proper basis for the decision to discontinue treatment and care.[145]

Certainly, the tests of "no therapeutic purpose" and "no benefit" leave considerable room for differences of opinion among doctors, One wonders how long such latitude can prevail in an area so dominated by *ethical* rather than *clinical* considerations.[146] Nevertheless, doctors clearly focus on the interests of the individual patient in question, rather than on the many others who could benefit from access to the same resources.

Lord Keith distinguished between futile and other treatment: "[I]t would not be lawful for a medical practitioner who assumed responsibility for the care of an unconscious patient simply to give up treatment where continuance of it would confer some benefit on the patient."[147] Lord Browne-Wilkinson, recognizing the difficulties presented by competing demands for scarce resources, posed the following question:

> Given that there are limited resources available for medical care, is it right to devote money to sustaining the lives of those who are, and always will be unaware of their own existence rather than treating those who, in a real sense, can be benefited, e.g. those deprived of dialysis for want of resources?[148]

He answered this by saying "it is not legitimate for a judge in reaching a view as to what is for the benefit of the one individual whose life is in issue to take into account the wider practical issues as to allocation of limited financial resources."[149] This suggests that managerial imperatives ought not to contradict clinical ones, but in reality, the notion of "benefit" is more complicated. Doctors have lists of patients to

---

142 *See id.*

143 *See id.*

144 *Id.* at 896 (per Lord Mustill).

145 Bolam v. Friern Hosp. Management Comm., 1 W.L.R. 582 (1957); *see also Airedale*, 1 All E.R. 861 (1993).

146 Compare the importance attached to the patient's own wishes in *Cruzan v. Director, Missouri Dep't of Health*, 497 U.S. 261 (1990). *See* NEWDICK, *supra* note 34, at 276–88; Tom Tomlinson & Diane Czlonka, *Futility and Hospital Policy*, HASTINGS CENTER REP., May/June 1995, at 28 (recommending procedural, rather than substantive guidelines in this area).

147 *Airedale*, 1 All E.R. 861 (per Lord Keith).

148 *Id.* at 879.

149 *Id.*

312 AMERICAN JOURNAL OF LAW & MEDICINE VOL. XXIII NOS. 2&3 1997

treat and must manage their time and resources to do so; and the business of managers is to promote the best interests of patients as a whole, by promoting the best clinical practices. Might circumstances arise in which the potential benefit to the patient is so marginal that it might still be regarded as futile. For example, is it futile to keep the patient in the hospital under observation for an extra few days or perform additional diagnostic tests that will almost certainly be negative? This issue is discussed next.

2. The Management of Marginal Treatment

In *Bland*, Lords Goff and Keith refer to the idea of therapeutic "purpose" or "benefit."[150] How sensitive is this notion: Is it absolute or relative? No one suggests that this commitment to doing what is best for the patient should encourage the waste of NHS resources. As the British Medical Association says, "[w]astage of resources is unethical because it diminishes society's capacity to relieve suffering through the other uses that could be made of the wasted resources. Doctors working within the NHS need to be aware of cost-effectiveness as well as clinical effectiveness in the care provided for the patient."[151]

Take the example of the diagnostic test designed to detect cancer of the bowel, which is reported to have cost $47 million for every case detected![152] For the overwhelming majority who tested negative, one suspects that the benefit was so marginal that it cannot have represented good value for money. Putting it another way, the small benefit notwithstanding, the resources were wasted by reference to those with more urgent clinical needs who received no treatment at all.

An analysis of this nature might have been relevant in the case of *R. v. Cambridge D.H.A., ex parte B*, in which a ten year-old girl with leukemia was refused the resources required to provide her with remedial (as opposed to palliative) treatment that might have prolonged her life.[153] An application to secure resources on her behalf was denied on the grounds that: (1) the doctors responsible for treatment considered it to be so untested that it was "experimental"; (2) its prospects of success were very small, i.e. between one and four percent overall; (3) it would have debilitating side-effects which, given her prospects, were not in her best interests; and (4) given her prospects, the total cost of the two stages of procedures (some £75,000) could not be justified.[154] The unanimous clinical view of the doctors was that the procedure should not be carried out. In accepting that view, the health authority, confirmed that the decision had been taken in light of "all the clinical and other relevant matters . . . and not on financial grounds."[155] Thus, although there was the possibility of some benefit, it was insufficient to justify treatment; it would have been wasteful in the circumstances of the case.

This demonstrates that clinical benefit is a far from absolute notion and the case of *Bland* must be understood in this light. But how relative is it? Compare the views

---

150 *See id.* at 861.

151 BRITISH MEDICAL ASS'N, *supra* note 135, at 300.

152 *See* Duncan Neuhauser & Ann M. Lewicki, *What Do We Gain from the Sixth Stool Guaiac?*, 293 NEW ENG. J. MED. 226 (1975).

153 2 All E.R. 129 (1995).

154 *See id.*

155 *Id.* at 138. The patient died of her illness about a year later. *See id.* For a comparable application concerning a liver/bowel transplant for a baby, but offering greater prospects of a successful outcome, see *McLaughlin v. Williams*, 801 F. Supp. 633 (S.D. Fla. 1992).

of doctors and managers to this issue. The medical profession is trained to promote the interests of individuals. By contrast, health economists and managers are concerned with groups of patients. It may be that substantial benefit could be conferred on an individual, but still create such vast opportunity costs as to be unacceptable by reference to the numbers denied care as a result. Concern is expressed, for example, at the costs associated with cardiopulmonary resuscitation,[156] but the question also extends to expensive medicines. Children with growing disorders need hormone treatment costing around £7,000 for a six month course of treatment.[157] Essential treatment of renal failure may cost £12,000 per year.[158] One product which reduces mortality in patients with gram negative septicemia costs £2,200 for a single dose.[159] In every case, it would be possible to divert the resources involved to benefit larger numbers of patients. If the full logic of opportunity costs is accepted, however, we must accept that the present duty of the doctor to his or her patient will become secondary to the welfare of the community or economic efficiency. How would the principle operate?; Which patients, or diseases, would command priority?; Who would be last on the list? This is a much more complicated issue with profound political and economic implications. In such circumstances, would patients retain any rights at all worthy of the name?[160]

This extended notion of opportunity costs as a method for allocating resources deserves three brief comments. First, scientific evidence is often insufficient to provide clear conclusions as to the benefits of a particular treatment.[161] It may be incomplete, ambiguous, or uncertain, and provide ample justification for disagreement both among doctors and managers as to whether treatment is worthwhile.[162] In such a case, which opinion should take precedence?; and What standard of agreement should be required before treatment is considered necessary or beneficial? Should it be the standard of *a* reasonable doctor or a responsible *body* of doctors or a wider *community* standard? Should *medical* standards be paramount at all or should managers or the courts reserve the power to arbitrate over the issue?[163]

Second, even when the scientific evidence is complete, there may be disagreement about the proper response to it. Take the example of a patient with a firm diagnosis of a pre-cancerous syndrome that may cause no ill effects. However, it has a fifty percent chance of developing into a very dangerous form of breast cancer. The evidence is complete; and in one sense, the patient is not ill at all. Should she un-

---

[156] *See* Donald Murphy & Thomas Finucane, *New Do-Not-Resuscitate Policies: A First Step in Cost Control*, 153 ARCHIVES OF INTERNAL MED. 1641 (1993); Tony Hope et al., *Not Clinically Indicated: Patient's Interest or Resource Allocation?*, 306 BRIT. MED. J. 379 (1993).

[157] *See Unlicensed Uses for Growth Hormone*, 32 DRUGS & THERAPEUTICS BULL. 53 (1994).

[158] *See* Roger Gabriel, *Picking up the Tab for Erythropoietin*, 302 BRIT. MED. J. 248 (1991).

[159] *See* M. Orme, *How to Pay for Expensive Drugs*, 303 BRIT. MED. J. 593 (1991); *see also* R. Williams, *Can We Afford Medical Advances?*, 27 J. ROYAL C. PHYSICIANS 70 (1993).

[160] For attempts to develop concepts of rights within this "macro" approach, see Troyen A. Brennan, *An Ethical Perspective on Health Care Insurance Reform*, 19 AM. J.L. & MED. 46 (1993), and Mark A. Hall, *Rationing Health Care at the Bedside*, 69 N.Y.U. L. REV. 693 (1994).

[161] *See* David M. Eddy, *Variations in Physician Practice: The Role of Uncertainty*, HEALTH AFF., Fall 1984, at 74.

[162] *See id.*

[163] For a spectrum of judicial responses to the question, see Wendy K. Mariner, *Patients' Rights After Health Care Reform: Who Decides What is Medically Necessary?*, 84 AM. J. PUB. HEALTH 1515 (1994).

314 AMERICAN JOURNAL OF LAW & MEDICINE VOL. XXIII NOS. 2&3 1997

dergo a mastectomy to remove the future risk?[164] Similar questions are provoked by the treatment of incurable and debilitating conditions such as Alzheimer's disease when the memories and personality of the patient appear to have been largely destroyed.[165] Clearly, the decision in such a case is driven as much by considerations of ethics and economics as by clinical merits. Matters of this nature have yet to reach the courts in England. For the future, the burden of these unenviable decisions might have to be more widely distributed so that other professional and lay interests are also represented.[166]

Lastly, contemporary medical training does not include the subject of health economics, and doctors have no special knowledge that permits the responsible adoption of such a principle in clinical practice. Arguably, therefore, contemporary legal standards should be reluctant to permit doctors to include matters of this nature as a basis for denying treatment to patients who are capable of obtaining significant benefit. Further, if such a system of allocating resources were to develop in the future, and the doctor's primary duty to the patient were to be replaced, the common law would have to develop a much more sophisticated principle of informed "denial" of health care in order for patients to react to their circumstances in a responsible manner.[167]

3. Evidence-Based Medicine Clinical Guidelines

A practical application of some of the concerns expressed above is contained in the idea of evidence-based medicine. Evidence-based medicine is described as "the process of systematically finding, appraising, and using contemporaneous research findings as the basis for clinical decisions."[168] The Department of Health has expressed concern that wide and avoidable variations in standards of health exist between sections of the population based on occupational class, region, sex and ethnic group.[169] The Department of Health believes these variations cannot be explained by clinical factors.[170] "What is now needed is for the NHS at local level to undertake a more systematic identification of local health variations, and to design and implement measures to tackle them. Future interventions must be rigorously evaluated, particularly for cost-effectiveness, and the findings of evaluations should be disseminated widely."[171]

164 The example is taken from *Katskee v. Blue Cross/Blue Shield*, 515 N.W.2d 645 (Neb. 1994). Both the doctor and patient wanted the operation to proceed. *See id.* at 647–48. The court approached the problem under principles of contract law and interpreted the ambiguous provision in the contract of insurance in the plaintiff's favor. *See id.* at 821.

165 *See In re* Conroy, 486 A.2d 1209 (N.J. 1985). In the absence of her own clear wish that treatment should not be continued (the subjective test, e.g., in a living will), or the trustworthy evidence of someone else to the same effect (the limited-objective test), or that the burdens of treatment outweighed its benefits (pure-objective test), treatment should not be withdrawn. *See id.* at 1231–33.

166 *See* Robert M. Veatch & Carol Mason Spicer, *Medically Futile Care: The Role of the Physician in Setting Limits*, 18 AM. J.L. & MED. 15 (1992).

167 *See* Frances H. Miller, *Denial of Health Care and Informed Consent in English and American Law*, 18 AM. J.L. & MED 37 (1992).

168 William Rosenberg & Anna Donald, *Evidence Based Medicine: An Approach to Clinical Problem-Solving*, 310 BRIT. MED. J. 1122 (1995).

169 *See* DEPARTMENT OF HEALTH, VARIATIONS IN HEALTH—WHAT CAN THE DEPARTMENT OF HEALTH AND THE NHS DO? ¶ 4.60 (1995).

170 *See id.*

171 *Id.*

To this end it has funded a number of centres to collect and collate the most recent international research findings.[172] Their objective is to screen the most respected clinical opinion throughout the world as a means of creating reliable clinical guidelines for doctors.[173] This, it is hoped, will reveal which procedures are most effective, clinically and economically, and so assist doctors and managers in decisions as to which should be encouraged and discouraged.[174] The significance of this new approach is that it shifts the judgment whether to provide health are away from a doctor's individual opinion and past practice toward scientific proof and hard evidence as a guide to decision making.[175] In the future, doctors will need to have greater access to guidelines as a reason for action. For those of us who still retain faith in clinical intuition or instinct—the touch that doctors develop in relation to their practice—such a development, which diverts attention away from patients and toward computer screens, is a mixed blessing. It will also tend to dilute the trust that has founded the traditional doctor-patient relationship.

The movement toward this form of decision making is slow, and its contemporary significance should not be over-emphasized. By their nature, guidelines, however reliable, tend to be based on aggregates of population, and individual physicians should always retain the discretion in relation to those who fall outside the framework. And, as we have seen, the evidence itself is often unavailable or unhelpful, in the sense that it has not yet been collated and consolidated into practical guidelines.[176] Indeed, the Department of Health has compared the relative success rates of a range of clinical treatments in Scottish hospitals.[177] The study shows significant variations in success rates between them.[178]

Nevertheless, bare statistics about variations do not explain why they occur, although they may invite further research by way of explanation. The Clinical Outcomes Working Group emphasized that:

> no conclusions can or should be drawn from the comparisons in this report about the quality or the efficacy of the treatment provided . . . or for patients admitted to different hospitals. Despite the standardisation for age and sex, and in many cases for deprivation and comorbidity as well, it is still just as likely that the observed differences in outcome are due to differences in patients, or in diagnostic criteria, as they are due to differences in treatment.[179]

Assuming these difficulties can be overcome, however, one ought to expect far greater influence from hospital managers in decisions as to the techniques to be used in treatment in the hospital units, and even which doctors should provide them. Such a process could be imposed by the use of clinical guidelines based on hard evidence of practice. Precisely this opportunity is available to health authorities by means of NHS contracts with hospitals which could specify details of this nature. This may provide a more systematic response to the enterprise of health care, but it would also

---

172 *See* Lisa Bero & Rennie Drummond, *The Cochrane Collaboration*, 274 JAMA 1935 (1995).

173 *See id.*

174 *See id.*

175 *See* JOHN APPLEBY ET AL., ACTING ON THE EVIDENCE 5 (1995).

176 *See* R. Smith, *The Poverty of Medical Evidence*, 303 BRIT. MED. J. 798 (1992).

177 *See* DEPARTMENT OF HEALTH, CLINICAL OUTCOMES WORKING GROUP, CLINICAL OUTCOME INDICATORS 4 (1995).

178 *See id.*

179 *Id.*

involve a radical transfer of discretion making from doctors to health service managers.

One of the more chilling conclusions from a recent study of the costs and benefits of medical care is provided in a report on the use of intensive care facilities.[180] Given that many of those treated in such units will not survive, what proportion of a hospital's budget should be devoted to intensive care? The report comments that it is difficult to assess whether some patients will benefit from intensive care and the only appropriate course will be to admit them for assessment.[181] With respect to others, however, "since organ-system support often defers but does not always prevent death, it is important that patients should not be offered treatment inappropriately. Intensive care can infringe on the patient's dignity, and, where the outcome is poor, can prolong the suffering for patients and their families."[182]

In other words, intensive care should not be provided and the patient should be allowed to die. "Dignity" is certainly relevant to such a situation. One is concerned, however, that the real motivation for the advice is cost. A patient's dignity and the cost implications of his or her treatment are very different things, consideration of which may lead to opposing recommendations as to clinical outcome. Evidence-based medicine will offer guidance on a wide range of cases, but we should be very careful to distinguish the clinical from the financial components of such an exercise.

IV. CONCLUSION—A STANDING COMMISSION ON PRIORITIES?

For the present, the government is reluctant to embroil itself in the details of the priorities debate and faces a number of directions at the same time. It acknowledges that "[t]here will always be a gap between all we wish to do and all we can. Setting priorities is a fact if life."[183] On the other hand,

> To attempt to draw up a national list of treatments which will and will not be provided would be an exercise fraught with danger. No one list could ever hope to accommodate the range and complexity of the different cases which clinicians face all the time. There would be a real risk of taking decisions out of the hands of doctors.[184]

Equally, clinical discretion is not absolute because clinicians may not always understand the economic consequences of their decisions. Thus, as part of its policy to increase efficiency within the system, the government encourages "[h]ealth authorities . . . to make better use of effectiveness and cost-effectiveness data . . . [and] to increase investment in interventions known to be effective and to reduce investment in interventions which have been identified as less effective."[185] With this background, what are the basic objectives of the system and how does it seek to achieve them?

As *ex parte Hincks*, *ex parte Collier*, and *ex parte Seale* demonstrate, health service managers and economists have inevitably acquired greater influence over the

---

180 *See* DEPARTMENT OF HEALTH, GUIDELINES ON ADMISSION TO AND DISCHARGE FROM INTENSIVE CARE AND HIGH DEPENDENCY UNITS ¶ 3.5 (1996).

181 *Id.*

182 *Id.*

183 GOVERNMENT RESPONSE TO THE FIRST REPORT FROM THE HEALTH COMMITTEE, 1995, Cmnd. 2826, ¶ 4.

184 *Id.* ¶ 7.

185 *Id.* ¶ 8.

manner in which resources should be distributed. It is this feature of planning, about which so little information and guidance exists, that people find unsettling because of the threat it presents to the fidelity between doctor and patient. With respect to local planning, The Royal College of Physicians warns that there is

> anxiety over the methods by which objectives and priorities are set by bodies that are managerial rather than expert and are overwhelmingly subject to political and fiscal pressures. . . . Even if such bodies contrive to resist the temptation to let resources determine priorities rather than serve them, the processes of decision are too opaque to gain the confidence of the public.[186]

One solution to the search for authority in decisions concerning health priorities is to include a democratic component. The Department of Health encourages this policy,[187] but it is not a complete answer. For example, lay people may attach more importance to high-technology medical interventions in preference to long-term care for elderly people and services for those with mental illnesses. Such a policy would focus resources on many fewer people than at present.[188] There is also the concern that public opinion could be manipulated to endorse rather than inform professional, or another group's, opinion.[189]

An alternative proposal is the creation of a National Council for Health Priorities with responsibility for involving, educating and informing the public, the professions and government of ways of improving priority setting. Precisely such advisory committees have reported to the Swedish and Dutch governments.[190] For example, in 1995, the Swedish Parliamentary Priorities Commission published *Priorities in Health Care* which identified the following category as commanding top priority: "[a] Care of life-threatening acute diseases and diseases which, if left untreated, will lead to permanent disability or premature death. [b] Treatment of severe chronic diseases. [c] Palliative terminal care. [d] Care of People with reduced autonomy."[191]

And in *Choices in Health Care*, the Dutch Committee recommended that a basic health care package should be concentrated on care that is necessary, effective, efficient and beyond the individual's own responsibility.[192] Thus, for example, in vitro fertilization, homeopathic medicines and adult dental care were thought not to be within the basic insurance package.[193] The costs of which, incidentally, have a rather modest overall impact on the distribution of resources. With both reports, however, a significant gap exists between the principle and the practice—of what treatments should actually be excluded from the system. It may be that in creating such bodies to determine priories we are searching for a holy grail that can never be

---

186 ROYAL COLLEGE OF PHYSICIANS OF LONDON, SETTING PRIORITIES IN THE N.H.S. ¶ 3.15 (1995).

187 *See* NATIONAL HEALTH SERVICE EXECUTIVE, LOCAL VOICES: THE VIEWS OF LOCAL PEOPLE IN PURCHASING FOR HEALTH (1992); *see also* Leonard Fleck, *Just Health Care Rationing: A Democratic Decisionmaking Approach*, 140 U. PA. L. REV. 1579 (1992).

188 *See* Chris Ham, *Priority Setting in the NHS*, 307 BRIT. MED. J. 435 (1993).

189 *See* D. HUNTER, RATIONING DILEMMAS IN HEALTH CARE 27 (1993).

190 *See, e.g.*, *Priorities in Health Care*, Swedish Government Official Reports, 5:1995, 136; *Choices in Health Care*, Government Committee on Choices in Health Care, The Netherlands, 1991.

191 *Priorities in Health Care*, *supra* note 190, at 136.

192 *See Choices in Health Care*, *supra* note 190.

193 *See id.* at 87–90.

318 AMERICAN JOURNAL OF LAW & MEDICINE VOL. XXIII NOS. 2&3 1997

found. When the very basis of our understanding of the concepts of "health" and "disease" is ambivalent,[194] and the significance of the scientific evidence on which clinical decisions are based is subject to such wide differences of professional opinion,[195] we must not be over-ambitious in constructing grand theories on which resources should be allocated. As one distinguished commentator has said, there is no "technological fix" or scientific method for determining priorities:

> The debate about priorities will never be finally resolved. . . . As medical technology, the economic and demographic environment, and social attitudes change, so almost certainly will our priorities. And we have to recognise that much medicine is about the management of uncertainty, where research may roll back the frontiers of ignorance but is never likely to eliminate totally the need for clinical discretion and the use of judgment in interpreting the evidence about efficacy and outcomes.
>
> Our aim must be therefore to build up over time our capacity to engage in continuous, collective argument. This means, in turn, devising institutions that encourage, rather than discourage, challenge. . . . In short, we should be at least as much concerned with the structure of our institutions, and the way in which they work, as with the development of techniques. The politics of priority setting (in the widest sense) matter as much as the methodologies used.[196]

Many will find this reassuring. A system in which health service managers, who have never seen the patient, became dominant in the decision about whether, and how, to provide treatment could not inspire confidence. Equally, given the developments that enable doctors to see more clearly the effectiveness of their decisions in both clinical and economic terms, neither should they expect their decision-making to be immune from review. But if this is right for clinicians, so it is for politicians and health service managers. What policies do they seek to achieve and what strategies have they adopted to do so? Of course, such a habit of dialogue will not produce radical change in the NHS. There will be a process of evolution rather than revolution. A standing commission, with these less ambitious objectives, could assist the development of realism and understanding in the system by tackling the most intractable problem in the health service: the balance between clinical and economic efficacy in the allocation of health resources.

---

194 *See* Katskee v. Blue Cross/Blue Shield, 515 N.W.2d 645 (1994) (whether a genetic predisposition to cancer is an illness, even before the condition becomes manifest).

195 *See* Albert G. Mulley & Kim A. Eagle, *What Is Inappropriate Care?*, 260 JAMA 540 (1988).

196 Rudolph Klein, *Dimensions of Rationing: Who Should Do What?*, 307 BRIT. MED. J. 309 (1993).

[19]

Health Care Rationing in the Courts: A Comparative Study

By TIMOTHY STOLTZFUS JOST

> The claim of the legally insured person against his insurer for medical treatment encompasses not just traditional medicine, but also the particular schools of alternative medicine. . . . This is in accordance with constitutional requirements. The obligatorily insured patient has a right of self determination for his medical treatment pursuant to the right of personality, in connection with the [constitutionally protected] right of bodily integrity. . . . With payment of his health insurance premiums, he has also gained a property-like right to comprehensive insurance protection.[1]

> The augmentative communication device the State will provide Fred C. will reportedly cost about six thousand penurious dollars. Mindful of the practical need to reduce medical costs, the Court nevertheless has before it no evidence that Texas Medicaid will now be required to fund untold numbers of ACDs . . . . The Court declines the invitation to reach the callous result of denying one forty-seven year old an augmentative communication device which would routinely be provided were he under the age of twenty-one.[2]

> I feel extremely sorry for the particular applicants in this case who have to wait a long time, not being emergency cases, for necessary sur-

---

* Newton D. Baker, Baker and Hostetler Chaired Professor, College of Law and Professor, College of Medicine and Public Health, The Ohio State University, Guest Professor, Universitaet Goettingen, 1996-97. The author wishes to thank Professor Dr. Erwin Deutsch, in whose institute much of this article was written, the Fulbright Foundation, which funded my research during 1996-97, and the DAAD, which funded earlier research on this topic in 1994. Numerous persons in Germany provided helpful information that contributed to this article, but the author would particularly like to thank Drs. Engelmann and Udsching of the German Supreme Social Court; Professors Ebsen, von Maydell, Heinze, Steinmeyer, Gitter, and Schulin; and Drs. Gerhard Brenner, Franz Knieps, and Dieter Barth for their help. David Hughes was very helpful with keeping me up to date with British developments. If I misunderstood anything my informants told me, the fault is all mine.

1. LSG Niedersachsen, 8/30/95, L 4 Kr. 11/95, 3 Breithaupt 1996, No. 42.

2. Fred C. v. Texas Health and Human Serv. Comm'n, 924 F. Supp. 788, 793 (W.D.Tex. 1996), *vacated by* 117 F.3d. 1416 (5th Cir. 1997).

gery. They share that misfortune with thousands up and down the country. I only hope that they have not been encouraged to think that these proceedings offered any real prospects that this court could enhance the standards of the National Health Service, because any such encouragement would be based upon manifest illusion.[3]

I. Introduction

This Article is a comparative study of the law's role in rationing health care in the United States, Germany, and Britain. More particularly, it examines the role of the courts and of other institutions through which these countries resolve disputes and protect rights in the context of health care resource allocation. It begins with a consideration of the role of law in health care relationships as a prologue to a discussion of law's role in resolving claims to health care resources. It next presents the problem of allocation of health care resources in the face of uncertainty and growing demands, and introduces the part law plays in this process. The focus then turns to the unique role of legal processes in each of the systems: the German social insurance system based on negotiated allocation of resources in a framework of legal obligations and rights; the British National Health Service, based on discretionary allocation of a fixed budget by payors and providers; the American public insurance system based on legal entitlements; and the American private insurance system based on contract with an ever more significant statutory overlay. It concludes with general reflections on the role of the courts and other dispute resolution mechanisms in health care resource allocation.

II. The Legal Dimension of Health Care Relationships

The relationships through which health care is provided and received have three important dimensions. Most obviously, perhaps, health care is delivered within professional relationships. One person, a professional, ministers to another person, a patient. The professional is entrusted with extensive authority over and responsibility for the patient, both on the basis of special education, training, and experience which allows the professional to understand and treat the patient's medical problems and because the ethical framework in which the professional operates is supposed to as-

3. R v. Secretary of State for Social Services, ex parte Hincks, 1 BMLR 93 (Ct. of App. 1980) (Opinion of Bridge, L.J.).

sure the professional's allegiance to the patient.[4] Traditionally the patient was, as the word indicates, the passive party in the relationship. The patient trusted and was ministered to.[5] In recent years the patient has become, at least in theory, a more active participant in the relationship. The patient is supposed to be educated regarding proposed interventions and their alternatives, and to consent to interventions before they occur.[6] The patient has more control over his life and over the timing of his death. In reality, however, in the context of the professional-patient relationship, the professional still is largely in control.[7]

Second, the relationships through which health care is provided are also economic.[8] The provider of health care is a merchant selling goods and services. The patient is a consumer. The patient, or the patient's insurer or employer, or the government, is a purchaser. Health care is a product provided in a market. Health care markets are governed by the laws of economics. Providers respond to incentives, providing more care when they are paid on a fee-for-service basis, and less when they are paid on a capitated or salary basis.[9] This has always been so, but we in the United States have become much more acutely aware of health care's economic aspect in recent years.[10] Other countries are also discovering this

---

4. *See* PAUL STARR, THE SOCIAL TRANSFORMATION OF AMERICAN MEDICINE, 4-17 (1982). Historically, health care institutions were also entrusted with the care of patients. They were sponsored by churches or by communities and supported by charitable contributions. They existed to provide a context in which professionals could provide care, not to make profit.

5. *See* Bradford H. Gray, *Trust and Trustworthy Care in the Managed Care Era*, 16 HEALTH AFF., Jan.-Feb. 1997, at 34, 35.

6. BARRY R. FURROW, ET AL., 1 HEALTH LAW §§ 6-9, 6-11 (1995) [hereinafter "1 HEALTH LAW"].

7. *Id.* at §§ 6-17, 6-19.

8. The literature on health economics is vast and rapidly growing. The classic source is Kenneth Arrow, *Uncertainty and Welfare Economics of Medical Care*, 53 AM. ECON. REV. 941 (1963).

9. *See* Alan Hillman, Mark Pauly, & Joseph Kerstein, *How do Financial Incentives Affect Physicians' Clinical Decisions and the Financial Performance of Health Maintenance Organizations*? 321 NEW ENG. J. MED. 86 (1989). Health care institutions are also driven by the profit motive: for-profit entities seek profits for their shareholders; non-profit entities strive for prestige and growth and make sure their managers and medical staff are well provisioned.

10. *See* STARR, *supra* note 4, at 420-36; *see*, among the many proposals for reforming health care, acknowledging its economic dimension, ALAIN C. ENTHOVEN, HEALTH PLAN (1990); Mark V. Pauly, et al., *Incremental Steps Toward Health System Reform*, HEALTH AFF., Spring 1995, at 125.

dimension of health care, although their responses to health care markets are very different from our own.[11]

In the market environment, the purchaser of services has considerable power. The purchaser is often not the consumer (the patient), however, but the consumer's employer, or an insurer, or the government.[12] The interests of the purchaser are independent of, and not always aligned with, those of the patient. While the sick patient may want every medical intervention that may be of benefit, for example, the insurer, who actually pays for medical care, must marshall its resources carefully to assure that all of its insureds can be served, its premiums remain competitive, and its managers and shareholders are well compensated.[13] Providers may be less powerful as sellers than they are as professionals, but they are far from powerless. They have a valuable commodity to sell, and often sell it under restricted market conditions where they are not exposed to the full force of competition.[14] Under some market structures, moreover, the consumer is also not powerless, although the consumer is often the weakest participant in health care markets.[15]

Health care provision relationships also exist, finally, in a third dimension—they are legal relationships. In every country, legislatures have adopted a complex web of statutes that establish the framework in which health care is delivered. These statutes, for example, govern the licensing of professionals and institutions, the financing and expenditures of social insurance or national health service programs, the funding of health care education and research, and the protection of public health.[16] In nations

11. *See, e.g.*, HEALTH CARE REFORM (Chris Ham, ed. 1997); LAURENE A. GRAIG, HEALTH OF NATIONS: AN INTERNATIONAL PERSPECTIVE ON U.S. HEALTH CARE REFORM (1993) (discussing health care reforms currently underway in other developed countries, including market-based reforms).

12. In 1995, 20.8% of personal health care expenditures were out-of-pocket. Private health insurance paid 31.5% of health expenditures, the government 44.6%. Katharine R. Levit, et al., *National Health Expenditures, 1995*, 18 HEALTH CARE FINANCING REV. 175, 205 (1996). During 1994, 85.5% of privately insured Americans were insured through employer-related coverage. *See* HEALTH INSURANCE ASSOCIATION OF AMERICA, SOURCE BOOK ON HEALTH INSURANCE DATA, 1996, 13 (1997) [hereinafter "HIAA"].

13. This conflict has been recognized by the federal courts in private health insurance coverage litigation in the United States. *See* cases cited *infra* at notes 411 through 417.

14. *See* OCCUPATIONAL LICENSURE AND REGULATION, 7-9 (Simon Rottenberg ed., 1980).

15. *See* ENTHOVEN, *supra* note 10, and Pauly et al., *supra* note 10, for proposals to empower consumers in health care markets.

16. *See Medical Law*, INTERNATIONAL ENCYCLOPEDIA OF LAW (Herman Nys, ed.) (national monographs discussing how these issues are addressed in various nations).

with federal government structures, such as the United States and Germany, health laws exist at both the national and state level, and interact with each other in complex ways. In some countries, constitutions cabin the discretion that lawmakers have for designing these systems.

Administrative agencies also play an active role in most health care systems, regulating professionals and institutions and managing public programs for health care purchasing and provision. Agencies issue rules and make adjudications that govern health care relationships. Finally, in most countries the courts also oversee health care relationships by reviewing and enforcing the decisions of administrative care agencies, interpreting and enforcing contracts, and protecting those who suffer tortious or criminal injury.[17]

It is not surprising that health care relationships have a legal dimension. Even the most private relationships, those within families, have a public, legal dimension. The extent and density of legal intervention in health care, however, is sufficiently remarkable to require explanation. The law intervenes in health care relationships because of deficiencies that exist in professional-patient or market relationships.[18] The courts are available to hear malpractice claims, for example, because professionals sometimes culpably harm rather than help patients. Licensing laws exist, at least in theory, because not all persons who would hold themselves out as professionals in fact meet minimal standards of competence and ethical conduct. Laws establish public health care financing programs because markets are only capable of making medical goods and services available to those who have money to exchange for those goods and services. Fraud and abuse laws penalize excessive and inappropriate responses of providers to the incentives offered by economic arrangements.

The legal structures through which diverse countries organize their health care systems vary greatly. They are products of different histories and different policy desiderata, and respond to different professional and

17. In many countries, including the United States, quasi-public entities exercise delegated power in governing or resolving disputes in health care relationships. The Joint Commission for Accreditation of Healthcare Organizations, for example, is one of the most important regulatory agencies in the American health care system, while the German *Krankenkassen* and *Kassenärztliche Vereinigungen*, although technically not government agencies, run the statutory health insurance system.

18. *See* Timothy S. Jost, *Oversight of the Quality of Medical Care: Regulation, Management, or the Market?*, 37 ARIZ. L. REV. 825 (1995); Timothy S. Jost, *The Necessary and Proper Role of Regulation to Assure the Quality of Health Care*, 25 HOUS. L. REV. 525 (1988). Alternatively, laws exist because those who lack power in professional-patient relationships or economic relationships sometimes possess political power or are able to appeal to a court or agency's sense of justice.

economic arrangements. Nevertheless, legal institutions in various countries are more or less comparable; the problems and issues they address in health care are in many respects similar, and the legal structures and techniques nations have developed for addressing these problems and issues share regular patterns. Cross-national comparative analysis of legal structures in health care is both possible and instructive.

Among the most important functions that law serves in societies generally are resolution of disputes and articulation and protection of the rights of individuals. These functions are of course closely related, as disputes involve conflicting assertions of rights. In most countries courts are primarily responsible for these functions. It is the task of courts to attend to particular disputes, while legislatures and rulemaking bodies concern themselves with policymaking in general.[19] However, other fora, such as administrative courts or arbitration or mediation panels, also play an important role in some nations in dealing with particular disputes. This Article focuses in particular on the role of courts and alternative dispute resolution mechanisms in health care systems. More specifically, it focuses on the part these institutions play in resolving disputes regarding resource allocation.

III. Law and the Allocation of Health Care Resources

One of the most important tasks facing modern health care systems is resource allocation. Health care resources must be allocated within health care systems in a context of scarcity and uncertainty. Health care resources are allocated through both professional and economic decisions. But the results reached through these mechanisms often cause disputes. These disputes are frequently resolved through legal institutions, and through the courts in particular.

By definition, all valuable resources are scarce, but awareness of scarcity in health care has become more acute in recent years as the demand for health care has increased. The proportion of national wealth that most developed nations spend on health care has increased in the past two decades.[20]

The most important factor driving health care cost increases throughout the world, and particularly in the United States, is the continual prog-

19. *See* Lon Fuller, *The Forms and Limits of Adjudication*, 92 HARV. L. REV. 353 (1978).

20. George J. Schieber, Jean-Pierre Poullier, & Leslie M. Greenwald, *Health System Performance in OECD Countries*, 1980-1992, 13 HEALTH AFF., Fall 1994, at 100, 101.

ress of medical technology.[21] Health care is very labor intensive, often demanding expensive, skilled labor. Unlike other industries, capital investment and technological development rarely result in substantial savings of labor costs in the health care industry. The demand for health care technology is likely to continue to increase.

Another important factor inexorably driving the increase in the demand for medical care in the long run is the aging of the population. In developed countries, two trends are simultaneously increasing the average age of the population: people are living longer, and the birth rate is declining; thus at any one time there are more older people and fewer younger people.[22] Assuming that most persons require periodic medical care, a longer life means a greater aggregate need for medical care. The chronic and degenerative conditions that accompany old age also result often in a greater need for medical care later in life, including in many instances the need for long term nursing care. Death is itself expensive, especially if it is repeatedly staved off. Moreover, the aging of the population not only increases the cost of a health care system, but also decreases its income, because older persons are less likely to be paying social insurance premiums or taxes to finance the services that they consume in ever-increasing volume. This inevitably leads to an imbalance of payments and income in social insurance funds or national health services, and to increased premium or tax levels.

Finally, other factors also contribute to health care cost increases. Administrative costs in health care are high and continually growing. Waste and abuse are costly and difficult to control.[23] For all of these reasons, demand for resources in health care is likely to continue to increase.

There seem to be limits, however, to the extent to which developed nations are willing to dedicate resources to health care. Virtually every

---

21. Joseph P. Newhouse, *An Iconoclastic View of Health Care Cost Containment*, 12 HEALTH AFF., Supp. 1993, at 152; Einer Elhauge, *The Limited Regulatory Potential of Medical Technology Assessment*, 82 VA. L. REV. 1525 (1996).

22. *See Gesundheitswesen in Deutschland, Kostenfaktor und Zukunftsbranche*, *in* SACHVERSTÄNDIGENRAT FÜR DIE KONZERTIERTE AKTION IM GESUNDHEITSWESEN (Sondergutachten ed., Nomos Verlagsgesellschaft, 1996). Aging of the population is a less important factor in explaining health care cost growth in the United States, but as the baby-boom generation reaches retirement age in the early twenty-first century, it is likely to become a more significant factor. Daniel N. Mendelson and William B. Schwartz, *The Effects of Aging and Population Growth on Health Care Costs*, 12 HEALTH AFF., Spring 1993, at 119.

23. *See* Jerry L. Mashaw & Theodore R. Marmor, *Conceptualizing, Estimating, and Reforming Fraud, Waste, and Abuse in Healthcare Spending*, 11 YALE J. REG. 456 (1994).

developed nation is currently engaged in a more or less urgent debate regarding "health care reform," i.e., how to control the escalating costs of health care.[24] Inevitably this discussion turns to how to allocate increasingly constrained resources within health care systems.

For the past two generations, scarce resources have been allocated both to and within health care systems on the basis of professional judgment.[25] Health care professionals, and in particular physicians, have determined, on the basis of their professional training and experience, what diagnostic and treatment modalities would benefit their patients. In the era of fee-for-service medicine, which existed both in the United States and Germany until the recent past, the decision of a physician that a patient required a service usually meant that the service would be provided. Even British National Health Service resource allocation decisions, within the context of the national health budget, were until recently largely controlled by professionals.[26]

These decisions regarding allocation of scarce health care resources, however, have been and continue to be made in a context of uncertainty. Though medicine is scientifically based, many medical procedures are not scientifically validated. There are significant variations in the use of medical procedures from country to country and from community to community within countries.[27] Even the way in which diseases are conceptualized varies from country to country.[28] Although outcomes studies are being pursued and practice guidelines formulated to reduce this variation, they still leave much of the territory of professional practice uncovered, and can offer only statistical probabilities, not specify what care is appropriate in particular cases.[29] Professional judgments regarding resource al-

24. *See* sources cited *supra* note 11.

25. *See* Elhauge, *supra* note 21, at 1536-47; Clark C. Havighurst & James F. Blumstein, *Coping with Quality/Cost Trade-Offs in Medical Care: The Role of PSROs*, 70 NW. L. REV. 6, 25-30 (1975).

26. S. Harrison, *A Policy Agenda for Health Care Rationing, in* RATIONING HEALTH CARE 885, 889 (R.J. Maxwell, ed. 1995).

27. LYNN PAYER, MEDICINE & CULTURE: VARIETIES OF TREATMENT IN THE UNITED STATES, ENGLAND, GERMANY, AND FRANCE (1988); John E. Wennberg, *Dealing with Medical Practice Variations: A Proposal for Action*, 3 HEALTH AFF., Summer 1984, at 6, 9.

28. *See* PAYER, *supra* note 27.

29. Arnold M. Epstein, *The Outcomes Movement-Will it Get us Where we Want to go?*, 323 NEW ENG. J. MED. 266 (1990); David M. Eddy & John Billings, *The Quality of Medical Evidence: Implications for Quality of Care*, HEALTH AFF., Spring 1988, at 19. *See also* Sandra J. Tanenbaum, *Knowing and Acting in Medical Practice: The Epistemological Politics of Outcomes Research*, 19 J. HEALTH POL., POL'Y & L. 27 (1994) (noting that doctors do not think in terms of statistical probabilities in making decisions).

location do not, therefore, reach predictable or even consistent results. Professional judgment as the basis of resource allocation tends to benefit some patients, but slights the needs of others.[30] Perhaps more importantly, professional judgments also err on the side of providing more, rather than fewer, procedures, as there is virtually no limit to the resources that can be allocated to health care with some beneficial effect.[31] In the end, therefore, professional judgment must be supplemented, limited, and directed by other forms of decision-making that serve other ends.

Decisions allocating health care resources allocation are also, and ever more prominently, economic decisions. In most sectors of the economy, innumerable individual purchasing decisions determine the ultimate allocation of resources. These purchasers, applying their own value calculations, make discrete purchases, which in aggregate determine resource allocation within an economy. Uncertainty as to value is, therefore, a problem for individuals, not for society. It has long been believed, however, that individual purchasing decisions also have their limits as a resource allocation tool in health care markets.[32] For this reason, markets have traditionally played only a limited role in health care resource allocation.

For market forces to work, purchasers must be relatively well informed. They must be able to evaluate the capacity of the product to meet their needs and to weigh comparatively a range of products with differing prices and values. Most consumers have a limited ability to judge their need for medical care and an even more limited capacity for evaluating

---

30. A fascinating example of this is the waiting lists of the national health service. It is well known that in Britain scarce health resources are allocated by the assignment of patients to waiting lists through professional judgment. Year after year, however, these waiting lists tend to limited to patients with "varicose veins, hernias, painful or immobile joints, cataracts and enlarged tonsils, or they are women awaiting sterilization." STEPHEN FRANKEL AND ROBERT WEST, RATIONING AND RATIONALITY IN THE NATIONAL HEALTH SERVICE: THE PERSISTENCE OF WAITING LISTS 6 (1993). What these conditions have in common is that they are of little interest to doctors—the procedures that address them are routine, boring, and have little research potential. *Id.* at 7-12. They are thus continually shoved behind more glamorous and interesting conditions and procedures. *See also* David Hughes & Lesley Griffiths, *"Ruling in" and "Ruling Out": Two Approaches to the Micro-Rationing of Health Care*, 44 SOC. SCI. MED. 359 (1997) (describing doctor's decision-making behavior in deciding who gets cardiac surgery or neurological rehabilitation services in British NHS units.)

31. *See* Elhauge, *supra* note 21, at 1547.

32. *See* CONGRESSIONAL BUDGET OFFICE, ECONOMIC IMPLICATIONS OF RISING HEALTH CARE COSTS (1992) [hereinafter "CBO"] (discussing basic failures in health care markets.)

particular medical goods and services.[33] Not only, as noted above, are objective standards often lacking to this end, but even the standards that exist are not readily understandable by consumers. In fact, consumers have traditionally depended on providers, especially physicians, to act as agents in advising them what and how much medical care they need.[34] It is only to be expected, however, that permitting suppliers to direct purchasing decisions will result in excess demand. An additional obstacle to relying on the decisions of individual consumers to reach an efficient allocation of health care resources is the prevalence of health insurance.[35] Individual instances of the use of medical care are often very expensive, and are uncertain in frequency and extent. The high cost of medical care makes it difficult for most persons to pay for anything other than routine health care out of current income.[36] Moreover, most persons are risk averse, and are willing to pay sizable insurance premiums to avoid the uncertain risk of catastrophic liability for medical care costs. Further, most nations have concluded that individual health is a benefit to the state and that because poor health is a risk to which all are exposed, its costs should be borne by all.[37] Thus, in all developed countries, health care is to a greater or lesser degree financed by society or by the state. For all of these reasons, medical care tends in most countries to be covered by insurance, either social insurance provided by the community or by commercial insurance.

Insurance, however, permits individuals to obtain health care at less than market cost (often without cost altogether). This results in moral hazard: insureds obtain health care of questionable value, that they would probably not purchase themselves at full cost, because the care is essentially free.[38] But it is not free, of course. All insureds must collectively

33. *Id.* at 13.

34. *Id.* at 13-14.

35. *Id.* at 17-18.

36. The uncertain occurrence and tremendous and unpredictable variation of medical care costs make financing through individual savings problematic. In 1996 and 1997, Congress adopted legislation encouraging experimentation with medical savings accounts (MSAs) to stimulate market competition in health care by encouraging consumers to pay for health care out of special savings accounts. Whether MSAs in fact will result in a reduction of medical costs, however, is strongly contested. Compare Pauly, *supra* note 10, with J. SHIELS, ET AL., CHANGES IN MEDICARE PROGRAM SPENDING UNDER ALTERNATIVE MEDICAL SAVINGS ACCOUNT MODELS (1995). Debt financing of health care, though common in the United States, puts providers at high risk, particularly when they provide care for the elderly.

37. DIANE LONGLEY, HEALTH CARE CONSTITUTIONS 1 (1996).

38. *See* Arrow, *supra* note 8 at 961-62; CBO, *supra* note 32 at 17-18. Insured persons face incentives to use more health care than they actually "need" either because they do not understand how to use health care appropriately or because the insured may derive

pay for it. The availability of insurance also lowers the cost to the individual of non-compliance with treatment requirements, again often imposing costs on the community. On the provider side, insurance encourages professionals to expand the demand for their services—to resolve uncertainty in favor of action—particularly where insurance pays the provider on a per-service basis.[39] Where insurance pays on a charge or cost basis (as was formerly often the case in many countries) not only the volume of services, but also the price of services expands continually.[40] In sum, the prevalence of insurance builds on the other market failures already present to weaken the incentives that individual consumers face for limiting their own demand for services, while at the same time creating incentives for providers to encourage increased demand for health care resources.

The limited ability of individual consumers to assure the efficient use of health care resources is only one problem with relying on markets to allocate resources in health care.[41] Another problem is that markets cannot, without more, reach an equitable allocation of health care resources. Markets require purchasers with purchasing power. Insured consumers have such power (within the limits of their insurance policies), but in most countries a significant proportion of the population lacks the money that would be needed to pay the full premiums of insurance out of their own funds. In the United States, for example, nineteen percent of the adult population currently lack health insurance, and most of these are not insured because they cannot afford it.[42] All developed countries, therefore, have created either social insurance systems or national health insurance systems to assure equitable access to health care. In the United States, over one quarter of the population are covered by public health insurance programs.[43]

an advantage from the medical service beyond its actual benefit for improving health (such as paid release from work, gratification of a drug dependency, satisfaction of an abnormal psychiatric need for medical treatment, for example).

39. Havighurst & Blumstein, *supra* note 25, at 27-28.

40. PHYSICIAN PAYMENT REVIEW COMMISSION, REPORT TO CONGRESS: MEDICARE PHYSICIAN PAYMENT REFORM: AN AGENDA FOR ACTION 26-28 (1987) [hereinafter "PPRC"].

41. *See*, discussing other concerns regarding market-based approaches to reforming health care delivery and finance, Thomas Rice, *Can Markets Give us the Health System we Want?*, 22 J. HEALTH POL., POL'Y & L. 383 (1997); Robert G. Evans, *Going for the Gold: The Redistributive Agenda behind Market-Based Health Care Reform*, 22 J. HEALTH POL., POL'Y & L. 427 (1997).

42. Karen Donelan, et al., *Whatever Happened to the Health Insurance Crisis in the United States*, 276 JAMA 1346 (1996).

43. HIAA, *supra* note 12, at 13.

Even if we cannot, in the end, rely totally on the decisions of individual consumers to allocate resources in health care, markets nonetheless play a key and ever more important role in resource allocation. As noted earlier, the real purchasers of health care are often not patients, but employers who purchase health insurance and insurers, managed care organizations, or health benefit plan administrators who purchase health services. These purchasers are increasingly aware of their market power and increasingly savvy in bringing it to bear on resource allocation decisions.[44] The interests of purchasers, however, are not necessarily congruent with the interests of consumers (patients), on the one hand, and are often contrary to the interests of providers, on the other. Economic resource allocation decision-making, therefore, often result in conflicts that must be resolved through other means.[45]

In developed nations, professional judgment and economic decisions interact in complex ways to yield health care resource allocation decisions. Many actors play a role in resolving uncertainty in health care. First, and most obviously, individual professionals continue constantly to make decisions as to the appropriateness and necessity of the use of health care resources in particular situations, based of course on professional judgment, but also with an eye to economic limitations and incentives. Second, health care institutions make resource allocation decisions, both by deciding how to allocate resources among particular types of equipment or facilities, and, in many countries, by allocating resources among particular patients.[46] Again, these decisions are influenced both by economic concerns and by pressure from the professionals that practice within the institutions. Third, purchasers and insurance administrators make resource allocation decisions.[47] In the United States, for example, employers that

44. *See, e.g.*, PHYSICIAN PAYMENT REVIEW COMMISSION, ARRANGEMENTS BETWEEN MANAGED CARE PLANS AND PHYSICIANS (1995) (describing arrangements through which managed care organizations purchase services from physicians); Elizabeth W. Hoy, et al., *A Guide to Facilitating Consumer Choice*, 15 HEALTH AFF., Winter 1996, at 9 (describing health care purchasing arrangements of major corporations).

45. *See, e.g.*, discussing conflict resolution issues in managed care, Eleanor D. Kinney, *Resolving Consumer Grievances in a Managed Care Environment*, 6 HEALTH MATRIX 147 (1996); Marc A. Rodwin, *Managed Care and Consumer Protection: What are the Issues?*, 26 SETON HALL L. REV. 1007 (1996).

46. This is obviously true in public health systems such as the British National Health Service, but is also true in the United States as well. *See* ANSELM STRAUSS, ET AL., SOCIAL ORGANIZATION OF MEDICAL WORK 189 (1985) (describing resource allocation processes in American health care institutions).

47. *See* Emily Friedman, *Managed Care, Rationing and Quality: A Tangled Relationship*, 16 HEALTH AFF., May-June 1997, at 174.

provide health insurance as an employment benefit negotiate policy coverage with health insurers and managed care organizations.[48] In most countries, governments are major purchasers of health care services, and make resource allocation decisions accordingly. In Britain, District Health Authorities and Fundholding General Practices establish resource allocation priorities by negotiating coverage contracts with hospitals.[49]

Governments also make resource allocation decisions, however, in their role as legislators, administrators, and adjudicators. That is to say, law also plays a major role in resource allocation decisions. The serious limitations of both professional judgment and economic decision-making necessitate the existence of legal frameworks to address and protect concerns otherwise slighted.

One of the most important functions of governments in the resource allocation context is to address the disputes that inevitably arise when resource allocation decisions are made by professionals or purchasers. Insurers deny coverage for services that patients desire or deny payment for services that doctors have provided. Hospitals lack facilities that some patients consider essential. Government national health services fail to provide services that patients believe they need. In these circumstances, claims often end up before courts. In some countries, other fora are also available to consider these disputes. How these courts and other fora respond to these disputes in three different countries is the focus of concern in this Article. Before we turn to the details, however, we will first briefly describe the health care systems of the countries we will study.

IV. National Models for Financing Health Care

The countries we will consider represent the three major models of health care financing found in developed nations. Historically, the earliest model is the social insurance model, exemplified here by the German health insurance system.[50] Under this model, employers and employees are required to pay premiums (payroll taxes) to statutory insurance funds, which in turn pay for medical care. By this means, more or less universal insurance coverage is extended to employees and to related groups, such as

48. *See* Gail A. Jensen, et al., *The New Dominance of Managed Care: Insurance Trends in the 1990s*, 16 HEALTH AFF., Jan.-Feb. 1997, at 125 (describing employers arrangements with insurers and managed care plans).

49. *See* JOHN ØVRETVEIT, PURCHASING FOR HEALTH (1995).

50. *See generally* RICHARD KNOX, GERMANY'S HEALTH SYSTEM: ONE NATION, UNITED WITH HEALTH CARE FOR ALL (1993); John K. Iglehart, *Health Policy Report: Germany's Health Care System*, 324 N. ENG. J. MED. 503, 1750 (1991).

employees' dependents and former employees who are now retired, disabled, or unemployed.[51] Framework laws normally guide social insurance programs by defining program coverage and regulating payments to providers. This Article examines, as exemplars of legal approaches to conflict resolution within social insurance systems, four of the most common types of disputes that arise within the German health care system: disputes involving the coverage of medical equipment,[52] disputes involving coverage of alternative (complementary) medicine,[53] disputes involving utilization review of the services provided by individual physicians,[54] and disputes involving the fixing of budgets for physician and hospital services.[55]

A second possibility is provision of tax-financed medical care by the state, exemplified here first by the British National Health Service.[56] Direct provision could be accomplished through government ownership of health care facilities and employment of health care professionals. This is not necessary, however, and in tax-financed systems a mixture of public and private provision often exists.[57] The direct payment model commonly involves the state most intensely in direction of the payment and provision of medical care. This Article will consider resolution of coverage disputes involving individual patients and institutional providers in the National Health Service.[58]

This article also examines coverage disputes in the American Medicare and Medicaid programs as further examples of public health care financing.[59] Medicare resembles closely European social insurance systems, while Medicaid is a tax-financed system. These programs are unlike both

---

51. *See* Eckhard Bloch, *Kreis der versicherten Personen, in* HANDBUCH DES SOZIALVERSICHERUNGSRECHTS, BAND 1, KRANKENVERSICHERUNGSRECHT 485 (Bertram Schulin ed., 1994) (describing covered groups) [hereinafter "HANDBUCH SVR"].

52. *See infra* text accompanying notes 108-29.

53. *See infra* text accompanying notes 130-60.

54. *See infra* text accompanying notes 161-219.

55. *See infra* text accompanying notes 220-44.

56. Although this Article refers throughout to the British National Health Service, there are some differences in administration of the NHS between England and the rest of Britain, and, where these exist, we describe the English variant. *See*, describing the NHS, JUDITH ALLSOP, HEALTH POLICY AND THE NHS TOWARDS 2000 (2d ed. 1995); CHRISTOPHER HAM, HEALTH POLICY IN BRITAIN (3rd ed. 1992).

57. In Britain, for example, the NHS is financed from central tax revenues, purchasing decisions are made at the district level by government health authorities, secondary and tertiary care are provided by non-profit "NHS trusts," and primary care is delivered by private general practitioners who contract with the government.

58. *See infra* text accompanying notes 261-84.

59. *See infra* text accompanying notes 287-380.

the German and British systems, however, in that coverage is an entitlement, not limited by a budget. This affects the nature of coverage disputes.

The third approach considered here is commercial or private health insurance. Private health insurance is available in virtually all developed nations. However, few nations (most notably the United States), rely on commercial insurance as a primary means of providing health care for the population generally. While commercial insurance exists technically by virtue of private arrangements, the relationships between insurers, insureds, and providers (including, under some circumstances, premium rates) are usually regulated by the government and commercial insurance is in some countries tax subsidized.[60] This Article examines one of the most common contexts in which commercial insurance disputes come before legal tribunals: the resolution of coverage disputes involving private health insurers in the United States, focusing in particular on disputes regarding the necessity or experimental nature of treatment.[61]

V. Germany: Social Courts and Arbitration Panels

The German health insurance program is an employment-based social insurance system. When Bismarck originated the system in the nineteenth century, its goal was to provide support for sick workers.[62] Over the past century, however, the system has evolved into a comprehensive health insurance program, financing not only the health care needs of workers, but also of their dependents and of formerly employed persons, be they retired, disabled, or simply unemployed. All workers who earn less than DM 72,000 per year in the former western zone or DM 61,200 per year in the former eastern zone (1996 figures) are legally obligated to be insured.[63] About eighty-eight percent of the population is currently enrolled in the social insurance system, seventy-five percent being mandatory enrollees

60. In 1995, employer-provided health benefits were subsidized in the United States to the extent of $90 billion. Alain C. Enthoven & Sara J. Singer, *Market-Based Reform: What to Regulate and by Whom*, HEALTH AFF., Spring 1995, at 105.

61. *See infra* text accompanying notes 381-435.

62. Iglehart, *supra* note 50, at 504-05; PETER ROSENBERG, THE ORIGIN AND DEVELOPMENT OF COMPULSORY HEALTH INSURANCE IN GERMANY, IN POLITICAL VALUES AND HEALTH CARE: THE GERMAN EXPERIENCE 105 (Donald W. Light and Alexander Schuller, eds. 1986).

63. Reinhard Busse, et al., *The Future Development of a Rights Based Approach to Health Care in Germany: More Rights or Fewer?* in HARD CHOICES IN HEALTH CARE, 21, 26 (Jo Lenaghan, ed. 1997).

and their families and thirteen percent voluntary enrollees.[64] Nearly nine percent of the population is covered by private health insurance and two percent by government programs, and less than one percent are uninsured.[65] Health insurance premiums for employees are paid half by the worker and half by the employer.[66]

The health insurance program is administered by self-governing, quasi-public, non-profit health insurance funds (*Krankenkassen*, here referred to as KKn, or KK in the singular). There are several hundred KKn, some of which are firm-specific (similar to our self-insured ERISA plans), some occupation-specific (such as special funds for craft-workers, miners, sailors, farmers), and some specific to particular geographic areas.[67] Historically Germans had only a limited ability to choose among these funds, but as of 1996, they have virtually unlimited freedom to choose among available insurers.[68] The populations insured by the various funds still vary significantly in terms of their age, income, and health status. Although Germany instituted a risk adjustment scheme several years ago to transfer income among the funds to compensate for this variance, premiums still vary from fund to fund.[69] The funds are organized at the state and federal level into associations.

Providers are also organized in corporate bodies. In particular, all doctors who provide services to members of the sickness funds are members of their state *Kassenärztliche Vereinigung* (KaV, plural KaVn), the union of insurance doctors,[70] and all dentists are organized into the *Kassenzahnärzliche Vereinigung* (KzV).[71] The hospitals are also organized at

64. Friedrich Schwartz and Reinhard Busse, *Fixed Budgets in the Ambulatory Sector: the German Experience*, *in* FIXING HEALTH BUDGETS, 93, 95 (Friedrich Schwartz, et al. eds., 1996) [hereinafter, "Fixing Health Budgets"].

65. BUNDESMINISTERIUM FÜR GESUNDHEIT, DATEN DES GESUNDHEITSWESENS, 1995, 278.

66. § 249(1) SGB V (Sozialgesetzbuch chapter 5).

67. Busse, et al., *supra* note 63, at 26.

68. § 173 SGB V.

69. Busse, et al., *supra* note 63, at 27; *see*, describing the German risk adjustment system, Ashley Files & Margaret Murray, *German Risk Structure Compensation: Enhancing Equity and Effectiveness*, 32 INQUIRY 300 (1995). During the first 6 months of 1996, DM 10.4 billion was transferred through the risk adjustment mechanism, mainly from the white collar insurance funds to the local, blue-collar, funds. *See* H. Korzilius, *Risikostrukturausgleich behindert Wettbewerb*, 93 DEUTSCHES ÄRZTEBLATT A-2440 (1996).

70. §§ 77, 95 SGB V.

71. § 77 SGB V.

the state and national level.[72] The genius of the German system is that resources for health care are allocated through the means of negotiations between these corporate entities representing providers on the one side, and the KKn, their organizational entities on the other, within a statutory framework but without direct government intervention.

Three principles are at the base of German coverage and payment policy. The first is a principle of comprehensiveness: the insurance system covers a comprehensive list of preventive and curative health care services, described below. The second is the *Sachleistungsgrundsatz*, or principle of direct payment of providers by the KKn or by the provider corporate organizations which are in turn paid directly by the KKn.[73] Until a 1997 amendment to the law, which is now being implemented, patients treated by a doctor received no information as to what services the doctor had billed for or how much he had billed. The level of these direct payments are established through negotiations between the corporate organizations and the KKn.[74] These negotiations take place in the context of the third principle, *Beitragsstabilität*, or premium stability.[75] Health insurance premiums are not supposed to rise faster than the incomes on which they are based. Payments to providers, therefore, should not be more generous than those that can be funded through stable premiums.

The German system of paying for health care is a result of the interaction of these principles. The principle of direct payment makes possible the use of budgets. For the major sectors of health care (ambulatory physician care, hospital care, drugs, and dental care), resources are allocated through budgets between representatives of the health insurance funds and representatives of the providers. The regional KaVn, for example, have, for the past twenty years, annually negotiated budgets with the sickness funds for funding all physicians' services within the region. At first these budgets were voluntary, and then from 1989 until 1997 they were mandatory.[76] The budgets are negotiated with reference to the principle of premium stability, within guidelines established by the Concerted Action in

72. § 108a SGB V. This provision was added by the second *Neuordnunggesetz* of 1997. Prior to that time the hospital associations were private and had no legal status.

73. §2(2) SGB V. This principle is not absolute however, and various exceptions are provided for indemnification. *See Rechtliche Grundprinzipien der gesetzlichen Krankenversicherung und ihre Probleme*, *in* HANDBUCH SVR, *supra* note 51, at 177, 211-24.

74. *See, e.g.*, describing this process with respect to physician payment, Schwartz & Busse, *supra* note 64.

75. §§ 71, 141(2) SGB V.

76. Schwartz & Busse, *supra* note 64, at 96-100.

Health Care organization, an organization representing all of the major interest groups in health care, established to guide these negotiations.[77]

The KaVn pay doctors from these budgets on a fee-for-service basis based on a national relative value scale, the *Einheitlicher Berwertungsmaßstab für ärztliche Leistungen* (EBM), which assigns a point value to each procedure.[78] The weight of points for particular services or specialties is further modified by each regional KaV using its own *Honorverteilungsmaßstab* (HVM) to reach a total quarterly point value for each member physician.[79] These point numbers are summed to yield a total number of points for all services billed during the quarter by all physicians, which is then divided into the quarterly budget to yield a point value.[80] This point value is then multiplied by the number of points billed by each doctor to determine the amount each particular doctor is paid. Under the EBM implemented in 1996, payments are also limited on a per patient basis by what are known as *praxisbudgets*, subject to a variety of exceptions.[81]

Hospitals are also paid on a negotiated basis. The operating costs of German hospitals have in recent years also been financed through budgets negotiated with the KKn, while the capital costs have been financed by the states.[82] Operating costs are funded in part through diagnosis-determined

77. *Id.* at 97; § 87 SGB V.

78. Winfried Funk, *Vertragarztrecht*, *in* HANDBUCH SVR, *supra* note 51, at 852, 888-90. Traditionally the EBM was further modified under the *Bewertungmaßstab für ärztliche Leistungen* (BMÄ) for the primary sickness insurance funds, which essentially covered blue collar workers, and the *Ersatzkassen Gebührordnung* (E-GO) for the substitute funds, which provided somewhat more generous payments for the coverage of white collar workers. Reimbursement is now essentially identical for both types of insurance.

79. *Id.* at 892. Each regional KaV establishes its own HVM for dividing up its own budget, and in some regions separate sub-budgets are established for various specialties, resulting in different specialists receiving more or less per point billed than others. *See* GÜNTHER SCHNEIDER, HANDBUCH DES KASSENARZTRECHTS 435-41 (1994).

80. Klaus-Dirk Henke, et al., *Global Budgeting in Germany: Lessons for the United States*, HEALTH AFF., Fall 1994, at 7-21. In the recent past, moreover, attempts have been made to improve compensation for primary care physicians and to decrease payment for technical services. There has also been a movement toward grouping some services, which are billed together for a lump sum.

81. *See* Thomas Ballast, *Mengenbegrenzung im EBM: Praxisbudgets*, DIE ERSATZKASSE, Dec. 1996, at 440.

82. A brief English description of the program is found in U.S. GENERAL ACCOUNTING OFFICE, 1993 GERMAN HEALTH REFORMS 32-34, 45-46 (1993). For an exhaustive description of the system, *see* KARL HEINZ TUSCHEN & MICHAEL QUAAS, BUNDESPFLEGESATZVERORDNUNG: KOMMENTAR MIT EINER UMFASSENDEN EINFÜHRUNG IN DAS RECHT DER KRANKENHAUSFINANZIERUNG (3. Auflage 1996).

per-case (*Fallpauschal*) and procedure-specific (*Sonderentgelt*) payments.[83] The classification scheme for these payments is established through negotiations between the hospitals and regional KKn at the national level, while the payment level is based on KKn/hospital association negotiations.[84] Hospital expenses for patients not covered by the case or procedure specific payments, and other expenses, are covered by flexible budgets negotiated between the individual hospitals and the KKn.[85] When negotiations are unsuccessful in establishing budgets, disputes are often submitted to arbitration panels, known as *Schiedsstellen*, discussed below.

The German health insurance system is actively supervised by a system of special courts, the *Sozialgerichte*, or social courts. Individual disputes regarding coverage of services or payment of providers and arbitration panel decisions are often appealed to the social courts.[86] Sixty-nine social courts of the first instance, which hear social insurance disputes, exist throughout Germany.[87] Appeals from decisions of these disputes are made to the *Landessozialgerichte*, which exist in each of the sixteen German states.[88] In some instances, appeals from the *Landessozialgerichte* can be taken to the *Bundessozialgericht* (BSG), which sits in Kassell.[89] In 1996, 131 of the 775 appeals resolved by the BSG involved sickness insurance claims, and another ninety-eight involved the claims of insurance doctors, making health insurance issues the second largest category of cases decided by the BSG after pension cases.[90] Germany is a civil law country, and court decisions do not have precisely the same precedential weight and effect that they have in the United States. Nevertheless, the decisions of the social courts, and of the BSG in particular, are taken very se-

83. *See* TUSCHEN & QUAAS, *supra* note 82, at 72.

84. *Id.*

85. *Id.* at 73-75.

86. *See* Peter Kummer, *Das sozialgerichtliche Verfahren*, *in* SOCIALRECHTSHANDBURCH 603 (Bernd Baron von Maydell and Franz Ruland eds., 1996). Germany has a number of systems of special courts, in addition to its general jurisdiction civil and criminal courts (headed by the *Bundesgerichtshof*) and its constitutional court (the *Bundesverfassungsgericht*). These courts have jurisdiction over tax law, employment law, administrative law and social law. *See* GESCHÄFTSVERTEILUNGSPLAN DES BUNDESSOZIALGERICHTS FÜR DAS JAHR 1997, *reprinted in* 50 NEUE JURISTICHE WOCHENSCHRIFT [NJW] 35* (1997).

87. Kummer, *supra* note 86, at 609-11.

88. *Id.* at 611-13.

89. *Id.* at 613-15.

90. DIE TÄTIGKEIT DES BUNDESSOZIALGERICHTS IM JAHRE 1996: EINE ÜBERSICHT 29 (Bundessozialgericht ed., 1997).

riously and play a major role in defining the contours and boundaries of German health insurance law.

Panels of judges preside over the social courts. In the courts of the first instance there are usually three judges, a professional judge and two lay judges.[91] In disputes regarding insurance coverage, one of the lay judges represents insureds, and the other represents the employers.[92] In matters concerning the relationship between health insurance companies and insurance doctors, one of the lay judges represents the insurance companies, the other the doctors; in matters concerning the internal relationships of insurance doctors, both represent the doctors.[93] At the state and national social court level, the panel consists of three professional judges and two lay judges.[94] The BSG is divided into a number of panels of judges, called senates, each of which has jurisdiction over a particular body of cases. The Sixth Senate, for example, hears disputes involving insurance doctors.

The courts hold oral proceedings in which the parties are often, though not always, represented by attorneys. The judges take an active role in the proceedings, interrogating the parties and their attorneys. They have, in fact, an obligation to investigate the facts thoroughly, and to assist the parties in effectively presenting their cases.[95] Access to the social courts has traditionally been free (though public law entities such as insurance companies must pay a fee), and the victorious claimant has the possibility of receiving his litigation costs from the losing insurance company.[96] Disputes involving social insurance programs end up, therefore, in court with great frequency.[97]

In general, the social courts have been very receptive to the claims of insureds and providers. Benefit coverage claims, however, only come before the courts in marginal cases. As noted above, the KKn are required by law to offer a comprehensive range of services. Social Insurance is governed by *Sozialgesetzbuch* V (the fifth Social Law Book, abbreviated SGB V). Section 2 SGB V requires the Social Insurance Funds to make avail-

91. § 12(1) SGG (*Sozialgerichtgesetz*).

92. SGG § 12(2).

93. SGG § 12(3).

94. SGG §§ 33, 40.

95. Kummer, *supra* note 86, at 657-59.

96. *Id.* at 695-700.

97. During 1994, 178,636 complaints were filed in the social courts of the first instance, 17,954 appeals filed in the *Landessozialgerichten*, and 713 appeals and 1511 requests to file an appeal were filed in the BSG. Kummer, *supra* note 86, at 611, 612, 615. Only a minority of these, of course, were health insurance cases.

able to their insureds (usually through direct arrangements with providers) the services listed in chapter 3 of SGB V.[98] The first section of chapter 3[99] specifies as covered under the insurance program services for the prevention, early diagnosis, and treatment, as well as rehabilitation services needed to prevent or reduce a handicap or need for nursing care. The chapter goes on to identify specifically medical care, dental care, medications, dressings, various therapists and treatments, medical devices, hospital care, and rehabilitation or occupational therapy as covered services for the treatment of illness.[100] The statute imposes a general limitation that services must be necessary and economically provided and must correspond with the general state of medical knowledge and attend to medical progress.[101] Additional sections impose a host of limitations on particular procedures, including cost-sharing obligations that have increased significantly under recent legislation. Payment for dental prostheses in particular has been increasingly limited in recent years.[102]

The structure of the German health care system, as described above, minimizes opportunities for disputes between insureds and insurers or between patients and providers over benefit coverage issues. The fee-for-service physician payment system, for example, rewards physicians for delivering as many services as possible to their patients. The physician has until recently also faced only limited incentives for controlling prescribing. From 1993 until 1996, the law imposed budgets (first fixed, thereafter negotiated) on prescribing by region.[103] These prescribing limits only applied to physicians as a group, however. Although they were substantially exceeded in 1996,[104] sanctions for exceeding the limits have not in fact yet been imposed.[105] Physicians who substantially exceed their peers in providing services or prescribing medications risk cutbacks in their payments under the German utilization review system, discussed below. This only

98. § 2(1) SGB V.

99. § 11 SGB V.

100. § 27(1) SGB V.

101. § 2 SGB V.

102. § 30 SGB V.

103. GENERAL ACCOUNTING OFFICE, PRESCRIPTION DRUG SPENDING CONTROLS (1994); Reinhard Busse & Chris Howorth, *Fixed Budgets in the Pharmaceutical Sector in Germany: Effects on Costs and Quality*, *in* FIXING HEALTH BUDGETS, *supra* note 64, at 109, 114-16.

104. Josef Maus, *Massive Ärzteproteste zeigen Wirkung*, 93 DEUTSCHES ÄRZTEBLATT A-3235 (1996).

105. For a discussion of the difficulties of imposing the sanctions, *see* Wolfgang Spellbrink, *Rechtsfolgen der Budgetüberschreitung nach § 84 SGB V*, 15 MEDIZINRECHT 65 (1997).

occurs after relatively extreme limits are reached, however, and the income-maximizing strategy of the individual physician is to provide the greatest possible number of services up to point where utilization review is triggered.

Other factors in addition to the payment system also limit conflicts over insurance benefit coverage. Patients have essentially free choice of physician. Any patient refused services by a physician is free to find another. All insureds, moreover, have free choice of insurer as of January 1, 1996, and white collar employees have had free choice for much longer.[106] In the past, insurers have competed in terms of serving their insureds, including making services available, rather than by limiting premiums.[107] Insurance companies, therefore, deny coverage requests only relatively infrequently.

A. *Coverage Disputes:* **Hilfsmittel**

Coverage disputes do arise, however, even in the German system. One of the most common objects of coverage disputes is *Hilfsmittel*, which is covered by statutory health insurance under SGB section 33. *Hilfsmittel* is roughly analogous to the category of durable medical equipment in the United States, but includes more broadly, "[v]ision and hearing aids, prostheses, orthopedic and other medical equipment, that in particular cases is necessary to assure the success of treatment of the sick or to compensate for a disability, so long as the equipment is not an article used generally by people in daily life (or excluded by other code sections)."[108] Examples from recent opinions include hand-held devices that detect color for the blind or fax machines for the deaf.[109] The BSG issued twenty published decisions regarding *Hilfsmittel* between 1990 and 1996, making this area one of the most hotly contested areas considered by the BSG.

Cases normally come to the court when an insured requests coverage of a particular device from a KK and the request is denied. Because KKn rarely deny coverage with respect to other treatments and services, it is cu-

106. *See* Johann Behrens, *Die Freiheit der Wahl und die Sicherung der Qualität (Versuch einer Antwort auf [nicht nur] amerikanische Fragen), in* GESUNDHEITSSYSTEMENTWICKLUNG IN DEN USA UND DEUTSCHLAND 197, 199 (Johann Behrens et al. eds., Nomos Verlagsgesellschaft 1996).

107. *See* Sabine Richard & Karl-Heinz Schönbach, *German Sickness Funds under Fixed Budgets, in* FIXING HEALTH BUDGETS, *supra* note 64, at 187, 191 (describing competition among sickness funds to offer more services).

108. § 33 SGB V.

109. BSG, 1/17/96, 3 RK 39/94, SozR 3-2500, § 33, No. 19 (fax machine); BSG, 1/17/96, 3 RK 38/94; SozR 3-2500, § 33, No. 18 (color detection apparatus).

rious that denials arise so often in this area. Disputes frequently involve very expensive equipment, however, which often might be useful to sizable categories of disabled persons (the blind, deaf, paralyzed, and so forth).[110] *Hilfsmittel* disputes can be seen as test cases, therefore, involving potentially large sums of money, and when the KKn believe that a denial is justified, appeals of the denial will be vigorously resisted by the KKn.[111]

The insureds win a surprising proportion of appellate decisions involving *Hilfsmittel* claims, and in many cases where the lower court upholds the KK denial of coverage, the appellate court remands for reconsideration of additional factors not attended to by the lower court. The social court decisions give only cursory attention to several statutory coverage requirements. Although SGB V, section 128, requires the sickness funds to publish jointly a list of covered *Hilfsmittel*, together with maximum prices to be paid for each item, the courts routinely treat this list as advisory rather than as binding; the fact that a specific item is not on the list is of no consequence.[112] Second, although SGB section 33(1) on its face requires that a device have curative potential and or completely compensate for a handicap, the courts find this requirement satisfied if a device will partially compensate for a handicap.[113]

Disputes normally center around three other *Hilfsmittel* coverage requirements. First, the statute excludes coverage for objects requested by handicapped persons that non-handicapped persons use regularly in their daily life.[114] The question here is not whether the item is widely used—glasses and hearing aids, for example, are covered despite the fact that millions of persons use them.[115] Rather, the question is whether the item is widely used for non-medical purposes. The court tends to take a statistical approach to this question. Computers (sought as perception or communi-

110. *See, e.g.*, BSG, 2/6/97, 3 RK 1/96 (unpublished) (computer systems costing DM 9100 sought as communications device for handicapped child) (on file with author).

111. In some cases the KKn also resist paying for a piece of equipment, not because it is not needed, but because some other entity (most often vocational rehabilitation insurance) is responsible for paying for it. *See, e.g.*, BSG, 7/26/94, 111 RAr 115/93, SozR 3-2500 § 33, No. 10 (orthopedic shoes used only for work not covered by sickness funds).

112. *See* BSG, 1/17/96, 3 RK 16/95, SozR. 3-2500, § 33, No. 20.

113. *See id.* (fact that air filter only made one room in dwelling suitable for handicapped person not decisive if room was bedroom and made it possible for person to sleep.) The fact that the device does not directly substitute for a body part is also not important, if the device in fact compensates indirectly for the loss of a bodily function); BSG, 1/17/96, 3 RK 38/94, Breithaupt 633 (1996) (color recognition device that does not cure or totally compensate for blindness, but assists a blind person to perceive things).

114. § 33(1) SGB V.

115. BSG, 1/17/96, 3 RK 39/94, SozR 3-2500, § 33, No. 19.

cation devices by the handicapped) were owned by twelve percent of the population in 1995, and were thus held to be objects widely used in daily life.[116] Fax machines (sought by a deaf person for communication) were owned by only 2.3% of private persons in 1994, and were therefore held not to be excluded.[117] Obviously, the extent of use of objects such as computers and faxes changes over time, generally in the direction of moving objects from covered to uncovered status as they become more widely used by the general public. The coverage exclusion for widely used devices is itself subject to two exceptions, however. First, even items that are in wide use may be covered, at least in part, if they are very expensive and thus not affordable by the insured.[118] Second, to the extent that items are similar to items in general use, but cost more because they have been adapted for the handicapped, such as hypoallergenic mattresses and pillows, the additional costs will be covered.[119]

A second requirement, found in SGB V section 12, provides that coverage is extended only to items the coverage of which are cost-effective. In applying this requirement, the BSG tends to perform a cost-benefit analysis, considering both the cost of the item and how useful it would actually be to the handicapped person in practice.[120] The fact that costs for ever more sophisticated devices for aiding the handicapped have dropped dramatically in recent years is relied on by the courts to support a continual expansion of coverage for these devices. Indeed, sometimes the BSG explicitly acknowledges that it ruled against coverage of a particular device when it was earlier disputed, but that costs have now dropped to the extent that coverage is warranted.[121] Also relevant in some of these cases are issues of whether the item is in fact necessary, or whether it might be a luxury. The BSG tends to interpret "need" expansively, however, finding that

---

116. BSG, 8/23/95, 3 RK 7/94, SozR 3-2500, § 33, No. 16. The BSG followed this determination in a later case, 2/6/97, 3 RK 1/96 (unpublished).

117. BSG, 1/17/96, 3 RK 39/94, SozR 3-2500, § 33, No. 19.

118. BSG, 10/15/95, 1 RK 18/94, SozR 3-2500, § 33.

119. BSG, 1/17/96, 3 RK 39/94, SozR 3-2500, § 33, No. 19 (though fax paid for by insurance, costs of using it are similar to ordinary telephone costs, and must be paid by insured); BSG, 1/25/95, 3/1 RK 63/93, SozR 3-2500, § 33 (bed adapted for handicapped child covered).

120. BSG, 11/21/91, 1 RK 43/89, SozR 3-2500, § 33 No. 4 (electric reading device that costs DM 5900). In some of these cases this consideration is almost mechanical. In the color detection device case, the court found that the object would be used 10 times a day, and was thus justified given its cost of DM 1470. BSG, 1/17/96, 3 RK 38/94.

121. *See* discussion of coverage of writing telephones for the deaf in BSG, 10/25/95, 3 RK 30/94; SozR 3-2500, § 33, No. 17.

the blind have a right to be able to read,[122] that persons who are deaf have a right not to be isolated from others,[123] and that persons who are paralyzed have a right to move freely in the environment.[124] The BSG has also found, moreover, that disabled persons have a right to have equipment provided to compensate for their handicaps rather than to be expected to rely on family members or others around them for help.[125] Sometimes the BSG invokes the human rights sections of the Constitution as a source of these rights.[126]

Finally, the BSG inquires under SGB V section 34 whether the items are so inexpensive that they are readily affordable without insurance assistance, or whether their therapeutic value is disputed.[127] Here again, the court tends to be generous, rejecting, for example, the policy of a KK that excluded a breast milk pump that cost DM 255 from coverage as an item of minimal cost.[128] On the other hand, the BSG has upheld exclusion of hearing aid batteries, which are cheap enough to be affordable by most insureds, and are covered by welfare for those who truly cannot afford them.[129]

In sum, the decisions of the social courts have continually supported expansion of coverage in this area. This may explain, in part, why *Hilfsmittel* costs have been one of the fastest growing areas of insurance coverage.

B. Coverage Disputes: Alternative and Experimental Medicine

The decisions of the BSG also appear to be a factor in expanding coverage of experimental and alternative medicine. On their face, the health insurance sections of the German Social Code would appear to strictly limit the services for which the health insurance funds are required to pay.

122. BSG, 8/23/95, 3 RK 7/95, SozR 3-2500, § 33, No. 16. The court also observed in this case that to force a blind person to rely on others to read to him would violate his constitutional right to privacy in communication.

123. BSG, 10/25/95, 3 RK 30/94, SozR 3-2500, § 33, No. 17.

124. BSG, 6/8/94, 3/1 RK 13/93, SozR 3-2500, § 33, No. 7.

125. BSG, 1/17/96, 3 RK 38/94, SozR 3-2500, § 33, No. 18. The Court also considers whether the device is necessary for assisting the handicapped for leading normal lives in general, or whether it is rather needed to permit the pursuit of a particular vocation. If an item is vocation specific, it is not the responsibility of the sickness funds, but might be paid for by the vocational rehabilitation insurance program.

126. *See* BSG, 2/26/91, 8 Rkn 33/90, SozR 3-2500, § 33, No. 3 (constitutional right of freedom of movement justifies payment for adaptive seat for auto).

127. § 34(4) SGB V.

128. BSG, 9/28/93, 1 RK 37/92, SozR 3-2500, § 34, No. 2.

129. BSG 6/8/94, 3/1 RK 54/93, SozR 3-2500, §33, No. 9.

Section 2, which defines the scope of services generally, provides that services must be provided effectively and economically, and only to the extent necessary,[130] further specifying that quality and efficiency of services must comply with the general state of medical knowledge.[131] Section 12 states even more emphatically that providers may not provide, insureds request, or insurers pay for services that are unnecessary or that are not economically provided, a directive repeated in sections 70 and 72.[132] Section 28 again obligates doctors to provide services according to the standards of medical practice, while section 34 excludes payment for ineffective medications.[133] Finally, section 135 provides that new diagnostic and treatment methods may not be ordered at the cost of the sickness funds until the Federal Commission of Insurance Doctors and Health Insurance Funds at the request of a KaV or the federal organization of KKn has made recommendations regarding the recognition of the new procedure and qualifications for doctors who may deliver it.[134] Under 1997 amendments to the health insurance law, these recommendations must consider the medical necessity and efficiency of the procedure as well as its effectiveness.[135]

The legislative history of the SGB supports a restrictive interpretation of these provisions. The report accompanying the 1989 Health Reform Law, the last major revision of coverage provisions, emphasized that payments by the health insurance funds must be limited to truly needed services, specifically excluding services

> . . . that are provided with methods that are not generally accepted. New procedures, that are not sufficiently researched, or exotic treatment methodologies (paramedical procedures), that are recognized, but that have not been proved, are not within the responsibility of the health insurance funds. It is not the task of the health insurance funds to finance medical research. This is also true when new methods in particular cases can lead to a healing of the disease or to a diminution of a disability.[136]

---

130. § 2(4) SGB V.

131. § 2(1) SGB V.

132. §§ 12(1), 70(10, 72(2) SGB V.

133. §§ 28(1), 34(2) SGB V.

134. § 135(1) SGB V; *see* ANDREAS SCHMIDT-RÖGNITZ, DIE GEWÄHRUNG VON ALTERNATIVEN SOWIE NEUEN BEHANDLUNGS-UND HEILMETHODEN DURCH DIE GESETZLICHE KRANKENVERSICHERUNG 92-93, 96-97 (1996).

135. Horst Dieter Schirmer, *Das Kassenarztrecht im 2. GKV-Neuordnungsgesetz —BGBl. 1997 I S. 1520 -*, 15 MEDIZINRECHT 431, 447 (1997).

136. Bundestag Print, 11/2237, 148, 157.

In practice, however, the restrictions imposed by SGB V, as interpreted by the BSG, are far less onerous than would first appear. As long as a code exists under the EBM, the codebook under which procedures are billed, a service can be provided and the doctor paid for it; it is subject only to retrospective review for excessive provision of care under the *Wirtschaftlichkeitsprüfung* process described below.[137] The EBM applies primarily to traditional medicine, however, and only covers new and experimental treatments to the extent they have been reviewed under the section 135 new diagnostic and treatment procedure approval process.

Where services are either experimental or non-traditional, and thus not yet recognized in the EBM, coverage policy becomes more complicated, although the service may still ultimately be paid for by the KKn.[138] First, section 2 SGB V states that alternative therapeutical modalities cannot be excluded from coverage.[139] Section 34, which deals with covered drugs, refers to "alternative therapeutic modalities such as homeopathy, phytotherapy, and antroposophy" and requires drugs from these therapeutic modalities to be evaluated according to the standards of these modalities.[140] This section does not explicitly limit alternative therapeutic modalities to these three schools, however, and other schools of treatment may be covered by sections 2 and 34. A provision in the recently adopted 1997 health reform law goes even further, amending section 135 to provide that new procedures are supposed to be reviewed according to the state of knowledge "in the particular school of therapy."[141] This provision was clearly added to encourage the extension of coverage to non-traditional medicine.

The rulings of the BSG interpreting the coverage of alternative or experimental medicine have been complex and contradictory. For a decade, the Third Senate of the BSG, which decides issues of coverage policy, has

137. *See* Bertram Schulin, *Alternativ Medicin in der gesetzlichen Krankenversicherung*, 40 ZEITSCHRIFT FÜR SOZIALREFORM 546, 553 (1994).

138. *See generally* SCHMIDT-RÖGNITZ, *supra* note 134.

139. § 2(1) SGB V.

140. § 34(2) SGB V; *see also* § 92(2) SGB V (requiring drug guidelines for drugs from the separate therapy modalities to be evaluated by experts from these modalities). For a description of these modalities, *see* Rüdiger Zuck, *Der Standort der Besonderen Therapierichtungen im deutschen Gesundheitswesen*, 44 NEUE JURISTISCHE WOCHENSCHRIFT 2933, 2934 (1991).

141. Zweites Gesetz zur Neuordnung von Selbstverwaltung und Eigenverantwortung in der gesetzlichen Krankenversicherung (2.GKV-NOG), § 50, to be codified at § 135(a)(1).1 SGB V. Alternative medical procedures, however, must be evaluated in terms of their effectiveness, necessity, and efficiency, and must be evaluated in terms of comprehensible scientific knowledge. Schirmer, *supra* note 135, at 447.

recognized the extension of coverage to alternative or experimental treatment methods in cases of severe illness of unknown origin where traditional treatment methods are ineffective or where recognized treatments are not appropriate for the particular case.[142] In either case, the court has required a plausible case to be made that the treatment can be effective.[143] The court has been willing to order the sickness fund to indemnify the patient, however, where a disputed treatment proves in fact to be effective.[144] The 14a Senate also supported alternative medicine in a decision rejecting the discipline of a dentist who refused to use amalgam fillings with mercury in them because of his adherence to natural healing.[145] The BSG relied in this decision on the constitutional arguments discussed below. A recent decision of the social appeals court for Lower Saxony went even further, recognizing coverage for plausible alternative treatment, even though the disease is not life threatening and traditional treatment may be available.[146]

Arguments that SGB V should be interpreted to cover alternative and experimental treatments not yet evaluated under the section 135 procedures are based in part on the structure of the Social Code. SGB V governs both the relationships between insurers and their insureds and between insurers and providers. It is argued that provisions like section 135 may limit payment of providers to particular procedures, but do not limit the independent and higher right of insureds to receive other procedures where such procedures are otherwise covered by SGB V.[147] Even though providers may not bill directly for services not covered by the EBM, it is argued, patients may receive such services and then claim indemnification from their insurer.[148] In short, the commentators argue that the direct payment principle is subordinate to the comprehensiveness principle.

142. SCHMIDT-RÖGNITZ, *supra* note 134, at 98-99, 107; Rolf-Ulrich Schlenker, *Die Außenseitermedizin und das System der gesetzlichen Krankenversicherung*, 39 DIE SOZIALGERICHTSBARKEIT 530 (1992); Matthias von Wulffen, *Besondere Therapiemethoden in der Rechtsprechung des Bundessozialgerichts*, 43 DIE SOZIALGERICHTSBARKEIT 250 (1996).

143. SCHMIDT-RÖGNITZ, *supra* note 134, at 100-01.

144. Stephan Biehl and Heinz Ortwein, *Sind Außenseitermethoden Maßnahmen außerhalb des Leistungskataloges der gesetzlichen Krankenversicherung (GKV)?*, 38 DIE SOCIALGERICHTBARKEIT 529, 531-32 (1991).

145. BSG, 9/8/1993, 14a RKa 7/92, SozR 3-2500, § 2, No. 2.

146. LSG Niedersachsen 8/30/95, L 4 Kr 11/95, Breithaupt 191 (1996).

147. *See* SCHMIDT-RÖGNITZ, *supra* note 134, at 104-06; Schulin, *supra* note 136, at 558-59.

148. SCHMIDT-RÖGNITZ, *supra* note 134, at 101.

Further, some commentators have argued that the German Constitution would be violated if SGB V were interpreted to permit decisions of a commission of doctors and insurers to establish rules that would limit the rights of insureds.[149] The delegation doctrine is much more robust in Germany than in the United States, and the German Constitution limits the entities to which authority for making generally binding rules can be delegated and the forms such rules can take. It has been forcefully argued that the commission that reviews experimental procedures is not an agency that can constitutionally limit the rights of insureds.[150]

It is also more broadly argued that a total ban on coverage for services not listed in the EBM would violate other constitutional rights. First, it would arguably violate the constitutional right of doctors to professional freedom.[151] Second, it would violate the constitutional right of self determination and personal integrity of persons who are required by law to be insured.[152] Finally, it has been argued that the property and equal protection rights of persons required by law to be insured would be violated if there were major gaps in their coverage, because supplemental commercial insurance is neither affordable nor available to fill the gaps.[153] A recent decision of the German constitutional court, holding that the constitutional right to self-determination, although applicable in the health insurance setting, is subject to the statutory responsibility of the health insurers to limit access to medication to promote efficiency, calls these arguments into question.[154] Nevertheless, they continue to be plausible.

In sum, the law has traditionally supported the claims of insureds to alternative and experimental medicine, and the limitations found in SGB V have been largely ineffective. Belief in alternative medicine is widespread in Germany, and some believe that the costs of alternative medicine impose a significant cost on the German health care system.[155]

There may, however, be a trend toward greater restriction of coverage of alternative and experimental treatment. In recent years, the BSG has

---

149. Thomas Clemens, *Verfassungsrechtliche Anforderungen an untergesetzliche Rechtsnormen*, 14 MEDIZINRECHT 432, 438-39 (1996).

150. Raimund Wimmer, *Verfassungsrechtliche Anforderungen an untergesetzliche Rechtsetzung im Vertragsarztrecht*, 14 MEDIZINRECHT 425 (1996); *cf.* Horst Dieter Schirmer, *Verfassunsrechtliche Probleme der untergesetzlichen Normsetzung im Kassenarztrecht*, 14 MEDIZINRECHT 404 (1996).

151. *See* Zuck, *supra* note 140, at 2933.

152. Art. 1 & 2 GG; *see* Zuck, *supra* note 140.

153. Schulin, *supra* note 137, at 562.

154. *See* BVerfG 3/5/97, 1 BvR 1068/96, 15 MEDIZINRECHT 318 (1997).

155. *Rückfall ins Mittelalter*, DER SPIEGEL, May 20, 1997, at 22; Schlenker, *supra* note 142, at 530.

become less receptive to alternative medicine, requiring at least a plausible understanding of the method of operation of a particular medical intervention.[156] A 1995 decision of the First Senate went further, requiring statistical evidence of effectiveness.[157] The most important development, however, is a 1996 decision of the Sixth Senate, which holds that claims of insureds are in fact limited by the section 135 coding rules.[158]

The Sixth Senate of the BSG is responsible for reviewing the claims of insurance doctors. As claims for coverage of alternative or experimental treatment have usually been brought by insureds, it has been generally silent on these issues. In 1996, however, it considered a case involving a doctor who had been refused permission to treat an addicted patient with Methadon because the drug's treatment guidelines were not met in the particular case. The decision is long and carefully argued, and reaches the conclusion that insureds are entitled only to receive insurance funds for services for which providers are authorized to bill, and that this situation does not violate the constitutional rights of insureds or providers or constitutional limitations on delegation.[159] The decision has been sharply criticized,[160] but has been followed in another Sixth Senate decision, which upheld the refusal of a KK to pay for extracorporeal shockwave lithotripsy outside the hospital before it was approved for ambulatory coverage under the new therapy guidelines.[161]

It remains to be seen whether these decisions will extend beyond the situations they addressed, where a federal commission representing both providers and insurers (and thus derivatively insureds and employers) had either already considered a particular treatment and issued guidelines regarding it or, alternatively, first issued guidelines regarding the therapy after the service was rendered for which the claim was submitted. It also remains to be seen whether other senates of the BSG will follow the decisions of the Sixth Senate. The fundamental argument of the decision, however, is compelling. The legislature is not capable of reviewing every

156. BSG, 2/9/89, 3 RK 19/87; BGG 2/10/93, 1 RK 17/91, *noted in* Wolfgang Wölk, *Paramedizinsche Therapie und Rechtsprechung*, 13 MEDIZINRECHT 492 (1995).

157. BSG, 7/5/95, 1 RK 6/95, 14 MEDIZINRECHT 373 (1996), *noted in* von Wulffen, *supra* note 142, at 252.

158. BSG 3/20/96, 6 RKa 62/94, *noted in* 15 MEDIZINRECHT 123 (1997).

159. *Id.* at 129.

160. Raimund Wimmer, *Substitution mit Methadon nach den NUB-Richtlinien*, 15 MEDIZINRECHT 224 (1997). In another recent decision involving methadon, the First Senate denied coverage because it was being used for a drug addiction maintenance program, not for the treatment of a sickness. BSG, 3/12/96, 1 RK 33/94, Breithaupt 824 (1996).

161. BSG, 11/13/96, 6 RKa 31/95 (unpublished) (on file with author).

treatment that could possibly be covered by the social insurance funds and deciding on a case by case basis whether or not it should be covered. This decision must either be delegated or left to the courts. It makes a great deal of sense to delegate it to a commission that represents providers, insureds, and those who pay for insurance. Judicial review must continue, but only with respect to the reasonableness of decisions made by the experts best capable of deciding. Whether the German social courts will take this approach, however, or whether they will continue to independently review the coverage of experimental and alternative medicine is not yet clear.

C. Efficiency Review Cases

In terms of sheer number of cases, probably the greatest involvement of the social courts in health care financing is with respect to the process of *Wirtschaftlichkeitsprüfung* (WP), or economic monitoring, established by section 106 SGB V. WP is essentially what we would think of as utilization review. In contrast to the cases just considered, it does not address the claims to particular types of coverage by individual patients, but rather the aggregate provision or ordering of services for patients by particular doctors. It is a process through which doctors and dentists who perform unnecessary procedures or who order unnecessary drugs or therapy are first warned and then, if they persist, have their payments reduced or are subjected to fines.[162] Committees composed of representatives of the KKn and the KaVn assess these penalties, which are subject to appeal to the social courts.[163] Decisions are frequently appealed and are frequently reversed by the social courts or settled after appeal. The WP process generates a great deal of work for lawyers, and a host of books have been written describing the WP process.[164]

The process of WP can only be understood in the context of the German system of sector-specific medical care budgets. For two decades, first

162. §106(5) SGB V. This discussion focuses primarily on the process as it is applied to physicians. The process as it is applied to dentists is in most instances almost identical.

163. *Id.*

164. ALEXANDER P.F. EHLERS, ET AL., PRAXIS DER WIRTSCHAFLICHKEITSPRÜFUNG (1996) [hereinafter "EHLERS, ET AL."]; ALEXANDER P.F. EHLERS, DIE WIRTSCHAFLICHKEITSPRÜFUNG IM VERTRAGARZTRECHT (looseleaf, 1993); DIETER RADDATZ, DIE WIRTSCHAFTLICHKEIT DER KASSENÄRZTLICHEN UND KASSENZAHNÄRZTLICHEN VERSORGUNG IN DER RECHTSPRECHUNG—WKR (1993); WOLFGANG SPELLBRINK, WIRTSCHAFLICHKEITSPRÜFUNG IM KASSENARZTRECHT NACH DEM GESUNDHEITS—STRUKTURGESETZ (1994); Thomas Clemens, *Honorkürzung wegen Unwitschaftlichkeit, in* HANDBUCH SVR, *supra* note 51, at 910-60.

voluntarily and then under the compulsion of law, the German sickness funds and insurance doctors have negotiated annual budgets for physicians' services.[165] In recent years, budgets have also been established for prescribed drugs and therapies.[166] The regional KaVs pay their physicians on a quarterly basis, with their payments depending on the number of points they billed for services during the quarter based on the point values assigned to services by the EBM.[167]

The obvious incentive created by this system is for each doctor to bill as many points as possible to obtain the largest possible slice of the fixed pie. Thus, a doctor's billings are reviewed by the KaV, to determine, first, whether they are honest and accurate, and, second, whether they are for services that are truly necessary. The honesty and accuracy of a doctor's billings are reviewed through the *sachlich-rechnerische Richtigstellung*, which reviews whether a service billed could in fact legally have been provided by the billing doctor considering his specialty and type of practice, whether the service is correctly coded, and, at the margins, whether it was in fact rendered.[168] The doctor's bills are also reviewed using a daily profile program that assigns a plausible minimum number of minutes to each of the services billed by physicians and reviews billing to determine whether the number of services billed by the doctor could in fact have been provided in a reasonable working day.[169] Doctors also have an obligation not to serve so great a number of patients that they cannot reasonably care for each patient, and doctors with unreasonably large practices may have their payments reduced accordingly.[170] These reviews are performed by the KaVn prior to the point when formal WP begins.

Doctors (and dentists) have an obligation under the SGB to provide services sufficiently, effectively, and economically, and in no greater volume than necessary.[171] Section 106 SGB V, and the extensive body of caselaw interpreting section 106 and earlier provisions of the *Reichsversicherungsordnug* (RVO) which preceded it, provide a variety of methods

165. *See supra* text at notes 76 through 77, Schwartz & Busse, *supra* note 64.

166. *See supra* text accompanying notes 103-05; Busse & Howorth, *supra* note 103.

167. *See supra* text accompanying notes 78 through 81.

168. *See* Thomas Clemens, *Sachlich-rechnerische Richtigstellung*, *in* HANDBUCH SVR, *supra* note 51, at 899-909.

169. *Id.* at 904-07; *see* Hermann Müller, *Allgemeinarzt war mit 25, 2 Stunden pro Tag der Spitzenreiter beim Abkassieren*, ÄRZTE ZEITUNG, Feb. 28, 1997, at 23 (reporting on doctors who billed for obviously impossible numbers of points during the second quarter of 1996).

170. Funk, *supra* note 78, at 892-93.

171. §§2(4), 12 SGB V.

that the KaVn and KKn may use to assure that services are economically provided. The favored approach to economic monitoring for billing for doctors' services is currently statistical review.[172] The key variable in this review is cost per patient, i.e., the average amount the doctor bills per patient.[173] A doctor's billings are reviewed to determine how many points the doctor has billed for each patient. For comparison purposes, doctors are grouped by specialty and locality.[174] The group must be both sufficiently homogenous and sufficiently large to permit meaningful statistical comparison.[175] Doctors are also generally compared by patient group, specifically considering separately older, retired patients and younger patients.[176] Doctors with extraordinarily high billings are subject to sanctions.

The statistical comparison usually encompasses a doctors' total billing, but it can be limited to particular services or categories of services.[177] Two different statistical approaches have been taken for comparison. Originally the comparison focused on percentage deviation from the average. Under this approach, doctors whose total billings exceed the average of their comparison group by fifty percent are considered to be obvious outliers, subject to sanctions unless they can explain the deviation.[178] Doctors whose billings lie in the twenty to fifty percent range are subject to scrutiny for uneconomic conduct.[179] Physicians whose billings lie less than twenty percent above the mean are considered to be within the range of random variation, and are not subject to further examination.[180] Where the review focuses on individual services or groups of services, rather than on total billings, a wider range of deviation is permitted, recognizing that ranges of variance will be broader with respect to individual services than for an entire practice.[181]

In recent years, the percentage deviation approach has been called into question. Some have argued that a more accurate approach is to consider distribution around the mean, i.e., location on the so-called Gausian

172. BSG, 11/15/95, 6 RKa 43/94, SozR 3-2500, § 106, No. 33.
173. SPELLBRINK, *supra* note 164, at 195-212.
174. *Id.* at 212-15.
175. *Id.* at 215-16.
176. RADDATZ, *supra* note 164, at 254-55.
177. SPELLBRINK, *supra* note 164, at 198-203.
178. *Id.* at 239.
179. *Id.*
180. *Id.*
181. BSG, 4/8/92, 6 RKa 34/90, SozR 3-2500, § 106, Nr. 11.

curve.[182] This approach recognizes that in very homogenous groups, a doctors' billings could be exceptional even though they lie only a small percentage above the norm, while in less homogenous groups a much larger percentage deviation could be unexceptional. Under this approach the determining factor is the number of standard deviations from the norm, with physicians whose billings lie over 1.6 standard deviations above the norm considered obvious outliers.[183] Neither the statute nor the decisions of the BSG endorse either approach. In a series of recent decisions, however, the BSG has criticized lower courts that have strictly relied on the Gausian distribution approach without further evidentiary evaluation.[184]

A doctor who is found to be a statistical outlier has two primary lines of defense. First, and most importantly, the doctor may argue that there are exceptional circumstances respecting his or her practice that justify the deviation.[185] The possibilities here are rather limited because (1) some exceptional circumstances are accounted for in the original comparison process (high proportion of elderly patients, for example, is not an excuse since elderly patients are compared separately); (2) others are accounted for by the permitted deviation from the mean (exceptionally sick patients); and (3) still others are not acceptable excuses as they are precisely the problem at which WP is aimed (particularly frequent use of expensive equipment). Some exceptional circumstances, however, are regularly recognized, such as the fact that a doctor is just beginning a practice and must perform an exceptional number of initial interviews and examinations, or that the doctor practices in a particular subspecialty or with a particular method that results in the treatment of more expensive patients.[186] Doctors such as pathologists who perform services primarily on a referral basis may also argue that they were simply performing services requested by other doctors.[187]

Second, doctors subject to sanctions for deviation from the norm with respect to particular services or groups of services may claim that the high

182. *See* WILHELM GAUS, PRÜFUNG DER WIRTSCHAFTLICHKEIT DER BEHANDLUNGS-UND VERORDNUNGSWEISE DES KASSENARZTES (1988).

183. Clemens, *supra* note 164, at 935.

184. BSG, 3/15/95, 6 RKa 37/93, reported at 49 NEUE JURISTISCHE WOCHENSCHRIFT 2448 (1996); Wolfgang Noftz, *Wirtschaflichkeitsprüfung im Vertrags(zahn)arztrecht zwischen Statistik und Intellektualität?—Aktuelle Tendenzen der neueren Rechtsprechung*, NEUE ZEITSCHRIFT SOZIALRECHT 207 (1997).

185. RADDATZ, *supra* note 164, at 374-444; SPELLBRINK, *supra* note 164, at 137, para. 274.

186. Clemens, *supra* note 164, at 937-38; SPELLBRINK, *supra* note 164, at 278-80.

187. SPELLBRINK, *supra* note 164, at 286-87.

use of certain services is compensated for by low usage in other areas.[188] Doctors may argue, for example, that they gave a high number of injections because they prescribed fewer oral medications.[189]

The individual cases of doctors may also be subjected to review on a case by case basis. For a long time, the BSG held up individual case review as the preferred form of economic review,[190] but it quickly became obvious that it was generally not practical. The BSG decided quite early that for an individual review to be truly accurate and reliable, it would have to go beyond the doctor's records, perhaps including an actual examination of the individual patient to determine the patient's actual condition.[191] Moreover, the examination would have to focus not on the patient's condition at the time of the review, but on the patient's condition at the time of the treatment. Individual review is difficult because the WP commissions do not have the resources to perform such examinations, and have no means to require patients to submit to them.[192] Individual review based on the doctor's records is permitted but is regarded skeptically by the courts. Extrapolations based on individual reviews are also permitted, allowing sanctions to exceed the levels warranted by the individual cases reviewed but only once a relatively large group of cases have been reviewed.[193] Only in the dental area, where review can readily be performed on the basis of x-rays, does individual review play a major role.[194]

188. RADDATZ, *supra* note 164, at 330-73.

189. Clemens, *supra* note 164, at 941-42.

190. RADDATZ, *supra* note 164, at 146.

191. *See* BSG, 6/2/87, 6 RKa 19/86, SozR 2200, § 368n, No. 54; Hans-Siegmund Danckwerts, *Kassenzahnärztliche Versorgung: Überwachung der Wirtschaflichkeit durch Einzelfallprüfungen*, 70 DIE ORTSKRANKENKKASSE 458 (1988).

192. SPELLBRINK, *supra* note 164, at 315-16.

193. At least 100 cases or 20% of the total, with a discount from the extrapolated result of 25% to account for uncertainty. SPELLBRINK, *supra* note 164, at 320-21.

194. SPELLBRINK, supra note 164, at 315. The 1989 health reform law introduced a new form of economic monitoring based on sampling. § 106(2)2 SGB V. The idea grounding this random review is that doctors who avoid being obvious outliers often also have uneconomical practices, and should be subject to review. Under the sampling review, two percent of non-outlier physicians are supposed to be randomly selected each quarter for review. § 106(2) SGB V; *see* Ursula Spiolek, *Das Wirtschaftlichkeitsgebot des SGB V und die beiden neuen Formen der Wirtschaflichkeitsprüfung—Stichproben- und Richtgrößenprüfung—nach § 106 II 1 SGB V*, 38 ZEITSCHRIFT FÜR SOZIALREFORM 209 (1992). Statistical review is not appropriate as a method for sampling review, both because sampling review is by definition a statutory alternative to statistical review, and because sampling is used precisely because the doctors it affects are not statistical outliers. Comprehensive case by case review of individual patients, on the other hand for two percent of all doctors would quickly exhaust the resources of the economic review

Not only are services provided by doctors subject to economic monitoring, but prescriptions, bandages, and therapy are also reviewed.[195] These reviews are normally carried out, again, through a statistical review of prescriptions.[196] They result in sanctions much less frequently than billing reviews,[197] but are of more interest to the KKn as they result in actual recoveries by the KK, not simply in reallocation of funds among doctors. Under the 1992 reform law, reviews are also supposed to be performed based on deviations from prescribing volume guidelines to be agreed to by the KaVn and KKn.[198] Between 1994 and 1997, however, implementation of these guidelines would have resulted under the terms of the law in termination of the prescribing budgets imposed by the 1992 law, and was resisted by the KKn who preferred to preserve fixed budgets.

Economic review committees consisting of an equal number of members from the KKn and the KaVn initially perform economic review.[199] A doctor who is sanctioned may have a hearing before an appeal committee, the *Beschwerdeausschuß*, which also contains members drawn equally from the KKn and KaVn.[200] If the sanction stands, the doctor may go to court.[201]

On the whole, doctors face fairly substantial incentives to appeal WP decisions. Access to the social court is free,[202] and a doctor whose com-

---

commissions. SPELLBRINK, *supra* note 164, at 325. Sampling review, therefore, has to date played virtually no role in EHLERS, ET AL., *supra* note 164, at 92.

195. § 106(2)1 SGB V.

196. SPELLBRINK, *supra* note 164, at 333.

197. Statistics regarding the use of WP nationwide are not available generally in Germany. The author wrote to all KVn in Germany, therefore, requesting information regarding WP statistics. A number of KVn responded, but most did not have the requested data available. A fee of the KVn provided data with response to the relative frequency of sanctions involving fee claims compared to those involving prescribing. In 1994, one KV had 36 prescribing WP cases, 123 fee WP cases; a second had 19 prescribing and 76 fee cases; a third in 1995 had 61 drug prescribing and 325 fee cases.

198. §§ 84, 106(2)1 SGB V.

199. § 106(4) SGB V.

200. § 106(5) SGB V.

201. *Id.* In the responses returned to the author's questionnaire, noted supra note 196, one KV stated that in 1995 during the first quarter of 1995 it sanctioned 213 doctors for excessive fees, 138 of which appealed internally, and 21 of whom ended up appealing to the social court. A second KV sanctioned 361 doctors during the first quarter of 1995, of whom 108 appealed internally and eight appealed to the social court. A third KV had 127 internal appeals in 1995, followed to date by six social court appeals. Finally, a fourth small KV had nine to eleven sanctions per quarter during 1995, of which two to four were appealed internally in each quarter, and one case was filed in the social court in each of three quarters.

202. § 183 SGG (*Sozialgerichtsgesetz*).

plaint is successful is entitled to have costs incurred in the appeal, including the costs of a necessary attorney, reimbursed.[203] Although since 1993 the doctor who loses a WP proceeding is obligated to reimburse a WP panel for necessary attorney costs it has incurred, panels do not usually retain attorneys unless a case goes to court, and they are not entitled to reimbursement for their administrative costs or the costs of internal legal staff.[204] On the other hand, an appeal to court does not generally stay the imposition of the sanction,[205] and therefore if a considerable sum of money is involved, a doctor may be better served by a settlement than by an appeal, which could last several years. Thus, doctors appeal WP decisions relatively often, but then settle the case on appeal.

In reading WP cases, one cannot help but be struck with the intensity of judicial supervision of the process. Section 106 of SGB V, which governs WP, is relatively short. Yet the BSG has developed an extensive body of caselaw governing in minute detail the methods that are available for WP, in what order they must be applied, the statistical methods that must be employed, the defenses doctors may raise, and the procedures through which the whole process is applied. As noted above, early decisions of the BSG imposed such rigorous demands on individual case review as to make this form of review, perhaps the most common form of utilization review in the United States, not viable. More recent decisions involving statistical review involve highly technical mathematical questions, difficult for the layman to understand.[206] This body of judge-made law applies nationwide, and cannot be varied by agreement by the regional KKn and KaVn.[207]

In the end, doctors have rights—rights enshrined in the Constitution, though these cases rarely advert to the Constitution. Article 12, section 1 of the Constitution protects the freedom of professionals to practice their profession, while Article 19, section 4 guarantees access to the court by those whose rights are violated by public institutions. Individual doctors must be treated fairly—the level of arbitrariness common in American utilization review decisions would not be tolerated in Germany.[208] This does not mean that doctors always bring or win WP appeals. Appeals are

203. EHLERS, ET AL., *supra* note 164, at 118-20.

204. *Id.* at 120-21.

205. *Id.* at 135-42.

206. *See, e.g.*, BSG, 8/5/92, 14a/6 RKa 4/90, SozR 3-2500, § 106, Nr. 13.

207. *See* BSG, 11/30/94, 6 RKa 16/93, SozR 3-2500, § 106, Nr. 25.

208. *See* Donald Light, *Life, Death, and the Insurance Companies*, 330 N. ENG. J. MED. 498 (1994); William P. Peters & Mark C. Rogers, *Variation in Approval by Insurance Companies of Coverage for Autologous Bone Marrow Transplantation for Breast Cancer*, 330 N. ENG. J. MED. 473 (1994).

often brought by the KaVn or KKn, and they often win. The more recent cases have emphasized the expertise and discretion of the WP panels, and have loosened the grip that some of the social courts were imposing on their decisions.[209] But one has the impression that the many demands and requirements imposed on WP by the courts have made it difficult both for doctors to know what to expect from the process and for the panels to know how to apply it. In the end, more and more cases are settled either before the *Beschwerdeausschuß* or at the first level of judicial review, probably leaving both the doctors and the payors feeling that the best result was denied.

Economic review has not been very successful in limiting unnecessary services or prescribing. First, it effects only a relatively small number of doctors, and an even smaller proportion of expenditures.[210] Because sanctions are generally limited to statistical outliers, the system has no effect on unnecessary services so long as most doctors provide them.[211] If it is true, as is generally believed, that doctors use practice computers to protect themselves from becoming outliers, the effect of sanctions on controlling the use of unnecessary procedures or prescribing is even less significant.[212] Even when doctors are sanctioned, the sanctions are quite mild. If the doctor is a first time offender, the most likely sanction is a warning.[213] When financial sanctions are imposed, the doctor's payments are usually only reduced to the level of obvious outlier status,[214] and thus the doctor remains well-paid. Doctors can lose their permission to practice as insurance doctors for repeated offenses, but this rarely occurs.[215]

As long as the tight physicians services and prescribing budgets of the 1992 reform law were in place, the KKn had fairly minimal interest in the WP process, which mainly involved reallocation of restricted budgets among providers. The significant increase in service billing that accompa-

209. *See supra* text accompanying note 184; Wolfgang Spellbrink, *Die "Intellektuelle Wirtschaftlichkeitsprüfung,"* 3 MEDIZINRECHT 125 (1996).

210. In response to the author's questionnaire, *supra* at note 196, one large KV reported reviewing between 5.61% and 6.31% of its doctors in each quarter in 1995, but in each quarter cut only between .53% and .6% of total payments to doctors through WP. Another KV reported reviewing between 2.1% and 3.9% of its doctors during four quarters in 1993 and 1994. A third reviewed between 9.81% and 12.16% of its doctors during the four quarter of 1995.

211. SPELLBRINK, *supra* note 164, at 306-08.

212. RADDATZ, *supra* note 164, at 167; *but see* SPELLBRINK, *supra* note 164, at 308-13.

213. § 106(5) SGB V.

214. *See* SPELLBRINK, *supra* note 164, at 302.

215. §§ 81(5), 95(6) SGB V; EHLERS, ET AL., *supra* note 164, at 255-63.

nied the fall of the point value during 1996 unleashed a flood of WP sanctions. Under the second *Neuordnungsgesetz* (NOG2), which took effect on June 12, 1997, fixed global budgets for both provider services and drugs were abolished, though more flexible budgeting will continue.[216] Praxis Budgets instituted for provider service billing effective July 1, 1997, basically capitate most services on an individual patient basis, diminishing the importance of WP, but the KaVn have committed themselves to abolishing Praxis Budgets, probably returning to a fee-for-service system.[217] Doctors have also fought hard for a fixed-point value based system, which is recognized to a degree by the NOG.[218] The NOG2 also requires prescribing volume guidelines to be put into place, and abolish the prior fixed budgets.[219] These prescribing guidelines are supposed to be specialty-specific. Doctors whose prescribing varies more than fifteen percent above the guidelines are supposed to be subjected to review automatically; those whose prescribing lies twenty-five percent above the average must pay the KKn for the difference, unless they can justify their prescribing based on exceptional circumstances peculiar to their practice.[220] This provision is likely to result in a flood of economic monitoring proceedings.

Fixed point value billing would make a vigorous WP system absolutely essential to the KKn. The institution of drug prescribing guidelines will also require tight WP oversight. It is likely that the importance of WP will greatly increase in the not too distant future. The question remains, therefore, whether the courts will permit the development of an effective WP process or whether they will interpret the statute narrowly and technically, making utilization review difficult.

D. Review of the Decisions of Arbitration Panels

To this point we have been discussing the role of the courts, especially the social courts, in resolving disputes regarding the allocation of resources in the German health care system. The primary means of resolving resource allocation disputes in the German health care system, however, is negotiation. In Germany, resource allocation policy over a wide range of issues, and in particular budgets that determine resource allocation to particular health care sectors, are determined through negotiations involving

216. 2 GKV-NOG, *supra* note 141 at § 20, to be codified at § 85(2) SGB V and § 27 to be codified at § 84 SGB V.

217. Josef Maus, *Praxisbudgets: Nur noch ein Modell für den Übergang*, 93 DEUTSCHES ÄRZTEBLATT A-1536 (1997).

218. 2 GKV-NOG, *supra* note 140, § 28 (amending § 85(2) SGB V).

219. *Id.* at § 27 (amending § 84 SGB V).

220. § 106(5a) SGB V.

the KKn on one side and provider organizations on the other.[221] Payments for hospitals, for example, are determined through negotiations between the representatives of the insurance funds and of the hospitals.[222] Budgets for payment of physicians have been negotiated between the KaVn and the state KKn associations.[223] In the past, drug budgets have been negotiated between the KaVn and the associations of *krankenkassen* (or *ersatzkassen*); in the future these same institutions will negotiate prescribing guidelines.[224] A wide range of issues other than budgets are also settled through institutional negotiations.[225]

If disputes must be settled through negotiations, however, there is always the problem of what to do when negotiations break down—when the parties can not or do not reach an agreement. The mechanism provided generally in German health insurance law is the *Schiedsstelle*.[226] *Schiedsstelle* are essentially arbitration panels. They exist at both the national and Land level in Germany, and address a wide variety of issues and problems both within and outside of the health insurance sector.[227] They impose a solution to disputes when the parties who are supposed to negotiate a solution are unable to do so. During 1996, for example, ten of the seventeen negotiations to establish the conversion value for the case and procedure payments for hospitals, discussed above, ended up before *Schiedsstelle*.[228]

Schiedsstelle generally have two types of members, partisan and nonpartisan. Each side of the contract dispute has an equal number of partisan members, who represent the interests of their institutions. The number of partisan members is usually determined by the number of sorts of insur-

221. *See* Marian Döhler & Philip Manow-Borgwardt, *Korporatisierung als gesundheitspolitische Strategie*, 3 STAATSWISSENSCHAFTEN UND STAATSPRAXIS 64 (1992).

222. § 18 KHG (*Krankenhausfinanzierungsgesetz*).

223. §§ 82, 83, 85 SGB V.

224. § 84 SGB V.

225. *See, e.g.*, § 87 SGB V, describing the contents of the national structural contract that is to be negotiated between the KaVn and the KK national association to establish the framework of health insurance medical practice.

226. *See, e.g.*, §§ 89, 114 SGB V; § 18 KHG; *see generally* Ruth Düring, *Das Schiedswesen in der gesetzlichen Krankenversicherung*, 21 ARBEITS-UND SOCZIALRECHT (1992); WOLFGANG GITTER AND MEINHARD HEINZE, DIE SCHIEDSSTELLE DES KRANKENHAUSFINANZIERUNGSGESETZS (1989).

227. *See, e.g.*, Timothy Jost, *Schlichtungsstellen and Gutachterkommissionen: The German Approach to Extrajudicial Malpractice Claims Resolution*, 11 J. ON DISPUTE RES. 81 (1996) (describing the use of *Schiedsstelle* in medical malpractice cases).

228. TUSCHEN & QUAAS, *supra* note 82, at 84-85. All of the *Schiedsstelle* decisions in these cases were appealed to the administrative courts.

ance funds affected by the negotiations, with an equal number of representatives of the provider or provider organizations. *Schiedsstelle* generally have three "non-partisan" members, including a chair, who are supposed to be appointed by both sides by agreement.[229] Neither the partisan nor the non-partisan members are bound by the instructions of those who appoint them—all are technically free agents.[230] If the parties cannot agree on an impartial chair, one is chosen by lot from the nominees of both sides.[231] As a practical matter, each side usually picks one sympathetic "impartial" member, and the chair—usually an eminent professor or retired judge—is the only member who is truly impartial.

Schiedsstelle proceedings are initiated when the parties reach an impasse in negotiations, or, with respect to hospital budget negotiations, when six weeks pass without negotiations resulting in agreement.[232] *Schiedsstellen* must act quickly—*Shiedsstelle* dealing with contracts between the KKn and doctors must resolve the issues before them and issue a final order within three months.[233] *Shiedsstelle* proceedings are not open to the public, although the parties may be present while evidence is taken.[234] Only the members of the *Schiedsstelle* are present for its deliberations, although the members may consult their constituents.[235] The *Schiedsstelle* conducts an oral hearing, hearing witnesses and experts and assembling evidence.[236] The parties have an obligation to work together with the *Schiedsstelle* and to expedite the proceedings.[237] Decisions are reached by majority vote, with each party having one vote.[238]

The chair plays a major role in the proceedings, clarifying the issues in a written opening summary, ensuring that the parties submit appropriate documents, overseeing the proceedings, and writing the decision of the panel, with appropriate justification.[239] The *Schiedsstelle* have jurisdiction only to decide issues to the extent that the parties cannot themselves reach

---

229. §§ 89(3), 114(2) SGB V. Under § 18 of the KHG, there is only one neutral party, the chair, who is appointed by agreement of the parties, or, failing that, by the Land.

230. § 18(3) KHG; § 114(3) SGB V.

231. §§ 89(3), 114(2) SGB V.

232. § 18(4) KHG.

233. § 89(1) SGB V.

234. Düring, *supra* note 226, at 108-09.

235. *Id.* at 111.

236. *Id.* at 107-08, 109-10; Meinhard Heinze, *Verfahren und Entscheidung der Schiedsstelle*, *in* GITTER & HEINZE, *supra* note 226, at 61, 66-67.

237. *Id.* at 65-67.

238. § 114(3) SGB V; § 18a(3) KHG.

239. GITTER & HEINZE, *supra* note 226, at 70-84.

agreement, and the chair and other nonpartisan members often propose settlements for the parties to consider themselves before proceeding to impose a settlement.[240] In the final vote, the partisan and party-affiliated nonpartisan members quite often take the position of their constituents, leaving the chair the deciding vote.

The decision of the *Schiedsstelle* must comply with governing law. Setting of budgets for doctors' compensation, for example, must observe the principle of premium stability, but must also assure adequate compensation.[241] The *Schiedsstelle's* decisions that set hospital budgets must first be approved by the state administration before they become legally binding.[242] In the end, decisions of the *Schiedsstelle* can be appealed to court: hospital budget decisions are appealed to the administrative courts because they affect the Länder; other health insurance decisions are appealed to the social courts. The *Schiedsstelle* have considerable discretion in reaching their decisions, however, and the bodies that review their decisions can only reject them if they violate the law.[243] *Schiedsstelle* decisions are appealed fairly often, but are usually affirmed at the trial court level and rarely appealed to higher courts.

The *Schiedsstelle* play a vital role in resolving disputes in the German health insurance system, and, ultimately in resource allocation questions. Their existence assures that negotiations will reach a conclusion. If one party fails to cooperate in the negotiation process, the dispute will go to the *Schiedsstelle* which will resolve it. Thus, parties are always under pressure to negotiate disputes when negotiation is possible. On the other hand, as budgets have become tighter in recent years, an ever increasing number of cases are ending up in the *Schiedsstelle* process.[244] The legitimacy of the process depends to a certain extent on it being a last resort. If *Schiedsstelle* resolution of disputes becomes the norm, and if disputes are consistently sufficiently divisive that most are resolved by the chair, the whole institu-

---

240. Interviews between the author and Günter Spielmeyer, head of the *Bundesschiedsamt*, June 9, 1997, and Professor Wolfgang Gitter, May 22, 1997.

241. Andreas Hustadt, *Blockieren oder Gestalten? Zur Entscheidungspraxis und Rolle der Schiedsämpter*, 77 DIE ERSATZKASSE 117, 118 (1997)

242. Gunter Kisker, *Verwaltungsrechtdogmatik zwischen Vereinbarungsprinzip und direktionsprinzip—Zur Rechtsnatur der Schiedsstelle und zur Kontrolle ihrer Entscheidungen durch Genehmigungsbehörde und Gericht*, *in* GITTER & HEINZE, *supra* note 226, at 21; Dieter Krauskopf, *Das Genehmingungsverfahren durch die Verwaltungsbehörde*, *in* GITTER & HEINZE, *supra* note 226, at 39.

243. BVerwG 6/22/95, 3 C 34-93; BVerG 1/21/93, 3 C 66.90; *see* Kisker, *supra* note 242, at 30-33.

244. A recent article reports that in 17 of 22 KzV regions, *Schiedsverfahren* were necessary to establish dental budgets in 1996. Hustadt, *supra* note 241, at 118.

tion may be called into question. One way in which *Schiedsstelle* can retain legitimacy is to limit their efforts to preservation of the status quo, to avoid innovation that would provoke controversy. The *Schiedsstelle* have indeed been criticized for their lack of creativity and for their dedication to status quo preservation.[245] Nonetheless, their contribution to maintaining a system of resource allocation based on corporate negotiation and for reducing dependence on litigation must not be overlooked.

E. Conclusion

In summary, the German courts take a very activist role in overseeing the German statutory health insurance system. On the whole, they have tended to expand coverage, as with *Hilfsmittel* and alternative and experimental treatment, and to protect the rights of individual insureds and providers, as is evidenced in judicial review of *Wirtschaftlichekeitsprüfung* decisions. When discretion is clearly and properly delegated to another decisionmaking body, as with the *Schiedsstelle*, or perhaps with the commission of doctors and insurers responsible for updating the EBM to account for new technology, the courts defer to the decisions of such bodies.

VI. The British National Health Service: Allocating by Administrative Discretion

The British National Health Service offers a striking contrast to the German systems of health care finance—in the simplicity of its organization, in its economy, and in its freedom from judicial oversight. The NHS has for five decades provided tax-financed health care in Great Britain. It is centrally organized, headed by the NHS Executive, a Branch of the Department of Health, which operates within the framework established by the Department of Health and the Policy Board.[246] Both of the latter are headed by the Secretary of State for Health, who in turn answers to Parliament.[247] Operationally, the NHS is administered through District Health Authorities located throughout Britain, which purchase health care with funds allocated to them by the NHSE.[248] The DHAs contract with local NHS Trust hospitals and with private providers to purchase secondary and tertiary health care services for their constituents, and in a very few in-

245. *Id.* at 119-20.

246. LONGLEY, *supra* note 37, at 110-13.

247. *Id.*

248. RUTH LEVITT, ANDREW WALL, & JOHN APPLEBY, THE REORGANIZED NATIONAL HEALTH SERVICE, 68-73 (1995).

stances manage their own provider units directly.[249] The DHAs have recently been merged with the Family Health Service Authorities (FHSAs), which contract with independent general practitioners (GPs) to provide primary care, either independently or as fund-holding general practices.[250] The NHS is slated for further reorganization under a plan recently put forth by the new Labor government, but will retain a separation between purchasers and providers, with purchasing power moving toward new, larger, groups of primary care providers.[251]

Resource allocation decisions are made at every level of the NHS, beginning with the initial government budgetary decision as to how much to allocate to the NHS as compared to other government departments, followed by allocations among the districts by means of a weighted capitation formula, then by distribution of funds among providers according to District priorities and purchasing arrangements, and finally rationing of resources among patients by hospital management, "consultants" or hospital doctors, and general practitioners.[252]

The NHS operates arguably one of the most efficient health care systems in the world. In 1995 Britain spent 6.9% of its GDP on health care, 5.9% in NHS spending, and 1% in private.[253] This is about one half the percentage of GDP that the United States spent on health care in the same year.[254] In terms of real spending, the difference is even more dramatic: in 1995 Britain spent $1300 per person, Germany $2840 per person, and the United States $3830 per person.[255] Every resident in the United Kingdom, however, has access to NHS care, which though it does not always meet public expectations or the standards found in countries that spend more, is on the whole adequate and in some sectors quite good. Health care in the United Kingdom must explicitly compete head to head with other public services for resources in the budget process. The NHS budget represents in a very real sense a choice taken by elected representatives of the public as to what share of the nation's resources should be dedicated to health care. By contrast, health care in the United States is paid for by a host of private and public sources (including hidden public subsidies such as tax

249. *Id.*; *see* Timothy Stoltzfus Jost, et al., *The British Health Care Reforms, the American Health Care Revolution, and Purchaser/Provider Contracts*, 20 J.HEALTH POL., POL'Y & L. 885 (1995) (examining the contracting process and contracts).

250. LONGLEY, *supra* note 37, at 124, 128-29.

251. *See* NATIONAL HEALTH SERVICE, NHS WHITE PAPER, THE NEW NHS (1997).

252. RUDOLF KLEIN, ET AL., MANAGING SCARCITY 45-48, 55-60 (1996).

253. *Britain: An Unhealthy Silence?*, ECONOMIST, March 15, 1997, at 37.

254. *Id.*

255. *Id.*

exclusions and deductions), making effective control over health care expenditures far more difficult.

The existence of and need for rationing is openly acknowledged and discussed in Britain, and much of rationing theory and technology stems from Britain.[256] One small indication of the rationality of the NHS is a recent study that found that ten of the fifty most often sold pharmaceutical products in Italy and France and six of the fifty most often sold products in Germany had no clear evidence of therapeutical effectiveness; none of the fifty most prescribed drugs in Britain fell in this category.[257]

Rationing is carried out in the United Kingdom through a host of explicit and implicit methods. Among the best known British tools for rationing are waiting lists (delay) and standards of practice that deny many persons, particularly elderly persons, services that would be available in other nations. Waiting lists for certain surgical services have existed in the United Kingdom since the foundation of the NHS, and are often seen simplistically by economists as evidence that excess demand is inevitable when supply is artificially constrained. A recent reexamination of the waiting list phenomena reveals a much more complex explanation, in which waiting lists result on the one hand from the fact that the patients on waiting lists (mostly elderly) and the conditions from which they suffer (hernias and hemorrhoids, for example) tend to be unattractive and uninteresting to hospital doctors, and on the other from the fact that physicians are often rewarded for maintaining long waiting lists by opportunities for private practice and by access to new resources.[258] Waiting lists are, nonetheless, an important tool for allocating scarce resources within the NHS.

Denial of some services, often by simple failure to mention their potential availability or usefulness, was first documented by Aaron and Schwartz in their 1984 comparison of medical practice in the United King-

256. *See, e.g.*, FRANKEL & WEST, *supra* note 30; KLIEN, ET AL., *supra* note 252; RATIONING HEALTH CARE (R.J. Maxwell, ed., 1995); BILL NEW & JULIAN LE GRAND, RATIONING IN THE NHS: PRINCIPLES AND PRAGMATISM (1996) (recent British publications discussing rationing). The classic American book which initiated discussion of rationing in the United States was a study of the NHS. HENRY J. AARON & WILLIAM B. SCHWARTZ, THE PAINFUL PRESCRIPTION: RATIONING HOSPITAL CARE (1984). The quality-adjusted life year (QUALY) approach to valuation of health care interventions was developed in England, and is now being considered throughout the world. *See, e.g.*, Arti Kaur Rai, *Rationing Through Choice: A New Approach to Cost-Effectiveness Analysis in Health Care*, 72 IND. L.J. 1015 (1997).

257. S. Garattini & L. Garattini, *Pharmaceutical prescriptions in four European Countries*, 342 THE LANCET 1191 (1993).

258. FRANKEL & WEST, *supra* note 30, at 1-14.

dom and the United States.[259] Particularly well-documented is the denial of renal dialysis to the elderly, but many coronary care units also limit admission on the basis of age.[260]

Under the internal market reforms introduced by the Conservative government in the early 1990s, rationing became more explicit. Allocations are being made under these reforms (still largely in place under the new Labor government) in the first instance by the district health authorities and reflected in their purchasing plans. Purchasing plans of the District Health Authorities increasingly explicitly exclude certain procedures, though they tend to be marginal procedures which are not major expenditure concerns, like tattoo removal and reversal of sterilization.[261] Extra-contractual referrals, referrals of patients to providers who do not have a contract with a DHA, must be approved by a DHA.[262] Though DHAs may not refuse ECRs in emergencies, the fact that they must be approved makes rationing again more explicit. Recent government proposals would do away with ECRs, but also affirm a commitment to planned purchasing.[263]

When services are denied British patients, the patients occasionally go to court. The response they meet in the courts, however, is very different from that encountered by German patients seeking judicial relief. Cases directly challenging resource allocation decisions in the NHS have almost always been unsuccessful.[264] The National Health Services Act of 1977 recognizes a principle of comprehensiveness much like that governing the German health insurance system. The Act imposes on the Secretary of State a:

> . . . duty to continue the promotion in England and Wales of a comprehensive health service designed to secure improvement (a) in the physical and mental health of the people in those countries, and (b) in the prevention, diagnosis and treatment of illness, and for that purpose to provide and secure the effective provision of services in accordance with this Act.[265]

259. AARON & SCHWARTZ, *supra* note 256.

260. KLEIN, ET AL., *supra* note 252, at 87-88.

261. *Id.* at 68-73, 140-42.

262. LONGLEY, *supra* note 37, at 139-40.

263. *See* THE NEW NHS, *supra* note 251.

264. *See* DIANE LONGLEY, PUBLIC LAW AND HEALTH SERVICE ACCOUNTABILITY 79-82 (1993); CHRISTOPHER NEWDICK, WHO SHOULD WE TREAT? 119-35 (1995) [hereinafter "Newdick, Treat"]; Christopher Newdick, *Resource Allocation in the National Health Service*, 22 AM.J.L.& MED. 291 (1997) [hereinafter "Newdick, Resource Allocation].

265. National Health Services Act, § 1 (1977) (Eng.) [hereinafter "NHSA"].

The Statutes further provides at section 3(1) that "[i]t is the Secretary of State's duty to provide . . . to such extent as he considers necessary to meet all reasonable requirements . . .," and then proceeds to list specific medical services, such as hospital accommodation, medical, dental, and nursing care, and other health services.

Although on its face the statute appears to impose upon the Secretary of State an obligation to provide medical services, the courts have generally rejected attempts to enforce the statute judicially. The first case to consider the question was *R. v. Secretary of State for Social Services, ex parte Hincks*,[266] which challenged the failure of the Health Services to construct a new orthopaedic unit in Birmingham, which had been approved by the Secretary of State in 1971 but postponed, and then abandoned in 1978. The plaintiffs alleged that the Secretary of State had failed in his duty to provide a comprehensive health service by not constructing the unit as approved. The Court of Appeals, by Lord Denning, affirmed at trial court judgment denying relief, noting that the courts could not direct the Secretary of State's decisions as to how to allocate resources among competing claimants.[267]

Subsequent cases have denied relief in cases in which: (1) a premature baby was denied an operation to repair his heart;[268] (2) a four year old boy, who needed an operation to repair his heart had had a desperately needed surgery scheduled and canceled three times;[269] and (3) a woman was denied in vitro fertilization because she was over thirty-five years of age.[270] The courts invariably in these cases review the decision of the health authority under a gross abuse of discretion standard,[271] and on this basis uphold the health authority's decision.

In the recent case of *R. v. Cambridge Health Authority ex parte B*, the lower court broke with previous deferential precedents, indicating its willingness to review the decision of a health authority. The health authority had denied B, a ten year old girl with leukemia, a bone-marrow

266. 1 BMLR 93 (1992) (decided in 1980).

267. *Id.* at 95-96.

268. R. v. Secretary of State, ex parte Walker, 3 BMLR 32 (1992) (decided 1987).

269. R. v. Central Birmingham Health Authority, ex parte Collier (unreported 1988), *reprinted in part in* IAN KENNEDY AND ANDREW GRUBB, MEDICAL LAW-TEXT AND MATERIALS 428 (1994)).

270. R. v. Scheffield Health Authority, ex parte Seale, 25 BMLR 1 (1994).

271. Under English law this is referred to as the Wednesbury standard of review. Professor Newdick describes a Wednesbury unreasonable decision as one "so unreasonable that no reasonable person addressing himself to the issue in question could have come to such a decision." Newdick, Resource Allocation, *supra* note 264, at 297.

transplant (her second), which would have cost £75,000. Judge Laws, writing for the lower court, rejected the claim of the health authority that it did not have the resources to fund the needed care, and remanded the case to the health authority to reconsider and explain its decision.[272] The case was appealed, however, to the Court of Appeals, which on the same day reversed the lower court judgment and upheld the decision of the health authority.[273] The Court of Appeals found that the medical evidence supported the Health Authority's judgment that the treatment had a low chance of success and was not advisable. The Court of Appeals maintained the tradition of limited judicial review of NHS decisions.

In *R. v. North West Thames Regional Health Authority ex parte Rhys William Daniels*,[274] the court went slightly further, holding that the action of a health authority had in fact violated the law. However, it then granted no relief. The case involved a three year old boy who needed a bone marrow transplant for the treatment of Batten's disease. The unit which was to do the transplant was closed before it could be done, and the family sued. The closure was technically illegal because the Health Authority had failed to consult the Community Health Council first, but the court further held that the closure was not irrational and that the patient's family did not have a right to be consulted before the closure. The court refused to order that the closure be reversed, or even to declare it illegal, because it held it had no power to do so.

Finally, in one recent case, *R. v. North Derbyshire Health Authority, ex parte Fisher*,[275] the court actually ordered a health authority to formulate and implement a policy making a particular treatment, Beta Interferon for Multiple Sclerosis, available. The court's decision, however, merely required the health authority to implement a circular issued by the national NHS stating that it was national policy to make the drug available, and did not challenge the health authority's discretion in making rationing decisions generally. It might indicate a greater willingness of the courts to challenge NHS rationing decisions, but it more likely means simply that in

---

272. 25 BMLR 5 (1995). Judge Laws relied in part on the European Convention on Human Rights, which requires public bodies to provide a substantial justification for decisions infringing human rights. The European Convention on Human Rights may in time prove a grounds for challenging health care rationing decisions in the United Kingdom, although this route is as of yet largely undeveloped. *See* Rhonda James and Diane Longley, *Judicial Review and Tragic Choices: Ex Parte B*, 1995 PUB. L. 367.

273. 2 All. E.R. 129 (1995).

274. Reported in *Down by Law*, HEALTH SERVICES J., August 26, 1993, at 33.

275. *Health Authority Operated Unlawful Policy*, THE TIMES (LONDON), Sept. 2, 1997, at 35. The hearing date was July 11, 1997.

making rationing decisions health authorities may not violate central resource allocation policy promulgated by the NHS through regulatory channels.

On the whole, however, the British courts, in contrast to the German courts, have refused to recognize the comprehensiveness principle as judicially enforceable with remarkable consistency. They do not interfere with rationing decisions. The courts also play no role in resource allocation disputes between payors and providers. Under the 1990 Conservative reforms, the Health Authorities, which previously had provided services through their own hospitals and other provider units, were reconstituted as purchasers. Hospitals, on the other hand, were spun off into independent NHS trusts.[276] The health authorities are now supposed to contract with the trusts (as well as with private institutions and institutions directly managed by health authorities) to purchase services.

Disputes often arise regarding the formation or interpretation of these contracts. The NHS statute states, however, that an NHS contract " . . . shall not be regarded for any purpose as giving rise to contractual rights or liabilities, but if any dispute arises with respect to such an arrangement, either party may refer the matter to the Secretary of State for determination."[277]

That is, NHS contracts are not enforceable in court, although they are subject to arbitration under the auspices of the Secretary of State. As disputes between health authorities and trusts are most severe during the contract negotiation phase (that is, they are more likely to involve the terms of the contracts being negotiated rather than enforcement of breached contracts) judicial enforcement of contracts would be of limited value in any event. In fact, not only are the terms of NHS contracts not litigated, they have only rarely resulted in formal arbitration. The Secretary of State has issued regulations establishing an arbitration procedure, but the procedure has almost never been used.[278] Rather, the parties usually rely on mediation, conciliation, or informal arbitration.[279] A major impediment to the use of arbitration seems to be the form of arbitration used—pendulum arbitration.[280] Under pendulum arbitration, the arbitrator must adopt either the solution offered by one side or that offered by the other. This approach

276. LONGLEY, HEALTH CARE CONSTITUTIONS, *supra* note 37, at 117-19.

277. NHSA, *supra* note 265, at § 4(3).

278. David Hughes, et al., *Settling Contract Disputes in the National Health Service: Formal and Informal Pathways, in* CONTRACTING FOR HEALTH 98, 106 (R. Flynn and Gareth Williams eds., 1997).

279. *Id.* at 104-10.

280. *Id.* at 111.

does not afford enough flexibility to reach the essentially management solutions necessary for resource allocation. Recent proposals for restructuring the NHS seem to contemplate even less formal arrangements between purchasers and providers, making judicial involvement even less likely.[281]

Although British courts are generally not open to complaints of patients who believe they have been improperly denied care, there are host of other avenues.[282] Procedures are available for complaints against general practitioners and there are separate procedures for complaints against hospitals.[283] The Health Service Commissioner is available as a general ombudsman when more specific complaint procedures do not apply.[284] Other specialized authorities are available for investigating other specific problems, such as mental health care.[285] The number of complaints to all sources has risen sharply in the recent past.[286]

The existence of complaint procedures underscores the fact that the NHS is a public service, answerable to the public. In some cases complaints have, in fact, made a difference. One complaint to the Health Services Ombudsman, for example, regarding a stroke patient who was refused long term care within the NHS and had to go to a private nursing home, resulted in the Ombudsman condemning the NHS policy, the health authority agreeing to pay for the cost of the patient's care, and a change in NHS policy accepting responsibility for caring for patients requiring specialist nursing care.[287] Complaint procedures, like conciliation and mediation procedures for resolving disputes with providers, allow health authorities to respond to resource demands without constraining them to respond to particular demands in precise particular ways.

The NHS also, in the end, remains accountable through malpractice litigation when resource shortages result in patient injury.[288] In *Bull v. Devon Health Authority*, for example, a hospital was found liable when lack of staffing in maternity care resulted in child suffering serious damage when its mother had to wait for over an hour for a doctor to arrive during a complicated delivery of twins.[289]

---

281. *See* THE NEW NHS, *supra* note 251.

282. *See* LONGLEY, PUBLIC LAW, *supra* note 264, at 66-79.

283. JUDITH ALLSOP & LINDA MULCAHY, REGULATING MEDICAL WORK 180-86 (1996).

284. *Id.* at 55-72.

285. *Id.* at 44-47.

286. *See* HEALTH SERVICE COMMISSIONER FOR ENGLAND, FOR SCOTLAND, AND FOR WALES, ANNUAL REPORT, 1996-97 (1997).

287. Newdick, Resource Allocation, *supra* note 264, at 305-06.

288. Newdick, Treat, *supra* note 261, at 77-118.

289. Eng. C.A. Feb. 2, 1989, *available in* LEXIS, Enggen Library, Cases File.

On the whole, however, the courts respect the discretion granted the NHS by Parliament to make its own rationing decisions free from judicial oversight. The courts defer to NHS decisions, retaining only the right, largely theoretical, to intervene if resource allocation decisions are indefensibly irrational.

VII. American Public Health Care Entitlements: Medicare and Medicaid

In contrast to the freedom the British National Health Service enjoys from judicial oversight, America's national health programs are more subject to judicial supervision. Although the United States is not commonly regarded as having "socialized medicine," it in fact operates two of the largest public health care financing systems in the world. Medicare is America's health care social insurance program. In 1995 Medicare insured about 38 million Americans, 33.4 million of who are over 65 and 4.6 million of whom are disabled, and spent about $187 billion.[290] Medicaid funds health care services for the poor: in 1995 it covered 36.3 million recipients and spent $133 billion.[291] Medicare and Medicaid program decisions limiting coverage are both subject to judicial review. The courts have taken a very different approach, however, to reviewing decisions under the two programs.

A. Medicare

Medicare is a social insurance program, resembling in many respects the social insurance programs of central Europe. It is, on the whole, more parsimonious than its European cousins. It is not based on a comprehensiveness principle: Part A (financed by payroll taxes) basically covers hospital care and related institutional services (home health, hospice services, very limited nursing facility care), and Part B (financed by general revenue funds and premiums) covers physician care, treatment by clinical psychologists or social workers, outpatient hospital care, dialysis, durable medical equipment and prosthetic devices, home health, and a few other services; but neither program covers dental care, vision care, or most prescription drugs.[292] A new Medicare Part C, established in 1997, recognizes a variety of "Medicare+Choice" managed care plans that might expand services for some Medicare beneficiaries, but are unlikely to dramati-

290. PPRC, *supra* note 40, at 126, 135.

291. Levit, et al., *supra* note 12, at 196.

292. *See* 1 HEALTH LAW, *supra* note 6, at §§ 13-5, 13-6.

cally expand coverage except insofar as they charge supplemental premiums.[293] Moreover, Medicare imposes much larger copayments than are common in Europe, as well as deductibles and length of hospital or nursing home stay time limits that are unknown in Europe.[294] Medicare is also, however, in a limited sense more generous: unlike the British National Health Service and certain sectors of the German health insurance system, it does not have a fixed budget—Medicare must pay for whatever covered services its beneficiaries consume. Medicare has thus proved very expensive.

The courts play a very limited role in the Medicare program.[295] The Medicare statute combines a strict exhaustion requirement (from which the Supreme Court has repeatedly and almost without exception refused to deviate) with an exhaustive array and exhausting sequence of administrative remedies, effectively keeping most disputes from ever reaching the courts.[296] A number of important issues, moreover, are simply removed from the jurisdiction of the courts by judicial review preclusion provisions.

Private insurers and data processors, called carriers in Part B and intermediaries in Part A, pay Medicare claims; they contract with the Health Care Financing Program to carry out this function.[297] A beneficiary or physician who has treated the patient on an assignment basis (i.e. has agreed to present the claim directly to Medicare) who is dissatisfied with a carrier decision must first request reconsideration from the carrier, and then, if $100 or more is at issue, appeal to the carrier hearing officer.[298] If the carrier's decision remains unsatisfactory, and if $500 or more is involved, the appeal can be taken to a Health and Human Services Administrative Law Judge, and ultimately to the HHS Appeals Council.[299] An in-

293. *See* Balanced Budget Act of 1997, Title IV, Pub. L. 105-33, 111 Stat. 251, 270, §§ 4000-4041 (1997).

294. Medicare beneficiaries spent $29.7 billion on Medicare copayments and deductibles for covered services in 1996, 12.9% of the total expenditures for covered Services. PPRC, *supra* note 40, at 136.

295. During 1996, the CCH Medicare and Medicaid Guide reported 109 Medicare-related cases, many of which involved fraud and abuse issues and most of which were trial court decisions. During the same year, the BSG entered judgments in 464 appeals (*Revisionen*). TÄTIGKEIT, *supra* note 90, at 24. As nearly 30% of the appeals considered by the court involved health insurance member or provider issues, *id.* at 32, the BSG almost certainly decided more cases than all reported Medicare decisions. Of course, the lower social courts decided thousands more.

296. 1 HEALTH LAW, *supra* note 6, at § 13-32.

297. 42 U.S.C. §§ 1395h, 1395u.

298. 42 C.F.R. §§ 405.807, .820.

299. 42 C.F.R. § 405.8.

dividual dissatisfied with a Part A decision can request reconsideration from the Health Care Financing Administration, followed by, if $100 or more is at stake, a hearing from an Administrative Law Judge and Appeals Council Review.[300] In most instances, an appeal can reach a federal court only after these administrative remedies have been exhausted and when $1000 or more is at stake.[301] Few do so.

Coverage disputes arise in a number of contexts under the Medicare program, three of which will be addressed here: coverage of new technology, medical necessity determinations, and determinations regarding long term care.[302] Every year, many new technologies—drugs, devices, and procedures—become available. The Medicare statute excludes from coverage services "not reasonably necessary for the diagnosis or treatment of illness or injury or to improve the functioning of a malformed body part,"[303] and has been interpreted to exclude experimental procedures.

Decisions as to whether to cover new technologies are in most instances made by carriers and intermediaries applying their own policies and criteria.[304] Decisions regarding a small number of major new technologies are made at the national level. A panel of HCFA physicians and health professionals reviews the technology and determines whether to (1) allow individual Medicare carriers or intermediaries discretion to cover or not to cover a service, (2) commission a special study (as was done with heart transplants), or (3) ask the Public Health Service to assess the technology.[305] If a technology is referred to the Public Health Service for assessment, the assessment is done by the PHS Office of Health Technology Assessment, which will publish a notice in the Federal Register asking for

300. 42 C.F.R. §§ 405.710, .720, .722, .724.

301. 42 U.S.C. §§ 405(h), 1395ff(b)(2), 1395ii; *see* Heckler v. Ringer, 466 U.S. 602, 606-07 (1984). Where only a constitutional challenge to a statute is involved, the appellant can proceed directly to federal court without exhausting remedies once the issue at stake as been presented to the government. 42 C.F.R. §§ 405.717 - 405.718e.

302. *See* 1 HEALTH LAW, *supra* note 6, at § 13-7.

303. 42 U.S.C. § 1395y(a)(1).

304. *See* Eleanor D. Kinney, *National Coverage Policy Under the Medicare Program: Problems and Proposals for Change*, 32 ST. LOUIS U. L.J. 869 (1988); PHYSICIAN PAYMENT REVIEW COMMISSION, REPORT TO CONGRESS, 1994, 113-34; GENERAL ACCOUNTING OFFICE, MEDICARE TECHNOLOGY ASSESSMENT AND MEDICAL COVERAGE DECISIONS (1994) [hereinafter "GAO MEDICARE"].

305. Louis Hays, *From the Health Care Financing Administration: Medicare Coverage*, 262 JAMA 2794 (1989). *See* Proposed Rule, Criteria and Procedures for Making Medical Services Coverage Decisions That Relate to Health Care Technology, 54 Fed. Reg. 4302 (Jan. 30, 1989).

comments, do a literature search, and reach a conclusion.[306] Although approval by the Food and Drug Administration of a drug or device does not guaranty that Medicare will pay for its use, HCFA published a rule in 1995 committing Medicare to cover devices not yet FDA approved but described as "non-experimental/investigational," i.e., devices that are modifications or improvements on existing approved devices and that are known to be safe and effective, if they otherwise meet Medicare payment requirements, such as reasonableness and necessity.[307]

Administrative and judicial review of national coverage determinations has been strictly limited since the Omnibus Budget Reconciliation Act of 1985. Administrative Law judges may not review the validity of national coverage determinations on administrative appeals.[308] Courts may not hold national coverage determinations to be invalid for failure to comply with the publication and comment requirements of the Administrative Procedure Act.[309] If a court determines that the record supporting a national coverage determination is incomplete or that information supporting the decision is otherwise lacking, the court must remand the case to HHS for further consideration, and can only determine that the item or service is covered on review of the supplemental record.[310] The cases reviewing national coverage decisions pursuant to these provisions have generally upheld the challenged coverage determination with minimal scrutiny.[311] For example, *Bosko v. Shalala*, a case challenging the refusal of HHS to reconsider its seven year old policy refusing coverage for autologous bone marrow transplantation, held that the HHS decision was supported by substantial evidence, claiming that "[t]he Medicare statute 'unambiguously vests final authority in the Secretary, and no one else, to determine whether a service is reasonable and necessary, and thus whether reimbursement should be made.'"[312] In a few cases, HCFA coverage policies not considered to be national coverage determinations have been set aside for failure

306. GAO MEDICARE, *supra* note 304. The staffing of the OHTA permits it to only do fewer than 10 studies a year.

307. 42 C.F.R. §§ 405.203, .205, .207, .209, .211.

308. 42 U.S.C. § 1395ff(b)(3)(A).

309. 42 U.S.C. § 1395ff(b)(3)(B).

310. 42 U.S.C. § 1395ff(b)(3)(C).

311. *See* Friedrich v. Secretary of Health and Human Services, 894 F.2d 829, 838 (6th Cir. 1990), Mathews v. Shalala, No. 93 Civ. 1408 DC, 1997 WL 124106, *5 (S.D.N.Y. Mar. 18, 1997); Bosko v. Shalala, No. 95-1608, 1996 WL 895356, *4 (W.D. Pa. Aug. 28, 1996).

312. *See* [1997-1 Transfer Binder] Medicare & Medicaid Guide (CCH) para. 45,139 at 53,524 (W.D. Pa. Aug. 28, 1996) (quoting New York v. Secretary of Health and Human Serv., 903 F.2d 122, 125 (2d Cir. 1990)).

to comply with the notice and publication requirements of the Administrative Procedure Act,[313] or a court has remanded a case to supplement the rule-making record.[314] Consistent with congressional intent, however, the courts have stayed on the sidelines with respect to Medicare determinations with respect to technology coverage.

A second category of coverage cases involves utilization review: review of the claims of professionals and institutions regarding the treatment of individual patients, often involving routine and non-experimental modalities. Carriers review claims made under Part B are reviewed, and Medicare Peer Review Organizations review claims regarding inpatient hospital care.[315] Claims are reviewed on both a pre- and post-payment basis, with denial resulting in non-payment for the service. Reviews are based on computer algorithms, and vaguely resemble the German efficiency review system. The appeal procedures and judicial review procedures outlined above are available for adverse utilization review determinations, and a handful of cases have ended with judicial review overturning the original denial.[316]

Two factors combine, however, to keep medical necessity issues out of both the appeal and judicial review process. The first is the "waiver of liability" provisions of the Medicare statute.[317] If a Medicare beneficiary receives services ultimately determined not to have been "reasonable and necessary," Medicare will still pay for the services if neither the beneficiary nor the person who provided the service "knew, or could reasonably have been expected to know," that the services were excluded from coverage.[318] Beneficiaries are presumed not to have knowledge of noncoverage absent written notice,[319] but providers are expected to know that services are excluded from coverage on the basis of "HCFA notices, including manual issuances, bulletins, or other written guides or directives from in-

313. *See* Linoz v. Bowen, 800 F.2d 871, 878 (9th Cir. 1986); Cedars-Sinai Med. Ctr. v. Shalala, 939 F. Supp. 1457, 1465 (C.D.Cal. 1996).

314. *See* American Lithotripsy Soc'y v. Sullivan, 785 F. Supp. 1034, 1037 (D.D.C. 1992).

315. *See* Timothy P. Blanchard, *"Medical Necessity" Denials as a Medicare Part B Cost-Containment Strategy: Two Wrongs Don't Make it Right or Rational*, 34 ST. LOUIS U. L.J. 939 (1990); Alice G. Gosfield, *Slouching Toward the Millennium: False Claims in Medicare Physician Billing*, *in* HEALTH LAW HANDBOOK, 1997, 51, 76-82) (Alice G. Gosfield ed.) [hereinafter "1997 Handbook"].

316. *See* Alice G. Gosfield, *Part B Physician Reimbursement Development, Limits, and Pitfalls*, *in* 1990 HEALTH LAW HANDBOOK 275, 308-09 (Alice G. Gosfield ed.).

317. 42 U.S.C. § 1395pp; 42 C.F.R. § 411.400.

318. 42 C.F.R. § 411.400(a)(2).

319. 42 C.F.R. § 411.404.

termediaries, carriers or PROs," Federal Register notices of national coverage decisions, or "acceptable standards of practice in the local community."[320] If the provider is deemed to have knowledge of noncoverage, but the patient is not, the provider may neither bill Medicare nor the patient for the cost of the service, and must refund any money collected from the patient.[321] A physician who believes that a service is not covered by Medicare may inform the patient of that fact, and provide the service at the patient's cost if the patient agrees to pay for it independently,[322] but there are, of course, risks in telling a patient that he or she must pay for a service because Medicare considers it unreasonable or unnecessary.[323] In the end, the most likely effect of the "waiver of liability" provisions is to create an incentive for physicians to err on the side of not providing, or even offering, services when necessity might become an issue.

This incentive is strengthened by a second phenomena, the recent dramatic increase in Medicare fraud prosecutions. Federal law provides a plethora of criminal, civil, and administrative penalties for false claims. A doctor who submits a false claim commits a felony,[324] is subject to both civil and administrative fines of three times the amount claimed plus $5000 to 10,000 per claim,[325] and, if convicted of a felony, can be excluded from the Medicare program and from other federal and state health care programs for five years or more.[326] Claims submitted for unnecessary services are false claims. The false claims acts are increasingly being used to police billing practices.[327] A recent Office of Inspector General investigation involving over 100 teaching hospitals challenged as fraudulent the hospital's billing for the use of investigational devices for treating Medicare patients.[328] There are undoubtedly many professionals and providers who continue to bill for services of questionable necessity; the payment system still rewards this. But the risks of doing so are increasing, as are the incentives to deny services. Patients denied care, however, because the doctor simply fails to mention the possibility of a service (because the doctor fears denial of payment and of liability waiver on the one hand or

320. 42 C.F.R. § 411.406(e).

321. 42 C.F.R. § 411.402.

322. 42 U.S.C. § 1395u(l)(C)(ii).

323. *See* Blanchard, *supra* note 315, at 1015-21.

324. 18 U.S.C. §§ 287, 1347; 42 U.S.C. § 1320a-7b(a).

325. 31 U.S.C. § 3729(a); 42 U.S.C. § 1320a-7a.

326. 42 U.S.C. §§ 1320a-7(a)(1).

327. *See* Gosfield, *supra* note 315, at 51.

328. Sanford V. Teplitzky and S. Craig Holden, *1996 Developments in Health Care Fraud and Abuse*, *in* 1997 HANDBOOK, *supra* note 310, at 35-36.

false claims prosecution on the other) cannot appeal the denial, much less seek judicial review. Thus, judicial review is likely to play a smaller role in these cases, except insofar as fraud cases become trials on medical necessity.[329]

The courts have been most active in the final category of disputes considered here: cases involving long term care. Medicare does not pay for "custodial care,"[330] and a host of cases have addressed the question of whether a beneficiary in a hospital or nursing home was simply receiving "custodial care."[331] These cases generally involve retroactive denials of large sums of money, and often both the provider and beneficiary have a strong incentive to appeal. The cases are fact intensive and depend on the patient's "total condition."[332] Courts tend to go along with the finding of the patient's physician that the patient needed skilled, and not simply custodial, care,[333] but other courts recognize that the treating physician often stands to gain from a decision for the patient and that his or her testimony must therefore be discounted.[334] A related issue is the meaning of a need for "part-time and intermittent care," a statutory requirement for home health services.[335] *Duggan v. Bowen*,[336] in which the court found HHS's restrictive definition of the term to be arbitrary and capricious and contrary to law, as well as promulgated in violation of the Administrative Procedure Act, is one of the most successful attempts to use the courts to extend Medicare coverage policy.[337]

Duggan and the custodial care cases, however, are the exception rather than the rule. By and large, restrictions on judicial review, layer upon layer of administrative remedies, incentives built into the system to

329. Recent fraud and abuse amendments provides civil penalties for false claims where there is a pattern of billing for services that "a person knows or should know are not medically necessary." 42 U.S.C. § 1320a-7a(a)(1)(E).

330. 42 U.S.C. § 1395y(a)(9); 42 C.F.R. § 411.15(g).

331. 1 HEALTH LAW, *supra* note 6, at § 13-7.

332. *See* Ridgely v. United States, 475 F.2d 1222, 1224 (4th Cir. 1973); Whitman v. Weinberger, 382 F. Supp. 256, 263 (E.D.Va. 1974).

333. *See* Ridgely, 475 F.2d at 1224; Breeden v. Weinberger, 377 F. Supp. 734, 737 (M.D.La. 1974).

334. *See* Goodrich v. Richardson [1974 Transfer Binder] Medicare and Medicaid Guide (CCH) para. 26,885 (E.D.Pa. 1974).

335. 42 U.S.C. § 1395x(m)(4).

336. 691 F. Supp. 1487, 1514 (D.D.C. 1988).

337. *See* Eleanor D. Kinney, *The Role of Judicial Review Regarding Medicare and Medicaid Program Policy: Past Experience and Future Expectations*, 35 ST. LOUIS U. L.J. 759, 783-84 (1991). OBRA 1997 enacts into law an expanded definition of coverage sought by the plaintiffs in *Duggan*. *See* Pub. L. 105-33, 111 Stat. 336, § 4012.

encourage providers to police coverage themselves, and the sheer mind-numbing complexity of the Medicare statute have operated in tandem to keep the courts from playing a significant role in Medicare coverage issues.[338] They have mainly operated at the margins, occasionally straightening out procedural deficiencies in Medicare decision-making, but have left to Congress and the administrative agencies the job of running the program.

B. Medicaid

Compared to the limited judicial involvement in Medicare coverage decision-making, judicial involvement in the Medicaid program has been quite generous, both in terms of its extent and its results. Medicaid is the federal/state program that finances health care for some of America's poor. Historically, Medicaid eligibility was tied to eligibility for cash welfare programs—the program covered the elderly, disabled, blind, and families with dependent children. Over time, however, Medicaid has been transformed into a program that increasingly pays for care for both elderly and disabled persons with serious and chronic medical conditions who require high cost care and poor children and pregnant women, who require relatively low cost, but cost-effective care.[339] The majority of program funding comes from the federal government, and federal statutes and administrative rules and issuances govern the state programs.[340] The states participate in the program voluntarily, contributing from about twenty to fifty percent of program cost, but none have been able or willing to forgo the federal money the program brings. The federal statute requires coverage of certain eligibility groups and the provision of particular benefits, but the states have considerable discretion in deciding whether or not to cover optional groups or to provide optional benefits.[341] In fact, Medicaid programs vary significantly in size and scope from state to state.[342]

338. They have played a somewhat more active role in payment issues, where the considerable resources of providers and their associations are more often brought to bear.

339. *See* BARRY FURROW, ET AL., HEALTH LAW 865-67 (3d ed. 1997); Sandra J. Tanenbaum, *Medicaid Eligibility Policy in the 1980s: Medical Utilitarianism and the "Deserving" Poor*, 20 J. HEALTH POL., POL'Y & L. 933 (1995).

340. FURROW, ET AL., HEALTH LAW, *supra* note 339, at 881.

341. *Id.* at 870.

342. A 1995 GAO report on Medicaid reported that Nevada served 284 Medicaid beneficiaries for every 1,000 poor or near-poor individuals in the state, whereas Rhode Island served 913 per 1,000. Similarly , Mississippi spent, on average, less than $2400 per person on Medicaid services, while New York spent an average of almost $7,300 per person. GENERAL ACCOUNTING OFFICE, MEDICAID, SPENDING PRESSURES DRIVE STATES TOWARD PROGRAM REINVENTION (1995).

The Medicaid statute requires states to cover a fairly short list of services: inpatient and outpatient hospital services; laboratory and X-ray services, nursing facility and home health services for adults, physicians' services, nurse-midwife and legally authorized nurse practitioner services, and early and periodic screening, diagnostic, and treatment services (EPSDT) for children, and a few others.[343] A wide range of optional services can be covered by the states, however, and because Medicaid recipients often have no other means to purchase health care services, and coverage of optional services brings federal dollars, many states cover a number of optional services.[344]

Although states have considerable discretion as to deciding what services to cover at the macro level, their discretion is much more limited with respect to provision of services to individual patients at the micro level. The federal courts, following dicta in an early Supreme Court decision, have consistently read the Medicaid statute as requiring coverage of available services deemed "medically necessary."[345] This has generally been interpreted to mean services deemed necessary by the recipient's treating physician.[346] Under the federal regulations, each Medicaid-covered service "must be sufficient in amount, duration, and scope to reasonably achieve its purpose."[347] A state "may not arbitrarily deny or reduce the amount, duration, or scope of a required service . . . to an otherwise eligible recipient solely because of diagnosis, type of illness or condition."[348] The EPSDT provisions explicitly define EPSDT, a mandatory service for children under twenty-one, to include "necessary health care, diagnostic services, treatment, and other measures . . . to correct or ameliorate defects and physical and mental illnesses and conditions discovered by the screening services, whether or not such services are covered

343. 42 U.S.C. § 1396a(a)(10)(A); 1396d.

344. *See* MEDICARE AND MEDICAID GUIDE, *supra* note 312, para. 15,500 for a state by state list of coverage.

345. *See* Beal v. Doe, 432 U.S. 438, 444-45, (1977) (stating that "serious statutory questions might be presented if a state Medicaid plan excluded necessary medical treatment from its coverage.").

346. *See* Pinneke v. Preiser, 623 F.2d 546, 550 (8th Cir. 1980) (stating that the decision of whether or not certain treatment or a particular type of surgery is "medically necessary" rests with the individual recipient's physician and not with clerical personnel or government officials"). *See also* Weaver v. Reagen, 886 F.2d 194, 200 (8th Cir. 1989); Rush v. Parham, 625 F.2d 1150, 1157 (5th Cir. 1980); Visser v. Taylor, 756 F. Supp. 501, 507 (D. Kan. 1990).

347. 42 C.F.R. § 440.230(b).

348. 42 C.F.R. § 440.230(c).

under a state plan."[349] Several courts have further held, however, that states cannot refuse to provide services to persons over twenty-one and that they must provide under EPSDT to those under twenty-one.[350] A provision in the federal statute requiring that "assistance shall be furnished with reasonable promptness to all individuals"[351] has been interpreted to mean that provision of necessary benefits cannot be deferred or delayed by the states.[352] Finally, some courts have simply held state Medicaid limitations to be "unreasonable."[353]

The most important factors influencing judicial involvement in Medicaid coverage disputes, however, may be jurisdictional rather than substantive. Unlike the Medicare program, where layer upon layer of administrative remedies must be exhausted before the beneficiary can get to court (if judicial review is available at all), the Medicaid recipient can go directly into federal court. The courts have long recognized the right of Medicaid recipients to sue state programs that have allegedly deviated from federal program requirements under 42 U.S.C. § 1983.[354] In *Wilder v. Virginia Hospital Association*,[355] the Supreme Court recognized the right of providers to sue directly as well. Some members of the Supreme Court seem eager to cut back on federal court jurisdiction over benefit program disputes,[356] and the latest Supreme Court precedents could be interpreted as undermining direct access to the courts.[357] However, a recent federal statute, although it is very poorly drafted, seems to support congressional intent to keep the federal courts open to recipients,[358] and attempts in the

349. 42 U.S.C. § 1396d(r)(5).

350. *See* Fred C. v. Texas Health & Human Serv. Comm'n, 924 F. Supp. 788, 792 (W.D. Tex. 1996) (durable medical equipment); Hunter v. Chiles, 944 F. Supp. 914, 919 (S.D. Fla. 1996); McDaniel v. Betit [1996-2 Transfer Binder] Medicare & Medicaid Guide (CCH) para. 44,473 (D.Utah 1996) (organ transplantation); Salgado v. Kirschner, 878 P.2d 659, 660 (Ariz. 1994) (organ transplantation).

351. 42 U.S.C. § 1396(a)(8).

352. *See* Smith v. Miller, 665 F.2d 172, 174 (7th Cir. 1981); McMillan v. McCrimon, 807 F. Supp. 475, 480-81 (C.D. Ill. 1992).

353. *See* Skubel v. Fuoroli, 113 F.3d 330, 336-37 (2d Cir. 1997).

354. *See* Maine v. Thiboutot, 448 U.S. 1, 5-6 (1980); Rand E. Rosenblatt, *The Courts, Health Care Reform, and the Reconstruction of American Social Legislation*, 18 J. HEALTH POL., POL'Y AND L. 439, 444-49 (1993).

355. *See* 496 U.S. 498, 524 (1990).

356. *See* Rosenblatt, *supra* note 354, at 456-68.

357. *See* Suter v. Artist M., 503 U.S. 347, 362 (1992).

358. 42 U.S.C. § 1320a-2; *see* Cherry v. Thompson, [1995-2 Transfer Binder], Medicare and Medicaid Guide (CCH) para. 43,485 (S.D. Ohio. 1995) (interpreting statute in Medicaid claim context); *see also* Brian D. Ledahl, *Congress Overruling the Courts:*

1995 federal budget bill to eliminate federal jurisdiction in Medicaid disputes failed to become law.[359]

The federal courts normally do not require exhaustion of state Medicaid program administrative remedies as a condition precedent to litigation.[360] Many benefit disputes, moreover, come before the federal courts on motions for preliminary injunctions, brought by desperate recipients who have been denied treatment that their treating physicians consider necessary.[361] These cases focus the court starkly on the irreparable injury the plaintiff faces, and often allow the plaintiff to obtain the desired service on a simple showing of likelihood of success on the merits.[362] Because the Eleventh Amendment prohibits damage awards against the states if benefits are improperly denied, the courts have all the more incentive to order the award of benefits prospectively to avoid the need for retrospective relief.[363]

Because Medicaid is a state as well as a federal program, recipients also have the option of suing in state court to obtain benefits. State court suits are most likely to be brought where state law or state judges are more sympathetic to the recipient's claim, and plaintiffs therefore win a significant proportion of these cases.[364] A number of state courts, for example,

---

Legislative Changes to the Scope of Section 1983, 29 COL. J.L. & SOC. PROB. 411 (1996).

359. *See* Balanced Budget Act of 1995, H.R. 2491, § 2154(e)(1) (1995) (prohibiting judicial review of state Medicaid plans under federal law except by the Secretary of HHS.) A recent court of appeals decision, however, holds that federal regulations requiring the states to provide particular Medicaid services not required by statute are not enforceable under 42 U.S.C. § 1983. *See* Harris v. Patton, 127 F.3d 993, 1012 (11th Cir. 1997).

360. *See* Tallahassee Mem'l Reg'l Hosp. v. Cook, 109 F.2d 693, 702 (11th Cir. 1997); Visser, 756 F. Supp. at 504.

361. *See, e.g.*, Mair v. Barton, [1987 Transfer Binder] Medicare & Medicaid Guide (CCH) para. 36,692, *available in* 1987 WL 108989 (D Kan. July 27, 1987).

362. *See, e.g.*, DeSario v. Thomas, 963 F. Supp. 120, 132 (D. Conn. 1997).

363. The courts also recognize that Medicaid recipients lack the financial capacity to pay for services up front and sue for reimbursement later. *See* Dodson v. Parham, 427 F. Supp. 97, 108 (N.D.Ga. 1977).

364. *Cf.* state court cases granting denied benefits: Jackson v. Stockdale, 264 Cal. Rptr. 525, 532 (Cal. Ct. App. 1989) (root canal treatment and crowns); Persico v. Maher, 465 A.2d 308, 322 (Conn. 1983) (orthodontic dental services for minor); McCoy v. Idaho,, 907 P.2d 110, 115 (Idaho 1995) (gastric bypass surgery for obesity); Biewald v. Maine, 451 A.2d 98, 102 (Me. 1982) (urine testing materials); Buhs v. State Dept. of Pub. Welfare, 306 N.W.2d 127, 132 (Minn. 1981) (chiropractic X-rays); Kirk v. Dunning, 370 N.W.2d 113, 115 (Neb. 1985) (periodontal treatment); Monmouth Med. Ctr. v. State Dept of Pub. Welfare, 403 A.2d 487, 494 (N.J. 1979) (hospital services); A.M.L. v. Dept. of Health, 863 P.2d 44, 48 (Utah 1993) (breast reduction for patient with lupus); with cases denying treatment: Holmes v. Kizer, 13 Cal. Rptr. 2d 746, 755 (Cal. App.

have held that Medicaid beneficiaries have a state constitutional right to abortion, even though federal funding for most abortions is banned.[365]

The federal courts have quite consistently supported recipient claims to Medicaid services. Federal courts have, for example, required state coverage of sex-change operations,[366] access to off-formulary drugs,[367] augmentive communication devices,[368] Clozaril for the treatment of schizophrenia,[369] and AZT treatment for AIDS.[370] Even when optional services are at issue, the courts hold that the states that have opted to offer a service cannot deny it to persons who need it. States that provide eye-glasses for post-cataract surgery patients, for example, must also provide them for patients with serious refractive error.[371] Courts have also reserved the right to review state determinations that a procedure is "experimental" and thus not covered.[372]

Where there are specific federal limitations on Medicaid coverage, the courts have tended to interpret these quite conservatively and to order states to provide coverage where it is not prohibited. Congress has repeatedly imposed strict limits on the availability of Medicaid funding for abortions, for example, but the federal courts have consistently required the states to fund medically necessary abortions to the extent not prohibited by federal law.[373] When Congress recently expanded Medicaid abortion

1992) (marijuana); Viveros v. State Dept. of Health and Welfare, 889 P.2d 1104, 1107 (Idaho 1995) (surgery to reduce and reshape child's ears); Anderson v. Dept. of Soc. Servs., 300 N.W.2d 921, 926 (Mich. 1981) (root canal).

365. *See* Right to Choose v. Byrne, 450 A.2d 925, 941 (N.J. 1982); Moe v. Secretary of Admin. and Fin., 417 N.E.2d 387, 485 (Mass. 1981); Committee to Defend Reprod. Rights v. Myers, 172 Cal.Rptr. 866, 886 (Cal. 1981).

366. *See* Pinneke v. Preisser, 623 F.2d 546, 550 (8th Cir. 1980).

367. *See* Dodson, 427 F. Supp. at 111.

368. *See* Hunter v. Chiles, 944 F. Supp. 914, 922 (S.D.Fla. 1996); Fred C., 924 F. Supp. at 792.

369. *See* Visser, 756 F. Supp. at 507.

370. *See* Weaver, 886 F.2d at 199-200; Mair, [1987 Transfer Binder] Medicare & Medicaid Guide (CCH) para. 36,692, *available in* 1987 WL 108989.

371. *See* Ledet v Fischer, 638 F. Supp. 1288, 1293 (M.D. La. 1986); *see also* White v. Beal, 555 F.2d 1146, 1152 (3d Cir. 1977); Simpson v. Wilson, 480 F. Supp. 97, 103 (D. Vt. 1979) (state programs that provide glasses for persons with eye diseases must also provide them for persons with refractive error).

372. *See* Miller v. Whitburn, 10 F.3d. 1315, 1320-21 (7th Cir. 1993); Meusberger v. Palmer, 900 F.2d 1280, 1283-84 (8th Cir. 1990); Weaver, 886 F.2d at 198.

373. *See* Elizabeth Blackwell Health Ctr. v. Knoll, 61 F.3d 170, 184 (3rd. Cir. 1995), *cert. denied*, 116 S.Ct. 816 (1996); Hern v. Beye, 57 F.3d 906, 913 (10th Cir. 1995), *cert. denied*, Weil v. Hern, 116 S.Ct. 569 (1995); Preterm v. Dukakis, 591 F.2d 121, 134 (1st Cir. 1979).

funding to cover abortions in rape and incest cases, for example, the courts required state expansion as well.[374]

Cases involving coverage of organ transplantation under EPSDT also illustrate this tendency. As discussed above, the EPSDT program requires the states to provide necessary medical treatment services to children, including presumably organ transplantation where necessary. 42 U.S.C. § 1396b(i)(1), on the other hand, requires the states, as a condition of federal funding, to promulgate written standards respecting coverage of organ transplantation that treat similarly situated individuals alike and that provide that restrictions on facilities and practitioners which may provide organ transplantation are "consistent with the accessibility of high quality care to individuals eligible for the procedures under the State plan." Several federal courts have interpreted these provisions as giving the states discretion over the extent to which their Medicaid programs will cover organ transplantation.[375] Other courts, however, have read these provisions as subordinate to the general requirement that Medicaid cover necessary organ transplants, and have ordered transplants not available under state law.[376] Still others have interpreted state standards as covering[377] or potentially covering[378] organ transplants in situations where the state had denied coverage.

State Medicaid agencies seeking to limit Medicaid coverage have been most successful in federal litigation challenging coverage limitations when they have imposed across-the-board utilization restrictions, for example, limiting length of coverage for hospital stays[379] or restricting coverage to three physician visits a month.[380] Although these usage restrictions could have an equally devastating effect on recipients as denials of specific

374. *See* Knoll, 61 F.3d at 184; Hern, 57 F.3d at 913.

375. *See* Dexter v. Kirschner, 984 F.2d 979, 987 (9th Cir. 1992); Ellis v. Patterson, 859 F.2d 52, 55 (8th Cir. 1988); *see generally* Lisa Deutsch, *Medicaid Payment for Organ Transplants: The Extent of Mandated Coverage*, 30 COL. J.L.& SOC. PROB. 185 (1997); C. David Flower, *State Discretion in Funding Organ Transplants under the Medicaid program: Interpretive Guidelines in Determining the Scope of Mandated Coverage*, 79 MINN. L. REV. 1233 (1995); David L. Weigert, *Tragic Choices: State Discretion over Organ Transplant Funding for Medicaid Recipients*, 89 NW. L. REV. 268 (1994).

376. *See* Pittman v. Florida Dept. Health & Rehab. Serv's, 998 F.2d 887, 892 (11th Cir. 1993); Pereira v. Kozlowski, 996 F.2d 723, 727 (4th Cir. 1993).

377. *See* Meusberger, 900 F.2d at 1283.

378. *See* Miller, 10 F.3d at 1320-21 (remanded to determine if liver-bowel transplant properly characterized as "experimental").

379. *See* Charleston Mem'l Hosp. v. Conrad, 693 F.2d 324, 330 (4th Cir. 1982); Virginia Hosp. Ass'n v. Kenley, 427 F. Supp. 781, 786 (E.D. Va. 1977).

380. *See* Curtis v. Taylor, 625 F.2d 645, 652-53 (5th Cir. 1980).

services, courts ultimately recognize the authority of states to place some limits on program expenditures, and tend to see this as a reasonable approach.[381] The Supreme Court has rejected challenges to such limitations based on their disproportionate effect on disabled persons.[382] Even in cases completely rejecting challenges to limitations of services by Medicaid agencies, however, courts have required state compliance with due process notice and hearing requirements to permit challenges to individual applications of the rule.[383]

Although recipients have enjoyed considerable success when they have brought judicial challenges to Medicaid coverage policy, such challenges are nevertheless relatively rare. By definition, Medicaid recipients cannot afford medical care, and they cannot afford legal representation either. Although legal services programs have represented some in the past, funding for legal services for the poor has become ever more restrictive. Medicaid is moving quickly to managed care, and is encouraged to do so by recent federal legislation.[384] Although Medicaid managed care plans must provide grievance and appeal procedures,[385] the structures and incentives of managed care plans will render less frequent the situation most likely to result in a favorable judicial decision: the patient and her doctor aligned against a state bureaucracy. Judicial activism in the Medicaid program has had a significant impact on the program, however, and is in marked contrast to the restrained role the courts have played in the Medicare program.

VIII. Private Insurance Coverage in the United States: From Contract to Administrative Law

The volume of litigation involving private insurance coverage in the United States, though not nearly as great as in Germany, is larger than the volume of public insurance cases, and rapidly increasing.[386] This litigation is unlike that involved in all other programs discussed so far, because it is, at least in theory, based on contract rather than on statutes and regulations.

381. *But see* Montoya v. Johnson, 654 F. Supp. 511, 514 (W.D. Tex. 1987) (rejecting $40,000 cap on inpatient hospital expense payments as impermissible).

382. *See* Alexander v. Choate, 469 U.S. 287, 308-09 (1985).

383. *See* Cherry v. Thompkins, [Transfer Binder 1995-2] Medicare and Medicaid Guide (CCH), para. 43,385 (S.D. Ohio March 31, 1995).

384. Pub. L. 105-33, 111 Stat. 278 , §§ 4701-4710 (1997).

385. 42 U.S.C. § 1932(b)(5).

386. *See* Mark Hall, et al., *Judicial Protection of Managed Care Consumers: An Empirical Study of Insurance Coverage Disputes*, 26 SETON HALL L.REV. 1055, 1060-61 (1996).

For the past decade, these cases have generally involved high cost therapies sought by patients with critical illnesses (often women with breast cancer), which therapies have been refused by insurers and claims administrators who assert that the therapies are experimental and of unproven value. The rationing issues raised by the cases (as well as the issues they present regarding the appropriate role of markets, regulators, and professionals in health care resource allocation, federalism, dispute resolution, and gender discrimination) have resulted in a considerable body of academic commentary.[387]

Historically, health insurance coverage disputes were litigated only rarely. They often involved marginal therapies or dubious medical value, as insurers would normally cover therapy if it was ordered by a reputable physician.[388] When disputes arose, they were generally decided under rather straightforward contract law principles.[389] The insured commonly won, even in some rather extreme cases, as the courts would apply the principle of *contra proferentum* to interpret vague and ambiguous contracts in the insureds favor, or interpret clauses in light of the insured's "reasonable expectations."[390] In some jurisdictions, the emerging law of bad faith breach of insurance contracts gave the insured the benefit of tort as well as

387. *See generally* MARK A. HALL, MAKING MEDICAL SPENDING DECISIONS: THE LAW, ETHICS, & ECONOMICS OF RATIONING MECHANISMS 68-73 (1997); RAND E. ROSENBLATT, ET AL., LAW AND THE AMERICAN HEALTH CARE SYSTEM 139-292 (1997); John H. Ferguson, et al., *Court-Ordered Reimbursement for Unproven Medical Technology: Circumventing Technology assessment*, 269 JAMA 2116 (1993); Margaret Gilhooley, *Broken Back: A Patient's Reflections on the Process of Medical Necessity Determination*, 40 VILL. L. REV. 153 (1995); Mark A. Hall & Gerard F. Anderson, *Health Insurers' Assessment of Medical Necessity*, 140 U. PA. L. REV. 1637 (1992); Comment, Barbara A. Fisfis, *Who Should Rightfully Decide Whether a Medical Treatment Necessarily Incurred Should be Excluded from Coverage under a Health Insurance Policy Provision Which Excludes from Coverage "Experimental" Medical Treatments*, 31 DUQ. L. REV. 777 (1993); Comment, J. Gregory Lahr, *What is the Method to Their "Madness?" Experimental Treatment Exclusions in Health Insurance Policies*, 13 J. CONTEMP. HEALTH L. & POL'Y 613 (1997); Richard S. Saver, *Reimbursing New Technologies: Why are the Courts Judging Experimental Medicine?*, 44 STAN. L. REV. 1095 (1992); Comment, Denise S. Wolf, *Who Should Pay for "Experimental" Treatments? Breast Cancer Patients v. Their Insurers*, 44 AM. U. L. REV. 2029 (1995).

388. *See* 1 HEALTH LAW, *supra* note 6, at § 11-2; Hall & Anderson, *supra* note 387, at 1645-46.

389. 1 HEALTH LAW, *supra* note 6, at § 11-2.

390. Hall & Anderson, *supra* note 387, at 1648-49; Saver, *supra* note 387, at 1100-03; Einer Elhauge, *The Limited Regulatory Potential of Medical Technology Assessment*, 82 VA. L. REV. 1525, 1549-52 (1996).

contract law, and raised the stakes for insurers who denied coverage.[391] In others, state insurance mandates denied insurers the discretion to refuse to cover certain services.[392]

In the late 1980s, however, several factors changed the nature of insurance contract disputes.[393] For one thing, the stakes got higher: disputes became focused on cutting edge therapies that cost tens, if not hundreds, of thousands of dollars.[394] As insurance markets became more competitive, insurers may have become more aggressive in denying coverage for such procedures.[395] Disputes also increasingly involved preadmission or preprocedure utilization review denials, rather than retrospective payment denials, and thus presented much more urgently and immediately the need for treatment.[396] Disputes began to focus less on therapies commonly regarded as quackery or as excessive and unnecessary, and more on therapies that came from the mainstream of medical practice, even if they remained arguably experimental in nature.[397] Finally, and most importantly, the disputes largely moved from state court, where they were litigated as contract and tort law claims, to federal court, where the disputes are litigated under the Employee Retirement Income Security Act of 1974.[398]

ERISA is a law adopted in the 1970s to protect the security of pensions.[399] Incidentally, however, the law regulates employee benefit as well as pension plans, including health benefit plans. ERISA preempts any state law that relates to an employee benefit plan.[400] State laws that regulate insurance, including insurance benefit mandates,[401] are saved from

391. *See* Aetna Life Ins. Co. v. Lavoie, 505 So.2d 1050, 1053 (Ala. 1987); Hughes v. Blue Cross, 263 Cal. Rptr. 850, 857-58 (Cal. Ct. App. 1989); 1 HEALTH LAW, *supra* note 6, at § 11-3.

392. 1 HEALTH LAW, *supra* note 6, at § 11-4.

393. *See* ROSENBLATT, ET AL., *supra* note 387, at 212-13; Hall & Anderson, *supra* note 387, at 1644-62.

394. The cost of Autologous Bone Marrow Transplantation for breast cancer, the most frequently litigated issue in recent years, ranges from $80,000 to $150,000 GENERAL ACCOUNTING OFFICE, HEALTH INSURANCE, COVERAGE OF AUTOLOGOUS BONE MARROW TRANSPLANTATION FOR BREAST CANCER 3 (1996) [hereinafter "GAO COVERAGE"].

395. Hall & Anderson, *supra* note 387, at 1658-62.

396. *Id.* at 1644-57.

397. *Id.* at 1651-57.

398. 29 U.S.C. §§ 1001 *et seq.*

399. *See* Daniel M. Fox & Daniel C. Schaffer, *Health Policy and ERISA: Interest Groups and Semipreemption*, 14 J. HEALTH POL, POL'Y & L., 239 (1989) (setting forth history of ERISA preemption).

400. 29 U.S.C. § 1144(a).

401. *See* Metropolitan Life Ins. Co. v. Massachusetts, 471 U.S. 724, 758 (1985).

preemption.[402] Self-insured employee benefit plans, however, are deemed not to be insurance for purposes of state regulation, and are thus solely regulated by federal law.[403] In large part because of this provision, sixty percent of employees in large firms are now in self-insured plans.[404] ERISA also totally preempts tort claims involving denials of insurance benefits.[405] These claims are regarded as based on state law that "relates to" benefit plans, and are thus preempted under ERISA. They are not, however, laws that "regulate insurance," and are thus not saved from preemption under ERISA's savings clause.[406] ERISA allows defendants to remove insurance claim benefit cases to federal court, where most courts have held that they are to be tried without a jury.[407] As most private health insurance in the United States is obtained as an employment benefit, insurance claims disputes are increasingly being tried in federal courts under ERISA.

Although many issues involving ERISA remain hotly contested, the outline of ERISA law as it affects insurance claims disputes is becoming clear. ERISA permits a beneficiary covered by ERISA plans to bring a civil action "to recover benefits due to him under the terms of his plan, to enforce his rights under the terms of the plan, or to clarify his rights to future benefits under the terms of the plan."[408] It does not permit recovery of extra-contractual or punitive damages, but does allow prevailing plaintiffs (or defendants) to recover costs and attorney's fees.[409] Beneficiaries must exhaust plan remedies before pursuing judicial remedies.[410]

Under the Supreme Court's decision in *Firestone Tire and Rubber Company v. Bruch*, benefit determinations made by plan fiduciaries and

402. 29 U.S.C. § 1144(b)(2)(A).

403. 29 U.S.C. § 1144(b)(2)(B).

404. Gregory Acs, et al., *Self-Insured Employer Health Plans: Prevalence, Profile, Provisions, and Premiums*, 15 HEALTH AFF., Summer 1996, at 266, 269.

405. *See* Pilot Life v. Dedeaux, 481 U.S. 41, 57 (1987). Malpractice claims, alleging substandard medical care, are not preempted by ERISA, and can be brought against managed care plans that provide medical care directly either on corporate negligence or vicarious liability theories free from ERISA preemption. *See* Dukes v. United States Healthcare, Inc. 57 F.3d 340, 354 (3rd. Cir. 1995) *cert. denied* 116 S.Ct. 564 (1995). However, benefit denials, even by managed care plans, are preempted, *see id.* at 356; Cannon v. Group Health Serv., 77 F.3d. 1270, 1274-75 (10th Cir. 1996).

406. *See* Dedeaux, 481 U.S. at 57.

407. *See* Turner v. Fallon Community Health Plan, 953 F. Supp. 419, 422-23 (D. Mass. 1997).

408. 29 U.S.C.A. § 1132(a)(1).

409. 29 U.S.C. § 1132(g)(1).

410. *See* Hall v. National Gypsum Co., 105 F.3d 225, 231 (5th Cir. 1997); Denton v. First Nat'l Bank, 765 F.2d 1295, 1300 (5th Cir. 1985).

administrators are generally subject to de novo review by the courts.[411] The Court adopted this standard because it saw ERISA plans as fiduciaries, and considered a de novo review standard as appropriate for judicial review of fiduciary decisions.[412] Where the terms of benefit plans, however, give plan administrators and fiduciaries "discretionary authority to determine eligibility for benefits or to construe the terms of the plan," however, the Supreme Court observed that a more deferential form of review was appropriate—plan decisions should be upheld unless they are "arbitrary and capricious."[413] Health plans are now customarily written, therefore, to allow substantial discretion to the health plan in determining benefits.[414] Health plans that retain discretion to make coverage decisions win significantly more coverage cases than those that do not.[415]

Even where the plan retains discretion in making benefit determinations, however, the Supreme Court in *Bruch* suggested that courts should review determinations more closely where the plan administrator or fiduciary faces a conflict of interest.[416] This proposition poses a conundrum. From one perspective, plan administrators always face a conflict of interest, as an important part of their job is to preserve plan assets to assure coverage for other plan beneficiaries, keep premiums low, and, in some instances, to make a profit for the plan.[417] Even if an administrator does not bear risk, it may deny claims because its continued position as a plan manager depends to some extent on its success in keeping the costs faced by

---

411. *See* Firestone Tire & Rubber Co. v. Bruch, 489 U.S. 101, 115 (1989). Questions of law, including interpretation of contracts, are also subject to de novo review. *See* Fuja v. Benefit Trust Life Ins. Co., 18 F.3d 1405, 1409 (7th Cir. 1994).

412. *See* Firestone, 489 U.S. at 113.

413. *See id.* at 113; *see, e.g.*, Maune v. International Bhd, 83 F.2d 959, 962-63 (8th Cir. 1996) (applying standard).

414. Where the contract does not expressly grant the health plan discretion, the courts apply the de novo review standard to health plan decisions. *See* Marro v. K-III Communications, 943 F. Supp. 247, 250-251 (E.D.N.Y. 1996). Courts also require that plan language clearly and unequivocally give the plan discretion. *See* Adams v. Blue Cross/Blue Shield, 757 F. Supp. 661, 666-67 (D. Md. 1991).

415. Hall, et al., *supra* note 386, at 1063.

416. *See* Firestone, 489 U.S. at 115.

417. *See* Pitman v. Blue Cross & Blue Shield, 24 F.3d 118, 123 (10th Cir. 1994); Brown v. Blue Cross & Blue Shield, 898 F.2d 1556, 1561 (11th Cir. 1990); *see*, arguing that insurer's interest conflicts are not a serious problem, Hall & Anderson, *supra* note 387, at 1668-70. Treating physicians, who normally testify for plaintiffs in coverage dispute cases, also usually face a conflict of interest, as they are unlikely to be paid for a procedure unless the insurer approves it. *See* Estate of Goldstein v. Fortis Benefit Co., *available in* 1996 WL 18977, *5 (N.D. Ill. Jan. 19, 1996); Hall & Anderson, *supra* note 387, at 1066-68.

the risk bearing employer under control and because it may not want to set a precedent for coverage for its risk-bearing business.[418] Courts have adopted several different approaches to resolving cases once a conflict is found.[419] Some courts have adopted a continuum approach, under which they consider the degree of conflict faced by the plan administrator or fiduciary and adjust the level of review accordingly,[420] while other courts have adopted a two step approach, first deciding whether a substantial conflict exists, then placing the burden on the fiduciary to prove that its decision was not tainted by self-interest.[421] The Second Circuit has recently applied yet another test, considering whether the conflict of interest in fact influenced the insurers decision.[422]

Ultimately, whatever standard a court applies, it is left with the job of interpreting a contract and applying its terms to the facts of the case. In doing so, some courts apply common law principles, such as *contra proferentum*,[423] or trust law principles, resolving ambiguities in favor of the beneficiary.[424] Other courts, however, have concluded that state common law of insurance contract interpretation is preempted by ERISA, including the principle of *contra proferentum*, and that the courts should read insurance contracts without favoring either party.[425]

Treating private insurance coverage disputes as contract disputes is problematic, however. Coverage cases are in most instances brought by patients who have not in fact negotiated the contract directly with the insurer. Normally the contract is between the insurer and the beneficiary's

418. *See* Reilly v. Blue Cross & Blue Shield United, 846 F.2d 416, 424 (7th Cir. 1988); ROSENBLATT, LAW & ROSENBAUM, *supra* note 387, at 240.

419. *See* Velez v. Prudential Health Care Plan, 943 F. Supp. 332, 340-41 (S.D.N.Y. 1996).

420. *See* Martin v. Blue Cross & Blue Shield, 115 F.3d 1201, 1206 (4th Cir. 1997); Doe v. Group Hosp. & Med. Servs., 3 F.3d 80, 87 (4th Cir. 1993); Van Boxel v. Journal Co. Employees' Pension Trust 836 F.2d 1048, 1052-53 (7th Cir. 1987).

421. *See* Brown, 898 F.2d at 1566-67; *see also* Atwood v. Newmont Gold Co. Inc. 45 F.3d 1317, 1322-23 (9th Cir. 1995).

422. *See* Whitney v. Empire Blue Cross & Blue Shield, 106 F.3d 475, 477 (2d Cir. 1997); Sullivan v. LTV Aerospace & Defense Co., 82 F.3d 1251, 1255-56 (2d Cir. 1996).

423. *See* Lee v. Blue Cross/Blue Shield 10 F.2d 1547, 1551 (11th Cir. 1994); Doe v. Group Hospitalization & Med. Serv, 3 F.3d 80, 89 (4th Cir. 1993); Heasley v. Beldern & Blake Corp., 2 F.3d 1249, 1257-58 (3rd Cir. 1993); Masella v. Blue Cross & Blue Shield, 936 F.2d 89, 107 (2d Cir. 1991).

424. *See* Blair v. Metropolitan Life Ins. Co., 974 F.2d 1219, 1222 (10th Cir., 1992).

425. *See* Brewer v. Lincoln Nat'l Life Ins. Co., 921 F.2d 150, 153-54 (8th Cir. 1990); Allen v. Adage, Inc., 967 F.2d 695, 701 (1st Cir. 1992); Hammond v. Fidelity & Guar. Life Ins. Co., 965 F.2d 428, 430 (7th Cir. 1992).

employer, and not infrequently the dispute involves a clause added in a rider or policy modification of which even the employer may not have been fully aware.[426] When providers sue, they are even more distant beneficiaries of the initial contract.[427] In making some decisions, insurers apply internal policies not in fact included in their contracts.[428] Even when an individual policy is involved, the dispute rarely involves truly negotiated terms, but rather interpretation of forms provided by the insurer.

The courts seem intuitively to recognize these facts. The cases increasingly resemble more judicial review of the reasonableness of regulatory actions imposed on beneficiaries than an attempt to interpret and apply negotiated contract terms.[429] Cases in which insureds prevail often involve arbitrary insurer conduct, much like that condemned in administrative review proceedings. The largest number of disputes, for example, concern autologous bone marrow transplantation (ABMT) for treatment of breast or other cancers.[430] Although insurers have more often than not approved ABMT claims,[431] insurers have often rejected claims for ABMT for breast cancer, one of the most common forms of cancer, while allowing it for treatment of less common cancers, where the success of using the ABMT might be better established, but also where fewer potential cases are involved, and thus the costs of the therapy over time are less. Therapy has been often rejected under open-ended criteria, which allow insurers to make these distinctions, but which appear suspicious to the courts.[432] Courts are also troubled when insurers provide minimal information to patients regarding denials, change the basis of a denial after it is challenged, or otherwise fail to address requests reasonably.[433] Also, conduct of insurers who deny ABMT to women with breast cancer, while approving its use

426. *See, e.g.*, Martin, 115 F.3d at 1202 (small employer claimed that Blue Cross had never provided it with a copy of the insurance contract); Bushman v. State Mutual Life Assurance Co., 915 F. Supp. 945 (N.D.Ill. 1996) (plaintiff claimed to have bought policy based on representations at marketing meeting that it was "equal to or better than" prior policy, and did not get copy of policy until three months after it was in effect.).

427. *See* 1 HEALTH LAW, *supra* note 6, at § 11-9.

428. *See* Pirozzi v. Blue Cross-Blue Shield, 741 F. Supp. 586, 590 (E.D.Va. 1990).

429. *See* Murphy v. Wal-Mart Assoc. Group Health Plan, 928 F. Supp. 700, 705 (E.D. Tex. 1996); *see*, advocating this approach, Hall & Anderson, *supra* note 387, at 1698-709.

430. *See*, listing many of the cases, Whitney v. Empire Blue Cross & Blue Shield, 920 F. Supp. 477, 482 n.5 (S.D.N.Y. 1996), *vacated & remanded*, 106 F.2d 475 (2d Cir. 1997); *see also* Saver, *supra* note 387, at 1111-18.

431. *See generally* Peters & Rogers, *supra* note 208.

432. *See* Whitney, 920 F. Supp. at 486; Wolf, *supra* note 387, at 2063-72.

433. *See* Velez, 943 F. Supp. at 341-43 (S.D.N.Y. 1996); Wolf, *supra* note 387, at 2072-74.

for men with testicular cancer, for example, raises interesting gender discrimination issues.[434] On the other hand, insurers that follow reasonable procedures and apply reasonable substantive criteria are likely to prevail. Health plans that use independent panels of experts for making decisions, or that rely on the decisions of external technology assessment bodies, or that have generous procedures for grievances and appeals are likely to win.[435]

Insurers seem to be winning more cases in federal court under ERISA than in the state courts under state contract and insurance law.[436] In particular, they do significantly better in the federal appeals courts, where the courts focus more on the law, which is on the whole favorable to the insurers, and less on the pathetic facts presented by individual dying patients.[437] At the trial court level, however, (and particularly where preliminary injunctions are sought) many courts are still concerned with the dire conditions of claimants, and put off by the callousness or ineptness of some insurers.[438] They are also impressed by persuasive expert testimony supporting the insured's claims.[439] Even when they rule for insurers, they often do so decrying the fact that statutory law forces them to do so.[440] But as private law coverage disputes rely less on contract law, and more on in-

434. Wolf, *supra* note 387, at 2086-89.

435. *See* Martin, 225 F.3d at 1207-09 (insurer extensively reviewed literature before denying claim); Santucci v. Hyatt Corp., 955 F. Supp. 927, 930 (N.D. Ill. 1997) (insurer used independent expert reviewers); Healthcare Am. Plans, Inc. v. Bossemeyer, 953 F. Supp. 1176, 1178-85 (D. Kan. 1996) (elaborate contract and review procedure); Bushman , 915 F. Supp. at 946-47 (contract specifically listed covered procedures, not including that sought). *See*, discussing ideal experimental treatment exclusion language, David Eddy, *Benefit Language: Criteria that will Improve Quality While Reducing Cost*, 275 JAMA 650 (1996). (Proposed treatment reviewed by panel of two highly qualified experts completely independent of insurance company). Courts will also enforce policy provisions requiring disputes to be submitted to arbitration. *See* Davenport v. Blue Cross, 60 Cal.Rptr. 2d 641, 648 (Cal. Ct. App. 1997).

436. *See* Hall, et al., *supra* note 386, at 1062; Wolf, *supra* note 387, at 2062.

437. Hall, et al., *supra* note 386, at 1064; *see, e.g.*, Parks v. Blue Cross & Blue Shield, 116 F.3d 485 (9th Cir. 1997) *available in* 1997 WL 303308, *3; Fuja, 18 F.3d at 1412; Maune v. International Bhd of Elec. Workers, 83 F.3d 959, 964 (8th Cir. 1996).

438. *See* Marro v. K-III Comm., 943 F. Supp. 247, 251-53 (E.D.N.Y. 1996); Hall and Anderson, *supra* note 387, at 1676; *see* Velez, 943 F. Supp. at 338 (holding that preliminary injunction ordering payment of benefits was prohibitory rather than mandatory, since it prohibited the insurer from "interference with vested contract rights.").

439. *See, e.g.*, Pirozzi, 741 F. Supp. at 591-93.

440. *See* Fuja, 18 F.3d at 1407; Bushman, 915 F. Supp. at 953-54; *see also* Andrews-Clarke v. Travelers, *available in* 1997 U.S. Dist. LEXIS 17390 (Oct. 30, 1997) (court in dismissing state law suit against an insurer for wrongful denial of claim removed into federal court describes ERISA as "ridiculous" and "disturbing").

terpretation of statutes, and review of the reasonableness of the decisions of increasingly sophisticated insurers, claimants seem to be losing with increasing frequency.

IX. Conclusion

All developed nations rely on some form of third party payment—social insurance systems, national health services, commercial insurance—for financing health care services. Because such services and the resources needed to purchase them are scarce, inevitably someone is denied services he or she desperately wants, and perhaps desperately needs. Providers are often, moreover, refused payment for services they have provided to their patients or believe that their patients need. Patients and providers denied services or the funds to purchase services often have plausible legal claims—statutory, regulatory, or contractual—to the denied services or funds. Sooner or later these claims end up in court. The victims of rationing turn to the judiciary as their last hope.

The vast majority of instances of rationing are never challenged in court, of course. Rationing is often effected by mechanisms that do not present a clear refusal or denial of a service that is subject to judicial review. These mechanisms include deterrence (potential patients are discouraged from seeking services by geographic inaccessibility or unfriendly receptionists, providers are discouraged from providing services by utilization reviewers whose phone and fax lines are always busy), deflection (patients are steered away from the service they need to less expensive services or to services that some other agency will pay for), delay (including queues for services and endless requests for more information), or dilution (patients get the rationed service, only less of it).[441] Only a very tiny fraction of express decisions to deny or to terminate services, moreover, are challenged in court, even in countries like Germany that have an active system of judicial review.

Judicial challenges to service denials, however, have a greatly disproportionate impact on subsequent resource allocation decisions. Although many decisions to deny ABMT for the treatment of breast and other cancers were challenged in court in the United States in the late 1980s and early 1990s, most insurers in fact approved payment for this service during that time,[442] and many did so to avoid potential litigation.[443] Judicial over-

441. *See* KLEIN, ET AL., *supra* note 252, at 11-12.

442. Peters & Rogers, *supra* note 208. In 1990, the national Blue Cross/Blue Shield organization agreed to fund clinical trials to be carried out under the auspices of the Na-

sight of the *Wirtschaftlichkeitsprüfung* system in Germany has largely determined the forms which that process has taken. Even in Britain, where the courts have in most instances refused to get directly involved in resource allocation decisions, the government has from time to time revised its policies once they were challenged.[444]

It is obvious, of course, that the courts under consideration here are not fungible. England has no written constitution, a strong civil service, and a relatively weak tradition of substantive judicial review or administrative decisions.[445] German social court tribunals include representatives of insureds or insurance doctors, are specifically constituted to decide social benefits questions, and operate in an environment of strong constitutional review. American courts draw on both a heritage of judicial independence and a tradition of deference to decisions made by contracting individuals, legislatures and even administrative agencies.

Even if the courts we have considered are not fungible, they are comparable. They are trying to accomplish the same task—reviewing the coverage decisions of payors. And they going about it the same way—determining contested facts and applying law (as found in statutes, regulations, or contracts) to the facts to resolve coverage disputes.

The role of courts in resource allocation decisions in the United States with respect to private insurance has been widely noted. A number of commentators have observed that the courts tend to support insureds at the expense of insurers, and that they tend to say "yes" rather than "no."[446] This study, examining the decisions of courts in a variety of health care systems in response to a variety of claims, reveals a more complex and textured picture.

It seems to be true that if courts are asked whether a service claimed by a patient or provided by a provider is "necessary" or "appropriate," they

---

tional Cancer Institute to study the effectiveness of ABMT. ROSENBLATT, ET AL., *supra* note 387, at 253-54.

443. *See* GAO, *supra* note 394, at 9; *see also* Claudia A. Steiner, et al., *Technology Coverage Decisions by Health Care Plans and Considerations by Medical Directors*, 35 MED. CARE 472, 480 (1997) (stating that potential legal challenges is a significant consideration in coverage decisions).

444. Newdick, Resource Allocation, *supra* note 264, at 303, 306.

445. *See* PETER SHEARS AND GRAHAM STEPHENSON, JAMES' INTRODUCTION TO ENGLISH LAW 136 (1996) (stating that to be reversed by a court on grounds of irrationality, an administrative decision must "be so outrageously unreasonable that no sensible person who had applied his mind to the question to be decided could have arrived at it.").

446. Elhauge, *supra* note 21, at 1550-56; Hall, *supra* note 386 at 68-73; Hall & Anderson, *supra* note 387, at 1674-81; Saver, *supra* note 387, at 1100-03.

tend to answer affirmatively.[447] In such decisions, the court has before it an ill or injured patient in a truly pathetic situation, whose immediate and pressing claim for services is to be weighed against the abstract and theoretical claims of persons not present, or of an impersonal organization that commands considerable resources.[448] Judges are, like other decisionmakers, more sensitive to the needs of identified than statistical persons.[449] Courts are also troubled by the conflicts of interest faced by payors, which are obligated to pay for care required by the claimant, but also are concerned with their own profits and the needs of other insureds. Courts are less likely to attend to the conflict faced by the treating physician, who testifies that care he offers the patient is urgently needed.

If, however, the courts are asked to defer to another decisionmaking body, they will in most instances willingly do so. The most obvious example of this is Britain, where the courts seem almost bewildered when asked to review NHS resource allocation decisions, given the high degree of discretion afforded the NHS in these matters.[450] Courts seem much less likely to intervene in Medicare decisions, where there are layers and layers of administrative review, than in decisions of the Medicaid program, where there is no exhaustion requirement. In Germany, courts are much less likely to reject decisions of the *Shiedsstelle*, which are granted broad discretion by law, than the decisions of the insurers themselves. While courts sometimes protest their impotence in these situations, they nonetheless defer as the law requires.[451]

Finally, and not surprisingly, courts are also capable of constraining their desire to help patients in need when a statute, regulation, or contract requires them to consider factors other than need. The German social courts, for example, have proved adept at applying complex criteria in deciding claims to *Hilfsmittel*; the American federal courts have enforced statutory limits on Medicaid abortion coverage and upheld state regulations limiting utilization of Medicaid services where federal regulations permit states this discretion.

447. Mark Hall's empirical study also found that insureds win well over half the time in coverage disputes. Hall, *supra* note 386, at 1062.

448. Hall & Anderson, *supra* note 387, at 1676-77.

449. *See* Max Mehlman, *Rationing Expensive Lifesaving Medical Treatments*, 1985 WISC. L. REV. 239, 253-56 (1985).

450. Hall's study of judicial review of insurance coverage in the United States, however, also found that the level of success of patients dropped dramatically when the insurer retained discretion in making coverage decisions. Hall, *supra* note 386, at 1063.

451. *See* cases cited *supra* note 440.

In the end, the most important question is what role courts should play in making coverage decisions. Institutionally, courts are particularly well adapted to particular tasks, such as resolving claims of right or involving the application of laws, regulations, or contracts to proposed conduct (e.g., is a particular medical device covered under the health insurance law) or disputes based on claims of fault involving the interpretation of past conduct (e.g., was a doctor's performance in the past "uneconomic").[452] Twenty years ago, Professor Lon Fuller in a germinal article noted that courts are less adept at resolving complex disputes regarding multiple parties and policy considerations, and "interacting points of influence," such as more global disputes regarding the allocation of resources within a health care system.[453] Such "polycentric" disputes involve intricate networks of many persons, facts, and issues and cannot readily be presented to or resolved by a court.[454] They are also focused on economic and political interests rather than on rights.[455] Resolution of some disputes or issues affects others; institutions and approaches are needed that can incorporate a more global perspective on the range and relationship of issues than can courts.

Such disputes are often resolved prospectively through legislative or regulatory processes.[456] Legislatures and regulatory agencies are equipped to hold hearings involving many parties and issues and to arrive at complex solutions addressing both factual and policy disputes. Each of the health care systems discussed in this article has developed administrative mechanisms for managing some resource allocation issues: the *Schiedsstelle* in Germany; the District Health Authority priority setting and negotiations processes in Britain; the Medicare technology assessment process or increasingly sophisticated technology assessment programs of major insurers in the United States.

Whether we should turn to such processes or to the courts for decisions depends on what we want to accomplish. If our primary goal is protecting the interests of patients, we should assure early and liberal access to the courts. The German statutory insurance system, imbued with a tradition of comprehensive coverage and service to patients, has traditionally embraced this alternative. If, on the other hand, we are more concerned

452. Henry H. Perrit, Jr., *And the Whole Earth was One Language: A Broad View of Dispute Resolution*, 29 VILL. L. REV. 1221, 1228 (1984).

453. *See generally* Fuller, *supra* note 19.

454. *Id.* at 394-395. The idea was borrowed by Fuller from the writings of Michael Polanyi.

455. Perrit, *supra* note 452, at 1229.

456. Fuller, *supra* note 19, at 398.

with limiting health care expenditures, then the role of the courts should be sharply limited, and managerial processes accentuated, as in Britain.

It is possible, however, both to retain and restrain judicial oversight of health care rationing decisions. This can be accomplished by creating expert review bodies that are responsible for reviewing denials of services in the first instance, requiring exhaustion of administrative remedies, but allowing judicial review in the end. It may be difficult to achieve the "right" level of judicial scrutiny, as courts have a tendency to withdraw from the field once administrative review becomes available, but our evidence also suggests that courts will carry out policy that is clearly articulated by legislation or contract.

This study suggests a host of models for intermediate review mechanisms: arbitration panels, complaint mechanisms, administrative law judges, and grievance panels to name a few. The technology is available. It is up to us, however, to make use of it, to construct a system that will allocate scarce resources, and that will do so justly.

Resource Allocation and Vulnerable Groups

[20]

LIFE STYLE, HEALTH STATUS, AND DISTRIBUTIVE JUSTICE

Robert L. Schwartz†

ONLY A FEW years ago the American system for providing health care was considered rather benign — an inevitable consequence of American values. Over the past few years, however, the increased amount of our resources allocated to health care — now about fourteen percent of the gross domestic product[1] — and the consistently high levels of those people not covered by even that very high expenditure — fifteen percent across the United States, and up to twenty-five percent in some states[2] — have made the system simply unacceptable. To put it simply, the cost of health care and the widespread lack of access to it have become a national

---

† Professor of Law, University of New Mexico. B.A., Stanford University; J.D. Harvard School of Law. The author appreciates the commentary and editorial assistance offered by Pam Lambert, Margaret Caffey-Moquin, Karen Kingen and Jessica Sutin.

1. George D. Lundberg, *National Health Care Reform: The Aura of Inevitability Intensifies*, 267 JAMA 2521, 2522 fig. 2 (1992). This is a remarkable increase over the 12% figure for the previous year. *See* E. BROWN, HEALTH USA: A NATIONAL HEALTH PROGRAM FOR THE UNITED STATES DEPARTMENT OF COMMERCE, 1991 UNITED STATES INDUSTRIAL OUTLOOK 44-1-11-6 (1991). Dr Lundberg, editor of the Journal of the American Medical Association, views the increase in the resources spent on health care as an "extreme" that is "unacceptable". Lundberg, *supra* at 2522. The amount of our national resources spent on health care has increased regularly and substantially over the past forty years.

> National expenditures on health care have increased from $12.7 billion in 1950 to $41.9 billion in 1965 to $647 billion in 1990. Per capita spending on medical care has grown from $82 per year in 1950 to $211 in 1965 to $2511 in 1990 . . . Between 1980 and 1988, the medical care component of the consumer price index increased 85% compared to a general increase of inflation of 43% . . . Americans spend more on health care than they spend on groceries, owner-occupied housing, or transportation.

BARRY R. FURROW ET AL., HEALTH LAW 661 (2d ed. 1991).

2. Medicaid, which is the primary program designed to cover the poor, covers fewer than half of the people under the federal poverty line. FURROW ET AL., *supra* note 1, at 529. *See also*, Geraldine Dallek, *Health Care for America's Poor: Separate and Unequal*, 20 CLEARINGHOUSE REV. 361 (1986). New Mexico, the state with the highest percentage of its population without any form of private or public coverage, only recently brought that percentage down to one-fourth of its residents. GOVERNOR'S HEALTH POLICY ADVISORY COMMITTEE, HEALTH FOR THE FUTURE: A PROPOSED HEALTH POLICY FOR NEW MEXICO 9 (1988). *See also*, KATHLEEN BROOK ET AL., HEALTH INSURANCE COVERAGE IN NEW MEXICO 10 (1991). When the underinsured are added to the uncovered, the number may rise to one-fourth the population of the entire country. Pamela J. Farley, *Who are the Underinsured?*, 63 MILBANK MEMORIAL FUND Q. 476 (1985).

scandal.[3]

As this scandal has unfolded, we have reacted to it just as we react to most other scandals that manifest themselves during political years; we have begun our search for scapegoats. Indeed, we have rounded up the usual suspects — some people blame the problems on insurance companies[4], others blame the problem on lawyers and the legal system[5], still others blame the problem on greedy, profit driven private enterprise and the existence of the market mechanism for the delivery of health care[6], and yet others blame it on bureaucratic government regulation of that market.[7] Doctors,

3. With the American Medical Association and the American Hospital Association joining virtually every other national organization that deals with health care financing in calling for dramatic health care reform, it is hard to find any support for the current structure. Presidential candidates are fighting with each other over the structure that ought to replace the current financing system, but there is no disagreement that the current system provides inadequate access at excessive cost. The only question is which kind of substantial change will be most effective. As Dr. Lundberg points out:

> At least 57 national and state legislative proposals for health care reform have been filed; major components of the Republican and Democratic platforms will deal with health care reform. Presidential contenders have already developed their postures regarding health care reform . . . With President Bush having entered the discussion, the reality of reform seems assured. The only questions now are what, how much, how soon, how incremental, how complete, how effective, and how long-lasting.

Lundberg, *supra* note 1, at 2521. He suggests that "[m]ajor political change in a democratic republic such as ours comes about when a cluster of forces temporally coalesces to form a critical political mass of sufficient strength to power that change," something that has now happened with our health care system. *Id. See also* Robert J. Blendon et al., *Making the Critical Choices*, 267 JAMA 2509 (1992) (discussing substantive questions that must be addressed by any new system).

4. *See, e.g.*, Kevin Grumbach et al., *Liberal Benefits, Conservative Spending: The Physicians for a National Health Program Proposal*, 265 JAMA 2549 (1991).

5. Not surprisingly, this is a central part of the American Medical Association's entry into the health care reform sweepstakes. *See* James A. Todd et al., *Health Access America — Strengthening the US Health Care System*, 265 JAMA 2503 (1991) (reviewing problems with current insurance availability in the United States and proposing reforms to improve access and quality of health care). Limited access to health care is also one of the myriad of social ills that President Bush blames on lawyers and the legal system. George Bush, The President's Comprehensive Health Reform Program 50 (1992).

6. *See e.g.*, Rand E. Rosenblatt, *Health Care, Markets, and Democratic Values*, 34 Vand. L. Rev. 1067 (1981); Bruce C. Vladeck, *The Market vs. Regulation: The Case for Regulation*, 59 Milbank Memorial Fund Q. 209 (1981); and Robert G. Evans, *Tension, Compression, and Shear: Directions, Stresses and Outcomes of Health Care Cost Control*, 15 J. Health Pol., Pol'y & L. 101 (1990). *See also* Arnold S. Relman, *What Markets Are Doing to Medicine*, Atlantic Monthly 98, 106 (1992) (warning that "if physicians continue to allow themselves to be drawn along the path of private entrepreneurship, they will increasingly be seen as self-interested businessmen and will lose many of the privileges they now enjoy as fiduciaries and trusted professionals").

7. *See e.g.*, James F. Blumstein, *Rationing Medical Resources: A Constitutional, Legal and Policy Analysis*, 59 Tex. L. Rev. 1345 (1981) and James F. Blumstein & Frank A. Sloan, *Redefining Government's Role in Health Care: Is a Dose of Competition What the Doctor*

medical schools, hospitals, drug companies — all have been alleged to be culpable for the scandal of our health care system.

The newest and most original scapegoat upon which we can place the blame for the high cost of health care are those whose life style choices puts their health or lives at risk. Of course, if our health care cost and access problems are a consequence of unhealthy choices made by autonomous individuals, we are relieved of the obligation of figuring out how to reform our health care delivery system. In that case, the solution to our health care problem is obvious — we merely need to impose appropriate penalties on those who make costly, immoral and unhealthy life style choices.

The call for some kind of mechanism that would make people pay for the health consequences of their life style choices is coming from a variety of sources. Some physicians have announced that they will automatically reject alcoholic liver transplant candidates, or put them lower on the priority list, because their moral fault — their alcoholism — caused them to need the transplant.[8] At least one state has attempted to deny Medicaid funding for liver transplants for former alcoholics unless they can prove abstinence for at least two years prior to the transplant.[9]

Employers are cashing in on this trend as a way to save insurance dollars. For example, Circle K stores proposed denying coverage for all employee health claims resulting from self-induced conditions; they would deny coverage for the results of drug or alcohol abuse, self-inflicted wounds, and AIDS (unless it can be proven that it was acquired by transfusion).[10] Several employers pay larger motor vehicle accident death benefits to an employee's family if the employee was wearing a seat belt during the fatal accident.[11] Some companies charge employees who smoke more than other employees to participate in their group health plan;[12] Turner

---

Should Order? 34 VAND. L. REV. 849, 852 (1981). *See also* CLARK C. HAVIGHURST, DEREGULATING THE HEALTH CARE INDUSTRY: PLANNING FOR COMPETITION (1982).

8. Gregory Tetrault, *The Morality of Transplantation*, 266 JAMA 213 (1991). *See also* Carl Cohen & Martin Benjamin, *Alcoholics and Liver Transplantation*, 265 JAMA 1299 (1991).

9. Allen v. Mansour, 681 F. Supp. 1232 (E.D. Mich. 1986).

10. *See* George Will, *Who Should Insure Our Lifestyle Choices?*, WASH. POST, Aug. 11, 1988, at A21 (discussing policy to deny employee coverage for certain ailments). *Also see*, Jaime Fernandez, *The Folly of Basing Health Insurance on "Lifestyle Choices"*, WASH. POST, Aug. 20, 1988, at A21 (responding to the article by George Will).

11. Laurie Cohen, *Wanted: Healthier Workers; More Companies Give Rewards for Staying Well*, CHI. TRIB., Jan. 6, 1992, at B1.

12. *Id.*

Broadcasting refuses to hire any employee who smokes;[13] and the United States Senate has considered a Medicare Part B premium surcharge for smokers.[14] Haggar Apparel Company pays only 60% of the cost of prenatal care (rather that the 100% otherwise standard) if the pregnant employee or family member delays seeking prenatal medical care after she becomes aware of her pregnancy.[15] The state of Delaware plans to implement a scheme later this year under which it would charge unhealthy state employees more for group health insurance than it charges other employees.[16]

The courts have already confronted some of these attempts to hold individuals responsible for their health status. Turner Broadcasting has not been required to hire smokers.[17] Michigan may not impose a two year sobriety rule to refuse liver transplants to Medicaid patients who were alcoholics. All Medicaid recipients must be treated on the basis of medical necessity.[18] Other attempts to make patients, employees, aid recipients, and the insured financially responsible for their medical conditions or to deny them care for these conditions altogether are certainly bound for Congress, state legislatures, the courts, and union-management negotiation tables.

I. THE RANGE OF LIFE STYLE CHOICES AND THEIR CONSEQUENCES ON HEALTH STATUS

If all of those whose life style choices have health consequences were required to bear the full burden of those consequences, there would be few of us (and few diseases or injuries) that would not be implicated. While the medical hazards of smoking and alcohol consumption are well known,[19] the medical consequences of other kinds of action are less established or less obvious. Helmetless mo-

13. Dan Cordtz, *For Our Own Good*, FIN. WORLD, Dec. 10, 1991, at 48.

14. David Durenburger, *Financing Health Care for an Aging Population*, WASH. POST, April 14, 1987, at Z14.

15. Cordtz, *supra* note 13.

16. Cohen, *supra* note 11.

17. Christine Woolsey, *Off-duty Conduct: None of the Employer's Business?*, BUS. INS., Feb. 17, 1992, at 10.

18. Allen v. Mansour, 681 F. Supp. 1232 (E.D. Mich. 1986).

19. The Office of Technology Assessment estimates the cost of smoking in the United States at over $65 billion per year, with $22 billion attributable to health care costs and $43 billion attributable to lost productivity. For an analysis of the costs of alcohol to society *see William R. Miller*, THE EFFECTIVENESS OF ALCOHOLISM TREATMENT MODALITIES: TESTIMONY TO THE U.S. SENATE COMMITTEE ON GOVERNMENTAL AFFAIRS, in 2 CAUSES AND CONSEQUENCES OF ALCOHOL ABUSE 158 (1989). Willard G. Manning et al., *The Taxes of Sin: Do Smokers and Drinkers Pay Their Way?*, 261 JAMA 1604 (1989) (discussing the consequences of smoking and alcohol use and their costs for society).

torcyclists[20] and bicyclists[21] and drivers who do not wear seat belts put their lives at risk;[22] obese and sedentary people put their health at risk.[23] Those who consume excess fat or insufficient fiber have increased risk of some kinds of cancers[24] (and, possibly, heart disease). Even former President Bush risks some kinds of cancer when he refuses his broccoli. On the other hand, those who eat too many carbohydrates run the risk of the most common disease, dental cavities.[25] Those who engage in unprotected sex run the risk of several different illnesses;[26] those who engage in protected sex run risks from certain types of protection;[27] those who engage in no sexual

20. Allen Short, *Collision Course: State Must Pass Helmet Law for Motorcyclists or Face Funding Cut*, MINN. STAR TRIB., Mar. 1, 1992, at A1 (citing estimates by the General Accounting Office that indicate that motorcycle riders with helmets have fatality rates as much as 70% lower than those without helmets).

21. According to one study done at Allegheny General Hospital in Pittsburgh, 50,000 children were injured in bicycle-related accidents in 1990, and over 1,000 died. Eighty five percent of the injuries could have been avoided through the use of bicycle helmets. *Asides and Insides in Healthcare*, CHI. TRIB., Dec. 8, 1991, at 44. *See also* Robert Thompson et al., *A Case - Control Study of the Effectiveness of Bicycle Safety Helmets*, 320 NEW ENG. J. MED. 1361 (1989). *See generally*, A JONES ET AL., COST OF INJURY IN THE UNITED STATES; A REPORT TO CONGRESS 115-16 (1989).

22. The Chairman of the National Transportation Safety Board has estimated that 18,087 lives were saved in 1990 as a direct result of mandatory seat belt laws. *See* Bill McAllister & Evelyn Richards, *Nine States Targeted on Seat Belt Laws*, WASH. POST, Sept. 20, 1991, at A25.

23. *See* W.B. Kannel & Tavia Gordon, *Physiological and Medical Concommitants of Obesity: The Framingham Study, reprinted in* OBESITY IN AMERICA 125 (George A. Bray, ed., 1979).

24. The increased risk is not just the risk of colon cancer, a risk that is fairly well known. *See* Kara Smigel, *Fewer Colon Polyps Found in Men with High-Fiber, Low-Fat Diets*, 84 J. NAT. CANCER INST. 80 (1992). There is an association between saturated animal fats and breast cancer, too. *See* David P. Rose, *Effect of Dietary Fat on Human Breast Cancer Growth and Lung Metastasis in Nude Mice*, 83 J. NAT. CANCER INST. 1491 (1991). *See also David P. Rose*, LIPIDS, OBESITY AND FEMALE REPRODUCTIVE CANCER, in LIPIDS AND WOMEN'S HEALTH (Geoffrey P. Redmond, ed., 1991). David I. Gregorio et al., *Dietary Fat Consumption and Survival Among Women with Breast Cancer*, 75 J. NAT. CANCER INST. 37 (1985).

25. *See* Rosie Schwartz, *It's Time To Put A Stop to Sugar-Filled Breakfasts*, OTTAWA CITIZEN, March 11, 1992, at E2.

26. The Centers for Disease Control reports that 11,609 people have contracted AIDS through heterosexual contact. The number who contracted it this way in 1990 (2,289) is up 30% from those who contracted it by heterosexual contact in 1989. In addition, the Executive Director of the American Social Health Association reports that 12 million new sexually transmitted disease cases are reported each year. See Beth Sherman, *Its A Scary New World for Those Re-Entering the Dating Scene after Divorce or Death of A Spouse*, NEWSDAY, Jan. 25, 1992, at 17.

27. *See* Sharon Snider, *The Pill — Thirty Years of Safety Concerns*, 24 FDA CONSUMER 8, 10 (1990). *See also* Robert Stein, *Spermicides Linked to Urinary Tract Infections*, UNITED PRESS INT'L, Jan. 2 1991., and Ridgley Ochs, *The Latest in Birth Control Methods: Research-*

activity may run yet another set of physical, emotional, and psychological risks.

People who choose to live far enough away from where they work or shop so that they have to drive to those sites substantially increase their chance of death or serious bodily injury in an automobile accident. Those who choose to work as miners or police officers or loggers run a greater risk of violent or accidental death than do the rest of us.[28] Although being unemployed also substantially shortens ones life expectancy.[29] Those who participate in certain sports (including skiing, boxing, hang gliding, and statistics suggest, baseball and football) risk severe injury.[30]

People who do not become vaccinated against measles are at

---

ers: Reliable, Safe Forms on the Market, NEWSDAY (Nassua and Suffolk), Apr. 28, 1992, at 61.

28. *See* RUTH GASTEL, OCCUPATIONAL DISEASE: INSURANCE ISSUES (1992) (discussing generally occupational illnesses).

29. Harold Gilliam, *Mend Your Ways or Count Your Days*, SAN FRANCISCO CHRON., June 9, 1991, at 13/Z1. Not surprisingly, health is also closely related to homelessness; the indigent homeless are worse off than the indigent with homes. *See* Lillian Gelberg et al., *Health, Homelessness and Poverty; A Study of Clinic Users*, 150 ARCHIVES INTERNAL MED. 2325 (1990).

30. Data from the National Athletic Injury-Illness Reporting System indicate that most drownings, many firearm fatalities, 10% of brain injuries, 7% of spinal cord injuries, and 13% of facial injuries are related to sports. Susan G. Gererich, *Sports Injuries; Implications for Prevention*, 100 PUB. HEALTH REP. 570 (1985). A Vermont study on cross-country skiing revealed an injury rate of 0.72 per 1000 skier days. Per Renstrom & Robert J. Johnson, 8 SPORTS MED. (6) 346 (1989). A study of elite Alpine skiers in Quebec estimated the injury rate at 17 per 1000 skier days. Ross E. Anderson & David L. Montgomery, *Physiology of Alpine Skiing*, 6 SPORTS MED. 4, at 210 (1988). A recent estimate ranked boxing fatality rates (about 0.13 deaths per 1000 participants annually) at or less than those for hang gliding. Robert G. Morrison, *Medical and Public Health Aspects of Boxing*, 255 JAMA 2475 (1986). A study conducted among high school athletes participating in male football, baseball, and soccer, and female basketball and track and field, reported injuries to 39.5% of the participants. R. Durant et al., *Findings from the Preparticipation Athletic Examination and Athletic Injuries*, 146 AM. J. DISABLED CHILDREN 85 (1992). On the other hand, rule changes in football, together with better training and coaching techniques, reduced the occurrence of permanent cervical quadriplegia from 34 in 1976 to 5 in 1984. Joseph S. Tong et al., *The National Football Head and Neck Injury Registry; 14-Year Report on Cervical Quadriplegia, 1971 Through 1984*, 254 JAMA 3439 (1985). Running, a sport widely engaged in for its fitness benefits, poses risks, although generally of a less serious nature. A study of 1,680 runners in two community road race events in Canada reported that 48% of the participants experienced at least one injury during the 12-month follow-up period; 54% of those injuries were new. Stephan D. Walter, *The Ontario Cohort Study of Running-Related Injuries*, 149 ARCHIVES INTERNAL MED. 2561 (1989).

All of the dangers of these athletic endeavors are exacerbated when the athletes look for a competitive advantage through the use of medicine. *See* Virginia S. Cowart, *Ethical, as Well as Physiological, Questions Continue to Arise Over Athlete's Steroid Abuse*, 261 JAMA 3362 (1989).

risk for that disease,[31] and those who forego their winter flu shots put themselves at greater risk of that sometimes fatal disease.[32] Those who allow themselves to live with high blood pressure put themselves at risk for a whole range of diseases.[33] Those who do not participate in a symptomatic screening for breast cancer, colon cancer, lung cancer, heart disease and other diseases are at greater risk of death from those diseases.

Poverty is a lifestyle with adverse health consequences.[34] Those who are poor are at much higher risk of illness than those who are rich. Those who choose to live in Chicago or New York City rather than Minneapolis or Salt Lake City are also choosing a life style that, according to statistics, is likely to result in a shorter life.[35]

The rich variety of life style choices for which individuals may bear moral responsibility and the various health consequences of those choices suggest that no analysis of the propriety of imposing that responsibility may apply to every person or every condition. Some relevant life style choices involve health care decision making; some involve career choices; some involve leisure time choices. Should we treat the responsibility that accompanies these different

31. The Centers for Disease Control reported 27,672 measles cases in the United States in 1990, a 52.1% increase over the incidence reported for 1989. Among the 1990 cases were 89 suspected measles-associated deaths. Division of Immunization, Center for Prevention Services, Centers for Disease Control, *Measles — United States*, 1990, 265 JAMA 3227 (1990). In 1983, the disease reached its nadir in the United States with 1,497 cases. The dramatic rise in incidence has been attributed to a failure to vaccinate. Laura L. Fisher & R. Gordon Douglas, *Infectious Diseases*, 265 JAMA 3130, 3131 (1991).

32. Annual deaths from influenza and its complications range from 20,000 to 40,000; yet only 30% to 40% of high-risk people are vaccinated each year. Kristin L. Nichol et al., *Influenza Vaccination: Knowledge, Attitudes, and Behavior Among High-Risk Outpatients*, 152 ARCHIVES INTERNAL MED. 106 (1992).

33. Hypertension (high blood pressure) currently places about 58 million Americans at increased risk for stroke, heart disease, and kidney failure. Morbidity and Mortality Weekly Report, Centers for Disease Control, *Progress Toward Achieving the 1990 High Blood Pressure Objectives*, 264 JAMA 2192 (1990).

34. *See* Gelberg et al., *supra* note 29, at 2325. Poverty appears to be one of the primary reasons African Americans are at a higher risk for cancer than Whites. *See* Suzanne P. Kelley, *Blacks at Higher Risk for Cancer; Myths, Mistrust and Poverty Are Among Factors*, STAR TRIB., Dec. 8, 1991, at B1.

35. This increase in longevity is thought to be due, in part, to the high proportion of Mormons in the population of Utah. Because of their abstinence from tobacco, alcohol and caffeine, together with good general health practices, active Mormons have been recognized as a population at very low risk for cancer. James E. Enstrom, *Cancer Mortality Among Mormons*, 36 CANCER INST. 805 (1975). *See also* James E. Enstrom, *Health Practices and Cancer Mortality Among Active California Mormons*, 81 J. NAT'L CANCER INST. 1807 (1989). Actually, the states with the longest average life spans are Minnesota and The Dakotas; Nevada (which also has a large Mormon population) has the shortest average life span. *See* Gilliam, *supra* note 29, at 13.

kinds of decisions differently? Is there more culpability attached to a leisure time choice that to an employment choice? Is there more culpability in making an "unhealthy" work choice than in making a risky decision about medical treatment?

To determine when, if ever, it might be appropriate to make someone pay for her self-induced health status, we should determine what the reasons for imposing such a responsibility could ever be.

II. ARE INDIVIDUALS RESPONSIBLE FOR THEIR HEALTH STATUS?

The idea that one is responsible for one's own health status is not new. It is recognized in virtually every form of ancient medicine, and it provides the basis of many systems of folk medicine.[36] For centuries people have believed that illness is a form of divine retribution, and that the unworthy are proven so by their disease state.[37] This historical approach is reflected in the current belief that "clean living" is the way to health (and, thus, ill health must be the consequence of unclean living).[38] If you are sick, it is likely to be because you deserve it. You got your cold, just as your

36. *See* Erik Eckholm, *AIDS and Folk Healing, a Zimbabwe Encounter*, N.Y. TIMES, Oct. 5, 1990, at A10 (describing one current example where the belief that one is responsible for personal health is present in folk medicine).

37. *See* Peter Sedgwick, *Illness — Mental and Otherwise*, in CONCEPTS OF HEALTH AND DISEASE: INTERDISCIPLINARY PERSPECTIVES 119, 125-26 (Arthur Caplan et al. eds., 1981). As Sedgwick points out, "[i]n a society where the treatment of the sick is still conducted through religious ritual, the notion of illness will not be entirely distinct from the notion of sinfulness or pollution." *Id.* at 126. *See also* Henry Cohen, *The Evolution of the Concept of Disease*, in CONCEPTS OF HEALTH AND DISEASE: INTERDISCIPLINARY PERSPECTIVES 209 (Arthur Caplan et al. eds., 1981).

38. Indeed, this twentieth century phenomenon is remarkably similar to nineteenth century developments. Presbyterian minister Sylvester Graham's mid-nineteenth century notions that we should avoid alcohol, meat, and overly refined grains — and that spiritual health is necessarily closely related to physical health — is reflected in the current interest in "natural" foods, even if the nineteenth century Christianity that provided the underpinning to Rev. Graham's theory is now replaced by a more general and less sectarian notion of spirituality. The cracker invented by Rev. Graham has its analogue in the shelves of whole grain crackers now available in the natural food stores. His spiritual and physical Puritanism also touched off a conviction to "biological living" in nineteenth century cereal magnates John Harvey Kellogg and C. W. Post, who espoused and expanded Graham's principles through writing, lecturing, and product development.

For a more thorough account of the relationship between religious movements and health movements in the nineteenth century, *see* James C. Whorton, *Traditions of Folk Medicine in America*, 257 JAMA 1632 (1987); JAMES C. WHORTON, CRUSADERS FOR FITNESS: THE HISTORY OF AMERICAN HEALTH REFORMERS (1982); and STEPHEN NISSENBAUM, SEX, DIET, AND DEBILITY IN JACKSONIAN AMERICA (1980). Indeed, the anti-medicine culmination of the nineteenth century "do it naturally" movement — Christian Science — may have

mother promised, because you walked out in the rain without a warm coat and rubbers, which, your mother assured you, was a moral failing. Radio talk shows hosts and their callers all know exactly which kinds of people have AIDS, and what kinds of immoral conduct gave rise to their affliction.

Are those who need medical care because of their moral choices less deserving of our health care resources than others? There are three ways that those who have made "unhealthy" choices could be required to bear the burdens of those choices. Those with "unhealthy" life styles could be denied health care (for the conditions their improper conduct abetted, or for all conditions); they could be given lower priority for scarce health care resources than those whose need is independent of their conduct; or they could be charged comparatively more than deserving others for their health care (either at the point of the health care services, or earlier through higher insurance premiums or additional taxes).

Whatever burden might be attached to "unhealthy" conduct is generally justified on three grounds. First, the additional burden deters others from making the same improper life style choices. Second, the burden appropriately punishes the morally wrongful conduct. Third, it is not equitable to distribute scarce health care resources to those who choose to create health risks (and who thus could choose to avoid them).[39] Each of these propositions is based on three presumptions; first, that the life style in question is truly voluntary; second, that the life style actually brought about the condition that now demands treatment; and third, that the life style is not warranted by other countervailing social interests. In fact, in most cases the voluntariness, causation and countervailing social interest elements are subject to a great many uncertainties.

III. VOLUNTARINESS

Before imposing any burden on those life style choices which result in the need for medical care, one must be sure that the life style choices are truly voluntary. It is impossible to deter conduct

its equivalent in the mistrust of medicine that seems to underlie the current interest in "natural" foods.

39. A fourth justification, that of efficiency, suggests that imposing the risk on one who can control it is the cheapest way of reducing that risk. In fact, this justification is really a combination of the justifications based on deterrence and the equitable distribution of scarce resources. For an excellent discussion of each of these justifications, and for the best analysis of how voluntary health risks might be considered by public policy, *see* Gerald Dworkin, *Taking Risks, Assessing Responsibilities*, HASTINGS CENTER REP., Oct. 1981, at 26. Much of the organization of this article is drawn from Professor Dworkin's excellent analysis.

that isn't within a person's control by imposing sanctions on that conduct; aging, for example, cannot be deterred by threats of punishment. No one would suggest that retributive justice permits the imposition of a punishment on one whose conduct was involuntary. Punishment requires moral responsibility, and moral responsibility is premised upon free will. Finally, principles of distributive justice require that people in like situations be treated in like ways. Two patients with identical medical conditions, each the consequence of a process beyond the patient's control, are in like situations with regard to their medical needs.

There are, however, few conditions that are purely voluntary. The choice to take a drink appears to be voluntary, but alcoholism, we know, is a product of several forces. Alcoholism does not occur in a vacuum. There is a genetic component, which may be race linked.[40] There certainly is a social component, and the alcohol use patterns of an alcoholic's family seem to have a substantial effect on the chances that one will become an alcoholic.[41] There is also a gender component of alcohol related diseases.[42] Alcoholism is more likely to lead to cirrhosis in women than in men, and any decision not to provide liver transplants to alcoholics will disproportionately impact women.[43]

Indeed, it is hard to find a life style "choice" or a health condition that is not, at least in part, a consequence of genetics, family environment, social environment, gender, life trauma, ethnicity, community, education (and, especially, health education) and, probably, most significantly, wealth. As one union official pointed out when his employer proposed a life style health insurance premium differential, the rich and the poor have different ways of dealing with stress. The rich may choose an occasional weekend in Barbados or on the slopes; the poor are more likely to choose "a six-pack and a smoke".[44] Is an impoverished person's choice to live in a poor neighborhood, miles away from the new suburban job belts, a voluntary act? Are the risks that arise from the eating habits of someone who has never been taught about the consequences of consuming fats, and who does not know what a complex carbohydrate

40. Cohen & Benjamin, *supra* note 8, at 1299.

41. *See* Miller, *supra* note 19.

42. Cohen & Benjamin, *supra* note 8.

43. *Id.* M. Berglund, *Mortality and Alcoholics Related to Clinical State at First Admission: A Study of 537 Deaths*, 70 ACTA PSYCHIATRICA SCANDINAVICA 407, 415 (1984).

44. *See* Cohen, *supra* note 11, at C1 (quoting Vance Sulsky, Chief Negotiator in Newcastle for the Delaware Public Employees Council 81 of the American Federation of State, County, and Municipal Employees).

is, voluntarily undertaken? Is a coal miner who knows no other way of feeding his family making a voluntary choice when he decides to go down into the mine? Is one who has become addicted to drugs or alcohol (or food or sex, for that matter) acting voluntarily while satisfying that addiction?

Obviously, there is some voluntary element to each of these kinds of conduct. Some kinds of conduct are more clearly the consequence of free choice than are others; arguably the failure to wear seat belts after a company-wide seat belt campaign is a truly voluntary act. Most life style choices, though, are the consequences of a variety of factors, and most commonly we do not know the significance of the different factors. The problem is not that we have yet to research the genetic, social, or family influences on alcoholism, for example, it is that we do not know the relative consequences of those influences despite our research. We do know that most life style choices — including those that have adverse health consequences — are the result of more than a series of simple voluntary choices.

IV. CAUSATION

One is responsible for one's health status only if it is actually (and perhaps approximately) caused by one's voluntary conduct. However, while it is possible to define general risks from identifiable kinds of conduct, it is difficult to draw a direct link between an example of that conduct and a particular health consequence.[45] We know that the use of seat belts generally decreases the risk of death in automobile accidents, but it is not so easy to determine that the use of a seat belt in a particular accident would save the life of the driver.[46] While we know of the connection between lack of exercise and heart disease, we also know that hundreds of thousands of physically fit people die of heart disease each year while hundred of thousands of the unfit live.[47] It is usually impossible to trace an individual's death to that individual's exercise habits. While homosexual sex carries with it a risk of HIV, so does heterosexual sex.[48]

45. For an excellent discussion of the relationship between causation, voluntariness, and moral responsibility in this arena, *see* Dworkin, *supra* note 39.

46. While the National Transportation Safety Board says that 18,087 lives were saved in 1990 because of mandatory seat belt laws, no one can determine precisely who was saved because of the existence of those laws. *See* McAllister, *supra* note 22, at A25.

47. Indeed, some of the generally encouraged "healthy" behaviors appear to have no effect on some kinds of risks. *See* I-Min Lee et al., *Physical Activity and the Risk of Developing Colorectal Cancer Among College Alumni*, 83 J. NAT'L CANCER INST. 1324 (1991).

48. *See* Sherman, *supra* note 26, at 17.

We can say that having seven lottery tickets gives you a better chance to win than having only one; it is harder to say that someone won the lottery because she bought seven tickets. Similarly, while we can define conduct that increases the risk of illness or injury (and we all engage in a variety of conduct that does so in many different ways), it remains very difficult to conclude that an identifiable health event was actually caused by a life style choice.

V. COUNTERVAILING SOCIAL INTEREST

Even where voluntary conduct relates in a causally proximate way resulting in an adverse health consequence, society may wish to encourage that arguably dangerous conduct. In some cases the justification for such conduct is quite obvious; we want soldiers, police officers, firefighters and others to undertake those occupations even though they face danger when they do so. Some justifications are less apparent, however. We acknowledge the talents of daredevil stunt artists, NFL tackles, and great boxers because of the pleasure those entertainers bring to the entire society; it is worth it for all of us for those with particular skills to undertake those health risks.

While driving across town to work is more dangerous than walking down the street to work, there is a social value in being able to choose your place of work and being able to maintain your home community and neighborhood even when you change your place of work. This social value may be a countervailing social interest that justifies the substantial voluntary health risks undertaken by commuters.

For many kinds of social justifications, the quality of the allegedly countervailing social interest is a matter of real and intense social debate. The first African Americans who risked integrating their schools also faced physical danger to themselves. This voluntarily undertaken risk is justified and appropriately applauded by our society. Civil rights workers in the 1960s faced real health risks when they marched in the South; we now think of those risks as justified by the nature of their cause and the ultimate outcome of their endeavors. Will we feel that way about others who now risk their own safety to demonstrate, for example, in support of the right to life or the right to choose?

How are we to treat the person who refuses to wear a seat belt because he views it as an inappropriate intrusion by government into his private realm of decision making? How are we to evaluate the motorcyclist who does not wear a helmet as a matter of political expression — as a part of the Hell's Angels uniform, for example?[49] While smoking, eating "unhealthy" foods, playing high risk sports, and participating in identifiable social activities are all leisure life-style choices, they also may have expressive political content. It is difficult to determine the appropriate level of generality upon which we would base a justification for voluntarily undertaking health risks.

Consequently, it is not easy to determine whether particular voluntary conduct which actually causes an adverse health result is justified on the basis of principles important to the rest of society.

VI. ARGUMENTS FOR ASSESSING INDIVIDUAL RESPONSIBILITIES

A. Deterrence

One argument for denying coverage for health care that is caused by voluntary conduct, or for charging more for such health care, is to deter undesirable conduct. We may wish to deter the conduct because it is costly or unpleasant for the one engaging in the conduct or her family. If someone knows that he will be denied treatment for lung cancer if he smokes, the argument goes, he will stop smoking. If someone knows that she will be denied bypass surgery if she is obese or has not exercised regularly, the argument continues, she will lose weight and begin an exercise regimen. If someone knows that health care is generally not available for HIV related conditions, the argument concludes, he will avoid intravenous drug use, and homosexual sex (and, perhaps, heterosexual sex).

In fact, there is no evidence that these kinds of incentives are of any value. It is hard to believe that the added cost of health care, or the risk that it will not be available, will add much to the deterrence value of the health risk itself. Lost health care coverage simply comes too late to be an effective deterrent, and, as a general matter, its consequences are too insignificant to add anything to the incentive of good health itself.[50] If the risk of death from lung and car-

49. LAURENCE H. TRIBE, AMERICAN CONSTITUTIONAL LAW 939-40 (1st ed. 1978) (raising the issue of where the appropriate level of government intervention into private lives should be drawn).

50. In applying deterrence theory to criminal behavior it has been asserted that "an individual will engage in proscribed conduct as long as the 'perception of the possibility that he . . . will suffer a sanction' is less that the 'expected private benefit' provided by that conduct." Thus, deterrence as a theory applied to life style choices, ranging from criminal activity to diet and health care, presumes that people engage in cost-benefit analysis before they

diovascular disease does not discourage a person from smoking, it is hard to believe that the cost or availability of treatment for these conditions will make a difference. For those who participate in behavior that puts them at risk of HIV infection, the nature of the health care available for that disease five or ten years hence is simply too removed to be a meaningful deterrent.

The argument that the absence of good health care for a disease leads people to avoid the risk factors of that disease also suggests that making health care more available for particular diseases will encourage people to run the risks of those diseases. The development of new and widely available techniques for treating heart disease has not encouraged people to engage in behavior that puts their heart at risk, however.[51] The attention this medical care has brought to the health risk has resulted in healthier behavior — presumably the result of greater knowledge of and concern about the health consequences of the behavior. Needle exchange programs do not lead to an increase in the number of people who use drugs; they have simply made it safer for those who already do so.[52] There simply is no example of a health status that has become more com-

act. *See* A. Morgan Cloud, *Cocaine, Demand and Addiction: A study of the Possible Convergence of Rational Theory and National Policy*, 42 VAND. L. REV. 725, 767 (1989).

The courts have recognized this principle in malpractice cases where the defense of comparative or contributory negligence of the patient is based upon the patient's unhealthy lifestyle and the resultant need for medical treatment. For example, in *Ostrowski v. Azzara*, 545 A.2d 148, 150 (N.J. 1988), the doctor alleged that the diabetic plaintiff had smoked cigarettes and had failed to maintain her weight, diet, and blood sugar at acceptable levels. The Supreme Court of New Jersey reversed the trial court decision allowing this evidence of pretreatment health habits to go to the jury on the issue of causation. *See also Sawka v. Prokopowycz*, 306 N.W.2d 354 (Ct. App. Mich. 1981), where the court determined that smoking did not constitute contributory negligence in an action for failure to diagnose lung cancer, and *Jensen v. Archbishop Bergen Mercy Hospital*, 459 N.W.2d 178. 187 (Neb. 1990), where the Supreme Court of Nebraska held that the failure to lose weight was not contributory negligence in an action for malpractice for treatment of the embolism, even though the failure to lose weight may have been causally related to the creation of the embolism. *But see Musachia v. Rosman*, 190 So. 2d 47 (Fla. Ct. App. 1966). For an analysis of these cases, *see* Madelynn R. Orr, Comment, *Defense of Patients' Contribution to Fault and Medical Malpractice Actions*, 25 CREIGHTON L. REV. 665 (1992). Of course, deterrence is not the only reason for the existence of the criminal law or tort law.

51. The death rate from major cardiovascular disease in the United States has fallen from 510 per 100,000 population in 1950 (its peak) to 410 per 100,000 in 1985 to 366 per 100,000 in 1990. DEPARTMENT OF HEALTH AND HUMAN SERVICES, NATIONAL CENTER FOR HEALTH STATISTICS, MORTALITY: DEATH RATES FOR SELECTED CAUSES, 1992 INFORMATION PLEASE ALMANAC ATLAS & YEARBOOK 1992 814 (1992). *See also* P. Gunby, *Cardiovascular Disease Remains Nation's Leading Cause of Death*, 267 JAMA 335 (1992).

52. *See* Philip J. Hilts, *AIDS Panel Backs Efforts to Exchange Drug Users' Needles*, N.Y. TIMES, Aug. 7, 1991, at A1. For an interesting perspective in the variety of needle exchange programs, *see* Arnold S. Trebach, *Lessons From Needle Park*, WASH. POST, Mar. 17, 1992, at A17 (discussing why some needle exchange programs are more effective than others).

mon because it has become more successfully treatable. Indeed, in some cases the result of this deterrent approach, which would provide treatment for those who did not cause their own health status but deny it to those who did, is nothing more that to drive underground the behavior or life style choice that created the problem.[53] Where the deterrent is not the denial of treatment, but rather, a surcharge on current health coverage costs, this consequence is likely to be exacerbated. One result of driving this behavior underground is that education and health promotion campaigns — which may effectively deter unhealthy conduct — cannot reach those with the greatest need.

The use of a higher charge for medical coverage for those who have voluntarily put their health at risk, and denial of health care for voluntarily acquired illnesses or injuries, is not likely to provide much of an incentive to engage in healthier behavior. These deterrents add little to the fear of the adverse health outcome and, in fact, they may undercut the success of health education, which is more likely to be of value. In any case, there is no reason to believe that they would be as effective as incentives as other more direct approaches — including paying people to stop smoking, making physical fitness activities more available to people where they work and live, and assuring that cars are equipped with adequate safety devices.

B. Punishment

The second argument for imposing the burden of voluntary health risks on those who create them is based in the notion of retributive justice. There are two parts to this argument — the first is that voluntarily acquiring illness or injury is punishable conduct, and the second is that the limitation of access to health care is an appropriate form of punishment.

Illness and injury are evidence of immorality, the argument goes, because we are the stewards of our own bodies, and it is immoral in some fundamental way for any person to despoil the body he has been given.[54] This is a moral responsibility recognized, for example, in the Bible: Do you not know that you are a temple of God, and *that* the Spirit of God dwells in you? If any man destroys the temple of God, God will destroy him, for the temple of God is

53. *See* Trebach, *supra* note 52.

54. *See* Sedgwick, *supra* note 37, and the accompanying text.

holy, and that is what you are.[55]

It is, of course, recognized in entirely nonreligious literature also. To the extent this unhealthy state is caused by voluntary conduct, it is as subject to punishment as any other culpable conduct. On the other hand, this ancient and new age sense of moral culpability for one's health status runs counter to another development over the past thirty years; for the most part we have stopped treating health status as criminal. Private drunkenness cannot be criminal,[56] being addicted to narcotics cannot be criminal[57] and we no longer bring attempted suicides to the police station and book them as soon as they are stabilized (although, until the 1950s, this was common).[58]

There can be little doubt that the deprivation of adequate health care is viewed as an appropriate part of criminal punishment, even when the underlying culpable conduct is not health related. The deplorable condition of our prison health systems is one way in which the morally culpable are provided with much lower quality medical care than the righteous majority.[59] The practice of providing virtually unlimited resources to treat innocent newborns, the only fully nonculpable among us, also suggests that moral status is a relevant consideration in the distribution of health care resources.[60]

Of course, there are problems in using the availability of health care as a punishment, whether for health-related quasi-crimes or for

55. 1 *Cor.* 3:16-17 (New American Standard Bible). A few chapters later in the same book includes a somewhat softer exhortation:

> Or do you not know that your body is a temple of the Holy Spirit who is in you, whom you have from God, and that you are not your own? For you have been bought with a price; therefore glorify God in your body.

1 *Cor.* 6:19-20 (New American Standard Bible). *See also* Gerald J. Gruman, *Death and Dying: Euthanasia and Sustaining Life — Historical Perspectives*, in ENCYCLOPEDIA OF BIOETHICS 261 (Warren T. Reich, ed., 1978).

56. Powell v. Texas, 392 U.S. 514 (1968). Although Justice Marshall, writing for a plurality, declined to find the Texas statute that criminalized public drunkenness unconstitutional, he emphasized that the Texas court's conviction was for a public, not a private, act.

57. Robinson v. California, 370 U.S. 660 (1962) (holding that a California statute which made it punishable for any person to be addicted to the use of narcotics cruel and unusual punishment in violation of the Eighth and Fourteenth Amendment).

58. For a good history of the legal treatment of suicide, *see* GEORGE PATRICK SMITH, FINAL CHOICES: AUTONOMY IN HEALTH CARE DECISIONS (1989).

59. *See* B. Jaye Anno, *The Role of Organized Medicine in Correctional Health Care*, 247 JAMA 2923 (1982), and Iris F. Litt & Michael I. Cohen, *Prisons, Adolescents and the Right to Quality Medical Care: The Time is Now*, 64 AM. J. PUB. HEALTH 894 (1974). *See also* Andrew Skolnick, *Government Issues Guidelines to Stem Rising Tuberculosis Rates in Prisons*, 262 JAMA 3249 (1989).

60. Child Abuse and Neglect Prevention and Treatment, 45 C.F.R. § 1340.15 (1991). *See also* Iafelice v. Zarafa, 534 A.2d 417 (N.J. Super Ct. App. Div. 1987).

other misdeeds. We do not deny any other necessities to those who have committed crimes; why should this necessity be denied to those who have not? Is the denial of treatment that is necessary to preserve life (or to make it more bearable) proportional to the immoral conduct? Are isolation and hastened death the right punishment for intravenous drug use or unprotected homosexual sex? Heterosexual sex? Would you impose a penalty on either? Would you impose the same penalty on both? Is death at the side of the highway, while the paramedics look on, the proper punishment for failure to wear a seat belt or a motorcycle helmet? Is the decision to deny affordable health care coverage to a family the proper punishment for a smoking employee? What, exactly, is the proper punishment for choosing to live outside of Utah?

If punishment is a justifiable reason for denying care to those who have created the need for medical care as a result of their voluntary conduct, we will have to develop a quasi-criminal system to define medical quasi-crimes and their appropriate punishments. Someone will have to define these quasi-crimes and determine when risks to health are justified by other concerns. In fact, some high risk activities seem to bring little moral condemnation in this society, and others are almost universally condemned. High risk activities of the rich and famous — skiing, high stress life styles, flying private planes, scuba diving — seem acceptable. High risk activities of the poor — smoking, overeating, drinking — seem to be morally unacceptable. We can presume that invidious discrimination that affects the rest of the health care system will also have an affect on the description and punishment of culpable health states. If race and gender seem to play some subtle role in the selection of liver transplant candidates when those attributes are formally irrelevant,[61] and if they play a very substantial role in the selection of bypass surgery candidates,[62] we should expect that they will play some role in determining those who are morally qualified to receive health care.

61. *See* Cohen & Benjamin, *supra* note 8. *See also* Phillip J. Held et al., *Access to Kidney Transplantation: Has the United States Eliminated Income and Racial Differences?*, 148 ARCHIVES INTERNAL MED. 2594 (1988).

62. Indeed, race seems to play a significant role in determining access to a whole range of medical interventions, from primary care through tertiary care. For a summary and account of the role in determining who has access to care, *see* Durado D. Brooks et al., *Medical Apartheid: An American Perspective*, 266 JAMA 2746 (1991). *See also* Stepan G. Rostand et al., *Racial Differences in the Incidence of treatment for End-Stage Renal Disease*, 306 NEW ENG. J. MED. 1276 (1982), and Council on Ethical and Judicial Affairs, *Black-White Disparities in Health Care*, 263 JAMA 2344 (1990).

In the end, defining health conditions that deserve punishment, and prescribing health-related punishments for those conditions, is unlikely to be done in a way that fairly will serve the underlying purposes of punishment in this society.

C. The Equitable Distribution of Health Resources

Probably the most often expressed and politically expedient reason for imposing the cost burden of voluntary health risks on those whose conduct gave rise to the risks is that it more equitably distributes scarce health resources by more equitably distributing their costs. It is only fair that a person who creates a health risk should have to pay for it. After all, people who choose to wear fancy clothes, drive fast cars, attend expensive colleges or influence important state legislators pay more for their pleasure; they pay more to get more. Those who choose to live in a way that requires the expenditure of additional health care resources ought to pay more because they are getting more.

While it is fair for society to pool its resources to pay for chance occurrences that afflict its members, it hardly seems fair to require those who take steps to avoid illness and injury to subsidize those who voluntarily undertake the risk of illness and injury. Those who choose to run health risks cost the rest of us money, and they should pay it back — either by paying larger health insurance premiums, or forgoing health care for their self-induced conditions.

Of course, these assertions presume that those with unhealthy life styles actually *do* cost us money and this attempt to shift costs to them is not simply an attempt to blame the increasing costs of health care on those with offensive looks or unpopular habits. In fact, there is good reason to believe that, at the very least, people with some unhealthy life styles actually save us much more than they cost. One unreleased 1971 British government study evaluated the financial consequences of imposing a large enough excise tax on cigarettes to substantially reduce smoking — one of the most socially unacceptable life styles.[63] The simplistic notion that former smokers would be healthier and require less care from the national health service proved true — to a point. At first, there would be an improvement in health status and health care resources would be preserved. But non-smokers get sick and die, too, and while they may live longer than smokers (on the average), there is no evidence

63. Howard Leichter, *Public Policy and the British Experience*, HASTINGS CENTER REP., Oct. 1982 at 32, 36-38.

that their final illnesses are less expensive than the final illnesses of smokers. While there is an initial savings, there is a substantial additional long term cost that arises out of the increase in the number of elderly patients and their delayed illnesses. The British study suggested that a twenty percent fall in smoking would save four million pounds (based on 1971 prices) ten years after it was put into effect, but would cost an additional two million pounds after thirty years.[64]

In addition, smoking may save society money in a host of other ways. The years smoking takes off of one's life always come off the back end; indeed, smoking leads to disease that is likely to cause death around the time the smoker ends her working life and about the time she begins retirement. The additional social security costs required to support a non-smoking society would be enormous; even in the short run they would probably exceed the financial savings provided to the health care system. In the United States the consequences of a dramatic reduction in smoking without an accompanying change in the age of retirement could include bankruptcy of the social security system, a politically unbearable increase in the cost of the Medicare program, and the failure of many retirement plans. Because much long term care for the elderly is provided through state Medicaid programs, that state expenditure, which is already the fastest growing item in most state budgets, would grow even faster if people were living longer. This

64. *Id.* at 36. There would be a substantially greater differential if there were a 40% fall in smoking. That would save 16 million pounds over a decade, but cost the British government 29 million pounds (still in 1971 pounds) after 30 years. The 29 million pound additional cost reflects a net increase in social security payments of 24 million pounds. The relative change in the cost of health care and social security associated with 20% and 40% falls in cigarette smoking are indicated in the following chart.

Estimated Changes in Health Care and Social Security Expenditure (based upon 1971 prices)

Fall in cigarette smoking	Net change in health care costs	Net change in social security payments	Net overall change (L million)
20 percent fall			
1981	−4	−4	−8
1991	−4	+1	−3
2001	+2	+10	+12
40 percent fall			
1981	−7	−9	−16
1991	−1	+5	+4
2001	+5	+24	+29

SOURCE: *Cigarette Smoking and Health*, Report by an Interdepartmental Group of Officials, London: October 1971.

would require either additional tax revenue or a further decrease in the availability of health services to the non-elderly poor.

As the British study points out, there are further financial consequences of a decrease in smoking. A decrease in smoking (which would decrease tax revenue derived from cigarettes, of course) would be accompanied by an increase in the purchase of other goods, many of which would be imported. This would lead to a further trade imbalance. If smoking were reduced by the imposition of an additional tax on cigarettes, the tax revenue from that source could remain stable, but the consumer price index would go up, and that would require additional government expenditures.[65]

It isn't surprising that the British analysis of this issue looked primarily to government costs, which include social security payments and costs incurred by the national health care system. Any analysis of the cost of smoking in the United States would be more complex. The only attempt to do this analysis looked at the external costs of smoking — those costs born by the society and not the smoker — in order to determine whether the current taxes on smoking were economically efficient.[66] The external costs considered in the study were derived from collectively financed programs, including health insurance, pensions, sick leave, disability insurance, and group life insurance. The study separately considered such external costs as property loss from fires associated with cigarette smoking and employer-paid sick leave occasioned by cigarette smoking.

The study found that "each pack of cigarettes increases medical costs by thirty eight cents, but saved one dollar and eighty two cents in public and private pensions . . . Over all there is a net savings of ninety one cents per pack in undiscounted costs."[67] If all costs are discounted at five percent, there is a net external cost per pack of about fifteen cents, considering both medical cost savings and the pension cost reduction.[68] As the study points out, "our estimate of the external cost of smoking, fifteen cents per pack, is well below the current average (state plus federal) excise and sales taxes of thirty seven cents per pack."[69] Only if lives lost to passive smoking and fires are included as external costs does the external cost of

65. *Id.* at 36-38.

66. Willard G. Manning et al., *The Taxes of Sin; Do Smokers and Drinkers Pay Their Way?*, 261 JAMA 1604 (1989).

67. *Id.* at 1606.

68. *Id.* at 1606-07.

69. *Id.* at 1608.

smoking approach the current tax on a per-pack basis.[70]

While this American study was designed to evaluate tax policy, not the imposition of other burdens on smokers, it suggests that smokers already bear a financial burden that compensates for any they impose upon the rest of society. Of course, this conclusion is based upon several variously supported assumptions about retirement age of smokers and non-smokers, other health habits of smokers, the under reporting of smoking, the discount rate on pensions and other costs, the distribution of external and internal costs, and the value of life, which was set at one million, sixty six thousand dollars, or about ten dollars per hour.[71]

In other words, smokers do not cost the rest of us money; in fact, they save us money. If fairness were to require that smokers be charged more for health insurance than non-smokers, then fairness also requires that non-smokers be charged more for social security and make larger contributions to retirement plans. Similarly, those with unhealthy eating habits or inadequate exercise habits may be the patriots who are saving our social security system and keeping the Medicare tax contribution financing scheme effective and politically acceptable.

70. *Id.* at 1605, 1607. An interesting summary of the consequences of alternative discount rates on the net external cost of smoking is provided in a table included in the publication of this study:

Table 2: External Costs per Pack of Cigarettes*

	Discount Rate		
External Costs	0%	5%	10%
Costs per pack $ Medical care**	0.38	0.26	0.18
Sick Leave	0.01	0.01	0.01
Group life insurance	0.11	0.05	0.02
Nursing Home	−0.26	−0.03	0.00
Retirement Pension***	−1.82	−0.24	−0.02
Fires	0.02	0.02	0.02
Taxes in earnings to finance above programs $	−0.65	−0.09	−0.02
Total net costs per pack $ §	−0.91	0.15	0.24
Life expectancy at age 20 y per pack, min	−137	−28	−6

* The number of packs of cigarettes are corrected for underreporting. Costs (in 1986 dollars) per pack are calculated by dividing by the discounted number of packs smoked.

** Includes all but maternity, well, and dental care.

*** Includes disability insurance.

§ The sum of costs minus taxes on earnings, e.g., costs at 5% equals 0.15 = 0.26 + 0.01 + 0.05 − 0.03 − 0.24 + 0.02 − (−0.09).

71. *Id.* at 1607-09 (concluding that the taxes on liquor do not come close to paying the external costs that the use of liquor imposes on society. Of course, this conclusion is based on another series of rather arbitrary assumptions).

While it is unclear that others with different unhealthy life styles provide the rest of us with a subsidy, as smokers do, it is hardly clear that they cost us anything as a consequence of their habits. Whether helmetless motorcyclists are imposing a financial burden on the rest of us by engaging in their risky behavior depends upon which stereotypical view of this subgroup of motorcyclists is closer to the truth; are they healthy young people entering their working prime, or ne'er-do-wells who are unlikely ever to contribute to society?

Of course, there may be some kinds of choices that clearly impose a cost on society — the failure to wear seat belts, perhaps. However, the principle that costs should be equitably distributed would not permit imposing an additional cost on those who engage in this probably costly behavior without also imposing an additional cost on those who engage in other probably costly behaviors like driving (rather than walking) to work or skiing or not smoking — behaviors unlikely to be made the subject of any sanctions.

VII. CONCLUSION

It is difficult to assess which health related life style choices are truly voluntary; in fact, it is a mistake to ask that question as if there were an unambiguous answer in any case. While some behaviors are more voluntary than others, most are a consequence of a combination of voluntary action and genetic predisposition, ethnic background, wealth, geographic location, and a host of other factors. Even if we could assess the voluntariness of health related behavior, we should not impose the cost of its consequences upon the actor unless we can conclude with some certainty that the unhappy result was actually caused by the identified behavior. However, causation is as ambiguous and as difficult to establish as is the element of voluntariness. Finally, we ought not impose the cost of health consequences actually caused by voluntary conduct on the person who decided to run the risk of the consequence if the risk was justified by a countervailing social interest. Whether there is a countervailing social interest is also marked by uncertainty, ambiguity and ambivalence in most cases.

Even if we could identify some truly voluntary conduct that were clearly and causally connected to some adverse health condition, and even if we could conclude that this conduct were not otherwise socially justified, we could not base an argument for imposing the cost of the conduct — whether it be by denying access to health care for that condition, by giving lower priority to that health care claimant, or by charging that person a higher premium for health insurance — on any of the three bases usually advanced to justify that result: deterrence, punishment, and the equitable distribution of resources. This form of incentive is not likely to deter the unhealthy life style choices to which it may be applied; it will unfairly and improperly punish those who are not deserving of punishment, and it will do so without any regard for a sense of proportionality; and, finally, it will not lead to the equitable distribution of scare societal resources.

In fact, the recent call to impose the costs of health care on those who voluntarily create risks that result in those costs is a way to blame patients for the increase in health care costs. It is a way to avoid dealing with the real reason for the rise in those costs — reasons that include an irrationally structured health care delivery system and a highly subsidized market that can command almost any amount of resources.[72]

It is hardly surprising that the punish-the-smoker mentality surfaced first in England and Canada when the costs of those centralized health care systems began to rise precipitously in the 1970s.[73] It is not surprising that the same mentality has arisen in this country at the same time that smoking, consuming a diet high is saturated fats, driving without a seat belt, and several other unhealthy life styles are on the decline. We should not allow ourselves to be drawn away from serious evaluation of the justice of our health care system by focusing on the life style of patients. We should not be diverted from dealing with patient and community education and other proven ways of promoting and encouraging good health (which is certainly a valuable social end, even if it *costs* money) by figuring out how to impose sentence on those with life style related health problems. Even is we could, we ought not make patients pay for their life style choices.

72. *See* Barry Furrow et al., *supra* note 1, at 661-66.

73. *See* Leichter, *supra* note 63.

[21]

De Facto Health-Care Rationing by Age

The Law Has No Remedy

Marshall B. Kapp, J.D., M.P.H.*

INTRODUCTION

Health-care rationing—the conscious denial of potentially beneficial medical interventions to particular patients for the purpose of conserving and redirecting scarce resources[1]—has gone in the last quarter century from the status of a taboo subject to being part of respectable contemporary health policy discourse.[2] As one medical-legal commentator has stated:

> The issue of rationing has remained generally submerged in discussions of medical care in this country. We have not wanted to face it, perhaps because it is antithetical

* Professor, Departments of Community Health and Psychiatry; Director, Office of Geriatric Medicine & Gerontology, Wright State University School of Medicine. Address correspondence to Professor Kapp at Wright State University School of Medicine, Box 927, Dayton, Ohio 45401-0927.

[1] *See generally* Ubel & Goold, *"Rationing" Health Care: Not All Definitions Are Created Equal*, 158 ARCH. INTERN. MED. 209 (1998); J. AREEN, P. KING, S. GOLDBERG, L. GOSTIN, & A. CAPRON, LAW, SCIENCE AND MEDICINE 839 (2d ed. 1996); Reagan, *Health Care Rationing: What Does It Mean?*, 319 NEW ENG. J. MED. 1149 (1988). Rationing, which concerns microlevel parceling out of available resources, is distinguishable from the process of allocation, which involves macro- or policy-level decisions about how much resources ought to be devoted to a particular category of activity (for example, what should be the size of the national health budget?). *See, e.g.*, White, *Budgeting and Health Policymaking*, in INTENSIVE CARE: HOW CONGRESS SHAPES HEALTH POLICY 53 (1995); Sheldon, *Formula Fever: Allocating Resources in the NHS*, 315 BR. MED. J. 964 (1997). For a discussion of the ethical implications of the distinction between resource allocation, on one hand, and rationing, on the other, see H. MOODY, ETHICS IN AN AGING SOCIETY 187-207 (1992); Pawlson, Glover, & Murphy, *An Overview of Allocation and Rationing: Implications for Geriatrics*, 40 J. AM. GERIATRICS SOC'Y 628, 629 (1992). Rationing also should not be confused with the emerging topic of futile medical intervention; the latter offers no reasonable hope of any meaningful patient benefit and ethically should be withheld even if resources were infinite. *See, e.g.*, L. SCHNEIDERMAN & N. JECKER, WRONG MEDICINE: DOCTORS, PATIENTS, AND FUTILE TREATMENT (1995). *See also infra* notes 92-98 and accompanying text.

[2] *See, e.g.*, R. BLANK, RATIONING MEDICINE (1988); M. HALL, MAKING MEDICAL SPENDING DECISIONS: THE LAW, ETHICS, AND ECONOMICS OF RATIONING MECHANISMS (1997); McCarrick & Darragh, *Scope Note 32—A Just Share: Justice and Fairness in Resource Allocation*, 7 KENNEDY INST. ETHICS J. 81 (1997) (annotated bibliography); Rothman, *Rationing Life*, 39 N.Y. REV. BOOKS 32 (1992) (essay reviewing eight books touching on the topic of health care rationing).

> to the constant growth in health care resources upon which the industry has relied, perhaps because Americans have been unwilling to accept the notion that access to health care must be limited. In any case, just doctoring demands explicit discussion of rationing.[3]

Logically, virtually any form of significant health-care rationing must disproportionately impact high users of health-care services, a category into which older persons as a group fall. At the same time, critics roundly have condemned suggestions enunciated over the past decade that various forms of health care be rationed categorically and explicitly by society—specifically, by government, private health insurers, corporate benefits managers, and other third-party payment control entities—according to the "bright line" test of chronological age.[4]

Despite these articulated criticisms to explicit, overt (hard) forms of rationing, there is a substantial emerging medical literature indicating that age-based rationing is *de facto* taking place every day on the basis of individual bedside decisions and actions by physicians and nurses regarding individual patients.[5] The evidence is overwhelming that this differential treatment among patients of different ages—implicit, covert (soft) rationing—takes place regardless of comparable diagnoses, prognoses, or other potentially explanatory factors besides the particular patient's age. Following an outline of explicit rationing-by-age proposals, this article reviews the medical literature showing actual but unacknowledged rationing by age, notes relevant ethical and economic implications, and then discusses the law's theoretical and practical limitations in protecting older patients from this form of *de facto* age discrimination.

I. EXPLICIT AGE-BASED RATIONING PROPOSALS

The most influential of the modern calls for some explicit age-based health-care rationing scheme is that propounded by philosopher Daniel

[3] T. BRENNAN, JUST DOCTORING: MEDICAL ETHICS IN THE LIBERAL STATE 177 (1991).

[4] This article does not deal with proposals for explicit health-care rationing predicated on categorical criteria other than chronological age. The most noteworthy of these proposals is the Medicaid waiver designed as an outgrowth of the 1989 Oregon Basic Health Services Act. *See, e.g.*, Bodenheimer, *The Oregon Health Plan—Lessons for the Nation* (pts. 1 & 2), 337 NEW ENG. J. MED. 651, 720 (1997); Erwin, *The Oregon Plan: An Ethical Solution to the Health Care Crisis?*, J. HEALTH & HOSP. L. 133 (1993); Rosner, Kark, & Packer, *Oregon's Health Care Rationing Plan*, 11 J. GEN. INTERN. MED. 104 (1996); Fleck, *Just Caring: Oregon, Health Care Rationing, and Informed Democratic Deliberation*, 19 J. MED. & PHIL. 367 (1994).

[5] *De facto* health-care rationing also is widespread based on factors other than age, such as ability to pay and geographic location. *See, e.g.*, R. ROSENBLATT, S. LAW, & S. ROSENBAUM, LAW AND THE AMERICAN HEALTH CARE SYSTEM 36-128 (1997).

Callahan in *Setting Limits: Medical Goals in an Aging Society.*[6] Callahan's bold aim is[7] to nudge American society toward a paradigm shift in thinking about aging, health care, and death. In this new conception, old age would derive meaning in individual human lives, not through an egoistic pursuit of long life through the voracious consumption of costly medical technological interventions, but instead through a spirit of sacrifice that makes resources more available for future generations. Communal values of continuity and interconnectedness would replace the traditional focus on every person's entitlement to the maximum wizardry that the contemporary health-care industry has to offer. For Callahan, the function of the elderly is to hand the world over to the next generation and then step aside.

Operationalizing this vision would entail limiting public entitlement program payments (most importantly, Medicare[8] and Medicaid[9]) for acute medical treatments oriented primarily toward extending life for persons who already have lived a "normal life span," which Callahan deemed to be somewhere around age 80. He would substitute for life-extending acute medical treatment for the elderly more comfort and palliative interventions and other measures designed to improve the physical and mental quality of their lives. In this manner, the "ends of medicine" for the aged would move away from a mindset of curing every defeatable ailment to the more modest one of supporting older persons in their struggle with chronic, debilitating ailments as they descend toward a decent, "tolerable death."[10]

Under a more drastic approach to explicit age-based rationing, the government could outlaw (rather than just refuse to pay for) the provision of specified medical services (for example, organ transplants) to identified groups of patients (such as people more than 65 years of age), at any price and regardless of who is willing to pay the bill. Neither the patient, physician, nor other gatekeeper would have any leeway in such a model. Some philosophical proposals for health-care rationing according to age—such as Robert Veatch's "egalitarian justice over a lifetime" theory, which posits a straight priority claim to medical resources in inverse proportion to chronological age[11] (the "Fair

---

[6] D. Callahan, Setting Limits: Medical Goals in an Aging Society (1987). Subsequently, Callahan wrote *What Kind of Life: The Limits of Medical Progress* (1990), which dealt with the need for health-care rationing more generally, rather than concentrating on the age-based aspect. For other age-based rationing proposals, see, e.g., L. Churchill, Rationing Health Care in America: Perceptions and Principles of Justice (1987); Should Medical Care Be Rationed by Age? (T. Smeeding ed. 1987).

[7] I write of Callahan's ideas on this subject in the present tense, because he has continued to articulate them in numerous forums. *See, e.g.*, Callahan, *Controlling the Costs of Health Care for the Elderly—Fair Means and Foul*, 335 New Eng. J. Med. 744 (1996).

[8] 42 U.S.C. § 1395.

[9] *Id.* § 1396.

[10] *See also* Lamm, *Misallocating Health Care and Societal Resources*, 3 Notre Dame J.L., Ethics & Pub. Pol'y 241 (1988).

[11] Veatch, *Justice and the Economics of Terminal Illness*, 18 Hastings Center Rep. 34, 35 (Aug.-Sept. 1988). Simply put, for Veatch, the older a person is, the more opportunity that individual already has

Innings" concept) and Norman Daniels' "Prudential Lifespan Account" for rationing by age group but not by cohort[12]—could be interpreted as supporting this approach.

Although proposals for explicit rationing of health care solely on the basis of patient age are considerably milder than some other suggestions regarding adverse treatment of the elderly,[13] these rationing proposals nonetheless have been attacked broadly and vehemently on social, ethical, and legal grounds.[14] Arguments opposing official, overt age-based rationing are predicated on the propositions that the elderly have special needs for health care, that society has special duties to the elderly, and that singling out the older population for less advantageous treatment in the health-care marketplace constitutes a malicious form of invidious discrimination.[15]

Among other things,[16] it is claimed that overt age-based rationing would label the elderly as scapegoats and symbolically devalue them socially.[17] Such

---

had to consume his or her share of resources, and therefore the weaker is that person's claim to future resources that ought to be shared equally. Compare that with the American College of Emergency Physicians' Policy Statement: "Emergency physicians should not allocate health care resources on the basis of a patient's . . . past use of resources." American College of Emergency Physicians, *Emergency Physicians Stewardship of Finite Resources*, 30 ANNALS EMERG. MED. 562 (1997).

[12] N. DANIELS, AM I MY PARENTS' KEEPER? AN ESSAY ON JUSTICE BETWEEN THE YOUNG AND THE OLD (1988); N. DANIELS, JUST HEALTH CARE (1985). For Daniels, if decisions were made behind a "veil of ignorance"—in other words, if none of us could predict what our own future economic or health status might be—then prudent deliberators would prefer a distributive scheme that improves their chances of reaching a normal life span to one that gives them a reduced chance of reaching a normal life span but a greater chance to live an extended span once the normal span is achieved. Daniels has argued that, because all people age, they all are subject to the distribution of beneficial goods over the whole course of a life span. If we can determine what it would be prudent to give people at each stage of life to provide them with an equal opportunity to reach the next stage, then we could discover what justice requires between age groups. Philosopher Eric Rakowski styles the prudential argument in terms of an argument for respecting personal autonomy—respecting the way that most people would choose to budget their health care over the course of an entire lifetime. Rakowski, *Should Health Care Be Rationed by Age? Yes*, in CONTROVERSIAL ISSUES IN AGING 103, 107 (A. Scharlach & L. Kaye eds. 1997).

[13] For example, Dr. William Osler in 1905 recommended chloroforming everyone at age 60. Johnson, *Osler Recommends Chloroform at Sixty*, 59 PHAROS 24 (Winter 1996). *See also* Battin, *Age Rationing and the Just Distribution of Health Care: Is There a Duty to Die?*, 97 ETHICS 317 (1987).

[14] *E.g.*, Rivlin, *Protecting Elderly People: Flaws in Ageist Arguments*, 310 BR. MED. J. 1179 (1995); SET NO LIMITS: A REBUTTAL TO DANIEL CALLAHAN'S PROPOSAL TO LIMIT HEALTH CARE FOR THE ELDERLY (R. Barry & G. Bradley eds. 1991); TOO OLD FOR HEALTH CARE? CONTROVERSIES IN MEDICINE, LAW, ECONOMICS, AND ETHICS (R. Binstock & S. Post eds. 1991); A GOOD OLD AGE? THE PARADOX OF *SETTING LIMITS* (P. Homer & M. Holstein eds. 1990); Smith & Rother, *Older Americans and the Rationing of Health Care*, 140 U. PA. L. REV. 1847 (1992).

[15] Smith, *Our Hearts Were Once Young and Gay: Health Care Rationing and the Elderly*, 8 U. FLA. J.L. & PUB. POL'Y 1 (1996); Jecker & Pearlman, *Ethical Constraints on Rationing Medical Care by Age*, 37 J. AM. GERIATRICS SOC'Y 1067, 1072-73 (1989).

[16] For instance, there are religious objections to the idea of age-based resource rationing. *See, e.g.*, Post, *Justice for Elderly People in Jewish and Christian Thought*, in TOO OLD FOR HEALTH CARE?, *supra* note 14, at 120-37.

[17] Kapp, *Rationing Health Care: Will It Be Necessary? Can It Be Done Without Age or Disability Discrimination?*, 5 ISSUES L. & MED. 337, 347 (1989), *reprinted as Rationing Health Care: Legal*

a policy would send a negative public message about the old and also might have deeper implications for the attitudes of young people toward their futures and toward their aging family members.[18] It would reinforce prevalent biases about the negative social worth of the elderly.[19]

In a related vein, explicit rationing according to age would threaten to fragment the ethical and social covenant binding different generations to each other at present,[20] replacing interdependence with officially sanctioned age-group competition.[21] The fraying of this social fabric is evidenced already by the political power exerted by the "intergenerational equity" movement, which takes as its rallying cry the proposition that a dollar spent on older persons (for health-care or any other reason) is a dollar harmfully diverted away from services devoted to other age groups, especially the young.[22] This attitude is epitomized by former Colorado Governor Richard D. Lamm's now famous admonition to the elderly in a speech before the Colorado Health Lawyers Association: "You've got a duty to die and get out of the way. Let the other society, our kids, build a reasonable life."[23]

Issues and Alternatives to Age-Based Rationing, in Set No Limits, *supra* note 14, at 71, 80-81; Thomasma, *Moving the Aged into the House of the Dead: A Critique of Ageist Social Policy*, 37 J. Am. Geriatrics Soc'y 169 (1989).

18 Cassel & Neugarten, *The Goals of Medicine in an Aging Society*, in Too Old for Health Care, *supra* note 14, at 75-91.

19 American Geriatrics Society Public Policy Committee, *Equitable Distribution of Limited Medical Resources*, 37 J. Am. Geriatrics Soc'y 1063 (1989); American Medical Association Council on Ethical and Judicial Affairs, Ethical Implications of Age-Based Rationing of Health Care (1988); 1 Code of Medical Ethics Reports of the Council on Ethical and Judicial Affairs of the American Medical Association 53 (1992); Hentoff, *The Pied Piper Returns for the Old Folks*, 14 Human Life Rev. 108 (Summer 1988).

20 Post, *Should Health Care Be Rationed by Age? No*, in Controversial Issues in Aging, *supra* note 12, at 109-10. Regarding the covenant among different generations, see generally E. Kingson, B. Hirshorn, & J. Cornman, Ties that Bind: The Interdependence of Generations (1986); T. Koff & R. Park, Aging Public Policy Bonding the Generations (1994).

21 *See* Clark, *The Social Allocation of Health Care Resources: Ethical Dilemmas in Age-Group Competition*, 25 Gerontologist 119 (1985).

22 On the intergenerational equity movement and the tensions between generations, see Justice Across Generations: What Does It Mean? (L. Cohen ed. 1993); Justice Between Age Groups and Generations (P. Laslett & J. Fishkin eds. 1992); P. Longman, Born to Pay: The New Politics of Aging in America (1987); S. MacManus, Young v. Old: Generational Combat in the 21st Century (1996); T. Penny & S. Schier, Payment Due: A Nation in Debt, A Generation in Trouble (1996). According to one analyst of health policy and politics:

> Any debate over setting limits to medical technologies, shifting resources to preventive care, or rationing health care must address the intergenerational redistribution of resources and the implications of any policy changes for the elderly. It is likely that as the issues [of resource scarcity] raised here become understood by the current younger generations (those persons now under 30) that a form of intergenerational warfare will ensue. Unfortunately the battle lines are becoming increasingly intransigent as the crisis looms and the stakes heighten.

R. Blank, The Price of Life: The Future of American Health Care 20 (1997).

23 *Gov. Lamm Asserts Elderly, If Very Ill, Have a "Duty to Die,"* N.Y. Times, Mar. 29, 1984, at A16, col. 5. *See also* Lamm, *Rationing of Health Care: Inevitable and Desirable*, 140 U. Pa. L. Rev. 1511 (1992). For a philosophical defense of Lamm's thesis, see Hardwig, *Is There a Duty to Die?*, 27 Hastings Center Rep. 34 (Mar.-Apr. 1997).

Perhaps most significantly, opponents of Callahan[24] and others attack age-based rationing proposals for erroneously treating the elderly as a physically and mentally homogeneous population group, ignoring the immense variability among different older individuals.[25] Age is a particularly unreliable predictor of the potential benefit that any specific patient may derive from any specific medical intervention,[26] thus making broad formal generalizations about the value of treatment on the basis of age especially ill-advised.

Proposals for explicit age-based health-care rationing also have been criticized for their inherently sexist impact. Because the majority of older persons are female, it is posited, women would bear the adverse consequences of these rationing schemes disproportionately.[27]

Additionally, commentators have suggested possible legal barriers to the design and implementation of an explicit, public program of rationing health care—either through payment restrictions or outright prohibitions on service purchase and provision—on the categorical basis of age.[28] These would include objections claiming substantive and procedural due process violations,[29] a deprivation of the equal protection of the laws,[30] governmental interference with freedom of contract,[31] and contravention of the rights established by Congress' passage of the Americans with Disabilities Act (ADA).[32]

The overt age-based health-care rationing schemes that have been propounded thus far may or may not possess elements of substantive merit. That point notwithstanding, the pragmatic reality is that no plan, however mild, overtly singling out the elderly for less generous medical benefits opportunities than they enjoy currently stands any chance of surviving through our political process[33] unless there is some national catastrophe, such as the

---

[24] Callahan's proposal for age-based rationing inspired many symposia in reaction. *See, e.g.*, HEALTH CARE FOR AN AGING POPULATION (C. Hackler ed. 1994).

[25] American Geriatrics Society, *supra* note 19; Kapp, *supra* note 17, at 348.

[26] *Infra* notes 83-85 and accompanying text.

[27] Jecker, *Age-Based Rationing and Women*, 266 J.A.M.A. 3012 (1991).

[28] *See* Dubler & Sabatino, *Age-Based Rationing and the Law: An Exploration*, in TOO OLD FOR HEALTH CARE, *supra* note 14, at 92-119; Kapp, *supra* note 17, at 343-46.

[29] U.S. CONST. amends. V & XIV.

[30] U.S. CONST. amend. XIV.

[31] Allgeyer v. Louisiana, 165 U.S. 578 (1897).

[32] 42 U.S.C. § 12101; 28 C.F.R. pt. 36. *See* Orentlicher, *Destructuring Disability: Rationing of Health Care and Unfair Discrimination Against the Sick*, 31 HARV. CIV. RTS.-CIV. LIB. L. REV. 49 (1996); Orentlicher, *Rationing and the Americans with Disabilities Act*, 271 J.A.M.A. 308 (1994).

[33] *See* Morone, *The Bias of American Politics: Rationing Health Care in a Weak State*, 140 U. PA. L. REV. 1923 (1992). After advocating at least consideration of rationing certain technological interventions according to age, one scholar laments: "It should be a sign of despair that the overuse of patient autonomy [as enforced through the irrational political process] has rendered these tests [of resource distribution] stillborn." R. EPSTEIN, MORTAL PERIL: OUR INALIENABLE RIGHT TO HEALTH CARE? 76 (1997).

unequivocal demise of the Medicare program,[34] that rewrites all of the political rules.[35] As Professor Wendy Mariner has perceptively warned:

> It is unlikely that Americans will come to any consensus about how to reduce health care expenditures or allocate health care resources fairly if they are not faced with a shortage of resources. A just distribution of health care resources is not likely to be pursued until there is scarcity in health care.... Real scarcity may be necessary before Americans are willing to say no.[36]

Robert Blank reminds us that "one can hardly expect most elected officials to publicly advocate an explicit rationing policy. Elections and careers are lost, not won, on such issues."[37] Consequently, rationing in general, and on the basis of patient age specifically, is much more likely for the foreseeable future to continue occurring in a hidden, covert manner by physicians[38] and nurses acting at the individual bedside, rather than explicitly by government regulation, or for that matter, by the terms of private insurance company contracts.

II. COVERT RATIONING ON THE BASIS OF AGE

For years, the practice of British physicians in limiting various forms of medical treatment to their patients—from dialysis[39] to coronary care unit admission,[40] hypertension medication,[41] and proper cancer treatment[42]—on the basis of chronological age has been one of the world's best known

[34] On the problems and future of Medicare, see, e.g., Angell, *Fixing Medicare*, 336 New Eng. J. Med. 192 (1997); R. Epstein, *supra* note 33, at 147-83. *See also* Kapp, *Taking a Long-Term View of Long-Term Care: Rightsizing Terms of the Discussion*, 1 Quinnipiac Health L.J. 123 (1997).

[35] *See* Editorial, *The Immortal American*, Wall St. J., May 31, 1995, at A14, col. 1-2. *See also* L. Thurow, The Future of Capitalism 88-144 (1996) (speculating that the inability of the American political system to cope effectively with uncontrolled spending for the elderly threatens the fundamental fabric of democracy's future).

[36] Mariner, *Rationing Health Care and the Need for Credible Scarcity: Why Americans Can't Say No*, 85 Am. J. Pub. Health 1439, 1444 (1995).

[37] R. Blank, *supra* note 22, at 99. *See also id.* at 44 ("To some extent this public refusal to accept limits is understandable since to date public officials have masked the truth. Like President Clinton, they have promised workable reform without hard choices.").

[38] On the physician's role in both implicit and explicit rationing of health services, see Lee & Miller, *The Doctor's Changing Role in Allocating U.S. and British Medical Services*, 18 Law, Med. & Health Care 69 (1990).

[39] Moss, *Dialysis Decisions and the Elderly*, 10 Clinics Geriatric Med. 56 (Aug. 1994).

[40] Dudley & Burns, *The Influence of Age on Policies for Admission and Thrombolysis in Coronary Care Units in the United Kingdom*, 21 Age & Ageing 91 (1992).

[41] Dickerson & Brown, *Influence of Age on General Practitioners' Definition and Treatment of Hypertension*, 310 Br. Med. J. 574 (1995).

[42] Fentiman, Tirelli, Monfardini, Schneider, Festen, Cognetti, & Aapro, *Cancer in the Elderly: Why So Badly Treated?*, 335 Lancet 1020 (1990).

secrets.[43] Although uniformly practiced, British age discrimination in medical care has been covert in the sense that deprivations of potential beneficial treatment to older patients have been justified by the physician to the particular patient and the public under the linguistic guise of medical "indications."[44] In addition, health authority funding formulas built on weighted capitation have had the effect of overemphasizing the effects of age.[45]

In the United States,[46] we too have scrupulously stayed away from the language of rationing, but physicians routinely engage in the practice of consciously making clinical compromises that result in some potentially beneficial treatment being withheld from their patients for financial reasons.[47] There is substantial evidence that much of this covert practice has the effect of discriminating at the bedside against patients who are elderly.[48] In commenting on a study, one physician noted: "Age was never overtly identified as the sole reason for limiting treatment even though almost half of these very old patients had some limitation placed on their care."[49]

Of course, many older patients or their decisionmaking surrogates choose less intrusive alternatives to intensive therapy in certain situations, when presented with a choice.[50] We are concerned here, however, with the apparently widespread practice of unilaterally withholding more expensive forms of

---

[43] Schwartz & Aaron, *Rationing Hospital Care: Lessons from Britain*, 310 NEW ENG. J. MED. 52 (1984). For an analysis of the ethical implications of the National Health Service legislation, see C. NEWDICK, WHO SHOULD WE TREAT? LAW, PATIENTS AND RESOURCES IN THE N.H.S. (1995).

[44] Hope, Sprigings, & Crisp, *"Not Clinically Indicated": Patients' Interests or Resource Allocation?*, 306 BR. MED. J. 379 (1993).

[45] Judge & Mays, *Allocating Resources for Health and Social Care in England*, 308 BR. MED. J. 1363 (1994).

[46] For a comparative analysis, see Castillo-Lorente, Rivera-Fernandez, Vazquez-Mata, Project for the Epidemiological Analysis of Critical Care Patients, *Limitation of Therapeutic Activity in Elderly Critically Ill Patients*, 25 CRIT. CARE MED. 1643 (1997) (older patients in Spanish ICUs receive less care than younger patients); Greer, *Rationing Medical Technology: Hospital Decision Making in the United States and England*, 3 INT'L J. TECH. ASSESS. HEALTH CARE 199 (1987). For a global perspective, see Symposium, *Caring for an Aging World: Allocating Scarce Resources*, 24 HASTINGS CENTER REP. 3 (Sept.-Oct. 1994).

[47] Asch & Ubel, *Rationing by Any Other Name*, 336 NEW ENG. J. MED. 1668 (1997); Strauss, LoGerfo, Yeltatzie, Temkin, & Hudson, *Rationing of Intensive Care Unit Services: An Everyday Occurrence*, 255 J.A.M.A. 1143 (1986).

[48] *See* Wetle, *Age as a Risk Factor for Inadequate Treatment*, 258 J.A.M.A. 516 (1987).

[49] Hesse, *Terminal Care of the Very Old: Changes in the Way We Die*, 155 ARCH. INTERN. MED. 1513, 1517 (1995).

[50] Fried & Gillick, *Medical Decision-Making in the Last 6 Months of Life: Choices About Limitation of Care*, 42 J. AM. GERIATRICS SOC'Y 303 (1994).

> Because the United States lacks the structural mechanisms and public will to set limits on allocation of health care resources we look to other more politically feasible approaches to rationing at the end of life. Recently, these have included encouragement of advance directives. ... Although advance directives have been created ostensibly to empower patients to take control over medical decision making on their behalf and ensure patient autonomy, the resource allocation dimension is readily apparent in the laws and in the literature.

R. BLANK, *supra* note 22, at 74-75.

medical care in the absence of, or even contrary to, the older person's or surrogate's own informed direction.

This phenomenon may occur, for example, when patient age is silently factored into individual caregivers' decisions to admit patients to the hospital, provide intensive care, terminate therapy, or initiate vigorous treatment.[51] One physician queries and then suggests:

> Why, in the United States, do we spend fewer Medicare dollars on the final two years of life for a 90-year-old than for a 70-year-old? One explanation is that physicians are appropriately less aggressive in hospitalizing their oldest patients and initiating tests and treatments for them. Despite publicity to the contrary, the lower costs of acute care for older patients in the last two years of life suggest that clinicians consider age (or factors associated with age, such as the patient's functional level or prognosis) in making decisions about treatment of the oldest members of our society.[52]

The same physician hastens to admonish, however:

> Such decisions should not be based on age but should take into account the patient's ability to function, his or her general health, and the likely benefits of acute care, independent of age. Physicians must be careful not to deny care on the basis of ageism cloaked as cost containment.[53]

Despite this advice, there is ample evidence in the medical sciences literature that individual bedside decisions about the distribution of health resources not infrequently are made by physicians on the basis of the patient's age, even when potential confounding variables such as prognosis and severity of illness have been controlled for in the analysis. Cancer is often treated less aggressively in older patients—both male and female—solely because of the age factor.[54] Older patients are more likely than their younger counterparts to be the recipients of Do-Not-Resuscitate (DNR) orders when all other conditions are equal.[55] When attempted resuscitation is initiated for

---

[51] Barondess, Kalb, Weil, Cassel, & Ginzberg, *Clinical Decision-Making in Catastrophic Situations: The Relevance of Age*, 36 J. Am. Geriatrics Soc'y 919 (1988).

[52] Kramer, *Health Care for Elderly Persons—Myths and Realities*, 332 New Eng. J. Med. 1027, 1028 (1995).

[53] *Id.* at 1028.

[54] Bennett, Greenfield, Aranow, Ganz, Vogelzang, & Elashoff, *Patterns of Care Related to Age of Men with Prostate Cancer*, 67 Cancer 2633 (1991); Greenfield, Blanco, Elashoff, & Ganz, *Patterns of Care Related to Age of Breast Cancer Patients*, 257 J.A.M.A. 2766 (1987); Hynes, *The Quality of Breast Cancer Care in Local Communities: Implications for Health Care Reform*, 32 Med. Care 328 (1994); Mor, Masterson-Allen, Goldberg, Cummings, Glicksman, & Fretwell, *Relationship Between Age at Diagnosis and Treatments Received by Cancer Patients*, 33 J. Am. Geriatrics Soc'y 585 (1985); Samet, Hunt, Key, Humble, & Goodwin, *Choice of Cancer Therapy Varies with Age of Patient*, 255 J.A.M.A. 3385 (1986). Screening for cancer is also less aggressive in the case of older patients. *See* Caplan, *Disparities in Breast Cancer Screening: Is It Ethical?*, 25 Pub. Health Rev. 31 (1997).

[55] Boyd, Teres, Rapoport, & Lemeshow, *The Relationship Between Age and the Use of DNR Orders in Critical Care Patients: Evidence for Age Discrimination*, 156 Arch. Intern. Med. 1821 (1996);

cardiopulmonary arrest, the elderly frequently receive shorter trials of advanced cardiac life support before death is declared.[56] Advanced age has been identified as an independent risk factor for discontinuation of dialysis[57] and undertreatment of acute heart attacks.[58] Similarly, a physician may be less likely to offer an older patient a diagnostic work-up for a gastrointestinal bleed.[59]

In addition, limits are placed on aggressive care in nursing facilities—where the resident population is predominantly elderly—in often poorly understood ways.[60] One experienced geriatrician admits that, "[m]any of those who die in nursing homes are tacitly allowed to die without further attempt at salvation.... Doctors and nurses frequently decide quietly to approach nursing home residents with benign neglect of medical problems."[61]

De facto age discrimination appears to be most pronounced in the case of the "oldest old." In the acute hospital setting, less is spent per admission on persons over age 80 than on younger elderly patients,[62] perhaps because the

Jayes, Zimmerman, Wagner, & Knaus, *Variations in the Use of Do-Not-Resuscitate Orders in ICUs: Findings from a National Study*, 110 CHEST 1332 (1996). *But see* Rosenfeld & Wenger, *Letter, Do-Not-Resuscitate Orders in the Elderly: Age Discrimination or Patient Preference?*, 157 ARCH. INTERN. MED. 1041 (1997) ("Higher rates or DNR orders represent provider responsiveness to elderly patients' own values and preferences ...."). *But see* Varon & Marik, *Letter, Cardiac Arrest in the Elderly: CPR or No CPR, That Is the Question!*, 112 CHEST 1147 (1997) ("[D]ecisions to withhold resuscitation should not be based on age alone, and resuscitation efforts should not be withheld from the elderly because of concerns of ineffectiveness."). *See also* Ghusn, Teasdale, & Boyer, *Characteristics of Patients Receiving or Forgoing Resuscitation at the Time of Cardiopulmonary Arrest*, 45 J. AM. GERIATRICS SOC'Y 1118 (1997) (patients and physicians deciding to implement a DNR order may be overly focused on medical diagnosis and less so on functional status).

56 Fried, Miller, Stein, & Wachtel, *The Association Between Age of Hospitalized Patients and the Delivery of Advanced Cardiac Life Support*, 11 J. GEN. INTERN. MED. 257, 260 (1996).

57 Neu & Kjellstrand, *Stopping Long Term Dialysis: An Empirical Study of Withdrawal of Life-Support Treatment*, 314 NEW ENG. J. MED. 14, 18 (1986).

58 Krumholz, Murillo, Chen, Vaccarino, Radford, Ellerbeck, & Wang, *Thrombolytic Therapy for Eligible Elderly Patients with Acute Myocardial Infarction*, 277 J.A.M.A. 1683 (1997); Whittle, Wickenheiser, & Venditti, *Is Warfarin Underused in the Treatment of Elderly Persons with Atrial Fibrillation?*, 157 ARCH. INTERN. MED. 441 (1997); McLaughlin, Soumerai, Willison, Gurwitz, Borbas, Guadagnoli, McLaughlin, Morris, Cheng, Hauptman, Antman, Casey, Asinger, & Gobel, *Adherence to National Guidelines for Drug Treatment of Suspected Acute Myocardial Infarction: Evidence for Undertreatment in Women and the Elderly*, 156 ARCH. INTERN. MED. 799 (1996); Krumholz, Friesinger, Cook, Lee, Rouan, & Goldman, *Relationship of Age with Eligibility for Thrombolytic Therapy and Mortality Among Patients with Suspected Acute Myocardial Infarction*, 42 J. AM. GERIATRICS SOC'Y 127 (1994); Topol & Califf, *Thrombolytic Therapy for Elderly Patients*, 327 NEW ENG. J. MED. 45 (1992).

59 Gillick, *Is the Care of the Chronically Ill a Medical Prerogative?*, 310 NEW ENG. J. MED. 190 (1984).

60 Holtzman & Lurie, *Causes of Increasing Mortality in a Nursing Home Population*, 44 J. AM. GERIATRICS SOC'Y 258 (1996).

61 Gillick, *Limiting Medical Care: Physicians' Beliefs, Physicians' Behavior*, 36 J. AM. GERIATRICS SOC'Y 747, 749 (1988); Gillick & Mendes, *Medical Care in Old Age: What Do Nurses in Long-Term Care Consider Appropriate?*, 44 J. AM. GERIATRICS SOC'Y 1322 (1996). *Cf.* Hamel, Phillips, Teno, Lynn, Galanos, Davis, Connors, Oye, Desbiens, Reding, & Goldman, *Seriously Ill Hospitalized Adults: Do We Spend Less on Older Patients?*, 44 J. AM. GERIATRICS SOC'Y 1043 (1996).

62 Perls & Wood, *Acute Care Costs of the Oldest Old*, 156 ARCH. INTERN. MED. 754 (1996).

oldest old patients are not offered aggressive care solely because of advanced age.[63]

There are a variety of plausible explanations for covert rationing by physicians on the basis of patient age.[64] Physicians may be well-intentioned, misjudging the likely outcome of medical intervention with older patients.[65] They may be responding to concerns about excessive health-care costs,[66] especially in light of the direct and indirect cost-containment incentives promoted by today's pervasive managed care environments to influence physician practice patterns.[67]

Finally, rationing by age at the individual bedside may be the result of the physician's own often unconscious bias and prejudice regarding the elderly—in other words, ageism,[68] acting alone or in combination with therapeutic miscalculations and/or financial incentives. "[A]ge discrimination may . . . be practised at a primitive, subcortical level, with aged patients being accorded substandard treatment simply through the exercise of knee-jerk responses based on blind prejudice."[69] Whatever the explanation, the practice of covert bedside rationing of potentially beneficial medical treatments on the basis of patient age entails significant ethical and economic implications.

---

[63] *Id.* at 758 (citing Adolph, *The Elderly, Very Elderly and Traditional Practice Patterns*, 16 J. Am. Coll. Cardiol. 793 (1990) and Wenger, *President's Column—Elderly Patients Deserve High-Quality Coronary Care*, 3 Am. J. Geriatric Cardiol. 47 (1994)).

[64] *See* M. Wicclair, Ethics and the Elderly 80, 105–11 (1993). According to two physicians: "Important considerations involve whether interventions are equally appropriate at age 65 and 85 years, and whether interventions should vary by chronological age or physiological age." Barrett-Connor & Stuenkel, *Questions of Life and Death in Old Age*, 279 J.A.M.A. 622 (1998).

[65] Blanchette, *Age-Based Rationing of Healthcare*, 20 Generations 60, 63 (Winter 1996-97); Jayes, *et al.*, *supra* note 55, at 1338; Mulley, *Myths of Ageing*, 350 Lancet 1160 (1997); Gordon, *Is the Best Yet to Be?*, 350 Lancet 1166 (1997). Physicians also may be uncertain about the likely clinical value of a particular medical intervention with older patients. *See* Gurwitz & Goldberg, *Coronary Thrombolysis for the Elderly: Is Clinical Practice Really Lagging Behind Evidence of Benefit?*, 277 J.A.M.A. 1723 (1997); Piccione, *Cardiac Surgery in the Elderly: What Have We Learned?*, 26 Crit. Care Med. 196 (1998).

[66] *Cf.* Avorn, *Benefit and Cost Analysis in Geriatric Care: Turning Age Discrimination into Health Policy*, 310 New Eng. J. Med. 1294 (1984). *But see* Weel & Michels, *Dying, Not Old Age, to Blame for Costs of Health Care*, 350 Lancet 1159 (1997).

[67] On managed care incentives and physician behavior, see, e.g., Levinsky, *Truth or Consequences*, 338 New Eng. J. Med. 913 (1998); Webster & Feinglass, *Stroke Patients, "Managed Care," and Distributive Justice*, 278 J.A.M.A. 161 (1997); Blanchette, *supra* note 65, at 63; Furrow, *Incentivizing Medical Practice: What (If Anything) Happens to Professionalism?*, 1 Widener L. Symp. J. 1 (1995); Mirvis, Chang, & Morreim, *Protecting Older People While Managing Their Care*, 45 J. Am. Geriatrics Soc'y 645 (1997); Conflicts of Interest in Clinical Practice and Research 238-42 (R. Spece, Jr., D. Shimm, & A. Buchanan eds. 1996); Wolf, *Health Care Reform and the Future of Physician Ethics*, 24 Hastings Center Rep. 28 (Mar.-Apr. 1994); Horn & Sharkey, *The Impact of Managed Care Cost-Containment Strategies on the Aging Population*, 1 Crit. Issues in Aging 40 (1997). For a particularly vociferous attack on the adverse ethical consequences of managed care's financial incentives for physician conduct, see M. Rodwin, Medicine, Money & Morals: Physicians' Conflicts of Interest 158-62 (1993).

[68] Editorial, *Do Doctors Short-Change Old People?*, 342 Lancet 1 (1993).

[69] *Id.*

III. ETHICAL AND ECONOMIC IMPLICATIONS OF COVERT RATIONING

Although idealistic members of the academic and political elite[70] and a handful of naive practitioners[71] continue to imagine away the unpleasant problem of finite health resources, there is an overwhelming—albeit predominantly reluctant[72]—acknowledgment by responsible commentators[73] and professional organizations[74] that some form of serious health-care rationing is inevitable and, therefore, the responsible thing to do. Given this reality, ethical arguments have emerged on behalf of both explicit (government[75] and private insurer-dominated) and implicit (dominated by the physician at the

---

[70] *E.g.*, Califano, Jr., *Rationing Health Care: The Unnecessary Solution*, 140 U. PA. L. REV. 1525 (1992); Cassel, *Issues of Age and Chronic Care: Another Argument for Health Care Reform*, 40 J. AM. GERIATRICS SOC'Y 404 (1992) (claiming that it is the structure of the United States health-care system, not resource scarcity, that creates the inaccurate illusion that we need to ration health care); Mehlman, *Rationing Expensive Lifesaving Medical Treatments*, 1985 WIS. L. REV. 239 (the costs of any rationing system likely exceed its benefits) [hereinafter Mehlman, *Rationing*]. *See also* Sasaki, Sekizawa, Yanai, Arai, Yamaha, & Ohrvi, Letter, *Medical Costs for Older People Are Not Unfairly Spent*, 45 J. AM. GERIATRICS SOC'Y 657 (1997) ("Since medical expenses for older people do not seem to be unfairly spent, prevention of disease with age would seem to be the primary strategy to achieve reduced medical costs."). *Cf.* Mehlman, *Health Care Cost Containment and Medical Technology: A Critique of Waste Theory*, 36 CASE W. RES. L. REV. 778 (1985-86) (even wasteful medical intervention cannot be effectively identified and eliminated). *Accord* Blustein & Marmor, *Cutting Waste by Making Rules: Promises, Pitfalls, and Realistic Prospects*, 140 U. PA. L. REV. 1543 (1992).

[71] O'Malley, *Age-Based Rationing of Health Care: A Descriptive Study of Professional Attitudes*, 16 HEALTH CARE MGT. REV. 83 (1991) (survey shows that gerontological professionals still do not understand the reality of scarcity).

[72] *See, e.g.*, Light, *The Real Ethics of Rationing*, 315 BR. MED. J. 112 (1997); G. CALABRESI & P. BOBBITT, TRAGIC CHOICES: THE CONFLICTS SOCIETY CONFRONTS IN THE ALLOCATION OF TRAGICALLY SCARCE RESOURCES (1978); Eddy, *Health System Reform: Will Controlling Costs Require Rationing Services?*, 272 J.A.M.A. 324 (1994) (answering his own question, "Unfortunately, it will"). Addressing a 1997 London conference entitled "Rationing in the NHS: Time to Get Real," Dr. Eddy, who is senior adviser for health policy and management at Kaiser Permanente, a large managed care organization in the United States, indicated:

> Rationing is not simply a matter of administrative efficiencies of control of price of drugs, supplies, and salaries. It means the withholding of a beneficial treatment because of its cost. This phrase captures more honestly the painful reality we face. Wherever there's a boundary, there's someone who could benefit on the other side.

Goldbeck-Wood, *"Smart" Rationing Is Possible*, 315 BR. MED. J. 146 (1997).

[73] *See, e.g.*, Eddy, *Principles for Making Difficult Decisions in Difficult Times*, 271 J.A.M.A. 1792 (1994); Haber, *Rationing Is a Reality*, 34 J. AM. GERIATRICS SOC'Y 761 (1986); M. HALL & I. ELLMAN, HEALTH CARE LAW AND ETHICS IN A NUTSHELL 42-52 (1990); W. KISSICK, MEDICINE'S DILEMMAS: INFINITE NEEDS VERSUS FINITE RESOURCES (1994); Pawlson, *et al.*, *supra* note 1; H. SHENKIN, CURRENT DILEMMAS IN MEDICAL-CARE RATIONING: A PRAGMATIC APPROACH (1996); Weale, *Rationing Health Care: A Logical Solution to an Inconsistent Triad*, 316 BR. MED. J. 410 (1998).

[74] *See, e.g.*, American Geriatrics Society Ethics Committee, *Rational Allocation of Medical Care: A Position Statement from the American Geriatrics Society*, 45 J. AM. GERIATRICS SOC'Y 884 (1997); Danis, *Reply to Letter—Rationing Intensive Care*, 272 J.A.M.A. 1481 (1994) (on behalf of the Society of Critical Care Medicine, defending the use of age in making intensive care unit triage decisions).

[75] Blank, *Regulatory Rationing: A Solution to Health Care Resource Allocation*, 140 U. PA. L. REV. 1573 (1992).

bedside)[76] supply-side schemes for determining how limited resources ought to be distributed.

"The question then is not whether we should ration medical care but how we can best assure a fair and equitable system of rationing."[77] Market-based (that is, demand-side) rationing proposals, in which consumers are economically empowered to make the key financial coverage choices prospectively, also have been set forth in reply to the methodological questions of who and how,[78] but a detailed dissection[79] of these proposals is beyond the scope of this article.

As already noted, explicit age-based rationing initiatives are not going to become a prominent feature in the foreseeable political future of the United States, at least directly.[80] At the same time, covert rationing of health services according to patient age now happens at the individual bedside and this practice is likely to expand.[81] A central question, then, is whether such covert rationing by age can be justified ethically.

---

[76] *See* Mechanic, *Dilemmas in Rationing Health Care Services: The Case for Implicit Rationing*, 310 Br. Med. J. 1655 (1995); Mechanic, *Professional Judgment and the Rationing of Medical Care*, 140 U. Pa. L. Rev. 1713 (1992); Ubel & Arnold, *The Unbearable Rightness of Bedside Rationing: Physician Duties in a Climate of Cost Containment*, 155 Arch. Intern. Med. 1837 (1995); Morreim, *Fiscal Scarcity and the Inevitability of Bedside Budget Balancing*, 149 Arch. Intern. Med. 1012 (1989). One set of authors has advocated implicit rationing because it hides from public scrutiny the "explicit ordering of sensitive priorities and overt interpersonal comparisons, which are bound to have demoralizing effects in an egalitarian democratic society." Havighurst & Blumstein, *Coping with Quality/Cost Trade Offs in Medical Care: The Role of PSROs*, 70 Nw. U.L. Rev. 6, 57 (1975).

[77] R. Blank, *supra* note 22, at xii.

[78] *See* R. Epstein, *supra* note 33; Elhauge, *Allocating Health Care Morally*, 82 Cal. L. Rev. 1449 (1994); M. Hall, *supra* note 2; Havighurst, *Prospective Self-Denial: Can Consumers Contract Today to Accept Health Care Rationing Tomorrow?*, 140 U. Pa. L. Rev. 1755 (1992); R. Herzlinger, Market Driven Health Care (1997). *But see* Ubel & Goold, *Does Bedside Rationing Violate Patients' Best Interests? An Exploration of "Moral Hazard,"* 104 Am. J. Med. 64 (1998) (arguing that physicians are ethically correct to reject some patient demands, because patients often request marginally beneficial health services even though it would be in their best interests to spend their money on more valuable things). In any event, an economic empowerment strategy would require that each older consumer have a minimally adequate amount of resources to spend on his or her own health care. *See* Stuart & Grana, *Ability to Pay and the Decision to Medicate*, 36 Med. Care 202 (1998) (older persons without economic resources choose to undermedicate themselves).

[79] For a fair, balanced analysis of this approach, see Eddy, *Rationing by Patient Choice*, 265 J.A.M.A. 105 (1991). For a vigorous attack on market-based approaches to health care, based on principles of equal access, see R. Rosenblatt, *et al. supra* note 5, at 27-35.

[80] Rationing initiatives that appear age neutral on their face can turn out in practice to have a very pronounced impact on the elderly by utilizing criteria, for example, Quality Adjusted Life Years (QALYs), that *de facto* discriminate by age. *See* Somerville, *Should the Grandparents Die? Allocation of Medical Resources with an Aging Population*, 14 Law, Med., & Health Care 158, 161 (1986); Avorn, *supra* note 66.

[81] *Cf.* Mehlman, *Rationing*, *supra* note 70, at 285:

> Due to the visibility and political unpopularity of an explicit government ELT [expensive lifesaving treatment] rationing scheme, however, ELT rationing is bound to be implemented, if at all, less overtly. The most likely scenario is that rationing will take place on an ad hoc basis or pursuant to internal, nonpublic guidelines as health care providers accommodate public cost control pressures.

In few circumstances will the physician at the bedside be able to satisfy this burden of justification. Besides being subject to most of the ethical objections outlined already in the context of official, explicit age-based rationing ideas,[82] the physician's use of patient age as an implicit, covert criterion for limiting resource consumption at the bedside fails the test of utilitarianism.

Despite the usefulness of aggregated population statistics to make predictions, ordinarily any particular patient's age is not a dependable proxy for prognosis about that patient's medical prognosis or future quality of life, long-term survival expectancy, cognitive ability, or ability to tolerate aggressive treatment.[83] As physician Norman Levinsky cautions, it is possible to push too far in the direction of educating physicians to abate aggressive medical treatment for critically ill patients, forgetting in the process that medical intervention can be beneficial for certain older patients.[84] Frequently, there is no satisfactory way to determine who among the very ill will survive and do well—that is, to benefit—except to provide the treatment and then observe what happens.[85]

Because old age by itself has no predictive value in individual situations, age-based health-care rationing cannot be justified on the basis of conserving scarce resources.[86] Even if it could otherwise be justified ethically, this practice fails to achieve its economic goals.[87]

Hence, old age by itself is not a contraindication for aggressive medical treatment. "There seems to be an adequate moral as well as economic basis for making prudent decisions on the basis of functional status rather than age alone."[88] As physicians Teri Manolio and Curt Furberg have admonished their colleagues:

> As physicians, we must discipline ourselves to look beyond a patient's age to consider his or her medical condition and potential for benefit, as well as the desires of patients and their families. . . . [W]e must apply this information free of misconceptions as to

[82] *See supra* notes 15-27 and accompanying text.

[83] *See, e.g.*, Chelluri, Pinsky, Donahoe, & Grenvik, *Long-Term Outcome of Critically Ill Elderly Patients Requiring Intensive Care*, 269 J.A.M.A. 3119 (1993); Gillick, *A Broader Role for Advance Medical Planning*, 123 ANNALS INTERN. MED. 621, 622 (1995); Hanson, Danis, & Lazorick, *Emergency Triage to Intensive Care: Can We Use Prognosis and Patient Preferences?*, 42 J. AM. GERIATRICS SOC'Y 1277, 1280 (1994); Sage, Hurst, Silverman, & Bortz, *Intensive Care for the Elderly: Outcome of Elective and Nonelective Admissions*, 35 J. AM. GERIATRICS SOC'Y 312 (1987); Wetle, *supra* note 48.

[84] Levinsky, *The Purpose of Advance Medical Planning—Autonomy for Patients or Limitations of Care?*, 335 NEW ENG. J. MED. 741 (1996).

[85] Webster & Berdes, *Ethics and Economic Realities: Goals and Strategies for Care Toward the End of Life*, 150 ARCH. INTERN. MED. 1795 (1990).

[86] *Cf.* Teno, Lynn, Connors, Jr., Wenger, Phillips, Alzola, Murphy, Desbiens, & Knaus, *The Illusion of End-of-Life Resource Savings with Advance Directives*, 45 J. AM. GERIATRICS SOC'Y 513 (1997).

[87] Jahnigen & Binstock, *Economic and Clinical Realities: Health Care for Elderly People*, in TOO OLD FOR HEALTH CARE?, *supra* note 14, at 13-43.

[88] Kavesh, *The Practice of Geriatric Medicine: How Geriatricians Think*, 20 GENERATIONS 54, 58 (Winter 1996-97).

> the duration or quality of life that can appropriately be expected at advanced ages. Such is the nature of sound clinical judgment. Not to exercise it is to abandon our responsibilities as physicians to the majority of patients under our care.[89]

IV. LEGAL IMPLICATIONS OF COVERT RATIONING BY AGE

If covert health-care rationing at the bedside cannot be justified as a matter of ethics and economics, then what is the legal status of this physician behavior? Stated differently, what, if any, specific legal rights are violated and specific legal remedies are called into play when potentially beneficial medical treatment is purposely withheld or withdrawn from particular patients for the exclusive reason that those patients have reached advanced years? Put most directly, to what extent can older persons in the United States reasonably look to the legal system to protect them against the real and potential harms caused by the covert rationing of medical care on the basis of age?

The short response to the last query is—probably very little. Realistically, the equitable remedies available to respond prospectively and to prevent covert, age-based rationing before it occurs are limited and weak, as are the legal remedies for compensating the victim after the fact and thereby discouraging similar medical practice in the future. Indeed, some advocates of covert rationing support it precisely because avoiding government involvement in an overt rationing scheme eliminates the kind of legal, external interference that they believe can seriously impede a necessary rationing process.[90]

A. Prospective Legal Interventions

Theoretically, the equitable remedy of declaratory and injunctive relief,[91] in the form of a court order declaring the respective rights and responsibilities of the different parties and commanding the physician (and/or other relevant health-care provider(s))—temporarily or permanently—to provide a patient with a particular form of medical intervention, may be available to an older patient who is in danger of having potentially beneficial medical treatment withheld or withdrawn inappropriately. Equitable relief of this nature would require a showing of imminent danger of serious, irreparable injury.

---

[89] Manolio & Furberg, *Age as a Predictor of Outcome: What Role Does It Play?*, 2 Am. J. Med. 1, 5 (1992). *See also* The Rational Use of Advanced Medical Technology with the Elderly (F. Homburger ed. 1994); Wong, Salem, & Pauker, *You're Never too Old*, 328 New Eng. J. Med. 971 (1993).

[90] Blumstein, *Rationing Medical Resources: A Constitutional, Legal, and Policy Analysis*, 59 Tex. L. Rev. 1345, 1356-85 (1981).

[91] For a general outline of nonmonetary remedies, see E. Richards & K. Rathbun, Law and the Physician: A Practical Guide 13 (1993). For a history of the equitable power of the courts, see C. Rembar, The Law of the Land: The Evolution of Our Legal System 272-319 (1980). For a discussion of injunctions and other equitable remedies as used in the health sphere, see generally F. Grad, The Public Health Law Manual 181-91 (2d ed. 1990).

The most analogous legal precedent derives from the spate of cases in which courts prospectively have required health-care providers to make available to the plaintiffs/patients forms of medical intervention that the providers had claimed would be "futile,"[92] or nonbeneficial, for the particular patients but which the patients' surrogates demanded anyway. However, there appear to be virtually insurmountable substantive and pragmatic barriers to the obtaining of timely and effective injunctive relief in any but the most exceptional of circumstances involving imminent age-based rationing of medical services.

Substantively, the number of cases comprising the corpus of legal precedent ordering health professionals to provide care considered by them to be inappropriate is minuscule. The best known case in this category is *In re Baby K*,[93] a vigorously criticized[94] decision in which a federal circuit court badly misinterpreted a specific federal statute, the Emergency Medical Treatment and Active Labor Act (EMTALA),[95] to require a hospital emergency department to attempt repeated resuscitation of an anencephalic infant brought to it in cardiopulmonary arrest. Even assuming arguendo that EMTALA may properly be applied beyond the purview of Congress' intent, which was to prevent patients being turned away from hospital emergency rooms because of economic discrimination, a very small percentage of older persons at risk of undertreatment would be able to fit their claims under the umbrella of a statute pertaining to emergency care in the hospital.

In the other highly publicized futility case, the husband of 86-year-old patient Helga Wanglie convinced a Minnesota trial court to reject a petition by Mrs. Wanglie's personal physician that he be appointed to replace Mr. Wanglie as Mrs. Wanglie's legal guardian with authority to make medical decisions for her.[96] The petition had been filed because Mr. Wanglie's

---

[92] On the concept of medical futility, see L. SCHNEIDERMAN & N. JECKER, *supra* note 1. *See also* Caplan, *Odds and Ends: Trust and the Debate over Medical Futility*, 125 ANNALS INTERN. MED. 688 (1996); Dunn & Levinson, *Discussing Futility with Patients and Families*, 11 J. GEN. INTERN. MED. 689 (1996); Kapp, *Futile Medical Treatment: A Review of the Ethical Arguments and Legal Holdings*, 9 J. GEN. INTERN. MED. 170 (1994); Kopelman, *Conceptual and Moral Dispute About Futile and Useful Treatments*, 20 J. MED. & PHIL. 109 (1995); Miles, *Informed Demand for "Non-Beneficial" Medical Treatment*, 325 NEW ENG. J. MED. 512 (1991); Schneiderman, Jecker, & Jonsen, *Medical Futility: Response to Critiques*, 125 ANNALS INTERN. MED. 669 (1996). For skeptical perspectives on the concept of futility, see, e.g., Scofield, *Medical Futility Judgments: Discriminating or Discriminatory?*, 25 SETON HALL L. REV. 927 (1995); Taylor & Lantos, *The Politics of Medical Futility*, 11 ISSUES L. & MED. 3 (1995).

[93] 16 F.3d 590 (4th Cir. 1994).

[94] *See, e.g.*, Annas, *Asking the Courts to Set the Standard of Emergency Care—The Case of Baby K*, 330 NEW ENG. J. MED. 1542 (1994); Dzielak, *Physicians Lose the Tug of War to Pull the Plug: The Debate About Continued Futile Medical Care*, 28 J. MARSHALL L. REV. 733 (1995); Smith, *The Critical Condition of the Emergency Medical Treatment and Active Labor Act: A Proposed Amendment to the Act After* In the Matter of Baby K, 48 VAND. L. REV. 1491 (1995).

[95] 42 U.S.C. § 1395dd.

[96] *In re* Conservatorship of Wanglie, No. PX-91-283 (Minn. Dist. Ct., Hennipen County, June 28, 1991). For discussions of this case, see, e.g., Angell, *A New Kind of "Right to Die" Case*, 325 NEW ENG. J. MED. 511 (1991); Capron, *In re Helga Wanglie*, 21 HASTINGS CENTER REP. 26 (Sept.-Oct. 1991).

decisions included a demand—accurately reflecting the patient's substituted judgment—for continued artificial respiration and feeding despite his wife's permanently vegetative status.[97] This judicial decision, which was never appealed (the patient dying three days after it was rendered), attracted substantial notoriety. Nonetheless, it does not stand for the broad proposition that a provider's judgment[98] must be subordinated to a patient's every demand. Instead, it represents a much more limited holding that a patient's devoted husband ordinarily should not be forcibly replaced as her guardian by her physician absent strong proof that the husband is violating his fiduciary responsibilities. This is a narrow doctrinal foundation upon which to base future equitable claims for relief in age-based rationing situations.

Perhaps more important than the weakness of a substantive basis for the older patient's right to demand particular forms of medical treatment over the physician's objection, multiple practical factors will act as serious pragmatic impediments to the patient's obtaining injunctive relief in the age-based rationing context. In the *Baby K* and *Wanglie* cases, the health-care providers announced clearly in advance that they intended to withhold (resuscitation attempts from Baby K) or withdraw (artificial respiration and feeding tubes from Mrs. Wanglie) forms of life-sustaining medical interventions, thereby giving the respective patients' surrogates ample time to object.

These are highly unusual situations. Patients or their surrogates very rarely will have such timely notice, or indeed any notice at all, that their physicians intend to impose on them conscious rationing strategies. In the vast majority of cases, individual patients and their advocates literally will not know what they are missing, at least (if ever) until after the intervention has been withheld or withdrawn. Put another way, few patients in these scenarios will be able to get to a court before specific medical treatment actually has been denied to the particular patient. Requests for prospective relief are unlikely to be sufficiently ripe for adjudication.[99]

This situation contrasts starkly with the opportunities that would be available to older persons, acting as a class, to sue to enjoin a governmental entity or private insurance company from enforcing an announced, explicit

[97] There is a strong ethical consensus today that it is an excessive use of resources to supply aggressive medical intervention to persons in a permanent vegetative state. *See, e.g.*, Hastings Center, Guidelines on the Termination of Life-Sustaining Treatment and the Care of the Dying 4 (1987); Society for Critical Care Medicine, *Consensus Report on the Ethics of Foregoing Life-Sustaining Treatments in the Critically Ill*, 18 Crit. Care Med. 1435 (1990).

[98] *See generally* Daar, *Medical Futility and Implications for Physician Autonomy*, 21 Am. J.L. & Med. 221 (1995).

[99] For a discussion of the requirement that there be a justiciable case and controversy and the prohibition against courts giving advisory opinions, as applied to the area of claims arising out of medical decisions, see Coordinating Council on Life-Sustaining Medical Treatment Decision Making by the Courts, Guidelines for State Court Decision Making in Life-Sustaining Medical Treatment Cases 32-38 (2d ed. 1992).

rationing policy that used age as a categorical classification for providing discriminatory treatment.[100] Unlike the bedside variety, explicitly adopted age-based rationing criteria would afford aggrieved older persons clear notice in time to organize and join together to seek injunctive protection against the potentially injurious policy.

Moreover, Baby K and Helga Wanglie had ready, forceful advocates who possessed the physical, emotional, and financial wherewithal to vigorously press their demands for maximal medical treatment. Sophisticated and indefatigable advocacy of this sort is practically all-consuming, and few older patients will have access to it at a level necessary to prospectively preempt medical decisionmaking authority. In a related context, because injunctive relief ordinarily does not entail any monetary damages, the contingency fee arrangement would not be available to finance legal representation for such actions.

Moreover, an injunction would tend to inject the court intimately into the health-care delivery process. Courts may shun a role in which they would need to maintain jurisdiction to oversee the patient's case and ensure that the court's order is being carried out.[101]

B. Retrospective Legal Remedies

Just as it is essentially impotent in terms of providing prospective relief from the threat of treatment denial based on patient age, the legal system also is likely to be unavailing of any meaningful remedies[102] after medical treatments have been denied to individuals as a part of age-based, bedside physician rationing decisions. Here, as in the previous discussion of possible injunctive interventions, older patients seeking compensation for medical treatments they were denied will encounter powerful substantive and practical difficulties.

The filing of traditional civil malpractice lawsuits against particular physicians[103] seeking monetary damages will seldom be a promising avenue for pursuing patient grievances in the age-based rationing context. As one perceptive analyst put it succinctly after examining the contention that individual

---

[100] *See supra* notes 28-32 and accompanying text (outlining legal arguments against explicit age-based rationing schemes).

[101] *See* Mehlman, *Rationing*, *supra* note 70, at 289.

[102] *See generally* S. FISCINA, M. BOUMIL, D. SHARPE, & M. HEAD, MEDICAL LIABILITY (1991).

[103] This article concentrates on potential legal remedies—and their weaknesses—available in situations where a physician engages in bedside rationing of care on the basis of the patient's age. For discussions of potential claims brought directly against a managed care organization or other form of third-party payer for creating financial incentives that may encourage individual physicians to engage in rationing behavior, see, e.g., B. FURROW, T. GREANEY, S. JOHNSON, T. JOST, & R. SCHWARTZ, HEALTH LAW 308-31 (1995); M. RODWIN, *supra* note 67, at 165-75; R. ROSENBLATT, *et al.*, *supra* note 5, at 996-1077. *See also* Douglas, *Renal Failure and the Law*, 330 LANCET 1319 (1985) (distinguishing between potential liability of the British National Health Service and that of the individual nephrologist for providing less than maximally aggressive treatment to a patient in renal failure).

patients will be protected from harmful treatment by state tort law: "This is far from clear."[104]

Preliminarily, the patient would have to prove by a preponderance of the evidence: (1) the existence of a duty owed by the physician to the patient, arising out of the physician/patient relationship; (2) a breach or violation of that duty through an unintentional deviation from the professionally acceptable standard of care under the circumstances (negligence);[105] (3) injury of the type that the law recognizes and compensates by awarding monetary damages;[106] and (4) a link of proximate causation between the physician's negligence and the damage suffered by the patient.[107] For most older persons, this burden of proof will be insurmountable when applied to attempts to rectify the implicit rationing of medical treatment, retrospectively.

To begin, despite the high degree to which older individuals consume various health services and are at enhanced risk of sustaining iatrogenic injuries,[108] the aged are statistically quite underrepresented as medical malpractice plaintiffs in civil lawsuits actually filed.[109] There are several possible explanations for the fact that older persons (at least the current cohort) tend to sue physicians at a much less frequent rate than their younger counterparts. These explanations include the following: greater deference to authority figures; less demanding expectations of medical encounters and therefore less surprise and disappointment with bad outcomes; a lack of physical and mental stamina to seek out attorneys and to litigate claims through to resolution;[110]

---

[104] Silver, *From Baby Doe to Grandpa Doe: The Impact of the Federal Age Discrimination Act on the "Hidden" Rationing of Medical Care*, 37 CATH. U.L. REV. 993, 1015 n.142 (1988).

[105] Tort law, of which negligence theory is one component, contrasts with "no-fault" approaches to the problem of compensation for iatrogenic injuries. *See* U.S. DEPARTMENT OF HEALTH AND HUMAN SERVICES, REPORT OF THE TASK FORCE ON MEDICAL LIABILITY AND MALPRACTICE 43-46 (Aug. 1987); P. WEILER, MEDICAL MALPRACTICE ON TRIAL 114-58 (1991).

[106] *See* F. MCCLELLAN, MEDICAL MALPRACTICE: LAW, TACTICS, AND ETHICS 101-35 (1994); E. RICHARDS & K. RATHBUN, *supra* note 91, at 40-49. Professional disciplinary bodies might be able to discipline physicians (for instance, by suspending a license to practice) who improperly shortchange older patients out of potentially beneficial medical treatments without needing to prove specific patient injury. This remedy, however, would provide no direct benefit to the discriminated-against patient.

[107] On the elements of medical negligence, see generally M. BOUMIL & C. ELIAS, THE LAW OF MEDICAL LIABILITY IN A NUTSHELL 1 (1995); B. FURROW, *et al.*, *supra* note 103, at 237-65 (1995); D. HASTINGS, G. LUCE, & N. WYNSTRA, FUNDAMENTALS OF HEALTH LAW 136-37 (1995); J. KING, JR., THE LAW OF MEDICAL MALPRACTICE IN A NUTSHELL 9 (2d ed. 1986); F. MCCLELLAN, *supra* note 106, at 29-44.

[108] On this enhanced risk, see P. WEILER, H. HIATT, J. NEWHOUSE, W. JOHNSON, T. BRENNAN, & L. LEAPE, A MEASURE OF MALPRACTICE: MEDICAL INJURY, MALPRACTICE LITIGATION, AND PATIENT COMPENSATION 47 (1993) ("[P]atients over 65 were at increased risk of receiving negligent care than were younger patients.").

[109] Kapp, *The Malpractice Crisis: Relevance for Geriatrics*, 37 J. AM. GERIATRICS SOC'Y 364 (1989); Sager, Voelks, Drinka, Langer, & Grimstad, *Do the Elderly Sue Physicians?*, 150 ARCH. INTERN. MED. 1091 (1990); U.S. GENERAL ACCOUNTING OFFICE, MEDICAL MALPRACTICE: MEDICARE/MEDICAID BENEFICIARIES ACCOUNT FOR A RELATIVELY SMALL PERCENTAGE OF MALPRACTICE LOSSES (1993).

[110] On the complexity of medical malpractice litigation, see Hoffman, *Civil Trials*, in LEGAL MEDICINE 81-87 (4th ed. 1998).

and lack of personal advocates in the form of willing and able family members and friends to assist them (especially those elderly who are socially isolated) through the rigors of the legal process.[111] Given the slow pace of civil litigation in most jurisdictions, there also is a frequent danger that the lawsuit would outlive the plaintiff.

Further, if the patient has had a substantial amount of his or her health care paid for by Medicaid,[112] then the state may exercise its right to be indemnified for Medicaid expenditures on the patient's behalf out of any proceeds of a civil judgment or settlement, leaving the plaintiff with only the remainder, if any.[113] This possible obligation to pay the state for past and future care creates an obvious financial disincentive for such patients to pursue even meritorious malpractice claims.

Probably the greatest stumbling block, however, is the difficulty most older patients have in meeting their burden of proof regarding the basic elements of a medical malpractice claim. This difficulty would arise with great force in most situations involving alleged age-based rationing, and would make it particularly arduous to obtain representation by a personal injury attorney working only on a contingency fee basis.[114]

First, it would seldom be simple for an older patient to establish persuasively that the physician deviated from acceptable professional standards under the circumstances in withholding or withdrawing particular aspects of potentially beneficial medical intervention. Ordinarily what is acceptable practice in any circumstance is defined by a range of approaches; suboptimal care is not necessarily negligent practice.[115] Because age-based rationing

---

[111] Many of these factors have been cited to explain why poor individuals, contrary to popular perception, also tend to be underrepresented statistically as medical malpractice plaintiffs. *See* Rosenblatt, *Rationing "Normal" Health Care: The Hidden Legal Issues*, 59 TEX. L. REV. 1401, 1411-16 (1981); U.S. GENERAL ACCOUNTING OFFICE, *supra* note 109.

[112] *See generally* R. ROSENBLATT, *et al.*, *supra* note 5, at 1170-91 (discussing Medicaid coverage for nursing home care).

[113] *See, e.g.*, GA. CODE ANN. § 49-4-149 (1997); MO. ANN. STAT. § 208.215 (1997); N. J. STAT. ANN. § 30:4D-7(k) (1998); TENN. CODE ANN. § 71-5-117 (1997); Shelton v. Fresno Comm. Hosp., 219 Cal. Rptr. 722, 726 (Cal. App. 1985) (interpreting CAL. WELF. & INST. CODE § 14009.5 (1984)); Department of Pub. Welfare v. Tyree, 512 N.E.2d 1114, 1119-20 (Ind. App. 1987) (interpreting the Indiana Medicaid Lien Statute).

[114] Writing of legitimate medical malpractice claims generally, one critic of the system notes:

> Many significant harms never result in a lawsuit because the expense of trying a case makes it uneconomical. Lawyers are usually paid for malpractice cases with a contingency fee. They recover between one-third and one-half of any judicial award or settlement. But since they are paid only if they receive a favorable result, they are cautious in bringing claims. Since the cost of going to trial is high, lawyers are reluctant to pursue cases in which the amount of money they can recover will be small in comparison to the expense of litigation.

M. RODWIN, *supra* note 67, at 174.

[115] *See generally* B. FURROW, *et al.*, *supra* note 103, at 250 ("Given a range of possible approaches to medical treatments, and disagreement within medical specialties as to the best approach, the courts have developed a variety of defenses to give physicians some leeway in defending their deviation from customary medical practice.").

decisions already are widely made and implemented in everyday medical practice, such decisions are probably a factor—albeit an implicit one—in defining the professionally accepted standard of care.[116]

Second, even assuming arguendo that negligence could be proven in a given case, establishing the elements of injury and proximate causation present often overwhelming evidentiary hurdles. The kinds of injuries for which the tort system is prepared to supply substantial monetary damages—this being the only retrospective remedy at the courts' disposal—are those that most older persons, especially if they come to the health-care system already frail and sick, would have difficulty proving. Such damages would include lost present and future earnings and many future years of additional expenses and pain and suffering.[117] The speculative dollar value of claims for age-based rationing in any singular case may not be robust enough to justify—either for the patient or the attorney—risking the definite litigation costs of pursuing the claim.

Moreover, proving a link of proximate causation between the physician's negligence and the patient's injury would be impossible in many situations involving bedside age-based treatment rationing. In most instances, a physician could successfully defend against a malpractice claim of this type by arguing that any injury befalling the old, sick patient was the direct result not of the physician's rationing actions, but rather the natural and foreseeable sequela of the medical problem(s) that converted the person into a patient in the first place. As stated by one expert on medical malpractice litigation:

> The causal connection must generally be established by expert testimony stating to a reasonable medical certainty that the injury was the result of the health care provider's negligence. This presents a serious problem, because in many cases a plaintiff's injuries can stem from multiple potential causes, including *the illness for*

According to the editor of the *New England Journal of Medicine*:

> Many people believe that even if professional ethics won't prevent the reduction of quality as physicians reduce the cost of their care, policing the quality of care will. I doubt it. Measures of quality now available are still too unsophisticated and unreliable, and though they will undoubtedly improve, the differences in quality [among individual cases] are so subtle that they are likely to elude even the most sophisticated measuring techniques of the future.

Kassirer, *Our Endangered Integrity—It Can Only Get Worse*, 336 New Eng. J. Med. 1666 (1997).

116 It is only in exceptional cases that a court might find the legal standard of care exceeds the general current practice of the medical profession under particular circumstances. *See* Helling v. Carey, 519 P.2d 981 (Wash. 1974).

117 With respect to lost earnings, it has been stated:

> [T]he personal characteristics that the law acknowledges to be the most important in projecting a person's future earning capacity are *age*, health, intelligence, education, work history, and personality. Together these characteristics provide a reasonable basis for projecting what the individual is capable of earning in a particular economy.

F. McClellan, *supra* note 106, at 127 (emphasis added). *See also* King, Jr., *Causation, Valuation, and Chance in Personal Injury Torts Involving Preexisting Conditions and Future Consequences*, 90 Yale L.J. 1353 (1981).

which she was being treated, and experts may therefore be reluctant to express an opinion at the level of certainty required by the law.[118]

For this constellation of reasons, civil lawsuits sounding in negligence are unlikely to be brought successfully by or on behalf of older persons for bedside age-based rationing. Claims alleging the intentional tort of abandonment[119] also hold little promise, because very rarely does implicit age-based rationing take the form of total, obvious patient "dumping" by the physician; the rationing ordinarily takes place more subtly within the context of an enduring physician-patient relationship. Breach of explicit or implied contractual promises[120] by the physician to the older patient similarly appears only to be of hypothetical interest here. Proving the existence and content of an actionable promise, as well as a substantial amount of measurable damages, would be a daunting task in all but the most exceptional situations.

Some commentators have posited a fiduciary duty on the physician's part to inform a patient (or a decisionally incapacitated patient's surrogate) every time that a decision to ration potentially beneficial medical intervention is contemplated. This presumably would give the patient or surrogate an adequate opportunity to object, to try to convince the physician to reverse intentions, or to seek out the potentially beneficial care from some other health-care provider. Under this argument, a physician's failure to volunteer information about potential rationing and its alternatives in a timely fashion could expose that physician to civil liability for the intentional tort of fraud and deceit (or even criminal prosecution for fraud and deceit)[121] or the negligent tort of breach of the patient's informed consent rights.[122]

A plaintiff bringing an age-based rationing claim under either of these legal theories would encounter problems. Civil suits and criminal prosecutions predicated on deceit allegations would depend on the ability to establish a clearly delineated duty owed by a physician. Under such a duty, the physician would be required to volunteer any and all potentially relevant information about alternative forms of medical intervention with any chance of providing

[118] F. MCCLELLAN, *supra* note 106, at 43 (emphasis added).

[119] On abandonment, see generally Flamm, *Medical Malpractice and the Physician Defendant*, in LEGAL MEDICINE, *supra* note 110, at 125-26.

[120] On the physician/patient contract theory, see generally B. FURROW, *et al.*, *supra* note 103, at 234-37. *See also* Green, *Minimizing Malpractice Risks by Role Clarification: The Confusing Transition from Tort to Contract*, 109 ANNALS INTERN. MED. 234 (1988). *Cf.* Meisel, *The Expansion of Liability for Medical Accidents: From Negligence to Strict Liability by Way of Informed Consent*, 56 NEB. L. REV. 51 (1977).

[121] *See* Brahams, *End-Stage Renal Failure: The Doctor's Duty and the Patient's Right*, 329 LANCET 386 (1984); Douglas, *supra* note 103, at 1320-21.

[122] On informed consent principles generally, see B. FURROW, *et al.*, *supra* note 103, at 265-79. For a discussion of these principles as applied in the health-care rationing context, see, e.g., Appelbaum, *Must We Forgo Informed Consent to Control Health Care Costs?*, 71 MILBANK Q. 669 (1993); Hall, *Informed Consent to Rationing Decisions*, 71 MILBANK Q. 645 (1993); Mehlman, *Rationing*, *supra* note 70, at 284, 286.

therapeutic benefit to the patient. The duty would apply even if the physician is not contemplating using those forms of intervention for that patient. Such a disclosure duty could be endless and boundless, and it is unlikely that it could be delineated with sufficiently reasonable precision upon which to base civil or criminal penalties. In addition, proving the physician's intent to deceive, as would be required in a criminal or intentional tort case, could be quite an onerous evidentiary burden.

Negligent violation of informed consent cases require proof (in addition to the elements of decisional capacity and voluntariness)[123] that the patient either consented to undergo a specific medical intervention[124] without adequate information[125] or refused to undergo a recommended intervention[126] without knowledge of the risks inherent in the refusal. In the case of an older patient whose physician has engaged in age-based bedside rationing by withholding or withdrawing some aspect of possible intervention, there has been neither a decision to accept nor to reject a specific medical intervention by the patient.

Even if the patient were held to have made an inadequately informed decision because the right to demand a specific intervention was impaired by the physician's silence,[127] a successful suit on this theory (which is a variant of negligence)[128] also would require proof of injury to the patient proximately caused by the lack of information.[129] These are difficult enough burdens[130] for a plaintiff to meet in most normal situations, because the same medical

[123] For the necessary elements of valid informed consent, see P. Appelbaum, C. Lidz, & A. Meisel, Informed Consent: Legal Theory and Clinical Practice 35-62 (1987); R. Faden & T. Beauchamp, A History and Theory of Informed Consent 23-43 (1986); 1 President's Commission for the Study of Ethical Problems in Medicine and Biomedical and Behavioral Research, Making Health Care Decisions (1982). *See generally* Shugrue & Linstromberg, *The Practitioner's Guide to Informed Consent*, 24 Creighton L. Rev. 881 (1991).

[124] *E.g.*, Canterbury v. Spence, 464 F.2d 772 (D.C. Cir. 1972).

[125] On the subject of how much, and what kind of, information is needed for valid consent, see, e.g., Bianco & Hirsh, *Consent to and Refusal of Medical Treatment*, in Legal Medicine, *supra* note 110, at 257, 260-64.

[126] *See, e.g.*, Truman v. Thomas, 165 Cal. Rptr. 308 (Cal. 1980), *discussed in* Note, *From Informed Consent to a Duty to Convince:* Truman v. Thomas, 18 Hous. L. Rev. 917 (1981); Note, Truman v. Thomas: *Informed Refusal in Simple Diagnostic Testing*, 14 U. Cal.-Davis L. Rev. 1105 (1981).

[127] *See generally* Morreim, *Economic Disclosure and Economic Advocacy: New Duties in the Medical Standard of Care*, 12 J. Legal Med. 275 (1991).

[128] Claims alleging lack of informed consent have shifted over the past half century from a battery to a negligence theory. *See, e.g.*, B. Furrow, *et al.*, *supra* note 103, at 268 ("A judicial sense that medical judgment should be allowed more leeway has led to a movement away from battery to negligent nondisclosure over the years."); Natanson v. Kline, 350 P.2d 1093 (Kan. 1960).

[129] *See* Bianco & Hirsh, *supra* note 125, at 261 (for the proposition that the information withheld must have been "material," that is, that knowing the information would have made a difference in the decision of a reasonable patient in similar circumstances). *See also* Weisbard, *Informed Consent: The Law's Uneasy Compromise with Ethical Theory*, 65 Neb. L. Rev. 749 (1986); Note, *Informed Consent and the Material Risk Standard: A Modest Proposal*, 12 Pac. L.J. 915, 920-25 (1981).

[130] On the bifurcation of the materiality and causation issues, see Merz, *On a Decision-Making Paradigm of Medical Informed Consent*, 14 J. Legal Med. 231, 249-60 (1993).

decision usually would have been made by the patient and the same clinical result achieved with or without the physician's provision of the disputed information.[131] These evidentiary burdens would be steeper yet in most cases involving patients who entered the therapeutic relationship old and sick in the first place, and for whom more information about alternatives rejected by the physician probably would have little meaningful impact.

Retrospective challenges to specific instances of age-based rationing of medical interventions also may be challenged under various federal civil rights statutes. The most obvious instrument for use in such a challenge is the Age Discrimination Act of 1975.[132] Modeled after Title VI of the Civil Rights Act of 1964, which broadly prohibits discrimination on the basis of race, color, or national origin in programs and activities supported with federal financial assistance,[133] section 6102 of the Age Discrimination Act provides: "[N]o person in the United States shall, on the basis of age, be excluded from participation in, be denied the benefits of, or be subjected to discrimination under, any program or activity receiving federal financial assistance."[134]

All of the practical impediments that limit access to the courts by older persons for whom medical care has been rationed at the bedside would arise with full force in the case of claims potentially brought under the Age Discrimination Act or other civil rights statutes. Substantively, it is unclear whether Congress intended that these laws function to permit federal scrutiny of individual clinical treatment decisions that involve technical considerations of relative medical benefit.

Traditionally, state law has set malpractice standards and governed the reasonableness of such decisions.[135] Even an active proponent of applying the Age Discrimination Act in the medical sphere concedes:

> This does not mean that federal law will intrude every time a physician considers the age of his or her patient in deciding upon an appropriate treatment. Individual medical decisions would not be subject to review. However, where physicians engage in a consistent practice of denying access to a medical treatment because of their age, the ADA can be invoked.[136]

[131] For an extensive argument that these elements of proof should be unnecessary, because breach of informed consent should be considered a dignitary tort (invasion of the patient's autonomy alone ought to suffice to establish liability), see Shultz, *From Informed Consent to Patient Choice: A New Protected Interest*, 95 YALE L.J. 219 (1985). *See also* Seidelson, *Medical Malpractice Actions Based on Lack of Informed Consent in "Full-Disclosure" Jurisdictions: The Enigmatic Affirmative Defense*, 29 DUQ. L. REV. 39 (1990).

[132] 42 U.S.C. §§ 6101-6107.

[133] *Id.* §§ 2000d to 2000d-6.

[134] *Id.* § 6102.

[135] *But see* Silver, *supra* note 104, at 1061-64 (rejecting these arguments against application of the Age Discrimination Act to covert age-based rationing).

[136] *Id.* at 1070.

How a plaintiff could prove "a consistent practice of denying access to a medical treatment because of age," short of the defendant(s) handing over an evidentiary "smoking gun" in the form of a formal, written discriminatory policy, is not explained. In any event, if such a discriminatory policy exists, of course, then the phenomenon it represents would be explicit, rather than implicit, health-care rationing.

A high percentage of older people are physically and/or mentally disabled in one or more significant ways.[137] Congress enacted the Americans with Disabilities Act (ADA) in 1990,[138] expanding to most of the private sector groundwork established by section 504 of the Rehabilitation Act of 1973.[139] In doing so, Congress intentionally created significant opportunities for disabled individuals to legally challenge specific facets of their medical treatment on the grounds of impermissible discrimination. Title III of the ADA provides, in pertinent part:

> No individual shall be discriminated against on the basis of disability in the full and equal enjoyment of the goods, services, facilities, privileges, advantages, or accommodations of any place of public accommodation by any person who owns, leases (or leases to), or operates a place of public accommodation.[140]

Hospitals and professional offices of health-care providers are explicitly enumerated in the ADA as covered public accommodations for the purposes of this statute.[141]

Assuming the physical and mental stamina as well as the other attributes necessary to gain access to the legal system in order to press a complaint, an older individual who knows in a timely manner and can prove that he or she was, or is about to be, discriminated against in the provision of medical services solely because he or she is disabled may be able to gain injunctive

---

[137] *See, e.g.*, LaPlante, *The Demographics of Disability*, in The Americans with Disabilities Act: From Policy to Practice 55, 61 (J. West ed. 1991). *See also* American Association of Retired Persons, Implementation of the Americans with Disabilities Act 17-37 (1992); *Theme Issue—Aging and Disabilities: Seeking Common Ground*, 16 Generations 1 (E. Ansello & N. Eustis guest eds. Winter 1992); Parry, *The ADA and Older Americans: Key Nonemployment Related Issues*, 6 Best Prac. Notes (Center for Social Gerontology) 2 (Nov. 1994); Vogel, *The Americans with Disabilities Act: A New Tool for Older Persons and Elder Law Attorneys*, 9 Elder L. Rep. 1 (May 1993).

[138] 42 U.S.C. § 12101-12213. *See generally* Implementing the Americans with Disabilities Act: Rights and Responsibilities of All Americans (L. Gostin & H. Beyer eds. 1993); The Americans with Disabilities Act: From Policy to Practice, *supra* note 137.

[139] 29 U.S.C. § 794. This section provides, in pertinent part:

> No otherwise qualified individual with a disability in the United States shall, solely by reason of her or his disability, be excluded from the participation in, be denied the benefits of, or be subjected to discrimination under any program or activity receiving Federal financial assistance.

[140] 42 U.S.C. § 12182.

[141] *Id.* § 12181. *See also* Gottlich, *Protection for Nursing Facility Residents Under the ADA*, 18 Generations 43 (Winter 1994).

and/or monetary relief[142] under the ADA. The ADA clearly applies to medical treatment decisions and practices affecting individual patients.[143]

However, the key in cases relying on the ADA would be the plaintiff's ability to prove that disability, rather than age per se, was the improper basis for medical decisions denying the patient equal treatment, because age is not included as a component of the statutory definition of protected people.[144] Thus, any older person is covered by the ADA only because, and only to the extent that, he or she also happens to be disabled under the statutory definition.

Additionally, a successful plaintiff would have the burden of persuading the fact-finder that the covert rationing of medical services unfairly deprived that plaintiff of an opportunity to achieve a real medical benefit. Otherwise, the claim could be defended on the basis of the "bona fide medical judgment standard" that justifies disparate treatment when the patient is evaluated by the physician as unable to benefit from treatment because of his or her disability.[145] Put differently, a plaintiff may be required to show that he or she was otherwise qualified,[146] despite a disability, to receive the services that were withheld or withdrawn solely[147] on the basis of that disability.

CONCLUSION

De facto rationing of potentially beneficial medical interventions on the basis of a patient's age frequently occurs in this country and will continue and perhaps accelerate in the foreseeable future. This article argues that the American legal system, at least at present, is rather limited in its capacity either to effectively protect in advance individual older persons from being victimized by this form of age discrimination or to provide a suitable remedy

---

[142] Remedies for violation of the ADA are delineated at 42 U.S.C. § 12188, as those set forth in section 204(a) of the Civil Rights Act of 1964, codified at 42 U.S.C. § 2000-a(e).

[143] *See* Peters, Jr., *Health Care Rationing and Disability Rights*, 70 IND. L.J. 491 (1995); Orentlicher, *supra* note 32; Stade, *The Use of Quality-of-Life Measures to Ration Health Care: Reviving a Rejected Proposal*, 93 COLUM. L. REV. 1985 (1993).

[144] The ADA defines disability as:

> (A) a physical or mental impairment that substantially limits one or more of the [individual's] major life activities; (B) a record of such an impairment; or (C) being regarded as having such an impairment.

42 U.S.C. § 12102.

[145] *See, e.g.*, Glanz v. Vernick, 756 F. Supp. 632, 638 (D. Mass. 1991) (if a person's HIV-related disease decreases the person's ability to benefit from ear surgery, then the HIV disease may disqualify the person as a candidate for the surgery); Crossley, *Of Diagnoses and Discrimination: Discriminatory Nontreatment of Infants with HIV Infection*, 93 COLUM. L. REV. 1581, 1650-55 (1993); United States v. University Hosp., 729 F.2d 144, 146 (2d Cir. 1984).

[146] The "otherwise qualified" language of the Rehabilitation Act, Pub. L. No. 93-112, section 504, was not expressly repeated in the ADA.

[147] *See* B. TUCKER, FEDERAL DISABILITY LAW IN A NUTSHELL 44-47 (1994). Some cases have held that, when providers deny care for more than one reason, such as disability and poverty, section 504 provides no remedy. *See, e.g.*, Johnson v. Thompson, 971 F.2d 1487 (10th Cir. 1992).

to victims after care has been rationed. This limited capacity may be seen as a positive thing, in light of how ill-suited the courts are to decide the sorts of scientific questions involved in evaluating the potential medical benefits of a particular clinical intervention for a particular patient.[148]

Given the law's limitations,[149] the situation presents primarily an ethical challenge to the involved parties. A morally acceptable solution will depend mainly on the good faith and commitment to the ethical principles of patient autonomy (truly informed consent), beneficence (the fiduciary obligation to act in the patient's best interests), and fidelity (honesty and loyalty) of those who control particular medical decisions. Even the clearest of legal standards could not be self-executing; legal standards would require the individual physician to apply them at the bedside to specific patients. As stated (if less than artfully) by one law professor: "The law will never supercede bioethics because so much of the latter subject is concerned with actions taken by voluntary actions of patients, physicians, and health care institutions which are completely inside the current law."[150]

Rejecting both pure markets and government regulation to equitably distribute finite health-care resources, economist Victor Fuchs urges:

> There is room for, indeed need for, a revitalization of professional norms as a third instrument of control in health care. As long as physicians continue to perform priestly functions, as long as they are our ambassadors to death, as long as they control the introduction of new technology, they must be endowed with certain privileges and held to certain [moral] standards of behavior different from those assumed by the market or regulation models.[151]

In the final analysis, geriatrician Patricia Blanchette reminds us:

> Healthcare should be appropriate, not rationed. Appropriate care requires that (1) decisions to accept or reject care be truly informed with good data, (2) the tendency to an age bias be recognized and confronted, and (3) advance directives and health proxies or surrogate decision-makers be explained and recommended for adults of all ages. While there does not appear to be any move to institute overt rationing by age in the United States, the possibility of covert rationing is of serious concern. Health policy must be enlightened so that the possibility of overt or covert rationing to people of all ages who may need appropriate high-cost care will be acknowledged and rejected.[152]

---

[148] *See generally* Hall & Anderson, *Health Insurers' Assessment of Medical Necessity*, 140 U. Pa. L. Rev. 1637 (1992); P. Huber, Galileo's Revenge: Junk Science in the Courtroom (1993).

[149] On the law's limitations generally in the face of bioethical questions, see R. Dworkin, Limits: The Role of the Law in Bioethical Decision Making (1996). *But see* Editorial, *supra* note 68, at 2 ("if ethical considerations prove indecisive perhaps legal pressures might exert an untypically beneficial influence in persuading all doctors to give their patients the best professional counsel").

[150] 1 W.N. Keyes, Life, Death, and the Law 17 (1995).

[151] V. Fuchs, The Future of Health Policy 186 (1993).

[152] Blanchette, *supra* note 65, at 63.

Name Index

Printed and bound by CPI Group (UK) Ltd, Croydon, CR0 4YY
22/10/2024
01777637-0004